D0039352

DEC   2005

HOSPITAL FOR SPECIAL SURGERY MANUAL OF RHEUMATOLOGY AND OUTPATIENT ORTHOPEDIC DISORDERS: DIAGNOSIS AND THERAPY

Fifth Edition

MISERICORDIA COMMUNITY HOSPITAL
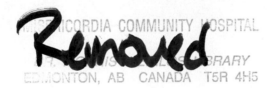
H. GWYNNE JONES LIBRARY
EDMONTON, AB   CANADA   T5R 4H5

Cheryl Blahut
780- 439 -6967
PT- Misercordia.

HOSPITAL FOR SPECIAL SURGERY MANUAL OF RHEUMATOLOGY AND OUTPATIENT ORTHOPEDIC DISORDERS: DIAGNOSIS AND THERAPY

Fifth Edition

Editors

Stephen A. Paget, M.D.
Joseph P. Routh Professor of Medicine
Weill Medical College of Cornell University
Physician-in-Chief
Division of Rheumatology
Hospital for Special Surgery-New York
    Presbyterian Hospital
New York, New York

Allan Gibofsky, M.D., J.D.
Professor of Medicine and Public Health
Weill Medical College of Cornell University
Attending Physician
Hospital for Special Surgery-New York
    Presbyterian Hospital
Professor of Law
Fordham University
New York, New York

John F. Beary III, M.D.
Clinical Professor of Medicine
University of Cincinnati
Attending Physician
Division of Rheumatology & Immunology
Veterans Administration Medical Center
Cincinnati, Ohio

Thomas P. Sculco, M.D.
Professor of Orthopedic Surgery
Weill Medical College of Cornell University
Surgeon-in-Chief
Department of Orthopedics
Hospital for Special Surgery-New York
    Presbyterian Hospital
New York, New York

Associate Editor

Doruk Erkan, M.D.
Assistant Professor of Medicine
Weill Medical College of Cornell University
Associate Physician-Scientist
Barbara Volcker Center for Women
    and Rheumatic Disease
Assistant Attending Physician
Hospital for Special Surgery-New York
    Presbyterian Hospital
New York, New York

International Editors

Josef S. Smolen, M.D.
Professor of Medicine
Chairman, Department of Rheumatology
Medical University of Vienna
Chairman, 2nd Department of Medicine
Rheumatic Disease Center, Lainz Hospital
Vienna, Austria

Stefano Bombardieri, M.D.
Professor of Rheumatology
Chief, Rheumatic Diseases Unit
University of Pisa
Pisa, Italy

Coordinator

Cookie Reyes
Clinical and Research Administrator
Hospital for Special Surgery
New York, New York

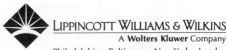
LIPPINCOTT WILLIAMS & WILKINS
A **Wolters Kluwer** Company
Philadelphia • Baltimore • New York • London
Buenos Aires • Hong Kong • Sydney • Tokyo

Acquisitions Editor: Sonya Seigafuse
Managing Editor: Nancy Winter
Project Manager: Nicole Walz
Senior Manufacturing Manager: Ben Rivera
Marketing Manager: Kathy Neely
Design Coordinator: Terry Mallon
Cover Designer: Becky Baxendell
Production Services: Laserwords Private Limited
Printer: RR Donnelley

Fifth Edition
© 2006 by Lippincott Williams & Wilkins
© 2000 by Lippincott Williams & Wilkins
530 Walnut Street
Philadelphia, PA 19106
www.LWW.com

All rights reserved. This book is protected by copyright. No part of this book may be reproduced in any form or by any means, including photocopying, or utilizing by any information storage and retrieval system without written permission from the copyright owner, except for brief quotations embodied in critical articles and reviews.

Printed in the United States

Library of Congress Cataloging-in-Publication Data

Hospital for Special Surgery manual of rheumatology and outpatient orthopedic disorders : diagnosis and therapy / editors, Stephen A. Paget ... [et al.] ; associate editor, Doruk Erkan ; coordinator, Cookie Reyes ; forewords, Sir Ravinder Maini, Charles L. Christian. — 5th ed.
    p. ; cm. — (Spiral manual series)
  Rev. ed. of: Manual of rheumatology and outpatient orthopedic disorders. 4th ed. c2000.
  Includes bibliographical references and index.
  ISBN 0-7817-6300-2
  1. Rheumatology—Handbooks, manuals, etc. 2. Orthopedics—Handbooks, manuals, etc.
I. Paget, Stephen A. II. Hospital for Special Surgery. III. Manual of rheumatology and outpatient orthopedic disorders. IV. Title: Manual of rheumatology and outpatient orthopedic disorders. V. Series: Spiral manual.
  [DNLM: 1. Rheumatic Diseases—diagnosis—Handbooks. 2. Ambulatory Care—Handbooks. 3. Bone Diseases—Handbooks. 4. Rheumatic Diseases—therapy—Handbooks. WE 39 H828 2006]
  RC927.M346 2006
  616.7'23—dc22

                  2005020653

Care has been taken to confirm the accuracy of the information presented and to describe generally accepted practices. However, the authors, editors, and publisher are not responsible for errors or omissions or for any consequences from application of the information in this book and make no warranty, expressed or implied, with respect to the currency, completeness, or accuracy of the contents of the publication. Application of this information in a particular situation remains the professional responsibility of the practitioner.

The authors, editors, and publisher have exerted every effort to ensure that drug selection and dosage set forth in this text are in accordance with current recommendations and practice at the time of publication. However, in view of ongoing research, changes in government regulations, and the constant flow of information relating to drug therapy and drug reactions, the reader is urged to check the package insert for each drug for any change in indications and dosage and for added warnings and precautions. This is particularly important when the recommended agent is a new or infrequently employed drug.

Some drugs and medical devices presented in this publication have Food and Drug Administration (FDA) clearance for limited use in restricted research settings. It is the responsibility of health care providers to ascertain the FDA status of each drug or device planned for use in their clinical practice.

The publisher has made every effort to trace copyright holders for borrowed material. If they have inadvertently overlooked any, they will be pleased to make the necessary arrangements at the first opportunity.

To purchase additional copies of this book, call our customer service department at (800) 638-3030 or fax orders to (301) 223-2320. International customers should call (301) 223-2300. Lippincott Williams & Wilkins customer service representatives are available from 8:30 a.m. to 6:30 p.m., EST, Monday through Friday, for telephone access. Visit Lippincott Williams & Wilkins on the Internet: http://www.lww.com.

                  10 9 8 7 6 5 4 3 2 1

With love, we dedicate this book to our families:

Sandra Paget, Daniel, Matthew, and Lauren
Karen Gibofsky, Lewis, Esther, and Laura
Bianca Beary, John Daniel, Vanessa, Webster, and Nina
Cynthia Sculco, Peter, and Sarah Jane

And to L. Robert Vermes, Jr.
"He who saves a single life saves the world entire."

-Talmud

And to our colleague and friend
Mary (Peggy) K. Crow, M.D.
Professor of Medicine
Weill Medical College of Cornell University
Attending Physician, Hospital for Special Surgery
President of the American College of Rheumatology 2005–2006

CONTENTS

I: MUSCULOSKELETAL DATABASE

II: THE STAT RHEUMATOLOGY AND ORTHOPEDIC CONSULTATION: YOUR GUIDE TO ACUTE CARE

III: CLINICAL PRESENTATIONS

IV: DIAGNOSIS AND THERAPY
A. CONNECTIVE TISSUE DISORDERS

B. SPONDYLOARTHROPATHIES

C. CRYSTAL ARTHROPATHIES

D. INFECTIOUS DISEASES INVOLVING THE MUSCULOSKELETAL SYSTEM

E. OSTEOARTHRITIS, METABOLIC BONE AND ENDOCRINE DISORDERS

F. OTHER RHEUMATIC DISEASES

V: ORTHOPEDIC SURGERY AND REHABILITATION: PRINCIPLES AND PRACTICE

VI: COMPLEMENTARY AND ALTERNATIVE MEDICINE   489

Gina Kearney and C. Ronald MacKenzie

VII: FORMULARY   497

Arthur M. F. Yee and Jane E. Salmon

VIII: APPENDICES

ACKNOWLEDGMENTS

We gratefully acknowledge our many friends, colleagues, and alumni of the Hospital for Special Surgery who have made helpful suggestions and contributions to this volume over the past quarter-century. We also gratefully appreciate the excellent assistance of JoAnn Vega in the preparation of this volume.

$\mathcal{T}$he composition and authorship of the *Manual of Rheumatology and Outpatient Orthopedic Disorders* continues to reflect the fact that rheumatology and orthopedic surgery have a seamless interface in pursuit of education and patient care goals relative to musculoskeletal disease. The inter-relationship of these two disciplines is a special and unique feature of the Hospital for Special Surgery, where many of the authors have trained or practiced.

The primary goal of this manual has been to serve the needs of students and physicians-in-training. Yet professionals of all ages (perhaps especially senior colleagues) find it useful for reviewing miscellaneous things not successfully committed to memory. These include: American College of Rheumatology Criteria for Diagnosis and Classification of Rheumatic Disease, neurologic dermatomes, molecular targets of autoantibodies, normal laboratory values, details in the formulary, etc. Between the fourth and fifth editions, there has been an explosion of the rheumatologic formulary; new anti-inflammatory drugs and biologic disease modifying antirheumatic drugs, some based on new insights relative to the pathogenesis of rheumatoid arthritis.

Over the span of our five editions, several new chapters have been added, reflecting our knowledge of recent advances: antiphospholipid syndrome, pregnancy, and connective tissue diseases, rheumatic associations with HIV infection, diagnostic imaging, patient education, perioperative management, ethical and legal considerations, measuring functional status, thinking like a rheumatologist, acute management of musculoskeletal and autoimmune disorders, and so on. In this edition, as in all previous ones, the emphasis remains the discussion of practical aspects of management of musculoskeletal disorders.

Charles L. Christian, M.D.
Physician-in-Chief Emeritus
Hospital for Special Surgery
New York, New York

$\mathcal{T}$his remarkable manual celebrates the publication of its fifth edition this year. Innovations in diagnosis, therapeutics, and management strategies that have emerged in the 5 years since the last edition make this update timely. The succinct, authoritative, and didactic style of presenting the rationale and practical information in this publication will doubtless continue to assist and guide physicians in their clinical practice.

The scope of the book is comprehensive, covering the full spectrum of therapy and practice of rheumatology. The broad church of the specialty covered extends to regional pain syndromes, fibromyalgia, diseases of bone, sports injuries, and the principles and practice of surgery and rehabilitation. New chapters in the general sections cover not only immunology, genomics, and proteomics but also ethical and legal issues and psychological aspects of rheumatic disease.

Making knowledge-based therapeutic interventions that maximize benefit and minimize risk has increasingly become part of rheumatological practice since publication of the last edition. The widespread use of anti-tumor necrosis factor (TNF) biologics added to methotrexate therapy has profoundly altered the health outcomes for patients with moderate-to-severe rheumatoid arthritis whose disease is not controlled by more effective regimens employing standard drugs as monotherapy or in combination. The recent emphasis on suppression of disease with judicious use of the available therapeutic armamentarium has permitted control of signs, symptoms, and joint damage in most patients. Not only has this permitted the maintenance of a good quality of life, but epidemiologic data also demonstrate that it has reduced cardiovascular complications and prolonged the life expectancy of these patients.

The use of currently available biologics, and those in the development phase, has been shown to be effective not only in rheumatoid arthritis but also in other inflammatory arthritides. The repertoire of targeted drugs that is now being developed shows promising results for systemic rheumatic disease and will enlarge the pharmacopoeia. However, these advances come at a price of unwanted side effects, such as increasing infection rates, in some patients. As another example, the widespread use of cyclo-oxygenase-2 (COX-2) inhibitors that control pain with an improved gastric tolerance profile has apparently led to an increase in cardiovascular occlusive events. This has sparked a debate on the safety and indications of all nonsteroidal anti-inflammatory drugs. The widespread public dissemination of this information has alarmed and confused patients at a time when the potential for the good of patients, resulting from technical and scientific developments, has never been greater.

The rheumatological practice landscape has changed and will continue to change with the advent of targeted biologic and chemical drugs and improvement in laboratory and imaging technologies. Managing this change will require a sharper focus and skill base in rheumatological practice. The responsibility and role of thought leaders and educationalists in this process has therefore become increasingly important. It is worth recalling that the origins of research with Coley's toxin that led to the discovery of TNF almost a century later originated at the Hospital for Special Surgery. The cooperation between surgeons and physicians and their allied health associates remains a hallmark of this institution in their quest for a better future for the health of patients. The editors and authors of this book, coming from this center of excellence in research and practice, have much to offer in this regard to the community of rheumatological practitioners worldwide. Their book deserves a place on the desk of trainees and established practitioners.

Professor Sir Ravinder Maini, B.A., M.B., BChir, Hon DSc, FRCP FRCP(E) FMed Sci
Emeritus Professor of Rheumatology
The Kennedy Institute of Rheumatology Division
Imperial College
London, W6 8RF
United Kingdom

$\mathcal{I}$n the 5 years since the last edition of *Manual of Rheumatology and Outpatient Orthopedic Disorders: Diagnosis and Therapy*, the clinical and investigative tectonic plates of rheumatology have shifted in a profound manner, all for the good of our patients. Through a combination of explosions in our knowledge about the basic mechanisms of disease, advances in our appreciation of the clinical "personalities" of autoimmune and musculoskeletal disorders, and the rapidity with which basic scientific wisdom is catapulted into therapeutic advances at the bedside, our patients are living longer and better lives. Nowhere is this sea change better seen than in the development of worldwide use of biologic drugs such as tumor necrosis factor (TNF)-α blockers. The three commercially available anti-TNF drugs have significantly and safely improved the lives of hundreds of thousands of patients with rheumatoid arthritis (RA), psoriatic arthritis, spondyloarthropathies, inflammatory bowel disease, and other systemic inflammatory disorders. Despite these advances, we are still treating the pathogenesis of diseases (such as RA) and not their etiology; although we can now block a centrally important proinflammatory cytokine, we are still unable to identify and destroy the etiologic agents that initiate the process of RA. However, just as systemic diseases such as rheumatic fever, polio, syphilis, and tuberculosis fell to the development of antibiotics in the last century, similar paradigm shifts will likely occur in the field of rheumatology.

We have moved from a "wait and see" attitude with regard to so many disorders to a "get tough and take no prisoners" approach, stimulated by the fact that illnesses such as RA, if not countered early and aggressively, are intrinsically joint damaging, life shortening, and work limiting. Rheumatologists have adopted the therapeutic approaches employed by our colleagues in the field of endocrinology and oncology. We now employ induction and maintenance treatment regimens in many diseases in order to optimally balance disease control with drug-related side effects, and we do so to achieve a "no evidence of disease" (NED) status. Just as endocrinologists aim for "tight control" of diabetes by decreasing glycosylated hemoglobin levels so as to avoid the development of neuropathy, nephropathy, and retinopathy, rheumatologists also "aim" at decreasing signs and symptoms of RA inflammation using sensitive and responsive clinical research tools such as the Health Assessment Questionnaire and the Disease Activity Score. Given the amazing effectiveness of anti-TNF medications, we have even resurrected the term disease remission and aim for it day by day in our care of our patients.

We have learned a great deal about both the diseases we treat and the medications we use to treat them. The former is possible through data obtained from randomized, controlled trials; observational studies; and use of and advances in clinical epidemiology and health services research. The latter has arisen from drug trials, postmarketing surveillance, and robust registries. In view of our newfound ability to really make a difference in the lives of our patients, early arthritis centers have risen, first in Europe and more recently in the United States, in an attempt to treat RA and other inflammatory disorders as close to their onset as possible. Studies have recently shown that with self-limited, 1-year courses of anti-TNF drugs, sustained remissions can be achieved.

Systemic inflammatory disorders such as RA and systemic lupus erythematosus (SLE) not only affect joints and kidneys, respectively, but are also associated with significant collateral damage in the form of premature atherosclerosis and osteoporosis. Life span is shortened in RA by approximately 10 years primarily due to ischemic heart disease. Therefore, treatment of these disorders demands a global approach, one that focuses not only on the characteristic disease manifestations themselves but also on those tissues affected by the "spill over" effect of systemic inflammation. We now treat RA and SLE like we would treat diabetes, with low-dose aspirin, aggressive lipid lowering, and smoking avoidance.

We have changed the look of our *Manual* to make it more user-friendly, added new chapters in order to keep the manual up-to-date in this rapidly changing field, and always kept in mind the need to deliver information in its most edible and rapidly digested form. We have carefully integrated the new science into each line of the *Manual* in an attempt to easily bring our increasing knowledge of the basic science to your patient. It is only with early disease recognition and the institution of the proper therapeutic approach that we can prolong our patient's lives and keep our patients diseasefree and damagefree, functional, and productive.

Stephen A. Paget, M.D.
Allan Gibofsky, M.D., J.D.
John F. Beary, III, M.D.
Thomas P. Sculco, M.D.

Juliet Aizer, M.D., M.P.H.
Rheumatology Fellow
Weill Medical College of Cornell University
Hospital for Special Surgery
New York, New York

John P. Allegrante, Ph.D.
Professor of Health Education
Department of Health and Behavior
    Studies, Teachers College
Department of Sociomedical Sciences,
    Mailman School of Public Health
Columbia University
Senior Scientist
Hospital for Special Surgery
New York, New York

Dalit Ashany, M.D.
Assistant Professor of Medicine
Weill Medical College of Cornell University
Assistant Attending Physician
Hospital for Special Surgery-New York
    Presbyterian Hospital
New York, New York

Joseph L. Barker, M.D.
Orthopedic Resident
Weill Medical College of Cornell University
Hospital for Special Surgery
New York, New York

Chiara Baldini, M.D.
Rheumatology Fellow
Department of Internal Medicine
University of Pisa
Pisa, Italy

Anne R. Bass, M.D.
Assistant Professor of Clinical Medicine
Weill Medical College of Cornell University
Assistant Attending Physician
Hospital for Special Surgery-New York
    Presbyterian Hospital
New York, New York

John F. Beary, III, M.D.
Clinical Professor of Medicine
University of Cincinnati
Attending Physician
Division of Rheumatology and
    Immunology
Veterans Administration Medical Center
Cincinnati, Ohio

Kristina Belostocki, M.D.
Assistant Professor of Medicine
Weill Medical College of Cornell University
Assistant Attending Physician
Hospital for Special Surgery-New York
    Presbyterian Hospital
New York, New York

Jessica R. Berman, M.D.
Assistant Professor of Medicine
Weill Medical College of Cornell University
Assistant Attending Physician
Hospital for Special Surgery-New York
    Presbyterian Hospital
New York, New York

David A. Bomback, M.D.
Orthopedic Surgeon
Connecticut Neck and Back Specialists
Danbury, Connecticut

Stefano Bombardieri, M.D.
Professor of Rheumatology
Chief, Rheumatic Diseases Unit
University of Pisa
Pisa, Italy

Barry D. Brause, M.D.
Professor of Clinical Medicine
Weill Medical College of Cornell University
Attending Physician
Hospital for Special Surgery-New York
    Presbyterian Hospital
New York, New York

Lisa R. Callahan, M.D.
Assistant Professor of Clinical Medicine
Weill Medical College of Cornell University
Assistant Attending Physician
Hospital for Special Surgery-New York
    Presbyterian Hospital
New York, New York

Daniel J. Clauw, M.D.
Professor of Medicine and Chief
Division of Rheumatology
Department of Medicine
Assistant Dean of Clinical and Transitional
    Research
University of Michigan Medical School
Ann Arbor, Michigan

Charles N. Cornell, M.D.
Professor of Orthopedic Surgery
Weill Medical College of Cornell University
Attending Physician
Hospital for Special Surgery-New York
    Presbyterian Hospital
New York, New York

Mary K. Crow, M.D.
Professor of Medicine
Weill Medical College of Cornell University
Director, Autoimmunity and Inflammation
    Program
Senior Scientist
Hospital for Special Surgery-New York
    Presbyterian Hospital
New York, New York

Sharon Danoff-Burg, Ph.D.
Associate Professor
Department of Psychology
State University of New York at Albany
Albany, New York

Edward F. DiCarlo, M.D.
Associate Professor of Clinical Pathology
Weill Medical College of Cornell University
Chief Surgical Pathologist
Director, Histology Laboratory
Hospital for Special Surgery-New York
    Presbyterian Hospital
New York, New York

Petros Efthimiou, M.D.
Assistant Professor of Medicine
University of Medicine and Dentistry of
    New Jersey
Attending Physician
The University Hospital
Newark, New Jersey

Keith B. Elkon, M.D.
Professor and Division Head
Division of Rheumatology
University of Washington
Seattle, Washington

Doruk Erkan, M.D.
Assistant Professor of Medicine
Weill Medical College of Cornell University
Associate Physician-Scientist
Barbara Volcker Center for Women
    and Rheumatic Disease
Assistant Attending Physician
Hospital for Special Surgery-New York
    Presbyterian Hospital
New York, New York

James C. Farmer, M.D.
Assistant Professor of Orthopedic Surgery
Weill Medical College of Cornell University
Assistant Attending Physician
Hospital for Special Surgery
New York, New York

Theodore R. Fields, M.D.
Associate Professor of Clinical Medicine
Weill Medical College of Cornell University
Director, Rheumatology Faculty
    Practice Plan
Associate Attending Physician
Hospital for Special Surgery-New York
    Presbyterian Hospital
New York, New York

Harry E. Figgie, III, M.D.
Deceased

Mark Figgie, M.D.
Associate Professor of Orthopedic Surgery
Weill Medical College of Cornell University
Chief, Surgical Arthritis Service
Associate Attending Physician
Hospital for Special Surgery-New York
    Presbyterian Hospital
New York, New York

Sandy B. Ganz, P.T., D.Sc., G.C.S.
Faculty, Division of Geriatrics and
    Gerontology
Weill Medical College of Cornell University
Director of Rehabilitation
Amsterdam Nursing Home
Associate in Research
Hospital for Special Surgery
New York, New York

Allan Gibofsky, M.D., J.D.
Professor of Medicine and Public Health
Weill Medical College of Cornell University
Attending Physician
Hospital for Special Surgery-New York
  Presbyterian Hospital
Professor of Law
Fordham University
New York, New York

Jo A. Hannafin, M.D., Ph.D.
Assistant Professor of Orthopedic Surgery
Weill Medical College of Cornell University
Director, Orthopedic Research
Director, Women's Sports Medicine Center
Assistant Attending Physician
Hospital for Special Surgery-New York
  Presbyterian Hospital
New York, New York

Louis L. Harris, M.D.
Senior Administrator and Director
Network Development and Planning
Burke Rehabilitation Hospital
White Plains, New York

Melanie J. Harrison, M.D., M.S.
Assistant Research Professor of Medicine
  and Public Health
Weill Medical College of Cornell University
Assistant Attending Physician
Hospital for Special Surgery-New York
  Presbyterian Hospital
New York, New York

John H. Healey, M.D.
Professor of Orthopedic Surgery
Weill Medical College of Cornell University
Chief, Orthopedic Service
Memorial Sloan-Kettering Cancer Center
New York, New York

Robert N. Hotchkiss, M.D.
Associate Professor of Orthopedic Surgery
Weill Medical College of Cornell University
Director of Clinical Research
Attending Physician
Hospital for Special Surgery
New York, New York

Robert D. Inman, M.D.
Professor of Medicine and Immunology
University of Toronto
Director, Arthritis Center of Excellence
Division of Rheumatology
Toronto Western Hospital
Ontario, Canada

Norman A. Johanson, M.D.
Professor and Chairman of Orthopedic
  Surgery
Drexel University College of Medicine
Hahnemann University Hospital
Philadelphia, Pennsylvania

Alan T. Kaell, M.D.
Professor of Clinical Medicine
State University of New York at
  Stony Brook
Stony Brook, New York
Chief, Division of Rheumatology
St. Charles Health System
Port Jefferson, New York

Lawrence J. Kagen, M.D.
Professor of Medicine
Weill Medical College of Cornell University
Attending Physician
Hospital for Special Surgery-New York
  Presbyterian Hospital
New York, New York

Stuart S. Kassan, M.D.
Clinical Professor of Medicine
University of Colorado Health Sciences
  Center
Colorado Arthritis Associates
Denver, Colorado

**Gina Kearney, M.S.N., R.N., C.S.,
A.H.N.-B.C.**
Holistic Nurse Practitioner
Integrative Care Center
Hospital for Special Surgery
New York, New York

Robert P. Kimberly, M.D.
Howard L. Holley Professor
  of Medicine
University of Alabama at Birmingham
Director, University of Alabama Arthritis
  and Musculoskeletal Center
Division of Clinical Immunology
  and Rheumatology
University Hospital
Birmingham, Alabama

Kyriakos A. Kirou, M.D.
Assistant Professor of Medicine
Weill Medical College of Cornell University
Assistant Attending Physician
Hospital for Special Surgery-New York
  Presbyterian Hospital
New York, New York

Alexander Krawiecki, M.D.
Hospital for Special Surgery
New York, New York

Joseph M. Lane, M.D.
Professor of Orthopedic Surgery
Weill Medical College of Cornell University
Attending Physician
Hospital for Special Surgery-New York
  Presbyterian Hospital
New York, New York

Henry Lee, M.D.
Dermatology Resident
Weill Medical College of Cornell University
New York Presbyterian Hospital
New York, New York

Thomas J. A. Lehman, M.D.
Professor of Clinical Pediatrics
Weill Medical College of Cornell University
Chief, Division of Pediatric Rheumatology
Hospital for Special Surgery-New York
  Presbyterian Hospital
New York, New York

David S. Levine, M.D.
Assistant Professor of Orthopedic Surgery
Weill Medical College of Cornell University
Assistant Attending Physician
Hospital for Special Surgery-New York
  Presbyterian Hospital
New York, New York

Michael D. Lockshin, M.D.
Professor of Medicine and Obstetrics
Weill Medical College of Cornell University
Director, Barbara Volcker Center
  for Women and Rheumatic Disease
Attending Physician
Hospital for Special Surgery-New York
  Presbyterian Hospital
New York, New York

Paul Lombardi, M.D.
Senior Clinical Associate in Orthopedic
  Surgery
Weill Medical College of Cornell University
Hospital for Special Surgery-New York
  Presbyterian Hospital
New York, New York

Michael E. Luggen, M.D.
Professor of Clinical Medicine
University of Cincinnati Medical Center
Rheumatology Consultants
Department of Internal Medicine
University Hospital
Cincinnati, Ohio

C. Ronald MacKenzie, M.D.
Associate Professor of Clinical Medicine
Weill Medical College of Cornell University
Associate Attending Physician
Hospital for Special Surgery-New York
  Presbyterian Hospital
New York, New York

Steven K. Magid, M.D.
Associate Professor of Clinical Medicine
Weill Medical College of Cornell University
Associate Attending Physician
Hospital for Special Surgery-New York
  Presbyterian Hospital
New York, New York

Lisa A. Mandl, M.D., M.P.H.
Assistant Professor of Medicine
Weill Medical College of Cornell University
Assistant Attending Physician
Hospital for Special Surgery-New York
  Presbyterian Hospital
New York, New York

Joseph A. Markenson, M.D.
Professor of Medicine
Weill Medical College of Cornell University
Attending Physician
Hospital for Special Surgery-New York
  Presbyterian Hospital
New York, New York

Richard R. McCormack, M.D.
Orthopedic Surgeon Emeritus
Hospital for Special Surgery
Weill Medical College of Cornell University
New York, New York

Stephen Ray Mitchell, M.D.
Director, Residency Program, Department
  of Medicine
Georgetown University
Washington, District of Columbia

Stephen A. Paget, M.D.
Joseph P. Routh Professor of Medicine
Weill Medical College of Cornell University
Physician-in-Chief, Division of
  Rheumatology
Hospital for Special Surgery-New York
  Presbyterian Hospital
New York, New York

Edward Parrish, M.D.
Associate Professor of Medicine
Weill Medical College of Cornell University
Attending Physician
Hospital for Special Surgery-New York
  Presbyterian Hospital
New York, New York

Helene Pavlov, M.D.
Professor of Radiology
Weill Medical College of Cornell University
Chief, Department of Radiology and
Imaging
Hospital for Special Surgery
New York, New York

Andrew D. Pearle, M.D.
Instructor in Orthopedic Surgery
Weill Medical College of Cornell University
Assistant Attending Orthopedic Surgeon
Hospital for Special Surgery
New York, New York

Paul Pellicci, M.D.
Professor of Orthopedic Surgery
Weill Medical College of Cornell University
Chief, Hip Service
Attending Physician
Hospital for Special Surgery-New York
Presbyterian Hospital
New York, New York

Andrea Piccioli, M.D.
Orthopedic Surgeon
Centro Traumatologico e Ortopedico
Rome, Italy

Tracey A. Revenson, Ph.D.
Professor of Psychology
The Graduate Center of the City
University of New York
New York, New York

Laura Robbins, D.S.W.
Associate Professor
Graduate School of Medical Sciences
Clinical Epidemiology and Health Sciences
Research
Weill Medical College at Cornell University
Vice President, Education and Academic
Affairs
Associate Scientist
Hospital for Special Surgery
New York, New York

Linda A. Russell, M.D.
Assistant Professor of Medicine
Weill Medical College of Cornell University
Assistant Attending Physician
Hospital for Special Surgery-New York
Presbyterian Hospital
New York, New York

Jane E. Salmon, M.D.
Professor of Medicine
Weill Medical College of Cornell University
Attending Physician
Hospital for Special Surgery-New York
Presbyterian Hospital
New York, New York

Lisa R. Sammaritano, M.D.
Associate Professor of Medicine
Weill Medical College of Cornell University
Associate Attending Physician
Hospital for Special Surgery-New York
Presbyterian Hospital
New York, New York

C. Michael Samson, M.D.
Co-Director, Uveitis Service
New York Eye and Ear Infirmary
New York, New York

Eric S. Schned, M.D.
Medical Director
Park Nicollete Clinic
Minneapolis, Minnesota

Robert Schneider, M.D.
Associate Professor of Radiology
Weill Medical College of Cornell University
Attending Physician
Hospital for Special Surgery-New York
Presbyterian Hospital
New York, New York

Sergio Schwartzman, M.D.
Associate Professor of Medicine
Weill Medical College of Cornell University
Associate Attending Physician
Hospital for Special Surgery-New York
Presbyterian Hospital
New York, New York

Rachelle Scott, M.D.
Associate Professor of Clinical
Dermatology
Weill Medical College of Cornell University
Assistant Attending Physician
New York Presbyterian Hospital
New York, New York

Thomas P. Sculco, M.D.
Professor of Orthopedic Surgery
Weill Medical College of Cornell University
Surgeon-in-Chief, Chairman
Department of Orthopedics
Hospital for Special Surgery-New York
Presbyterian Hospital
New York, New York

Nigel Sharrock, M.B., Ch.B.
Clinical Professor of Anesthesiology
Weill Medical College of Cornell University
Attending Physician
Hospital for Special Surgery-New York
Presbyterian Hospital
New York, New York

Monique Sheridan
Research Coordinator
Women's Sports Medicine Center
Hospital for Special Surgery
New York, New York

Animesh A. Sinha, M.D., Ph.D.
Assistant Professor of Dermatology
Weill Medical College of Cornell University
Attending Physician
Hospital for Special Surgery-New York
  Presbyterian Hospital
New York, New York

Robert F. Spiera, M.D.
Associate Professor of Medicine
Weill Medical College of Cornell University
Director, Vasculitis and Scleroderma
  Programs
Assistant Attending Physician
Hospital for Special Surgery-New York
  Presbyterian Hospital
New York, New York

Richard Stern, M.D.
Clinical Associate Professor
Weill Medical College of Cornell University
Attending Physician
Hospital for Special Surgery-New York
  Presbyterian Hospital
New York, New York

Edward Su, M.D.
Clinical Instructor of Orthopedic Surgery
Weill Medical College of Cornell University
Assistant Attending Physician
Hospital for Special Surgery-New York
  Presbyterian Hospital
New York, New York

Ioannis Tassiulas, M.D.
Assistant Professor of Medicine
Weill Medical College of Cornell University
Assistant Attending Physician
Hospital for Special Surgery-New York
  Presbyterian Hospital
New York, New York

Russell F. Warren, M.D.
Professor of Orthopedic Surgery
Weill Medical College of Cornell University
Surgeon-in-Chief Emeritus
Attending Physician
Hospital for Special Surgery-New York
  Presbyterian Hospital
New York, New York

Scott S. Weissman, M.D.
Adjunct Clinical Scientist
Columbia University College of Physicians
  and Surgeons
Attending Physician
Manhattan Eye, Ear, and Throat
  Hospital
Attending Physician and Director
Uveitis Service, New York Eye and Ear
  Infirmary
New York, New York

H. Hallett Whitman, III, M.D.
Assistant Professor of Clinical Medicine
Clinical and Research Associate
Cardiovascular Hypertension Center
Weill Medical College of Cornell University
Chief of Rheumatology
Summit Medical Group
Summit, New Jersey
Physician to the Outpatient Department
Hospital for Special Surgery
New York, New York

Thomas L. Wickiewicz, M.D.
Associate Professor of Orthopedic Surgery
Weill Medical College of Cornell University
Chief, Sports Medicine and
  Shoulder Service
Associate Attending Physician
Hospital for Special Surgery-New York
  Presbyterian Hospital
New York, New York

Riley J. Williams, M.D.
Associate Professor of Orthopedic Surgery
Weill Medical College of Cornell University
Sports Medicine and Shoulder Service
Associate Attending Physician
Hospital for Special Surgery-New York
  Presbyterian Hospital
New York, New York

Aviva Wolff, O.T.R., C.H.T.
Senior Hand Specialist
Department of Rehabilitation
Hospital for Special Surgery
New York, New York

Yusuf Yazici, M.D.
Assistant Professor of Clinical Medicine
New York University
Attending Rheumatologist
Hospital for Joint Diseases
New York, New York

Arthur M. F. Yee, M.D., Ph.D.
Assistant Professor of Medicine
Weill Medical College of Cornell University
Assistant Attending Physician
Hospital for Special Surgery-New York
   Presbyterian Hospital
New York, New York

Diana A. Yens, M.D.
Assistant Professor of Clinical Medicine
Weill Medical College of Cornell University
Assistant Attending Physician
Hospital for Special Surgery
New York, New York

John B. Zabriskie, M.D.
Associate Professor Emeritus
Clinical Microbiology and Immunology
Rockefeller University
Senior Physician
Rockefeller University Hospital
New York, New York

Musculoskeletal Database

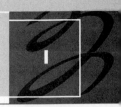

MUSCULOSKELETAL HISTORY AND PHYSICAL EXAMINATION

Stephen A. Paget, Charles N. Cornell, and John F. Beary, III

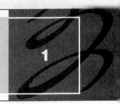

*T*he **musculoskeletal or locomotor system,** like other body systems, can be defined anatomically and assessed functionally. **Lower** extremities support the weight of the body and allow ambulation. They require proper alignment and stability. **Upper** extremities reach, grasp, and hold, thereby allowing self-care, feeding, and work. They require mobility and strength. Diseases and disorders of the musculoskeletal system disturb anatomy and interfere with function.

 MUSCULOSKELETAL HISTORY

A careful history is the most important and powerful of the information-gathering procedures used to define a patient's problems. In most musculoskeletal disorders, 80% of the diagnosis comes from this part of the clinical evaluation. The history of patients with rheumatic complaints should include the following: (a) reason for consultation and duration of complaints; (b) present medical care and medications; (c) chronologic review of present illness with emphasis on the locomotor system, consequences of time and disease, and present functional assessment; (d) past history—medical, surgical, and of trauma; (e) social history, emotional and work impact of the disorder, and environmental and work site factors; (f) family history, especially as it relates to the musculoskeletal system; and (g) review of systems. These queries cover the spectrum of rheumatic complaints: pain, stiffness, joint swelling, lack of mobility, physical handicap, and fear of future disability and handicap. The interviewer should be flexible and tactful and should avoid interrupting the patient with too many questions and merely guiding the flow of information. The objective of the interview is to define the patient's complaints and to identify patterns of disease and areas of musculoskeletal involvement that can be further scrutinized on physical examination.

I. **CHIEF COMPLAINT.** Note duration.
II. **PRIMARY PHYSICIAN.** Note name, telephone number, fax number, and e-mail address to assist in locating important data. A discussion with that physician may add

1

greatly to your assessment, may avoid the need to repeat expensive tests already performed, and will better define the course and tempo of the disorder.

III. **HISTORY OF RHEUMATIC DISEASES**

A. Determine the mode of onset, inciting events, duration, and pattern and progression of the musculoskeletal complaints.

   1. **Acute onset** is consistent with infectious, crystal-induced, or traumatic origin. It can also occur in the setting of a connective tissue disorder. Chronic complaints are seen with rheumatoid arthritis (RA), spondyloarthropathies, and osteoarthritis, or the chronic sequelae of traumatic or degenerative back problems.

   2. The **pattern of joint involvement** is very important in defining the type of joint disorder. Symmetric polyarthritis of the small joints of the hands and feet is characteristic of RA, whereas asymmetric involvement of the large joints of the lower extremities is most typical of spondyloarthropathies. A migratory pattern of joint inflammation is seen in rheumatic fever and disseminated gonococcemia. A monarticular arthritis is consistent with osteoarthritis, infectious arthritis, crystal-induced synovitis, or one of the spondyloarthropathies (e.g., psoriatic arthritis, reactive arthritis). An intermittent joint inflammation of the knee with remissions and exacerbations is typical of the tertiary phase of Lyme disease.

   3. **Location, pain characteristics, and associated findings** may all be important keys to the diagnosis. First, metatarsophalangeal joint inflammation of an acute and severe type is quite characteristic of gouty arthritis. Sudden onset of low back pain in the setting of lifting or bending with associated pain radiating down the lateral leg is a common presentation for a disk herniation with sciatica.

      Pain in the superolateral shoulder or upper arm occurring in the setting of playing tennis or painting a ceiling is typical of supraspinatus tendinitis or impingement syndrome.

B. Record the **severity of disease,** as revealed by a chronologic review of the following:

   1. Ability to **work** during months or years.
   2. Need for hospitalization or home confinement.
   3. When applicable, ability to do household chores.
   4. Activities of daily living and **personal care.**
   5. Landmarks or significant **functional change,** such as retirement from work, need for household help, assistance for personal care, and the use of a cane, crutches, or a wheelchair.

C. Assess **current functional ability.** This can be done in a question-and-answer format and quantified with the use of functional instruments such as the Health Assessment Questionnaire (HAQ) or the Arthritis Impact Measurement Scale (AIMS2), or functional ability can be measured with the use of a visual analog scale (0 representing no impact on function and 10 being the worst possible limitation in function).

   1. At home: independence or reliance on help from family members and others.
   2. At work: transportation and job requirements and limitations. Have the patient collect an hour-by-hour log of work activities, with an attempt to define actions that may cause or exacerbate musculoskeletal problems.
   3. At recreational and social activities: limitations and extent to which patient is house-bound.
   4. Review of a typical 24-hour period, with focus on abilities to transfer, ambulate, and perform personal care.

D. Obtain an overview of **management** for rheumatic disease.

   1. **Medications** used in the past, with emphasis on dosages, duration of treatments, efficacy response, and possible adverse reactions. Record the present drug regimen and how well the patient complies with it, and also the patient's understanding of the reasons for and potential complications of the medication.
   2. Instruction in and compliance with a **therapeutic exercise** program.
   3. **Surgical procedures** on joints, including benefits and liabilities. Record the name of the surgeon, date of the surgery, and the hospital. Operative pathology reports may be helpful.

   E. Determine the patient's understanding of the disease, therapeutic goals, and expectations.
   F. Record **psychosocial** consequences of disease.
      1. Anxiety, depression, insomnia. Obtain information about psychological/psychiatric intervention and a listing of psychotropic medications.
      2. Economic impact of handicap and present means of support.
      3. Family inter-relationships.
      4. Use of community resources.
IV. PAST HISTORY. Follow traditional lines of questioning, with attention to trauma and joint operations. Also question the patient about those specific medical disorders that could have a significant impact on, or association with, the joint disorder.
   Specific associations include psoriasis with psoriatic arthritis; ulcerative colitis or Crohn's disease with inflammatory disease of the spine or peripheral or sacroiliac joints; diabetes with neuropathic or septic joints, or osteomyelitis; hemochromatosis with severe osteoarthritis; endocrinopathies such as hypothyroidism with carpal tunnel syndrome or myopathy, hyperparathyroidism with pseudogout, and acromegaly with severe osteoarthritis. A complete medication list of the patient is essential, as well as an inquiry into prior medications. In this context, think about agents associated with drug-induced lupus, Raynaud's phenomenon associated with the use of β-blockers, eosinophilia-myalgia syndrome associated with L-tryptophan, or myositis associated with the use of "statin" drugs for hypercholesterolemia.
V. SOCIAL HISTORY. The physician must consider the following associations between the social history and types of musculoskeletal disorders:
   A. Work activities, including the possibility of joint or back trauma, exposure to toxins, or overuse syndromes. Specific examples include low-back syndromes, exposure to vinyl chloride leading to scleroderma-type skin changes, and carpal tunnel syndrome resulting from typing at a computer terminal.
   B. Sexual history, including sexual preference, sexual promiscuity, and the most recent sexual experience. Musculoskeletal disorders related to acquired immunodeficiency syndrome (AIDS) and venereal disorders such as gonococcal disease should be considered.
   C. Living site and conditions, including overcrowding (e.g., rheumatic fever), living in an area where Lyme disease is endemic, or a recent or distant history of tick bite.
   D. Emotional or physical stress, which could have an impact on the development or exacerbation of musculoskeletal disorders.
   E. The presence of **medical problems within the family,** including infectious disorders in children (e.g., fifth disease caused by parvovirus B19, rubella) and adults (e.g., hepatitis B and C, Lyme disease, tuberculosis).
   F. Recent travel, with specific emphasis on the development of dysentery caused by *Salmonella* or *Shigella* (e.g., reactive arthritis), or travel to an area where Lyme disease is endemic.
VI. FAMILY HISTORY. Inquiry about arthritis and rheumatic disease in parents and siblings may elicit vague and unreliable statements, but they are nonetheless important. The presence of severely handicapped relatives with RA or other severe rheumatic disease might result in a significant psychological impact on the patient and should be brought out in the interview. Such information may also be important in relation to the genetic background of arthritis in the family. The physician should inquire about the following musculoskeletal disorders, which clearly have a tendency to run in families: gout and uric acid kidney stones; RA and other connective tissue disorders; ankylosing spondylitis and other spondyloarthropathies; osteoarthritis, especially nodal disease in the fingers; and classic, heritable connective tissue disorders, such as Marfan's syndrome.
VII. REVIEW OF SYSTEMS. Emphasize diseases and systemic disorders related to rheumatic complaints and diseases of connective tissue. Especially inquire about eye disease (iritis, uveitis, conjunctivitis, dryness), mouth disorders (dryness, mouth sores, tightness), gastrointestinal problems (problems with swallowing, reflux symptoms, abdominal pain, diarrhea with or without blood, constipation), genitourinary complaints (including dysuria, urethral discharge, hematuria), and skin disorders (rash with or without sun sensitivity, nodules, ulcers, Raynaud's phenomenon, ischemic

changes). The presence of constitutional symptoms is also important, including complaints of weight loss, fatigue, fever, chills, night sweats, and weakness.

 ## PHYSICAL EXAMINATION WITH EMPHASIS ON RHEUMATIC DISEASES

Five aspects of the physical examination that should be recorded are (a) gait, (b) spine, (c) muscles, (d) upper extremities, and (e) lower extremities. The patient should be properly attired in a short gown, open at the back to allow examination of the entire spine. Examination should be methodic and start with observation of the patient's attitude, comfort levels, ease of undressing, method of rising from a chair and sitting down, and apparent state of nutrition. The patient is examined while standing, sitting, and supine. The examiner should rely mainly on inspection. When using palpation and manipulation, the examiner should be gentle and forewarn the patient of potentially painful maneuvers.

I. **GAIT.** Describe the gait, and note a limp or use of a cane or crutches. The normal gait is divided into the phases of stance (60%) and swing (40%). Clinically important gaits include the following:

    A. **Antalgic gait,** characterized by a short stance phase on the painful side.

    B. **Short-leg gait,** with signs of pelvic obliquity and flexion deformity of the opposite knee.

    C. **Coxalgic gait,** an antalgic gait with a lurch toward the painful hip.

    D. **Metatarsalgic gait,** in which the patient tries to avoid weight bearing on the forefoot.

II. **STANDING POSITION**

    A. Examining front and back, note **posture** (cervical lordosis, scoliosis, dorsal kyphosis, lumbar lordosis). Check if the pelvis is level by putting one finger on each iliac crest and noting asymmetry. Pelvic obliquity suggests unequal leg lengths. Note also if a tilt of the trunk to one side is present.

    B. Examine **alignment of the lower extremities** for flexion deformity of the knees, genu varum (bowlegs), or genu valgum (knock-knees).

    C. Observe **position of the ankles and feet** (varus or valgus heels, flat feet, inversion or eversion of feet).

    D. Check **back motion** on forward bending (with rounding of the normal thoracolumbar spine), lateral flexion to each side, and hyperextension. The extent of overall **spinal flexion** can be assessed with a metal tape measure. One end of the tape is placed at the C7 spinous process, and the other end is placed at S1 with the patient standing erect. The patient is then asked to bend forward, flexing the spine maximally. The measuring tape will reveal an increase of 10 cm with normal spine flexion; 7.5 cm of the total increase results from lumbar spine (measured from spinous process T12–S1) mobility in normal adults. The lumbar spine motion can be assessed by the Schober's test in an erect patient, wherein the examiner makes an ink mark at the lumbosacral junction and at a point 10 cm above. The patient is then instructed to maximally anterior flex, and the distance between the marks is recorded. Less than 5 cm of distraction is abnormal. These measurements are useful for the serial evaluation of patients with spondyloarthropathy.

III. **SEATED POSITION**

    A. Observe **head and neck motion** in all planes (Fig. 1-1).

    B. Examine **thoracolumbar spine motion** with the pelvis fixed. Observe rounding and straightening of back, lateral flexion to each side, and rotation to right and left.

    C. Check **temporomandibular joints.** Palpate, examine lower jaw motion, and measure the aperture between upper and lower teeth with the mouth fully open.

    D. Proceed with the rest of the routine examination of the head and neck; describe eye, ear, nose, and throat findings.

    E. **Upper extremities**

        1. **Shoulders**

            a. Note normal **contour** or "squaring" caused by deltoid atrophy. Palpate anteriorly for soft-tissue swelling and laterally under the acromion for tendon insertion tenderness.

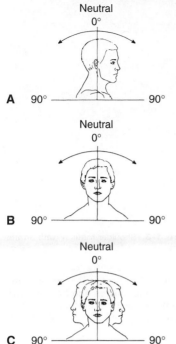

A 90° ———————— 90°
Neutral
0°

B 90° ———————— 90°
Neutral
0°

C 90° ———————— 90°
Neutral
0°

Figure 1-1. Neck motion. **A:** Flexion and extension. **B:** Lateral bending. **C:** Rotation.

    b. Function of the entire shoulder complex is evaluated by elevating both arms from 0 degrees along the sides of body to 180 degrees straight above the head. Quantify **internal** rotation by having the patient reach with the dorsum of the hands, the highest possible level of the back (Fig. 1-2); quantify **external** rotation by noting the position behind the neck or head that the hands can reach.

    c. Isolate the **glenohumeral joint motion** from the scapulothoracic motion by **fixing the scapula.** Holding both hands, assist the patient in abducting arms to the normal maximum of 90 degrees, and note restriction of

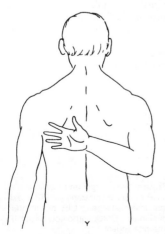

Figure 1-2. Internal rotation of shoulder, posterior view. Record range of reach: dorsum of hand to specific vertebral bodies.

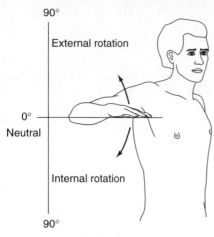

90°

External rotation

0°
Neutral

Internal rotation

90°

Rotation in abduction

Figure 1-3. Shoulder rotation (with arm in abduction).

motion on either side. To determine internal and external rotation of the glenohumeral joint on each side, the examiner **places one hand on the shoulder to prevent scapular motion** and, with the other hand, assists each arm to full external rotation of 90 degrees and full internal rotation of 80 degrees (Fig. 1-3).

2. **Elbows**
    a. Inspect each elbow for **maximum extension** to 0 degrees and full flexion to 150 degrees. Less than full extension is reported in degrees as flexion deformity or lack of extension.
    b. Inspection and palpation may reveal the presence of **olecranon bursitis** at the elbow tip or the soft-tissue swelling of **synovitis,** which is felt in the fossae between the olecranon and lateral epicondyle or between the olecranon and medial epicondyle.
    c. **Subcutaneous nodules and tophi** should be sought in the olecranon bursa and over the extensor surface of the elbow and forearm.
3. **Wrist and hands**
    a. Inspect and palpate wrists; metacarpophalangeal (MCP), proximal interphalangeal (PIP), and distal interphalangeal (DIP) joints of fingers; and carpometacarpal (CMC), MCP, and interphalangeal (IP) joints of thumbs (Fig. 1-4). Note shape and deformities: boutonniere, swan neck, and ulnar deviation.
    b. **Soft-tissue swelling** has a spongy consistency and should be sought on the dorsum of the wrist, distal to the ulna and over the radiocarpal joint.

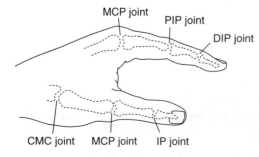

MCP joint

PIP joint

DIP joint

CMC joint   MCP joint   IP joint

Figure 1-4. Finger and thumb joints. MCP, metacarpophalangeal; PIP, proximal interphalangeal; DIP, distal interphalangeal; CMC, carpometacarpal; IP, interphalangeal.

On the volar surface, the normal step-down from hand to forearm may be obliterated by soft-tissue swelling. Volar synovitis may be associated with carpal tunnel syndrome. Tapping on the volar aspect of the wrist may elicit paresthesiae radiating into the radial three fingers, or even the forearm. This positive Tinel's sign is consistent with carpal tunnel syndrome. Thenar atrophy would further support this diagnosis.

    c. All **finger joints** should be examined by inspection and palpation for soft-tissue swelling, capsular thickening, and bony enlargement.

    d. **Average wrist motion** is dorsiflexion to 75 degrees, palmar flexion to 70 degrees, ulnar deviation of 45 degrees, and radial deviation of 20 degrees (Table 1-1).

    e. The **fist** is described as 100% when all fingers reach the palm of the hand and the thumb closes over the fingers. Halfway fist closing is recorded as 50%; less than 50% and 75% are other possible intermediate measurements. The distance from fingertips to palm can also be recorded.

    f. **Grip** is quantified by noting the patient's maximum strength in grasping two fingers of the examiner. **Pinch** is assessed by the force necessary to break the patient's pinch between index finger and thumb.

    g. **Pronation and supination** are combined functions of the elbow and wrist and are determined by having the patient hold the forearm horizontal and the thumb up. Pronation and supination are measured in degrees from the neutral position, with the hand turning palm up and palm down (Fig. 1-5).

F. While the patient is sitting, customary physical examination of the **neck and chest** should be performed; it should include examination of sternoclavicular joints and **measurement of chest expansion, which should be greater than 5 cm in the nipple line.**

IV. SUPINE POSITION

A. Start with the standard physical examination of the **abdomen,** and then proceed to the examination of the **lower extremities.**

B. Alignment of the **knees** is compared with the alignment noted on weight bearing (see section **II.B**). Palpate pedal pulses.

C. Low back

    1. Inspection, palpation, and assessment of range of motion (see section **II.D**).

    2. Neurologic examination. Look for radicular signs and root signatures (see section **I**).

    3. Traction maneuvers

        a. Straight leg-raising test to screen for lumbosacral nerve root symptoms; note angle of elevation that induces back or buttock pain.

        b. Gaenslen's maneuver to detect sacroiliac joint inflammation. Instruct the patient to lie supine on the examining table with knees flexed and one buttock over the edge. Ask the patient to drop the unsupported leg off the table. **This maneuver will elicit pain in the sacroiliac joint ipsilateral to the extended hip. The maneuver exerts a traction force on the sacroiliac joint, which opens it up.**

D. Hips

    1. Hip function is screened by gently log-rolling each lower extremity and noting the freedom of motion of the **ball-and-socket joint.** Rolling also allows measurement of the **internal and external rotation** of the hip joint in extension.

    2. With one hand fixing the pelvis, the other hand moves each hip to the normal 60 degrees of full **abduction** and to the normal 30 degrees of **adduction** while the hip is held in extension.

    3. Each hip joint is then examined in **flexion;** both lower extremities are flexed at knees and hips and carried toward the chest, which gives the maximum angle (120 degrees) of flexion of each hip.

    4. Normal hip **extension** is to −10 degrees. To avoid overlooking a hip flexion deformity for which accentuation of lumbar lordosis may compensate, the examiner keeps one lower extremity flexed over the chest, thereby flattening the lumbar spine, while instructing the patient to extend fully the opposite leg.

TABLE 1-1	Average Joint Motion for Young Adults

Joint motion	Normal value
Spine	
Cervical	
Forward flexion	40°
Lateral bending	30°
Extension	30°
Rotation	60°
Thoracic	
Rotation with pelvis fixed	45°
Chest expansion	>5 cm
Lumbar	
Forward flexion	90°
Lateral bending	30°
Extension	30°
Upper extremities	
Shoulder	
Abduction (arm at side and elevation above head)	180°
Forward flexion (a normal touchdown sign and good screener for rotator cuff dysfunction).	180°
Rotation (arm in abduction to 90°)	
Internal	80°
External	90°
Elbow	
Flexion	150°
Extension	0°
Forearm	
Pronation	90°
Supination	85°
Wrist	
Extension	75°
Flexion	70°
Ulnar deviation	45°
Radial deviation	20°
Fist (in percentage)	
Full fist	100°
Lower extremities	
Hip	
Flexion	120°
Extension	−10°
In flexion	
Internal rotation	25°
External rotation	35°
Abduction	45°
Adduction	25°
In extension	
Abduction	60°
Adduction	30°
Knee	
Flexion	130°
Extension	0°
Ankle	
Flexion	15°
Extension	35°
Hind foot	
Inversion–eversion (subtalar) (in percentage)	
Full motion	100°

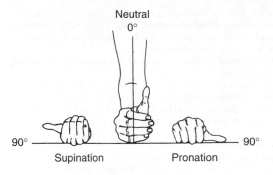

Neutral
0°

90° — Supination   Pronation — 90°

Figure 1-5. Forearm pronation and supination.

5. With the hip in 90 degrees of flexion, the joint is evaluated for internal rotation (25 degrees), external rotation (35 degrees), abduction (45 degrees), and adduction (25 degrees) (Fig. 1-6).

E. **Measurement of leg length** (see Chapter 23). If the discrepancy is greater than one-half inch, a heel lift for the shoe on the affected side should be ordered.

F. **Knees**

1. By inspection and palpation, note position and mobility of **patellae.** Knee extension–flexion range is 0 to 130 degrees. Also palpate for the presence of osteophytes at the tibiofemoral joint margin, which may also be tender.

2. **Soft-tissue swelling** is elicited by bimanual examination.

   a. Demonstrate intra-articular fluid by the **patellar click sign.** While compressing the suprapatellar pouch with one hand, push the patella against underlying fluid and the femoral condyle with the index finger of the other hand to elicit a click.

   b. For detection of a small amount of effusion, use the bulge sign. This maneuver is best executed by placing both hands on the knee so that the index fingers meet on the medial joint margin and the thumbs meet on the lateral aspect of the joint. Through a firm stroking motion of the fingers above

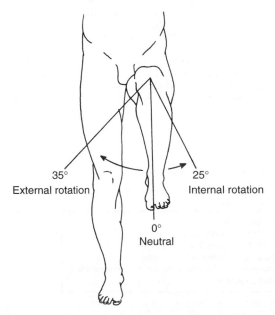

35°
External rotation

25°
Internal rotation

0°
Neutral

Figure 1-6. Hip rotation in flexion.

and below the patella, fluid is "milked" into the interior of the joint, and the **medial aspect of the joint becomes flat.** The thumbs are then pushed suddenly and firmly into the lateral joint margin, thereby producing a bulge of fluid on the medial side of the joint.

3. The **popliteal area** is examined for the presence of a synovial cyst. Standing makes the cyst more prominent.
4. **Knee stability** is evaluated by stressing medial and lateral **collateral ligaments.** Anteroposterior stability is assessed by holding the knee flexed with the foot firmly anchored on the bed and using both hands to pull and push the leg (drawer sign) to test the **cruciate ligaments.**

G. **Ankles and feet**
   1. **Synovial soft-tissue swelling** of the ankles at both malleoli should be distinguished from periarticular edema and fat pads.
   2. **Normal ankle motion** is 15 degrees flexion and 35 degrees extension.
   3. **Subtalar motion,** which allows inversion and eversion of the foot, is best reported as a percentage of normal, with 100% meaning full mediolateral motion.

H. **Toes.** By inspection and palpation, note the following:
   1. **Alignment** and deformity: hammertoes, claw toes, and hallux valgus.
   2. **Soft-tissue swelling** and presence of inflammation, which are best documented by mediolateral squeezing across the metatarsal joints; pain may be elicited.

I. **Muscle examination.** Proximally and distally, note the following:
   1. On inspection, muscle **wasting** and muscle **atrophy.**
   2. On palpation, muscle **tenderness.**
   3. On testing motion, muscle **strength** (Table 1-2).

J. **Neurologic examination**
   1. Standard evaluation of **tendon reflexes.**
   2. **Impairment of nerve root function** must be sought with care, and motor and sensory deficits recorded (see Chapters 19 and 20).
   3. Look for **nerve entrapment,** secondary to joint pathology (e.g., carpal tunnel syndrome).

V. **SYSTEMATIC EXAMINATION AND JOINT CHART**
   A. Inspection, palpation, and movement of joints may reveal swelling, tenderness, temperature and color changes over the joint, crepitation, and deformity.
      1. **Tenderness** on direct pressure over the joint and **stress pain** produced when the joint, at the limit of its range of motion, is nudged a little farther are important findings of inflammation. The number of tender and swollen joints can be recorded and compared with future joint counts after the institution of therapy.
      2. **Crepitation** is a palpable or audible sensation with joint motion caused by roughened articular or extra-articular surfaces rubbing each other. "Popping" sounds can also be heard and felt when tendons travel over bony prominences.
      3. **Bony enlargement, subluxation, and ankylosis in abnormal positions cause deformity.**

 TABLE 1-2   **Gradations of Muscle Weakness**

Grade	Muscle involvement
0	No muscle contraction
1	Flicker or trace of contraction
2	Active movement possible with gravity eliminated
3	Active movement possible against gravity
4	Active movement possible against gravity and resistance
5	Normal muscle power

B. **Quantification of findings**
1. **Range of motion** is reported in degrees and, when practical, in percentage of normal (i.e., fist and subtalar motions). See Table 1-1 for average values.
2. **Swelling and tenderness** are arbitrarily reported in grades 1, 2, and 3, which indicate size and severity, ranging from minimal to severe. Numbers of swollen and tender joints can be recorded (called a joint count) for future comparison after treatment has been instituted, and for use in controlled clinical trials.
3. Other physical signs of joint abnormality include **warmth and erythema over the joint** and should be expressed as grades 1, 2, or 3 (mild, moderate, or severe).

VI. **EXTRA-ARTICULAR FEATURES.** Examination is completed by recording specific findings important in rheumatic diseases, such as subcutaneous nodules, nail changes, rash, abnormal eye findings, sicca (dryness) signs of the eyes and mouth, lymphadenopathy, leg ulcers, and visceral involvement such as splenomegaly, pleural or pericardial signs, and neurologic abnormalities.

OVERALL ASSESSMENT OF JOINT STRUCTURE AND FUNCTION

The rheumatic disease history and systematic examination allow assessment of the following:

I. **DEGREE OF JOINT INFLAMMATION.** Number of acute joints (tender and swollen) and their location and degree of involvement.
II. **STRUCTURAL DAMAGE AND DEFORMITY** (malalignment, subluxation, and instability). Findings are reported by a count of joints deformed or limited in their motion.
III. **FUNCTION.** Assessment is based on the following:
A. **Joint range of motion.**
B. **Muscle strength** (grip strength, abduction of shoulders, straight leg raising, rising from squatting and sitting positions, and walking on toes). See Table 1-2.
C. **Activities of daily living.** Mobility, personal care, special hand functions, and work and play activities.
D. Function can be reported in **four classes** based on the American College of Rheumatology classification:

Class 1 **Normal function without or despite symptoms.**
Class 2 **Some disability but adequate for normal activity without special devices or assistance.**
Class 3 **Activities restricted; special devices or assistance required.**
Class 4 **Totally dependent.**

Other, more quantitative instruments are available for the evaluation and prospective assessment of function, performance of social activities, and emotional status. Specialized pain and function instruments are also available for clinical trials.

In conclusion, a comprehensive clinical evaluation (history plus physical examination) focused on the musculoskeletal system and psychosocial consequences of disease, followed by a complete physical examination with a detailed musculoskeletal and joint evaluation, is the clinical basis for the diagnosis and individualized management of rheumatic disease. Such an approach allows the professional to distill large amounts of information rapidly to reach a specific diagnosis and formulate an appropriate, focused, and effective therapeutic plan.

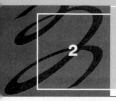

THINKING LIKE A RHEUMATOLOGIST
Arthur M. F. Yee

■ KEY POINTS

- **The diagnosis of many rheumatologic disorders is made clinically,** and so a detailed medical history and thorough physical examination are unequivocally central to the initial evaluation of the patient. A strong knowledge base of rheumatology streamlines the diagnostic process, enabling quicker development of management plans.

- **Always treat the patient, not the laboratory results.** Although laboratory, radiologic, and pathologic data can be very useful in the management of rheumatologic disorders, they should always be taken in the context of, and never supersede, the clinical picture. Appreciating the limitations of diagnostic tests optimizes their clinical utility.

- **Uncertainty is rife in rheumatology and must be accepted.** Management decisions must often be made even when the clinical picture is incomplete or atypical, or when clinical data is unavailable or inaccessible.

- **Rheumatologic disorders are often variable in course and severity.** The aggressiveness of therapy must be appropriate to the aggressiveness of disease, because both the treatment modalities and the illness carry potential dangers. The chronic nature of many conditions necessitates ongoing vigilance, even during periods of disease quiescence.

- **Better education of the patient,** especially with respect to the nature of illness and to therapeutic goals and expectations, and trust between the physician and patient optimize compliance and outcome.

*H*anging in my examination room are reproductions of two French impressionist paintings. The first is the famous *A Sunday on La Grande Jatte* by Georges-Pierre Seurat who pioneered the technique of juxtaposing small dots of different colors to create images that become apparent only when seen from a distance. Even then, however, smaller details can remain obscure and subtle. I use this painting to illustrate to patients how I often approach rheumatologic conditions. First, while I am generally called upon to evaluate a specific problem, I do not focus solely on one single "dot" but rather view it in the context of all the "dots" in order to see the whole clinical picture. Second, even if the picture is spotted with areas of fuzziness and uncertainty, it can still be fully appreciated and addressed with comfort.

FRAMING THE CLINICAL INVESTIGATION

Many rheumatologic conditions are clinical diagnoses and are systemic in nature, so it cannot be overstated that the skills most important to the rheumatologist are those that are also the most important to an astute internist. These include the ability to obtain an accurate medical history and conduct a thorough physical examination and to be comfortable with handling different organ systems. The review of systems, in particular, often provides crucial pieces of information that may not be spontaneously volunteered by the patient and also comprises a large part of my initial evaluations. This process, although seemingly exhausting, can be made very efficient by attaining familiarity with potentially relevant conditions. For example, an elderly man taking diuretics for hypertension who presents with recurrent acute inflammation of the first metatarsophalangeal joint need not necessarily be questioned for a history of sun sensitivity or a malar rash but should be questioned for a history of tophi or renal calculi. A young woman with a history of multiple osteoporotic stress fractures should probably be asked about symptoms suggestive of malabsorptive states. A large fund of knowledge *a priori* improves the diagnostic process by generating pertinent questions and discarding irrelevant ones.

ADDRESSING THE PATIENT, NOT STUDY RESULTS

Laboratory, radiologic, and pathologic studies can be extremely useful to the rheumatologist, but they should only be obtained in the appropriate setting. Inappropriate testing can often increase diagnostic confusion as well as become a source of unnecessary anxiety for the patient. The utility of diagnostic testing is highly dependent on the pretest probability of a particular condition; therefore, an astute clinical evaluation beforehand remains central. For example, the presence of circulating antinuclear antibodies (ANA) is highly sensitive for the diagnosis of systemic lupus erythematosus (SLE) but is also notoriously nonspecific. Therefore, in considering the diagnosis of SLE, a negative test result can be very useful in excluding this diagnosis, whereas a positive test result can best be used to support the clinical impression. Conversely, the anti-dsDNA antibody is highly specific but only moderately sensitive for SLE; therefore, it is less useful as a screening test and more useful (if positive) as a confirmatory test.

Tests such as the erythrocyte sedimentation rate (ESR) and C reactive protein (CRP) can provide useful information about the degree of activity of a systemic disease. However, one should never be swayed blindly by the results of these tests and should always take the overall clinical picture as the guide for developing the management plan. A patient with polymyalgia rheumatica (PMR) who has a slightly elevated ESR but who is feeling well does not need to have her corticosteroid dosage increased just to normalize the ESR. Conversely, a patient with PMR who complains of a recurrence of significant muscle stiffness in the morning should probably increase her corticosteroid dosage no matter what the ESR is.

LIVING COMFORTABLY WITH UNCERTAINTY

Because many rheumatologic diagnoses are made primarily on a clinical basis, one of the greatest challenges in training rheumatology fellows is to teach them to become comfortable with uncertainty. This can only be accomplished by maximizing clinical experience and maintaining a solid knowledge base.

Many criteria and classification schemes for the diagnosis of rheumatologic disorders have been published, but for the most part, these were developed for the purpose of clinical trials and population studies and not as the sole basis for making diagnoses in specific patients. Therefore, a young woman with a malar rash, glomerulonephritis, and a positive ANA should be treated as a patient with SLE, even if she does not fulfill a fourth criterion for diagnosis as established by the American College of Rheumatology.

Not infrequently, a patient may present with an obvious but undiagnosed systemic inflammatory condition which may be threatening a vital organ or even life, and awaiting a definitive pathologic diagnosis may carry unacceptable risks. An example of this may be an elderly woman presenting with fever, myalgias, and visual deficit of new vision loss, consistent with the diagnosis of giant cell arteritis (GCA). In this situation, therapy should not be delayed pending a temporal artery biopsy because the risk of permanent blindness far outweighs the risks of corticosteroid treatment. Moreover, a strong argument can be made for treating for presumptive GCA, even if the biopsy result is negative.

On another occasion, a patient may have an inflammatory condition such as an interstitial pneumonitis and show a steady decline in health status, but diagnostic testing has been reasonably extensive to exclude infection or malignancy although no definitive diagnosis has been arrived at. Here again, systemic anti-inflammatory or immunosuppressive therapy may be appropriate, provided continued vigilance is maintained for new or progressive problems.

TAILORING MANAGEMENT PLANS

Two important characteristics of many rheumatologic diseases are chronicity and wide variability in course and severity. SLE may be quite mild for many years, with easily managed intermittent arthritic or dermatologic flares, or may be aggressive and fulminant at any moment, with endangerment to vital organs or to life. It is important to remember to treat the patient at hand, and not the diagnosis. There is no one treatment regimen that is universally appropriate for any particular diagnosis, and the management plan needs to be as potent as the severity of a particular case dictates. Unlike oncologists who use very potent (and toxic) medications to treat a malignant neoplasm, that, if left untreated, would kill the patient, rheumatologists tend to walk a fine line between the threats imposed by the disease and the toxicities carried by the therapies. Close and vigilant monitoring for an indefinite period, to assess whether the patient requires medical treatment or not, is the rule.

PARTNERING WITH THE PATIENT

Rheumatologic conditions are often difficult to understand for the medical professional, let alone the patient. Therefore, every effort must be made to help the patient to the best of his/her ability to understand the nature of the illness and the goals of therapy and to establish a trusting doctor–patient relationship. Without understanding and rapport, compliance and, therefore, outcome are diminished.

The second painting hanging on my wall is *Two Young Girls at the Piano* by Auguste Renoir, who himself had severe arthritis and toward the end of his life required that his brushes be bound to his hands in order to paint. It is said by some that Renoir sometimes portrayed his subjects as having the arthritic changes of his own hands, and I can make out the synovitis on the hands of the two young girls in the painting. I can only imagine what more he could have produced if he were not so disabled. However, now with very effective treatments for our diseases, there is great promise to prevent their destructive consequences, and perhaps the full potential of all our patients can be protected and realized.

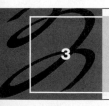

IMMUNOLOGY FOR THE PRIMARY CARE PHYSICIAN
Mary K. Crow

$\mathcal{T}$he function of the immune system is to limit damage to the host by micro-organisms. The immune response to an infection has two components:

I.   **The innate immune response** is the earliest phase of an immune response, triggered by microbial components such as lipopolysaccharide (LPS), heat shock proteins, bacterial DNA, and viral double-stranded (ds) RNA. It comprises phagocytes, including macrophages and neutrophils; natural killer (NK) cells; natural antibodies; soluble molecules, such as cytokines, chemokines, and immunomodulatory molecules (e.g., prostaglandins); and the complement system. Activation of the innate immune response is mediated by interaction of microbial components with members of the Toll-like receptor (TLR) family. A close connection exists between the innate and adaptive immune systems via interferon-α. This is an important concept because it is possible that an infection triggers an autoimmune disorder through this mechanism.

II.   **The adaptive immune response** develops several days after the initiation of a primary immune response and is mediated by lymphocytes expressing cell membrane receptors specific to the invading pathogen. Adaptive immunity is characterized by an increase in antigen specificity over time and development of immunologic memory.

      A. Specificity. Individual T and B lymphocytes bear cell surface receptors that recognize a defined molecular structure (epitope) on an antigen (i.e., a molecule on or in a bacterium or virus, or a peptide, that elicits an immune response). Each lymphocyte expresses a single receptor of unique structure and antigenic specificity.

T-cell receptors (TCRs) do not change upon antigen exposure, but B cells can modify their cell surface immunoglobulin (Ig) by somatic mutation.

B. Memory. Reintroduction of an antigen elicits an immune response more rapidly, and of greater magnitude, than that which occurred on initial exposure.

 CELLULAR AND MOLECULAR COMPONENTS OF THE IMMUNE RESPONSE

I. **The central players** in the generation of an adaptive immune response include an antigen, an antigen presenting cell (APC), an antigen-specific T lymphocyte, and a B lymphocyte capable of differentiation into a plasma cell that can secrete an antigen-specific Ig (antibody). Arguably, the most important structure in the immune system in terms of generation of a specific immune response is the trimolecular complex that includes the following:

A. Antigenic peptide.

B. Major histocompatibility complex (MHC) molecule on the surface of an APC.

C. TCR.

II. **APCs** are located at many sites throughout the body, especially skin, mucosal surfaces, lymph nodes, spleen, and liver. They are among the first cells to encounter infectious organisms. All APCs express cell surface MHC class I and II molecules.

A. **Types of APC**

1. **Activated B lymphocytes** specifically bind and process antigen via surface immunoglobulin (sIg) receptors or bind antigen-containing immune complexes via sIg reactive with the constant region of IgG (i.e., sIg with rheumatoid factor activity).

2. **Monocytes/Macrophages** bind and phagocytose intact or fragmented microorganisms, particulate or soluble antigens, or immune complexes via receptors for the Fc fragment of IgG or receptors for complement components (C4b/C3b and iC3b).

3. **Dendritic cells** are the most potent APCs because they express higher levels of MHC class II molecules and costimulatory (CD80, CD86) and adhesion [intercellular cell adhesion molecule-1 (ICAM-1)] molecules than other APCs. They have a capacity for "macropinocytosis"—"drinking" of the surrounding molecular constituents—and antigen processing. Dendritic cells can engulf apoptotic virus-infected cells and present the viral antigens to both CD4+ and CD8+ positive T cells. Follicular dendritic cells in lymphoid organs (a distinct cell type) may serve as a reservoir for presentation of preprocessed antigenic peptides to B cells. There are several subtypes of dendritic cells that may mediate different functions. Some derive from the myeloid lineage and others from the lymphoid lineage.

B. **Activation of an APC** occurs through uptake of antigen [through sIg or Fc receptor (FcR)], binding of microbial products to TLR, and binding of cytokines released after activation of the innate immune response [interferon-α (IFN-α), tumor necrosis factor-α (TNF-α)]. APCs are also activated by cell-mediated interactions with activated T cells (through CD40) and by T-cell–derived cytokines, such as interferon-γ.

C. **Function of APC**

1. Antigens generated in the intracellular compartment (e.g., virus-encoded proteins) are processed by enzymatic digestion in a "proteosome," chaperoned to the endoplasmic reticulum by members of the heat shock protein family of molecules, and incorporated into the binding site of MHC class I molecules as small peptides of approximately nine amino acids in length. These MHC class I-bound peptides are presented to CD8+ T cells.

2. Antigens taken in from the extracellular environment are enzymatically processed in specialized intracellular compartments enriched in MHC class II molecules. Antigenic peptides of variable length (13 to 18 amino acids) in the class II antigen-binding cleft are transported to the cell surface. These MHC class II-bound peptides are presented to CD4+ T cells.

3. Poorly understood intracellular processes favor the enzymatic cleavage and presentation of particular amino acid sequences within an antigen. This concept is termed "determinant selection." B cells that are activated by specific antigens

can take up those antigens through sIg and present a different set of epitopes than dendritic cells or monocytes. Presentation of such "cryptic" epitopes may break tolerance and lead to autoimmunity.

4. Dendritic cells can be "matured" by IFN-α or TNF-α, thereby increasing their capacity to activate T cells.

5. Activated APCs secrete cytokines, including IL-1, IL-12, TNF-α, and transforming growth factor-β (TGF-β), that help regulate the character of the T-cell response to antigen.

III. **T Lymphocytes** are the central regulatory cell in the immune system. Functional T-cell subsets include T helper cells, which produce either T helper 1 (T_H1) or T helper 2 (T_H2) cytokines and which support B cell, macrophage, or dendritic cell differentiation, or T cytotoxic/suppressor cells, which mediate death of target cells.

A. **Location.** Maturation and selection of the T-cell repertoire occurs in the thymus, whereas mature T cells are found in skin, lymph nodes, spleen, gut, lymph, and blood. Memory T cells may have different homing patterns than naïve T cells that have not been stimulated by antigens.

B. **Phenotype**

1. **TCR complex.** Most T cells express a TCR heterodimer composed of α and β chains. These chains contain constant and variable regions. The variable region of a given TCR-α or TCR-β chain is encoded by one of a number of variable genes, each characterized by particular nucleotide sequences. Variability among TCR is derived from transcription of different variable genes, insertions and deletions of nucleotides in the TCR chains, and variable pairing of α and β chains. The complementarity determining region 3 (CDR3) of the TCR chains constitutes the TCR structure that interacts with antigenic peptide in the MHC class I or II binding sites. A small T-cell population expresses a TCR heterodimer composed of γ and δ chains.

2. The **CD3 molecule** is composed of five chains that associate with the TCR in the T-cell membrane. It transduces activation signals to the T cell by triggering biochemical pathways, including protein kinases.

3. **Subset markers on the surface of T lymphocytes**

a. **CD4** is on 60% to 70% of T cells; it associates with MHC class II molecules on APC; and its expression correlates with helper/inducer function (meaning helping or inducing B cells to produce antibodies), although some CD4+ T cells can mediate cytotoxicity (meaning cell killing) through Fas ligand–Fas receptor interactions.

b. **CD8** is on 30% to 40% of T cells; it associates with MHC class I molecules on APC; and its expression correlates with cytotoxic/suppressor function (i.e., cell killing or suppression of an immune response).

4. **Accessory and costimulatory molecules that mediate binding to other cells and transmit activation or inhibitory signals**

a. **CD2 and lymphocyte function-associated antigen (LFA-1)** are adhesion molecules.

b. **CD28** ligation by CD80 or CD86 results in a T-cell stimulatory signal that augments TCR-mediated T-cell activation.

c. **CTLA-4** ligation by CD80 or CD86 leads to inhibitory signals to the T cell.

d. **ICOS** is a CD28-like molecule that appears to preferentially costimulate T_H2-like responses and memory T cells. Its ligand is B7RP-1.

e. **PD-1** is a CTLA4-like molecule that may transduce a negative signal to the T cell. A polymorphism in PD-1 has been associated with systemic lupus erythematosus (SLE).

f. **CD40 ligand (CD154)** is briefly expressed on the CD4 T-cell surface following TCR-mediated T-cell activation. It mediates ligation of CD40 on interacting B cells, macrophages, dendritic cells, activated endothelial cells, and activated fibroblasts. The connection between CD40 ligand and CD40 on B cells leads to class switching from IgM to IgG.

g. **Fas ligand** is briefly expressed on memory T cells following TCR-mediated T-cell activation. It mediates apoptosis of interacting cells expressing Fas receptor. This is one of many fail-safe mechanisms that help control and limit the immune response.

      h. Osteoprotegerin ligand (also called **TRANCE** or **RANK ligand**) stimulates osteoclast differentiation.

    5. **Receptors** include **IL-2R** (CD25), **IL-12R, IL-4R, IL-1R,** and **Fas.**

C. T-cell activation requires triggering of several biochemical pathways.

    1. Antigen-mediated signals. Antigenic peptide in the binding groove of MHC class I or II molecules binds to the CDR3 of TCR, resulting in triggering of the T cell via the TCR-associated CD3 complex. Activation of protein tyrosine kinases results in phosphorylation of intracellular regions of transmembrane and other associated molecules. Some of these important signaling molecules are ZAP-70, TCR zeta chain (TCR-ζ), and Lck. Additional biochemical events follow, including increase of intracellular calcium, activation of protein kinase C, and subsequent activation of transcription factors that move to the nucleus, bind to DNA, and activate transcription of genes encoding IL-2, CD40L, and other T-cell proteins. Microbial superantigens, soluble molecules that bind directly to MHC class II molecules, can also trigger T-cell activation through the TCR but bind to variable region sequences outside the CDR3 region of the TCR-β chain.

    2. Costimulatory signals. Ligation of CD28 by CD80 or CD86 transduces additional activation signals that extend and magnify those provided by TCR ligation.

    3. Many factors, including antigen dose, antigenic peptide structure, cytokines, and costimulatory signals, contribute to the character of the T-cell response that is elicited. Insufficient signal can lead to T-cell anergy (i.e., lack of immune responsiveness) or cell death.

D. T-cell function

    1. CD4+ T cells mediate delayed-type hypersensitivity and help in initiating antiviral responses. CD4+ T cells differentiate into either T_H1 cells or T_H2 cells, depending on the cytokines that they are exposed to. T_H1 cells produce IL-2 and IFN-γ and are effective in activating monocytes. T_H2 cells produce IL-4, IL-5, and IL-10 and promote allergic responses. Both T_H1 and T_H2 cytokines can support IgG production by B cells.

    2. CD8+ T cells mediate antigen-specific cytolysis (perforin- or granzyme-mediated) of virus-infected or tumor cells, act as suppressor cells, and produce cytokines.

E. T-cell regulation. T cells orchestrate and insure specificity of the immune response. The regulation of the T-cell repertoire and T-cell activity is essential. Tolerance means that we "tolerate" or do not react immunologically against our own tissues. Tolerance to self is critically important to the maintenance of health and the avoidance of disorders such as SLE and is maintained in the immune system by the following:

    1. Positive and negative (deletion/apoptosis) selection in the thymus—"central tolerance." This means that autoreactive cells that may exist early on in our lives are sensed and destroyed by the thymus.

    2. Clonal ignorance means that T cells do not recognize an antigen with sufficient strength to be either activated or deleted.

    3. Peripheral tolerance. Self-antigens often fail to activate potentially autoreactive T cells (their TCR may have insufficient affinity for self-antigen plus MHC to mediate full T-cell activation). T cells that have undergone excessive activation by self-antigens may undergo activation-induced cell death mediated by Fas ligand–Fas interactions or, in some cases, mediated by TNF-α. Inadequate growth signals from cytokines or costimulatory molecules may account for apoptosis of some self-reactive T cells. Suppressive cytokines (IL-10 or TGF-β) may inhibit expansion of self-reactive T cells. CD4+/CD25+ T cells and NK1 T cells may actively regulate autoreactive T cells that are present in the periphery.

IV. B LYMPHOCYTES

A. Location. B-cell development occurs in the bone marrow followed by homing to spleen, lymph nodes, and gut. The generation of specific antibody-secreting cells and memory B cells occurs in germinal centers in secondary lymphoid organs.

B. Phenotype

    1. sIg complex. Surface IgD and IgM are antigen receptors, and associated α and β chains transduce activation signals to the B cell.

2. Subset markers
   a. CD5+ B cells make "natural" antibodies. Their Ig genes usually secrete IgM isotype and low-affinity autoantibodies.
   b. Marginal zone B cells, surrounding the germinal centers, may be involved in production of autoantibodies. **CD21hi/CD23lo marginal zone B cells** may be involved in production of natural antibacterial antibodies that cross-react with self-antigens.
3. ICAM-1 is an adhesion molecule.
4. Receptors include FcγRIIb, which provides inhibitory signals to B cells, and BAFF/BLyS receptor, which provides survival signals to B cells.
C. B-cell activation
   1. Full activation of a resting B cell usually requires at least two signals, resulting in expression of lymphokine receptors and readiness to differentiate.
   2. Antigen-mediated signals through surface Ig. Binding of antigen by sIg results in activation of biochemical programs. The consequences of these include increased levels of intracellular calcium, activation of additional kinases (e.g., protein kinase C), and activation of transcription factors (e.g., NF-κB) that travel to the cell nucleus and initiate gene transcription.
   3. T-cell–mediated signals. T cells, activated through their TCR, briefly express an important accessory molecule, CD40 ligand. Engagement of B-cell CD40 by T-cell CD40 ligand results in activation signals to the B cell that promote B-cell survival, induce B-cell surface expression of activation molecules, as well as proliferation and isotype switch from IgM to mature Ig classes (IgG, IgA, and IgE). T-cell–derived cytokines bind to B-cell surface cytokine receptors and provide additional activation signals to the B cell. Some of these cytokine-mediated signals are transduced by molecules called JAKs and STATs, intracellular molecules that pass activation messages from cell surface receptors to the nucleus.
   4. When a B cell receives either sIg signals in the absence of CD40-mediated T-cell signals or CD40 signals in the absence of sIg signals, apoptosis (cell death) rather than full B-cell activation may result. CD40-triggered apoptosis is mediated through the Fas receptor, although sIg-triggered apoptosis is mediated through poorly defined non-Fas pathways.
   5. In addition to these antigen-specific mechanisms of B-cell activation, antigen nonspecific B-cell activation can be stimulated by Epstein-Barr virus (EBV), LPS, or microbial superantigens through TLR.
D. B-cell function. The primary function of B cells is to produce antibodies, the specific humoral factors that mediate the immune response to microbial infection. After receiving signal 1 (through sIg) and signal 2 (through CD40), the activated B cell proliferates and differentiates to memory B cells or antibody-secreting plasma cells. Antigen and T-cell signals also drive the process of somatic mutation of Ig genes, with B cells that express higher affinity antibody preferentially selected by antigen. The cytokines that stimulate the CD40-activated B cell help determine the isotype of the Igs secreted by the differentiated B cell. Activated B cells have the augmented capacity to act as APCs.
E. B-cell regulation. The capacity of Ig genes to undergo somatic mutation permits the generation of potentially damaging self-reactive Ig. The regulation of autoantibody secretion depends on the following:
   1. B-cell events. Deletion (apoptosis through sIg or Fas) or induction of anergy in self-reactive B cells following self-antigen ligation of sIg, downregulatory signals through B-cell FcγRII and other B-cell surface molecules, idiotype–antiidiotype networks.
   2. B-cell–independent events. Efficient T-cell tolerance (results in lack of autoantigen-specific T-cell help), "suppressor" T cells (including T-cell–mediated induction of B-cell apoptosis), and inhibitory cytokines.
V. CYTOKINES (PARTIAL LIST)
A. Immunoregulatory
   1. IL-2. Made by T cells, expands T and NK cells.
   2. IFN-γ. Made by T_H1 cells and NK cells; activates macrophages, NK cells.
   3. IL-4. Made by activated T_H2 cells; promotes T_H2 cell survival and induces class switch to IgE and IgG.

4. **IL-5.** Made by T_H2 cells; promotes differentiation of mast cells and eosinophils.

5. **IL-10.** Made by T_H2 cells; inhibits T_H1 cells; promotes B-cell proliferation and class switching.

6. **IL-12.** Promotes differentiation of T_H1 cells.

7. **TGF-β.** Made by activated T cells, monocytes; inhibits T-cell proliferation; promotes class switching to IgA.

8. **BAFF/BLyS.** B-cell survival factor produced by myeloid cells.

B. **Proinflammatory**

1. **IL-1.** Produced by monocytes; induces collagenase and stromelysin-1 production in synovial fibroblasts; high in rheumatoid arthritis (RA) synovium.

2. **TNF-α.** Produced by monocytes; allelic variations in promoter may influence susceptibility to some rheumatic diseases; induces cytokine production, cell activation; high in RA synovium.

3. **Granulocyte-macrophage colony-stimulating factor (GM-CSF).** Increases production of granulocytes, macrophages, and dendritic cells.

4. **IL-6.** Produced by monocytes, fibroblasts, activated lymphocytes; promotes plasma cell formation; high in RA synovium.

5. **IL-8.** A chemokine produced by monocytes, fibroblasts; attracts polymorphonuclear neutrophils (PMNs); high in RA synovium.

6. **Macrophage inflammatory protein-1 (MIP-1) α.** A chemokine produced by macrophages; attracts PMNs, induces secretion of inflammatory cytokines.

7. **RANTES.** A chemokine produced by activated T cells, fibroblasts; attracts T cells, monocytes, eosinophils.

8. **IL-15.** Produced by macrophages and fibroblasts; abundant in rheumatoid joint; promotes T-cell migration into joint and T-cell activation.

9. **IL-18.** Induces IL-1 and TNF-α; costimulant for T_H1 cytokines.

C. **Anti-inflammatory**

1. **IL-1 receptor antagonist.** Endogenous inhibitor of IL-1.

2. **IL-10.** Inhibits TNF-α and IL-2 production and stimulates production of IL-11; high levels of IL-10 in sera from patients with active SLE and RA.

3. **IL-11.** Made in rheumatoid synovium; synergistic with IL-10 in inhibiting TNF-α production; decreases matrix metalloproteinase (MMP) and increases tissue inhibitor of metalloproteinases-1 (TIMP-1) production.

4. **TGF-β.** Inhibits lymphocyte activation.

D. **Pleiotropic effects.** Some cytokines can be either pro- or anti-inflammatory, depending on the milieu and the timing in relation to antigen administration. For example, IL-10 is anti-inflammatory by virtue of its negative effect on APCs if given early in an immune response but can enhance proliferation of cytotoxic T cells when given later. Similarly, TNF-α is proinflammatory early in the immune response but downregulates T cells later in the response.

VI. **OTHER MEDIATORS**

A. **Complement components.** These are proteins that constitute the classic and alternative complement pathways that are activated by microbes or immune complexes. The products of the enzymatic activity of complement components generate chemotactic molecules that recruit inflammatory cells, promote phagocytosis of immune complexes, and stimulate death of microbes. Complement components also help clear apoptotic cells from the body. Deficiencies in complement components such as C1q, C2, or C4 can result in increased susceptibility to SLE, possibly because of impaired clearance of apoptotic cells or impaired solubilization of immune complexes.

B. **Endogenous inhibitors of complement**

C. **Prostaglandins**

 AUTOIMMUNITY

I. **FACTORS CONTRIBUTING TO DISEASE SUSCEPTIBILITY**

A. **Host factors**

1. **Genetic.** Polymorphisms in MHC class I or II, Fcγ receptors, complement components, costimulatory molecules (CTLA4 and PD-1), cytokines (possibly IL-10 or TNF-α), signaling molecules (PTPN22, IRF5, and Tyk2), and likely

many additional as-yet-to-be-defined genes contribute to susceptibility to autoimmune disease.

2. **Hormonal.** Mechanisms are not well defined.
3. **Immunologic.** Acquired or intrinsic molecular abnormalities in immune system function.

B. **Extrinsic triggers**
   1. Infectious agents.
   2. Drugs.
   3. Sunlight/DNA damage.

C. **Stochastic factors.** Chance.

II. **Immunogenetics** (see Chapter 5).

A. **MHC** is on human chromosome 6—highly polymorphic.
   1. Class I—HLA-A, B, C.
   2. Class II—HLA-DR, DP, DQ.
   3. Class III—C2, C4, factor B.
   4. Other genes in MHC include TNF-α, 21-hydroxylase, LMP, and TAP (molecules with functions related to antigen processing).

B. **MHC haplotypes associated with autoimmune disease**
   1. **DR4—rheumatoid arthritis.** The shared epitope hypothesis designates that a related group of human leukocyte antigen (HLA) alleles share a five amino acid epitope that confers susceptibility or determines severity of RA. This has been observed in whites but not in all ethnicities. The amino acids of the shared epitope are Q (glutamine), K (lysine), R (arginine), A (alanine), and A (alanine).
   2. **DR3—SLE**
   3. **HLA-B27—Ankylosing spondylitis**

C. **Proposed mechanisms by which MHC molecules might contribute to autoimmunity**
   1. Effect on generation of T-cell repertoire during maturation in thymus.
   2. Preferential binding of peptides derived from autoantigens.
   3. Disease susceptibility epitope itself may be processed and presented on self MHC molecules to T cells.

III. **POTENTIAL MECHANISMS OF SYSTEMIC AUTOIMMUNITY**

A. **APC**
   1. Increased availability of self-antigens due to decreased clearance of immune complexes or apoptotic cells.
   2. Increased endogenous "adjuvantlike" activity contributing to augmented APC function—CpG DNA, small RNAs.
   3. Altered presentation of antigen; presentation of splice variants; increased availability of caspase- or granzyme-cleaved self-antigens; post-translational modification of self-antigens.
   4. Altered selection of autoantigenic peptides.

B. **T cell**
   1. **Increased help.** Superantigens; altered threshold for activation; increased costimulatory signals or expression of CD40 ligand or helper cytokines.
   2. **Decreased suppression.** Including impaired Fas ligand-mediated apoptosis.
   3. Impaired T-cell repertoire selection or peripheral tolerance.
   4. Increased autocytotoxic cells.

C. **B cell**
   1. Secretion of autoantibodies based on polyclonal B-cell activation or antigen-driven B-cell responses—concepts of determinant spreading and molecular mimicry.
   2. Altered threshold for activation/impaired deletion of self-reactive B cells.

D. **Cytokines.** Altered expression or function of cytokines (IFN-α, IL-6, BAFF/BLyS, and chemokines).

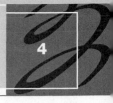
RHEUMATOLOGIC LABORATORY TESTS

Dalit Ashany, Anne R. Bass, and Keith B. Elkon

he laboratory studies outlined in this chapter are helpful in the diagnosis and treatment of rheumatic diseases. They should be interpreted in the context of a careful history and physical examination.

A test should be performed only if the results of the test will likely affect the diagnosis, prognosis, or therapy, and not if the results are of clinical or academic interest. Performing a large battery of screening tests, with no guidance from the specific clinical picture, will clearly lead to false-positive results and, possibly, incorrect diagnoses and treatments. One does not "chase" or "treat" a test but, rather, the patient and his or her entire clinical presentation. Tests are designated according to the context of an individual and his or her problems.

This chapter discusses erythrocyte sedimentation rate (ESR), C-reactive protein (CRP), autoantibody tests, complement tests, and other tests helpful in the serologic evaluation of rheumatic diseases.

ACUTE-PHASE REACTANTS

I. **ERYTHROCYTE SEDIMENTATION RATE.** The ESR (Westergren method) is a time-honored measurement of inflammation.

   A. Method of detection. The ESR measures the rate of fall, in mm/h, of red blood cells (RBCs) in a standard tube. Prolonged storage of the blood to be tested, or tilting of the calibrated tube, will falsely increase the ESR.

   B. Interpretation

   1. Normal Westergren ESR values are 0 to 15 mm/h for male subjects and 0 to 20 mm/h for female subjects. The ESR increases with age, and values up to 40 mm/h are not uncommon in the healthy geriatric individual. In inflammatory disorders, RBCs tend to form stacks (*rouleaux*), and these stacks cause the red cells to sediment more rapidly. This stacking may result from increased levels of fibrinogen.

   2. Measurement of the ESR can be helpful in evaluating the extent or severity of inflammation and in monitoring changes in disease activity over time. This test, however, cannot be used to definitely confirm or exclude any particular disease. Falsely low ESRs are found in sickle cell disease, anisocytosis, spherocytosis, polycythemia, and heart failure. Very high levels are seen in patients with monoclonal gammopathies.

II. **C-REACTIVE PROTEIN.** The CRP is an acute-phase reactant serum protein that is present in low concentration in normal serum. It was originally identified by its precipitin reaction with pneumococcal C polysaccharide.

   A. Method of detection. CRP is most commonly measured using an immunoassay or laser nephelometry.

   B. Interpretation

   1. CRP levels rise rapidly in response to an inflammatory stimulus (especially that provided by interleukin-6) and then fall when the inflammation subsides. Normal levels for healthy adults are less than 0.2 mg/dL, although levels of up to 1 mg/dL are not uncommon. Moderate elevations (1 to 10 mg/dL) in CRP levels can be seen in inflammatory conditions such as rheumatoid arthritis (RA) and giant cell arteritis. Elevations of greater than 15 to 20 mg/dL are generally seen in bacterial infections.

2. Although serum CRP levels are elevated in some patients with active systemic lupus erythematosus (SLE), most patients with lupus show only modest or no CRP elevation, even in the presence of active disease. Highly elevated CRP levels in patients with SLE should prompt consideration of a superimposed infection, although an elevated CRP level is not a definite proof of infection in these patients.

 AUTOANTIBODIES

I. **RHEUMATOID FACTOR (RF).** RFs are immunoglobulins with specificity for the Fc portion of immunoglobulin G (IgG). Multiple immunoglobulin classes have RF activity, but the RF detected by standard laboratory testing is an IgM antibody.
   A. **Method of detection.** There are many methods to measure RF. Those most commonly used include the enzyme-linked immunosorbent assay (ELISA), agglutination of IgG-coated latex particles, or nephelometry.
   B. **Interpretation.** Fifty percent to 75% of patients with RA have IgM RF, as do 3% to 5% of healthy subjects. RF positivity is associated with the HLA-DR4 haplotype and with more aggressive disease. Patients with extra-articular disease are invariably RF positive. IgM RFs are also commonly seen in patients with primary Sjögren's syndrome, and mixed cryoglobulinemia, as well as in patients with chronic infections such as subacute bacterial endocarditis and chronic hepatitis (Table 4-1).

II. **ANTICYCLIC CITRULLINATED PEPTIDE ANTIBODIES (ANTI-CCP).** Citrulline is formed by the deamination of the amino acid arginine. Antibodies directed against citrullinated peptides have been found in the serum of many patients with RA.
   A. **Method of detection.** ELISA detection of antibodies to citrullinated antigens is the technique that is most commonly utilized.
   B. **Interpretation.** The sensitivity of this test in patients with RA is 40% to 70%, but the specificity may be as high as 98%. In patients with undifferentiated arthritis, the

TABLE 4-1	**Frequency of Rheumatoid Factor as Measured by Latex Agglutination**

	Approximate frequency (%)
Sjögren's syndrome	90
Mixed cryoglobulinemia	90
Rheumatoid arthritis	75
Subacute bacterial endocarditis	40
Chronic interstitial pulmonary fibrosis	35
Pulmonary silicosis	30
Systemic lupus erythematosus	30
Waldenström's disease (macroglobulinemia)	28
Cirrhosis	25
Infectious hepatitis	25
Leprosy	25
Mixed connective tissue disease	25
Polymyositis	20
Systemic sclerosis (scleroderma)	20
Elderly patients (>60 y)	15
Tuberculosis	15
Trypanosomiasis	15
Juvenile idiopathic arthritis	10
Sarcoidosis	10
Syphilis	10

presence of anti-CCP antibodies is an important predictor for RA. Ninety-three percent of such patients will develop RA within 3 years. Some, but not all, patients with anti-CCP antibodies will also have a positive RF. Similarly, some, but not all, patients with a positive RF will have anti-CCP antibodies. The presence of both RF and anti-CCP best predict a poorer radiologic and functional outcome for patients with RA.

III. **ANTINUCLEAR ANTIBODIES (ANA).** The production of antibodies to a wide array of nuclear antigens is characteristic of lupus and the other connective tissue diseases. Because the ANA test detects any antibody binding to nuclear constituents, it is extremely useful as a screening test for these diseases.

   A. **Method of detection.** Indirect immunofluorescence assay (IFA) is the most common method of ANA testing. This technique employs a cellular substrate, now most commonly a human epithelial cell line (Hep-2), which is placed on a glass slide. The patient's serum is then applied (allowing autoantibodies to bind to the Hep-2 cells) and then tagged with a fluorescent-labeled anti-Fc IgG, which can then be visualized under a microscope.

   B. **Interpretation**
      1. ANA studies are usually reported according to the pattern (homogeneous, speckled, rim/peripheral or nucleolar) and by the titer, or intensity of fluorescence (1 to 4+). Titers of at least 1:40 are considered positive, but higher titers (>1:160) are usually present in patients with lupus or other connective tissue diseases. Up to 20% of healthy geriatric subjects, particularly women, have a positive ANA (usually <1:160). ANA titers do not correlate well with disease activity; therefore, once a positive ANA has been documented in a patient's serum, the test seldom needs to be repeated.
      2. The pattern of the ANA reflects the nuclear distribution of the antigen(s) being bound. A homogeneous pattern is common in lupus but is the least specific pattern for that disease. A rim pattern usually suggests the presence of antibodies to chromatin (DNA or histone proteins) and is seen in lupus, both systemic and drug-induced. Speckled ANAs may reflect antibodies to RNA-associated proteins and can be seen in lupus, mixed connective tissue disease (MCTD), and Sjögren's syndrome. Nucleolar ANAs are characteristic of scleroderma.
      3. A positive ANA can also be a nonspecific finding in a variety of other autoimmune conditions such as thyroiditis, juvenile arthritis, and psoriasis. Therefore, the ANA is a very useful diagnostic screening test, with high sensitivity for lupus and other connective tissue diseases but with very low specificity for those diseases, particularly when positive in only low titer.
      4. Extractable nuclear antigen (ENA) and DNA antibody testing (see the subsequent text) can be used to further evaluate the patient with a positive ANA. The prevalence and patterns of ANAs in various disease states are summarized in Table 4-2.

IV. **ANTI-DNA ANTIBODIES.** Antibodies against "native," or double-stranded DNA (dsDNA) are characteristic of patients with lupus. These antibodies bind to the deoxyribose phosphate backbone of DNA. Antibodies against single-stranded DNA (ssDNA), in contrast, bind to exposed purine and pyrimidine bases. Whereas anti-dsDNA antibodies are highly specific for lupus, antibodies to ssDNA can be seen in a wide variety of inflammatory conditions, such as drug-induced lupus and chronic hepatitis.

   A. **Method of detection**
      1. Until the 1990s, the Farr's assay was the most common method used to measure antibodies to dsDNA. This test has high specificity for lupus; however, because it requires the use of radiolabeled carbon, it has been supplanted by other assays that are safer to perform.
      2. The *Crithidia* assay uses the hemoflagellate, *Crithidia luciliae*, as a substrate for indirect immunofluorescence. The kinetoplast of this organism contains a concentrated focus of stable, circularized dsDNA, without contaminating RNA or nuclear proteins. This test is therefore sensitive and specific for antibodies to dsDNA.

TABLE 4-2	Frequency of Antinuclear Antibodies as Measured by Indirect Immunofluorescence Assay				
	ANA positivity (%)	Diffuse (homogeneous)	Pattern peripheral (rim)	Speckled	Nucleolar
SLE	≥90	++	++	+	0
MCTD	≥90	0	0	++	+
RA	30	+	0	0	0
Sjögren's syndrome	70	0	0	++	+
Scleroderma	≥70	+	0	+	++
Drug-induced SLE	≥90	+	+	0	0
Polymyositis	≥70	0	0	+0	0
Elderly patients (>60 y)	20	+0	+0	+0	+0
Chronic liver disease	20	+0	+0	+0	+0

+, common; ++, most common; 0, less common; +0, variable pattern. ANA, antinuclear antibody; MCTD, mixed connective tissue disease; RA, rheumatoid arthritis; SLE, systemic lupus erythematosus.

3. Many laboratories now use ELISA to measure antibodies to dsDNA because the test is inexpensive and easy to perform. Because purified DNA can denature in the plastic ELISA plate wells (exposing purine and pyrimidine bases), antibodies to ssDNA can at times lead to a false-positive result. (A "positive" result for the ELISA for antibodies to dsDNA in the presence of a negative ANA strongly suggests the presence of antibodies to ssDNA only.) Therefore, the specificity of this test for antibodies to dsDNA, and for lupus itself, is less than that of the Farr or *Crithidia* assay.

B. Interpretation. Anti-dsDNA antibodies occur in approximately 75% of patients with SLE but are rare in healthy subjects or in patients with other inflammatory and autoimmune conditions. In SLE, anti-dsDNA antibodies strongly correlate with the presence of nephritis, and their levels can rise and fall with disease activity. This makes the ELISA a useful, but not infallible, test for monitoring disease activity and response to therapy.

V. ANTIHISTONE ANTIBODIES. These antibodies are seen in more than 50% of patients with SLE, but they are seen in 100% of patients with drug-induced lupus. Therefore, a negative result is useful in ruling out drug-induced lupus.

VI. Antiphospholipid antibodies (most commonly the lupus anticoagulant test, anticardiolipin antibodies, and anti-β_2-gylcoprotein antibodies), which are seen in approximately 40% of patients with lupus, are associated with thrombosis and pregnancy morbidities. See Chapter 31 for a detailed discussion of this topic.

VII. EXTRACTABLE NUCLEAR ANTIGENS (ENA). Antinuclear antibodies are heterogeneous, and a variety of techniques have been used to determine the antigens to which these antibodies are directed. Early studies used techniques to separate nuclear components into those that were soluble [the "extractable" antigens (ENAs)] and those that were insoluble [chromatin (DNA and histones)].

A. Method of detection. Antibodies to ENAs were initially studied using a variety of techniques including immunodiffusion and counterimmunoelectrophoresis. Many of the specific antigens have now been identified and the proteins have been cloned. As a result, most laboratories now use ELISA to detect antibodies to particular ENAs.

B. Interpretation. Some of the antigens to which antibodies are commonly detected and their interpretations are listed below.

1. Smith (Sm). Antibodies to this antigen are not very sensitive for lupus (seen in only 20% to 30% of patients) but are highly specific for this disease.

2. **Ribonuclear protein (RNP).** Antibodies to this antigen are detected in 30% to 40% of patients with SLE, and very high titers are also characteristic of patients with MCTD.

3. **SS-A/Ro.** Antibodies to this antigen are detected in 40% of patients with lupus and are associated with photosensitivity, subacute cutaneous lupus, neonatal lupus, and Sjögren's syndrome.

4. **SS-B/La.** Antibodies to this antigen are detected in only 10% to 15% of patients with lupus. The antigen is strongly associated with Sjögren's syndrome, as well as neonatal lupus.

VIII. **ANTICENTROMERE ANTIBODIES.** These antibodies can be detected by IFA or ELISA. When an IFA is used, the substrate must include proliferating cells, so that centromere antigen is expressed. These antibodies are seen in 30% of patients with systemic sclerosis and are associated with the limited form of the disease (CREST syndrome).

IX. **ANTITOPOISOMERASE ANTIBODIES.** Also called anti-Scl 70 antibodies, these are seen in approximately 30% of patients with scleroderma and are associated with diffuse disease.

X. **ANTI-JO-1 ANTIBODIES.** This antibody, to histidine tRNA synthetase, is seen in approximately 25% of patients with myositis and is associated with interstitial lung disease.

XI. **ANTINEUTROPHIL CYTOPLASMIC ANTIBODIES (ANCA).** These antibodies, which are directed against cytoplasmic proteins, are helpful in the diagnosis of some forms of vasculitis.

A. **Method of detection.** These antibodies were first detected via an IFA that used alcohol-fixed neutrophils as the cell substrate. Two patterns of IFA were observed: a speckled cytoplasmic pattern, called c-ANCA, and a perinuclear pattern, called p-ANCA. In patients with vasculitis, these patterns were shown to reflect antibodies to either proteinase-3 (PR-3: c-ANCA) or myeloperoxidase (MPO: p-ANCA). Many laboratories now perform ELISA using these proteins as antigens.

B. **Interpretation.** c-ANCA is highly specific for Wegener's granulomatosis (present in approximately 80% of cases), whereas p-ANCA is seen primarily in microscopic polyarteritis nodosa, Churg-Strauss vasculitis, and crescentic glomerulonephritis. A positive p-ANCA by IFA can also be seen in other diseases, such as inflammatory bowel disease and tuberculosis. In these cases, the positive result is due to antibodies to cytoplasmic antigens other than MPO or PR-3, and ANCA testing by ELISA will yield a negative result. Therapeutic decisions and definitions of disease activity should be based on the clinical presentation and not solely on the ANCA titers.

 ## COMPLEMENT

The complement system is a major effector of the innate and humoral immune system. Activation of the system by immune complexes, polysaccharides, or oligosaccharides can occur through three pathways: the classical pathway, the alternative pathway, and the lectin pathway. All three pathways eventually cleave C3, with subsequent activation of the terminal components (C5b through C9). The complement system has three main physiologic functions: defending against bacterial infection, bridging innate and adaptive immunity, and disposal or clearance of cell debris and antigen–antibody complexes (Fig. 4-1).

I. **METHOD OF DETECTION.** Measurement of complement or its components can be performed by functional (i.e., hemolytic) assays or by antigenic assays that measure individual components.

A. Total hemolytic complement (CH50), measured in hemolytic units, evaluates the activity of a test serum to lyse 50% of a standardized suspension of sheep RBCs coated with rabbit antibody. All the nine components of the classical pathway (i.e., C1 through C9) are required for a normal result.

B. C3, C4, properdin, and factor B are measured by immunoassays including nephelometry and ELISA techniques.

II. **INTERPRETATION.** Evaluation of C3, C4, and CH50 is useful in patients with lupus, some of whom will have low values when their disease process is active and normal values when the disease is quiescent. CH50 measurements are also low in mixed

The complement cascade

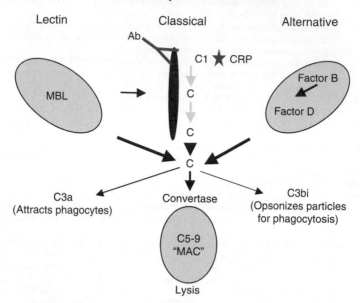

Lectin   Classical   Alternative

Figure 4-1. Complement pathways. The three pathways of complement activation: the MB-lectin (MBL) pathway, which is triggered by mannan-binding lectin, a normal serum constituent that binds some encapsulated bacteria; the classical pathway, which is triggered by antibody (Ab), by binding of CRP to C1q or by direct binding of complement component C1q to the pathogen surface; and the alternative pathway, which is triggered directly on pathogen surfaces. All of these pathways generate the effector molecules of complement. The three main consequences of complement activation are opsonization of pathogens mediated by C3bi, the recruitment of inflammatory cells mediated by C3a, and direct killing of pathogens through the membrane attack complex (MAC).

cryoglobulinemia and in urticarial ("hypocomplementemic") vasculitis. In contrast, most patients with other systemic autoimmune disorders do not have low complement levels.

III. **Complement deficiency states.** Deficiencies of early classic pathway components, C1, C4, and C2, are associated with SLE and SLE-like syndromes. Patients with lupus and with genetic complement deficiencies will never "normalize" that complement component level, despite quiescent disease. Deficiencies of terminal components C5 through C9 are associated with an increased incidence of infection, particularly with *Neisseria*. Deficiency of the inhibitor of C1 esterase is associated with hereditary angioedema, and deficiency of C3b inactivator is associated with increased incidence of infection.

CRYOGLOBULINS

Cryoglobulins are immunoglobulins present in the serum that precipitate in the cold and dissolve again on rewarming.

I. **TYPES.** Three different types of cryoblobulins have been defined.
   A. **Type I.** Monoclonal immunoglobulin—this type of cryoglobulin is typically seen in myeloproliferative disorders such as multiple myeloma and Waldenström's macroglobulinemia.
   B. **Type II.** Mixed cryoglobulin (immune complex of a polyclonal immunoglobulin and a monoclonal RF)—type II cryoglobulins are associated with hepatitis B or C in most cases.

C. Type III. Mixed polyclonal cryoglobulin (immune complex of a polyclonal immunoglobulin and a polyclonal RF)—this cryoglobulin is most often associated with autoimmune diseases, such as lupus and Sjögren's syndrome, and also with hematologic malignancies, hepatitis C, as well as other infections.

II. METHOD OF DETECTION

A. Blood to be studied for cryoproteins should be processed under carefully controlled conditions because if the sample is incorrectly processed, the result may be falsely negative. Blood being tested for cryoglobulins must be allowed to clot at 37°C, so that the cryoproteins remain soluble in the serum. (The cryoprotein will precipitate and become trapped in the clot if coagulation is allowed to occur at room temperature.) Subsequently, the serum can be separated by a brief centrifugation at room temperature.

B. After storage for 2 days at 0°C to 5°C, an aliquot is examined for the presence of a white precipitate in the bottom of the tube. The amount of cryoglobulins is quantified by performing a "cryocrit." This is performed by centrifuging the serum in a graduated tube at 4°C at 2,500 rpm, and then the percentage of cryoglobulins is calculated. Note that there is not a good correlation between cryocrit and disease activity or severity.

III. INTERPRETATION. Low levels of cryoglobulin (<30 μg/mL) can be found in a wide variety of inflammatory conditions (such as lupus) where they are of questionable significance. Cryoglobulins can also be pathogenic, such as in mixed cryoglobulinemia. In this vasculitic syndrome, cryocrit is usually in the 0.5% to 1.5% range. Sera with very large quantities of cryoprotein (cryocrit; 3% to 5%) usually contain monoclonal immunoglobulins and can be associated with Waldenström's macroglobulinemia or multiple myeloma.

IMMUNOGENETIC ASPECTS OF RHEUMATIC DISEASES

Allan Gibofsky

5

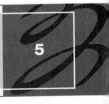

$\mathcal{T}$he efforts of numerous investigators during the last three decades have resulted in the recognition of a major histocompatibility complex (MHC) in humans, consisting of the alleles of at least seven closely linked loci on the short arm of autosomal chromosome 6. The antigens that the genes of this region code for were first detected on white blood cells and were, therefore, originally referred to as human leukocyte antigens (HLA). Initially, these antigens were of interest primarily to transplantation physicians because similarity between donor and recipient antigens seemed to influence allograft survival; soon, however, it was recognized that certain clinical conditions might be associated with one or more antigens of this system. A large number of diseases have been studied, and individual antigens or combinations of antigens have appeared with greater frequency than would be expected in the normal population. This increase in the frequency of occurrence of antigens is particularly true for rheumatic diseases and related syndromes with features of altered immunoreactivity, where, as will be discussed in subsequent text, the strongest and most significant associations have been demonstrated. Although it is recognized that many of the rheumatic diseases may occur as a result of multiple genetic factors, the strongest influences have been with the HLA genes of the MHC. This chapter reviews the basic concepts of immunogenetics, emphasizing the potential significance of the HLA system antigens in clinical rheumatology.

IMMUNOGENETIC NOMENCLATURE

Gene. Segment of DNA that directs the synthesis of a polypeptide chain or protein.
Allele. Alternative form of the same gene, resulting from mutation or duplication.
Locus. The position of a gene on any given chromosome.
Genotype. The genetic composition of an individual.
Phenotype. The observed expression of the genotype.
Haplotype. Closely linked loci, transmitted as a unit from each parent; two haplotypes constitute the genotype.
Alloantigen. Product of the A, B, C, or DR, DP, or DQ loci.

I. **LOCI DEFINITION.** Multiple closely linked loci have been defined by gene mapping techniques, and their products have been recognized by a combination of serologic and DNA typing methods. (A complete listing of the several hundred recognized alleles defined for the six loci can be found at www.ash1-hla.org.) These genes have been functionally assigned to several classes:

   A. Class I includes the products of the HLA- A, B, and C series.
   B. Class II includes the products of the HLA-DR, DP, and DQ series.
   C. Class III has recently been described and consists of the genes for various peptide transporters [e.g., Transporter Associated With Antigen Processing (TAP)], proteosome subunits (e.g., LMP), and other proteins involved in autoimmunity (e.g., DM, DO).

   Initial studies directed toward the development of serologic methods for the detection of HLA-D antigens resulted in the recognition of several additional gene products, preferentially expressed on the surface of B lymphocytes. These B-cell antigens have extensive biologic and chemical homologies with the I-region antigens of the murine histocompatibility system and are therefore also referred to as Ia antigens. These Ia alloantigens were primarily recognized with alloantibodies that developed as a result of immunization of the mother with paternal antigens during pregnancy or in the sera of renal transplant recipients who became immunized against nonmatching antigens present on the homograft. These human Ia antigens are highly polymorphic and have certain alloantigenic specificities related closely to HLA alleles. The gene products of the HLA-D region appear to be highly complex and polymorphic and have not yet been fully defined. Each product consists of a noncovalently associated combination of an α- and a β-chain. The α- and β-chains are substantially different from each other, and there is evidence for at least six α-chain genes and seven β-chain genes, all in the HLA region. These genes appear to be arranged in subsets corresponding to three distinct products, all of which are class II molecules: (a) DR molecules, (b) DQ molecules, and (c) DP molecules, which do not appear to be serologically defined. The α- and β-chain genes of each series' products are substantially more similar to each other than to genes of one of the other allelic series.

II. **GENETICS OF INHERITANCE.** The antigens of this system are inherited in the classic mendelian fashion. Unlike those phenotypic characteristics that exhibit dominant and recessive forms (e.g., eye color and ABO type), the HLA antigens are codominant; if a gene has been inherited from a parent, the corresponding HLA antigen will be expressed on the cell surface. Given the number of alleles at each locus, the number of possible phenotypic combinations is very large, indicating the enormous immunogenetic heterogeneity of an outbred population. Thereby, the finding of an altered frequency of a particular antigen in a patient group is likely to prompt intense interest in the biologic role of this system in the regulation of the immune response and disease susceptibility.

DISEASE ASSOCIATIONS

I.   Of the many conditions investigated thus far and shown to be associated with particular alleles of the HLA system, the rheumatic diseases have been the most important. Although the associations are high, they are neither absolute nor diagnostic;

the presence of an antigen is not the sole factor in disease pathogenesis because the antigen also occurs in diseasefree individuals. Nevertheless, the knowledge of the association may prove useful in permitting subdivisions of clinical groups within the larger population (e.g., pauciarticular juvenile chronic arthritis). This knowledge could facilitate the search for possible etiologic agents and could confirm or refute the following suggested mechanisms for HLA and disease associations:

   A. The HLA antigen may be structurally similar to the antigenic component of an infectious agent.

   B. The HLA antigen may be part of a neo-antigen that is formed in combination with an infectious agent.

   C. The HLA antigen may be a receptor for an infectious or environmental toxin.

   D. There may be linkage disequilibrium (i.e., the genes are located so closely together on the same chromosome that they are usually inherited together) between alleles at a particular locus and the HLA antigen associated with that disease (e.g., HLA-A3 and idiopathic hemochromatosis).

II. **ANKYLOSING SPONDYLITIS.** The most significant association of HLA antigen occurs in this disease. Between 85% and 90% of white patients have HLA-B27, which seems to be a marker for spondylitis in this group. Ethnic differences may also be important because the antigen occurs with different frequency in both patient and control nonwhite groups. The lower association in Pima Indians and American blacks, the groups in which the disease itself is less frequent, would suggest that B27 is not involved directly in pathogenesis but rather may be linked to the predisposing gene. Thus far, no HLA-DR association has been recognized, which suggests that susceptibility to ankylosing spondylitis may involve mechanisms different from those involved in the other rheumatic diseases such as rheumatoid arthritis (RA).

III. **REACTIVE ARTHRITIS (FORMERLY REITER'S SYNDROME).** Approximately 80% of white patients with the classic triad of manifestations (i.e., arthritis, urethritis, and conjunctivitis) have the antigen B27. This antigen is also seen in slightly lower frequency in their pure forms of this syndrome (i.e., fewer than all those manifestations.) It has been suggested that the reactive arthritis seen following infection with *Yersinia* or *Salmonella* is comparable to the form of Reiter's syndrome following bacterial dysentery. Also in these conditions, HLA-B27 level is increased.

IV. **RA.** HLA-DR4 (in particular, the subtype DR4B1*01) has been reported in 60% to 80% of white patients with classic adult seropositive RA, in comparison to 24% to 28% of controls. In contrast, no significant HLA association has been detected in adult patients with clinically similar seronegative disease, which suggests that seronegative and seropositive RA may have different immunogenetic bases.

V. **SYSTEMIC LUPUS ERYTHEMATOSUS (SLE).** Both HLA-DR antigens, DR2 and DR3, have been found to be increased in white patients with SLE. In addition, genes on other chromosomes have also been implicated in increasing susceptibility to SLE (see Chapter 30). This immunogenetic diversity would support the clinical variability seen in this disease. Some data have suggested that clinical subgroups of patients with SLE show an association with one or the other HLA-DR antigen (e.g., with DR3 in skin disease and with DR2 in vasculitis), but not necessarily with both.

VI. **SJÖGREN'S SYNDROME.** Primary Sjögren's syndrome in white patients shows a strong association with HLA-DR3. HLA-DR4 (in particular, the subtype DR4B1*01) is increased in frequency in patients with Sjögren's syndrome associated with a connective tissue disorder such as RA or SLE, which no doubt reflects the high incidence of RA seen in this population.

VII. **PSORIATIC ARTHRITIS.** The HLA antigens—A26, B38, Cw6, DR4, and DR7—have been reported to be increased in patients with psoriatic arthritis. In addition, B2 level has been reported to be increased in patients with axial skeletal disease. Different antigens have been associated with skin disease alone.

VIII. **INFLAMMATORY BOWEL DISEASE (IBD).** Patients with IBD and ankylosing spondylitis show an increased frequency of HLA-B27. No increase in the frequency of occurrence of this antigen is seen in patients with enteropathic peripheral arthritis as a manifestation of IBD.

IX. **BEHÇET'S DISEASE.** The HLA antigen Bw51 is increased in white patients with this condition. The association is even more significant in Asian and Asian American patients.

X. **LYME DISEASE.** The occurrence of HLA-DR2 and HLA-DR4 are increased in white patients with this disorder.

XI. **C2 DEFICIENCY.** The gene coding for the second component of complement is located on chromosome 6 and is part of the MHC. Several family studies of patients with C2 deficiency and an SLE-like illness in whom the deficient C2 gene segregated with the same haplotype (A10-B18) have been reported.

XII. **RHEUMATIC FEVER.** In several groups of patients with this disease, a B-cell alloantigen that is not related to HLA-D has been detected in virtually all patients tested. The relation of this alloantigen to other genes located within the MHC remains to be determined.

XII. **JUVENILE IDIOPATHIC ARTHRITIS (JIA).** HLA-B27 has been reported in 40% of patients with combined pauciarticular and axial disease. Associations with HLA-DR5 and HLA-DR8 have also been reported.

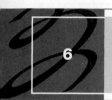

BONE, CONNECTIVE TISSUE, JOINT AND VASCULAR BIOLOGY, AND PATHOLOGY

Linda A. Russell and Edward F. DiCarlo

6

■ KEY POINTS

- Bone is composed primarily of an inanimate, calcified extracellular matrix with a small proportion of cells acting in a custodial role.

- Diseases of the bones are the result of disturbed cellular function that interferes with the maintenance of mechanical function.

- There are more than 14 types of collagen that comprise molecules in the extracellular matrix.

- Joints are organ systems whose functions depend on the competence of all of the component parts—bone, cartilage, ligaments/tendons, and synovium.

- Diarthrodial joints are composed of two articular surfaces that are bathed in synovial fluid and provide for stable and fluid motion.

- Osteoarthritis is a manifestation of the mechanical failure of a joint resulting from failure of at least one of the joint components.

- Rheumatoid arthritis (RA) is an example of the inflammatory destruction of a joint leading to stiffness and subsequent loss of function.

- Skeletal muscle permits motion by generating force and the diseases are either intrinsic to the muscle, such as in inflammation and the dystrophies, or secondary due to vascular or neurologic conditions.

- Several mechanisms are active in the development of vasculitis—but classification schemes are heavily dependent on clinical circumstances, the type and size of the involved vessels, and the type and degree of inflammation present.

*T*he musculoskeletal system comprises the organs that permit the human body to move in a coordinated and stable manner. Bones, tendons, ligaments, and muscles comprise the primary organs of the system, and ancillary structures such as blood vessels, fascias, and aponeuroses are included in the term "connective tissues"; all these structures have a connective tissue matrix that includes some form of collagen.

COLLAGEN

I.   **The collagens** comprise a set of molecules that provide the extracellular supporting framework for various tissues. More than 14 different collagens have been identified. Each collagen has a specific function. The **structure** of the collagen molecule is a triple helix.

II. Each **collagen type** has a specific amino acid sequence.
     A. Type I collagen comprises 90% of collagen in the body and is the major constituent of skin, tendon, bone, synovium, cornea, conjunctiva, and sclera.
     B. Type II collagen is found in cartilage.
     C. Type III collagen is often found with type I collagen in skin, synovium, and vascular wall tissues.
     D. Type IV collagen is found in basement membranes.
     E. Type V collagen is found surrounding fibroblasts, smooth muscle cells, and other mesenchymal cells.
     F. Type IX and XI collagens are found in cartilaginous tissues.

BONES

I.   **Bone** is primarily composed of an inanimate extracellular matrix, with a lesser component of living cells present in a custodial role. Bone, cartilage, and teeth have the unique ability to calcify. Bones are produced as a result of two processes:
     A. Endochondral ossification. Most bones are modeled in cartilage and develop by the orderly replacement of that cartilage with bone tissue. The processes of elongation and complex modeling of the ends of bones progress through endochondral ossification.
     B. Membranous ossification. Bones, or regions of bones that do not develop through endochondral ossification, are produced by the intramembranous (periosteal) deposition of bone. The midregions of flat bones (e.g., calvarium, mandible, ribs, and ilium) and the cortical shafts of long bones are produced through this process.

II. **Bone shape** depends on anatomic location and the forces applied to the bone. All bones change their shape (grow) through some combination of endochondral ossification and membranous ossification—through processes that take place in the epiphyses, in the apophyses (e.g., the greater and lesser trochanters), and at the periosteal surfaces.
     A. The ends of long bones and the complex edges of flat bones are composed of epiphyses and apophyses, which are modeled in cartilage, are capable of maintaining the complex shapes of the bone ends throughout development and growth, and are eventually replaced mostly by bone.
     B. Adjacent to the epiphyses and apophyses, the growth plate provides for growth of the bone through endochondral ossification. Most growth plates fuse in the late teenage years when normal human growth ceases.
     C. The midshaft of the long bones is the diaphysis and the transitional zone between the growth plate and the diaphysis is the metaphysis.
     D. The outer portion of a bone is composed of a cortex or compact bone and the inner portion is the medullary cavity that contains variable amounts of cancellous or trabecular bone. The bone marrow is in the medullary cavity.
     E. Within the diaphyseal shaft, the outer surface is referred to as the periosteum and the inner surface is called the endostium.
     F. The ends of long bones that form a joint are covered in a layer of articular cartilage that does not calcify and persists throughout life.

III. **The bone cells** are of three types. Osteoblasts are responsible for bone formation. Osteoclasts are responsible for bone resorption. Osteocytes play a role in mineral and bone homeostasis. Appropriate clinical markers for these cell types and their associated activity are presented in Table 6-1.

TABLE 6-1	Bone Cell Types with Appropriate Clinical Markers and Associated Activity	
Bone cell type	**Function**	**Marker of bone remodeling**
Osteoclast	Bone resorption	Urinary *N*-telopeptide, urinary *C*-telopeptide, deoxypyridinoline
Osteoblast	Bone formation	Bone alkaline phosphatase, osteocalcin
Osteocyte	Cell-to-cell communication	Unknown—none?

IV. **Bone remodeling** is a process that occurs throughout life and permits repair of injured bone and maintenance of serum calcium-phosphorus homeostasis.

V. **The bone matrix** is composed of collagen fibers (primarily type I) and noncollagenous proteins that in normal bone are arranged in orderly layers resulting in "lamellar bone." Crystals of hydroxyapatite are found on the collagen fibers and in the ground substance, which is composed of glycoproteins and proteoglycans.

VI. **Bone pathology** can be seen in several conditions including fracture, osteoporosis, osteomalacia, and Paget's disease.

    A. Fractures occur in the setting of high-impact trauma or in pathologic states such as the metabolic bone diseases, osteogenesis imperfecta, and both primary and metastatic neoplasms.

    B. Osteoporosis (see Chapter 53) is a systemic skeletal condition characterized by a reduction in the amount of bone to an extent that is sufficient to permit fracture during normal activity or after sustaining minimal trauma (i.e., fragility fracture). It leads to a condition where the rate of bone formation cannot keep pace with the rate of bone resorption, although both the rates may be reduced. This results in delicate, fragile trabeculae that are not well connected.

    C. Osteomalacia (Fig. 6-1) refers to any systemic skeletal condition that is characterized by an excessive amount of unmineralized bone tissue called "osteoid."

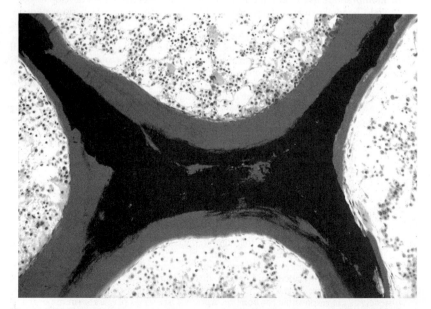

Figure 6-1. This photomicrograph of a nondecalcified section of bone in osteomalacia shows a bony trabecula whose surfaces are covered by a thick layer of osteoid (*grey tissue*). Only the central regions appearing in black are calcified (Von Kossa × 10).

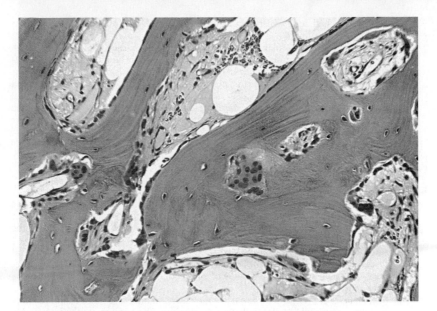

Figure 6-2. This photomicrograph of a decalcified section of bone in Paget's disease shows numerous, variably sized osteoclasts and uniform small osteoblasts aligned along the surfaces of irregular bony trabeculae. The result is derangement of the trabecular and matrix architecture with loss of mechanical integrity (hematoxylin–eosin, H&E × 25).

Osteomalacia appears with increased osteoid thickness and osteoid surface, coupled with a reduced or otherwise insufficient mineral apposition rate. Osteomalacia most commonly results from insufficient levels of calcium, phosphate, or vitamin D.

D. Paget's disease (Fig. 6-2 and Chapter 54) is a focal disorder of bone remodeling, possibly the result of genetic predisposition and viral activation, in which osteoclasts are morphologically abnormal (large, with many nuclei) and excessively active. This excessive osteoclastic activity, coupled with excessive osteoblastic activity, results in the formation of a primitive bone matrix (woven bone instead of lamellar bone), deranged bone tissue architecture (cortical and cancellous bone), and gross deformity of the affected bone. In the early stage, the bone is radiographically lytic and "hot" on the scan, whereas it is sclerotic and less active in the later stages.

 CARTILAGE

I. **Articular cartilage** provides for the smooth, fluid motion and equitable loading of a joint.

II. **COMPOSITION**
   A. A small proportion of cartilage is made up of chondrocytes, which are responsible for the synthesis and maintenance of the extracellular matrix and which comprises more than 95% of the substance of the cartilage tissue.
   B. The matrix consists primarily of collagen (type II) and proteoglycans.
   C. Proteogylcans provide the compressive and load-bearing properties of cartilage, being a complex of hydroscopic supramolecular aggregates that are held in place within the collagenous network of the cartilage.

III. **STRUCTURE**
   A. Cartilage has four loosely defined zones that blend into each other. From top to bottom, these zones are the superficial zone, the transitional zone, the radial zone,

and the calcified zone which attaches the cartilage to the subchondral bone at an irregular cement line.

B. Adult cartilage is avascular and its nutrition depends on the synovial fluid, which provides electrolytes and nutrients and removes waste products, all of which diffuse through the matrix to and from the chondrocytes. This is particularly important in the setting of infectious arthritis, in which chondrocytes, leukocytes, and bacteria compete for nutrients.

C. Cartilage is not innervated; therefore, these structures do not sense pain in disease states. Pain in a joint is actually sensed in the bone, the synovium, or the capsular and ligamentous structures, all of which are innervated.

 JOINTS

I. THREE PRINCIPAL TYPES OF JOINTS

A. Synarthrodial joints (synarthroses), as exemplified by the suture lines of the skull, are junctions between bones that do not move much relative to each other. Fibrous tissue interlocks these bones during growth. When growth ceases, the joints close.

B. Amphiarthrodial joints (amphiarthroses), as exemplified by the intervertebral discs, pubic symphysis, and upper part of the sacroiliac joint, are joints the movement of which is limited by fibrous or fibrochondral tissue that crosses from one bone to the next.

C. Diarthrodial joints (diarthroses) are the most common and most complex joints in the skeleton and are also called synovial joints. These joints are the least stable and allow for the greatest degree of unhindered movement, whereas ligaments, tendons, and capsular structures provide some support and stability. The bone ends of these joints are covered by cartilage and the surfaces are lubricated by synovial fluid.

II. Synovial fluid is produced by the synovial membrane and forms a thin film of lubrication covering the synovium and cartilage. During disease processes, the amount of synovial fluid may increase, resulting in an effusion. Synovial fluid is most commonly evaluated for cell count, Gram stain, culture, and crystal analysis. Cell counts are elevated in inflamed joints but not with osteoarthritis or after mechanical injury.

III. Synovium is the soft tissue that covers the nonarticulating surfaces of synovial or diarthrodial joints. The synovial surface is covered by a lining layer that is usually one to three cells thick and is supported by fatty tissue with collagen and has a bed of fenestrated microvessels, lymphatic vessels, and nerve fibers.

IV. Pathology of the joints is exemplified by two classic conditions—osteoarthritis, and rheumatoid arthritis.

A. Primary osteoarthritis (Fig. 6-3 and Chapter 51) results from the relatively slow degradation of cartilage, usually because of abnormal or prolonged normal stress on normal cartilage and is characterized by a loss of proteoglycans, disruption of the collagen architecture, necrosis and proliferation of the chondrocytes, and advancement of the calcified zone. Compensatory changes in the bone include sclerosis of the subarticular bone and marginal osteophytosis. Secondary osteoarthritis may result from any condition, including the inflammatory arthropathies in their late stages, that results in destruction of the cartilage or in compromise of the mechanical properties of the cartilage, leading to early and rapid failure of the joint.

B. Rheumatoid arthritis (Fig. 6-4 and Chapter 29) is an inflammatory disease that is characterized by thickening and hyperplasia of the synovial tissue, and usually intense but variable degrees of inflammation, which is composed of B and T lymphocytes and plasma cells with occasional germinal centers. Damage to the joint results from peripheral and, subsequently, from more central destruction of the cartilage and other intra-articular soft tissues by inflammatory pannus, with destruction of the subchondral bone by the inflammatory tissue and osteoclasts. This pattern of destruction prevents compensatory changes, such as osteophytosis and sclerosis, and results in an unstable and painful joint.

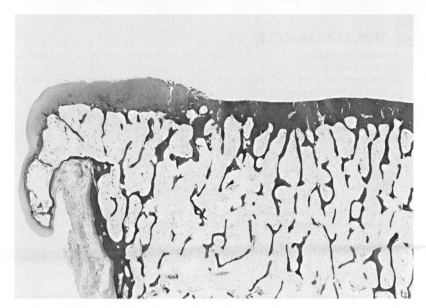

Figure 6-3. This photomicrograph of a decalcified section of a joint surface in osteoarthritis shows loss of the cartilage with a bandlike plate of densely sclerotic bone and a well-defined osteophyte at the margin (*left side*) (H&E × 2).

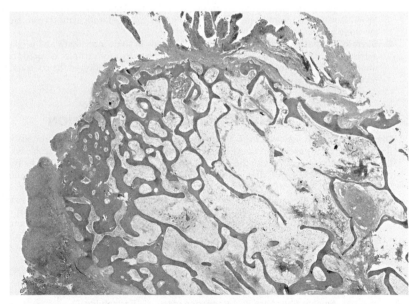

Figure 6-4. This photomicrograph of a decalcified section of a joint surface in rheumatoid arthritis shows destruction with loss of the cartilage and superficial bone due to the presence of erosive inflammatory pannus that appears as an irregularly thick and papillated covering over the surface of the bone (H&E × 2).

SKELETAL MUSCLE

I. **Skeletal muscle** permits motion by generating contractile force under the control of the nervous system.
    A. **Skeletal muscles** attach to the bones over broad surfaces or to specific points either by periosteal fibrous attachments or by tendons.
    B. **Muscles** are composed of fibers arranged in fascicles.
    C. **Muscle fibers** contain delicate filaments that are linearly arranged and connected to form the myofibrillary contraction apparatus.
    D. **Contraction and relaxation** of muscle requires the hydrolysis of adenosine triphosphate (ATP) and adequate amounts of calcium. Free fatty acids and glycogen are sources of ATP.
    E. **Muscle fibers** are of three principal types (Table 6-2). Type 1 fibers are slow to respond to electrical stimuli and are fatigue-resistant. Type 2b fibers respond more rapidly and with greater force, but fatigue more quickly. The response and fatigability of type 2a fibers are intermediate between type 1 and type 2b fibers.
    F. **A lower motor neuron** from the anterior horn of the spinal cord innervates several muscle fibers to form a motor unit.

II. **Muscle pathology** is very complex and results from local injury, such as in the compartment syndromes; primary disease, such as the muscular dystrophies and the inflammatory diseases; and secondary diseases, such as those related to medical treatments or neurologic abnormalities.
    A. **In polymyositis and dermatomyositis** (Fig. 6-5 and Chapter 32), the principal finding is inflammation that is composed of lymphocytes and macrophages involving individual or many muscle fibers, with variable degrees of myonecrosis, atrophy, and regeneration, eventuating in fibrosis and fatty infiltration.
    B. **Inclusion-body myositis** (Fig. 6-6) presents similar inflammatory features but with the addition of vacuoles rimmed by granular inclusions that are composed of densely aggregated membranous whorls or globular filaments containing various proteinaceous compounds, including acid phosphatase, α-1 antichymotrypsin, and cytokine factors.
    C. **Steroid myopathy** results from reaction to steroids in some individuals and is characterized by muscle weakness, with microscopic evidence of atrophy of predominantly type 2 fibers and with ultrastructural evidence of disruption of the contractile myofibrillary apparatus due to loss of thick myosin filaments.

 BLOOD VESSEL INVOLVEMENT IN INFLAMMATION

I. **Diseases of blood vessels** are a highly diverse group of conditions that produce inflammatory and degenerative changes that affect all or various parts of the vascular wall.
II. **Classification** schemes rely on the size and type of vessel that is involved and the type of inflammatory cells or inflammatory mediators that are present in the vascular lumen and wall.
    A. **Endothelial cells** are involved in vascular permeability, adhesion of platelets and white cells, regulation of cell trafficking, and regulation of coagulation. In addition, endothelial cells can directly secrete cytokines, such as platelet activation factor,

TABLE 6-2	Principal Types of Muscle Fibers	
Muscle fiber type	**Response rate**	**Fatigability**
Type 1	Slow	Fatigue-resistant
Type 2a	Intermediate	Intermediate
Type 2b	Rapid	Fatigues quickly

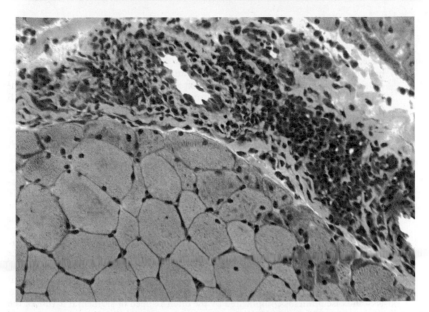

Figure 6-5. This photomicrograph of a muscle biopsy in dermatomyositis shows perimysial and perivascular chronic inflammation, composed mostly of lymphocytes, with well-defined perifascicular atrophy (fresh-frozen, H&E × 25).

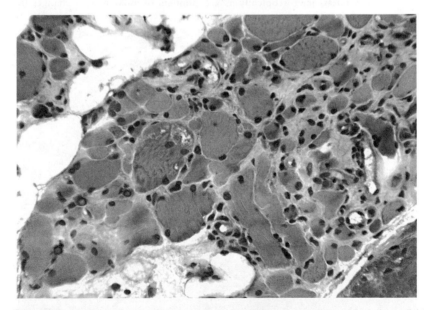

Figure 6-6. This photomicrograph of a muscle biopsy in inclusion-body myositis shows a slight degree of endomysial chronic inflammation with marked variation in the sizes of the muscle fibers. One of the large (*center*) fibers shows vacuolar degeneration with granular inclusions (fresh-frozen, H&E × 25).

prostaglandins, and adenosine nucleotides, and express cell surface molecules modifying immune responses.

  B. **Immune-complex** deposition, usually passively adsorbed onto endothelial cells, is the cause of vasculitic changes because of the associated changes in vascular permeability, inflammatory cell (neutrophils) attraction, and complement activation causing the vascular damage. Diseases such as hypersensitivity vasculitis, Henoch-Schönlein purpura, hepatitis C-related mixed cryoglobulinemia, and hepatitis B virus-associated polyarteritis nodosa (PAN) appear to be associated with immune-complex deposition.

  C. **Antibodies** play a role in the development of some forms of vasculitis.

  D. **Antineutrophil cytoplasmic antibodies** (ANCA) are present in patients with some forms of systemic vasculitides.

   1. c-ANCA binds to proteinase 3 and is implicated in Wegener's granulomatosis.

   2. p-ANCA binds to myeloperoxidase and is associated with Churg-Strauss vasculitis and microscopic polyangiitis.

   3. Antiendothelial antibodies may damage endothelial cells by antibody-dependent cellular cytotoxicity and complement activation mechanisms and may be relevant in Kawasaki's disease.

  E. **T_H1 lymphocytes** have been implicated in forms of vasculitis such as giant cell arteritis.

 III. **The pathology of blood vessels** results from the integral effect of local or systemic injury due to hypertension, atherosclerotic disease, inflammatory attack, and inflammatory attack directed against components of the vessel walls. The pathologic diagnosis of the vasculitides is complicated by the often skipped or segmental nature of the disease processes. The pathologic classification depends to a great degree on the type of inflammation present: polymorphonuclear neutrophil (PMN) leukocytes in PAN and leukocytoclastic vasculitis; giant cells in giant cell arteritis; necrotizing granulomas in Wegener's granulomatosis; and eosinophils in Churg-Strauss vasculitis.

  A. **PAN** (Fig. 6-7 and Chapter 37) involves small and medium arteries and arterioles and manifests microscopically as a continuum of inflammatory changes that

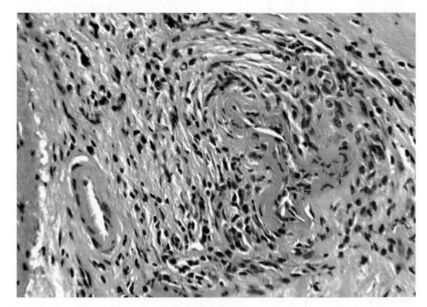

Figure 6-7. This photomicrograph of a small artery in polyarteritis nodosa shows obliteration of the entire mural structure with fibrinoid necrosis and a relatively sparse transmural infiltrate of lymphocytes. A small artery to the left is not affected, illustrating the patchy nature of this condition (H&E × 25).

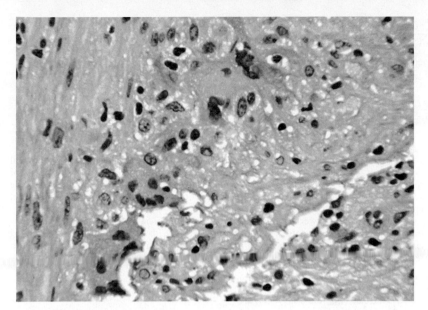

Figure 6-8. This photomicrograph of a temporal artery shows irregularly shaped and somewhat indistinct giant cells that are clustered in the vicinity of the now-destroyed internal elastic lamina. The intima to the right is thickened and hypercellular; other inflammatory elements are sparse (H&E × 25).

involve any and all layers of the affected vessels. The early lesion is characterized by edema or swelling of the media with focal fibrinoid necrosis followed by PMN and lymphocytic infiltration which eventually spreads through the entire wall including the adventitia. The inflammatory tissue resolves into focal mural fibrosis with eventual complete scarring. Lesions in all stages of activity, and even normal vessels, may be present in a single biopsy.

B. Giant cell arteritis (Fig. 6-8 and Chapter 35) in the superficial temporal artery and, occasionally, in other arteries of similar size manifests as destruction of the internal elastic lamina and an infiltrate of lymphocytes, macrophages, and giant cells.

C. Wegener's granulomatosis (see Chapter 37) has variable vascular changes depending on the organ involved, but a significant and diagnostic feature is the presence of a necrotizing granulomatous inflammation, which involves the vessel wall and the adjacent tissue, and a variable degree of infarction involving the adjacent tissue, especially when the lung is involved.

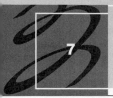

DIAGNOSTIC IMAGING TECHNIQUES

Robert Schneider and Helene Pavlov

*N*umerous diagnostic imaging techniques may be used to supplement history, physical examination, and laboratory tests in the evaluation of bone and joint disease. The choice of the imaging technique to be used and the sequence of usage of the techniques depend on the sensitivity and specificity of the technique for a particular problem; on the availability, cost, and risk involved; and on the experience in its use.

The goal is to answer the question raised by the clinician in the shortest time at the least cost and risk to the patient. A prior consultation with the radiologist and providing clinical information when ordering an imaging examination will help the radiologist and technologist to tailor their examination to the problem under investigation.

IMAGING TECHNIQUES

I. **Radiography** is usually the initial diagnostic imaging method in the evaluation of bone and joint pain because it is readily available and is of relatively low cost compared to other imaging methods. It provides excellent detail of bone anatomy and soft tissue calcification. Lucency, sclerosis, and periosteal reaction indicate bone abnormality. Cartilage, muscle, ligaments, tendons, and synovial fluid all appear with the same soft tissue density on radiography, which limits evaluation of abnormalities of these tissues. Cartilage destruction can be diagnosed if narrowing of the joint space is present (Fig. 7-1). Bone erosions can be seen around the joints. Determination of osteoporosis can be difficult because variations in technique can affect the apparent density on radiograms. Bony alignment can be determined and measured. Synovitis may be detected in the knee, elbow, and ankle because of the displacement of adjacent fat pads, but it cannot be reliably detected in the hip and shoulder. Other imaging methods, including magnetic resonance imaging (MRI), radionuclide scanning, and ultrasonography may pick up the bone and joint abnormality when radiograms are normal (Fig. 7-2).

Radiographic real-time imaging is done by fluoroscopy. C-arm fluoroscopes, which can be rotated and tilted, aid in localization during surgical procedures (e.g., internal fixation of fractures and osteotomies) and invasive radiologic procedures (e.g., myelography, nerve root, facet, and epidural spine injections, percutaneous needle biopsy, discography, joint aspiration and injection, and arthrography) (see Fig. 7-2C). Fluoroscopy with video recording can also be used for the evaluation of motion. Care must be taken to limit fluoroscopic time to avoid excessive radiation exposure.

II. **RADIONUCLIDE SCANNING**

A. **Bone scanning** with use of technetium 99m phosphate complexes has been used most frequently in the evaluation of metastatic disease to the skeleton and has largely replaced routine radiographic skeletal surveys for this purpose except for multiple myeloma. It is also used for the evaluation of benign bone disease because abnormalities that are not visible on radiograms may be detected. Bone scanning detects physiologic changes in the bone, as compared to the anatomic changes seen on radiograms. Increased uptake of radionuclide on a bone scan is caused mainly by increased osteoblastic activity associated with new bone formation and to a lesser degree by increased blood flow to bone. This can result from numerous causes, including infection, tumor, fractures, or synovitis. Although bone scanning is sensitive in detecting abnormalities of the bones and joints, it is

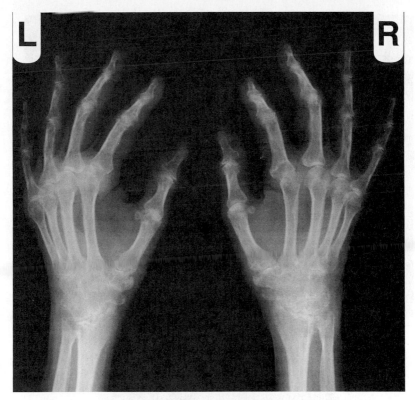

Figure 7-1. Oblique radiographs of the right and left hands and wrists in a woman with rheumatoid arthritis show narrowing of the radiocarpal, midcarpal, carpometacarpal, second metacarpophalangeal, and radioulnar joints, with periarticular osteoporosis and erosions.

not specific. Three-phase bone scanning, which includes blood flow and blood pool scans, as well as static images taken 2 to 4 hours or more after injection of the radionuclide, should be ordered for the evaluation of localized bone or joint pain. The early phases show vascularity, which may be helpful in diagnosing synovitis, infection, and soft tissue abnormalities. Single-photon emission computed tomography (SPECT) may provide more detail and can be helpful in diagnosing stress or traumatic spondylolysis and in detecting photopenic areas in avascular necrosis. Radionuclide bone scanning is most useful for screening the entire skeleton to localize the site of abnormality and also for detecting stress fractures, osteoid osteomas, and for evaluating painful joint prostheses.

B. Radionuclide infection scanning

1. Scanning with gallium citrate 67 shows increased uptake at sites of infection and some malignant neoplasms in the bones or soft tissues. It has a high sensitivity for bone and joint infection but is nonspecific because it may show increased uptake associated with other causes of increased bone turnover, including fractures or tumors, and may also show increased uptake in noninfectious inflammatory conditions, such as inflammatory arthritis. The specificity of a gallium scan for infection may be greater if it is compared with a bone scan. If the gallium scan shows more intense uptake than the bone scan at the affected site or if the uptake of gallium is not congruent with the uptake on the bone scan, then infection is likely. However, only one-third or even less of

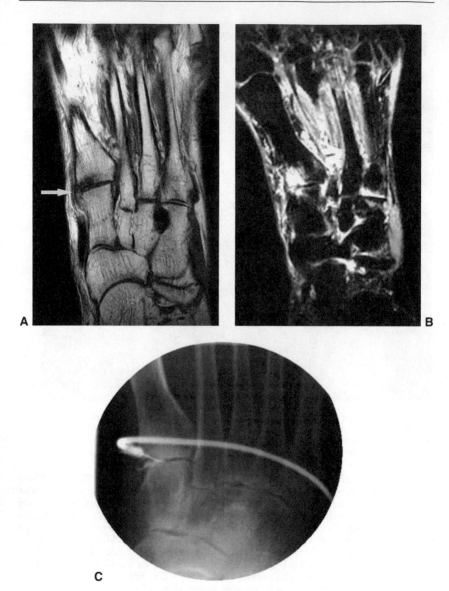

Figure 7-2. In a patient who had pain and swelling of the metatarsophalangeal joint of the great toe with normal radiographs, the proton density **(A)** and short tau inversion recovery (STIR) **(B)** sequence magnetic resonance imaging (MRI) showed osteoarthrosis with articular cartilage narrowing, bone marrow edema pattern, collapse of the subchondral bone, synovitis, and thickening of the medial ligaments (*arrow*). Using C-arm fluoroscopy the tube was tilted to make the joint tangential to the x-ray, allowing a needle to be inserted into the joint for aspiration and injection of local anesthetic and corticosteroids. Contrast was injected confirming the intra-articular position of the needle **(C)**.

bone infections meet these criteria. False-negative gallium scans may be seen in chronic infection or if the patient is treated with antibiotics before the scan is performed. Gallium scanning is preferred over white blood cell (WBC) scanning for diagnosis of infectious spondylitis, and for fever of unknown origin.

2. **Scanning with indium 111– or technetium 99m–labeled WBCs** can detect bone or joint infection because of migration of the radiolabeled WBCs to areas of infection or inflammation. Uptake of WBCs also occurs in noninfected bone marrow. Comparison of the WBC scan should be done with a bone marrow scan with radiolabeled colloid, such as ^{99m}Tc sulfur colloid, and uptake of WBCs not matched by the bone marrow scan is abnormal (Fig. 7-3).

The specificity of WBC scanning is greater than that of bone scanning or gallium scanning for bone and joint infection; however, mismatched uptake may also be seen in noninfectious inflammatory conditions.

C. **Positron-emission tomography (PET)** uses ^{18}F-fluorodeoxyglucose (FDG) as a scanning agent. FDG acts like glucose and is transported into cells and trapped. Malignant tumors and other conditions with high metabolic activity, such as infection, have increased glycolysis and increased uptake of FDG. PET CT (computed tomography) scan combines simultaneous PET and CT scan, allowing exact anatomic localization of areas of increased uptake of FDG. PET is highly sensitive for malignant soft tissue and bone neoplasms, however it has a lower specificity. It has a high cost, and reimbursement by medical insurance is limited to a relatively few indications at this time.

III. **Computed tomography (CT) scan** provides better bone detail than does radiography. Thin (1 mm or less) sections with multislice CT scanners provide high-resolution

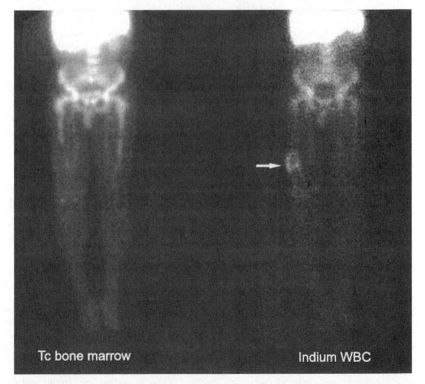

Tc bone marrow   Indium WBC

Figure 7-3. There is abnormal increased uptake of In-111 white blood cells in the right femur (*arrow*) and thigh not matched by a similar area on the ^{99m}Tc bone marrow scan, indicating active infection in this patient.

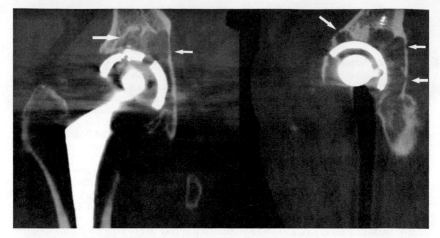

Figure 7-4. Reformatted coronal and sagittal images show large areas of osteolysis (*arrows*) around the acetabular component of a total hip prosthesis.

multiplanar (axial, coronal, and sagittal) images. This has almost completely replaced radiographic tomography. Three-dimensional images can also be created. Although CT scan provides better contrast for evaluation of soft tissue than does radiography, MRI is the superior scanning modality for soft tissue abnormalities. Some of the indications for musculoskeletal CT scan include evaluation of fracture displacement and alignment, bone tumors, and healing of fractures, joint arthrodesis, and surgical fusion of the spine. CT scans are routinely obtained immediately after myelography and discography. Metallic orthopedic hardware causes beam-hardening artifact on the scans; however, use of technique with high kilovoltage and high milliamperage, along with reformatted images, allows diagnostic images to be obtained in many cases (Fig. 7-4). CT guidance for interventional procedures allows exact needle placement for bone and soft tissue biopsies, radiofrequency ablation of osteoid osteomas and other neoplasms, and spinal injections that may be difficult to perform under fluoroscopy. Radiation exposure is higher for CT scan than for radiography; there is no radiation exposure with MRI and ultrasonography.

IV. **Magnetic resonance imaging (MRI)** has the advantage of providing multiplanar imaging with both anatomic and physiologic information that combines many of the capabilities of the other imaging modalities in one examination and also provides information for diagnosis of bone, joint, and soft tissue pathology, which is not available with other methods.

   A. **Technique.** The appearance of the MRI scan depends on the imaging sequence used. The spin echo technique is the most commonly used. T1-weighted images have a short echo time (TE), a short repetition time (TR); intermediate weighted or proton density (PD) images have a short TE and long TR; T2-weighted images have a long TE and long TR. Fluid is dark (low signal) on T1- and bright (high signal) on T2-weighted images. Fat is bright on TI- and of intermediate signal on T2-weighted images. Cortical bone has low signal on T1- and T2-weighted images. Bony abnormalities can be evaluated due to alterations in the marrow fat. Pathologic processes (neoplastic disease, infection, and fractures) will exhibit low or intermediate signal on T1-weighted sequences and high signal on T2-weighted images. Intermediate or PD images do not show differences in contrast of the tissues, as well as in T1 or T2; however, the resolution of the images is greater, allowing better evaluation of the morphology (see Fig. 7-2A). Fat suppression techniques such as short tau inversion recovery and chemical shift spin echo cause fluid to become very bright and fat dark, providing good contrast for detecting pathology (see Fig. 7-2B). High-resolution MRI images are needed to evaluate many abnormalities, such as labral tears of

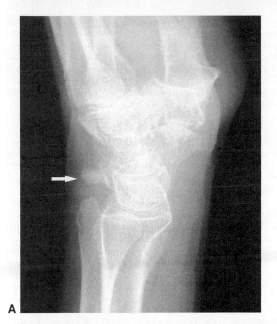

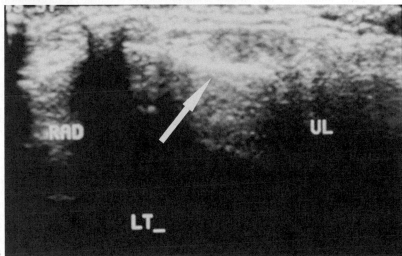

Figure 7-5. The lateral radiograph of the wrist **(A)** in a patient who had swelling and pain, without trauma, shows a calcific deposit in the dorsal soft tissues (*arrow*) representing calcific tendinitis of the extensor tendons. Under ultrasonographic guidance, a needle (*arrow*) was inserted into the calcific deposit **(B)**, which was aspirated and injected with corticosteroids. This resulted in relief of symptoms in less than 24 hours.

the shoulder and acetabulum, ligament tears in the wrist and elbow, and articular cartilage in the joints, and can be obtained by adjusting the scanning parameters using a smaller field of view and using surface coils instead of body coils for smaller structures. Various sequences are used for imaging of articular cartilage. Gadolinium diethylenetriamine penta-acetic acid (GD-DTPA) is an MRI contrast agent that, when used in typical doses (0.1 mmol/kg of body weight), acts primarily to shorten T1 relaxation times. Therefore, regions that readily enhance with contrast will appear bright on T1-weighted images. In the evaluation of the postoperative spine, contrast may help distinguish scar from recurrent disc herniation. Postoperative scar is felt to enhance with contrast by virtue of the rich vascularity of epidural granulation tissue. Conversely, the avascular adult disc will not demonstrate similar signal enhancement. A contrast-enhanced MRI examination performed long after surgery may not prove as reliable because scar tissue may become progressively fibrotic, with less discernible contrast enhancement. Inflammatory tissue will enhance with gadolinium, which may help define an abscess and differentiate from another form of fluid collection. Relative contraindications to GD-DTPA administration include hemolytic anemia because the agent may promote extravascular hemolysis. Because GD-DTPA is cleared via glomerular filtration, caution should be exercised in patients with impaired renal function. The most commonly reported adverse reaction is mild headache (<10% of patients).

B. Indications. MRI has become the imaging modality of choice for many abnormalities including evaluation of internal derangement of the knee (e.g., meniscal tears; cruciate, collateral, and quadriceps mechanism tears; and bone contusion), osteonecrosis, rotator cuff tears and glenohumeral instability, tendon, ligament, and muscle tears and other abnormalities, back pain, bone and soft tissue tumors, occult fracture, and for evaluation of the brain and spinal cord pathology. Articular cartilage abnormalities including chondromalacia, fissuring, and partial and full-thickness cartilage defects can be visualized on the MRI. Joint erosions and synovitis can be detected in patients with normal plain radiography (see Fig. 7-2C).

C. Contraindications to MRI include the presence of pacemakers, aneurysm clips, some prosthetic otologic and ocular implants, and some retained bullet fragments. Clinical concern increases when the metallic object is anatomically close to a vital vascular or neural structure. Most prosthetic heart valves are felt to be safe for MRI. In addition, most orthopedic materials and devices are considered safe, including stainless steel screws and wires. Prior knowledge of the specific type (manufacturer, material) of metallic implant is essential before the patient is exposed to a strong magnetic field. However, ferromagnetic metallic implants will cause image artifact, with large areas of signal void and adjacent high signal ("flare" response), which may interfere with accurate image interpretation. By using sequences designed for limiting metal artifact even in the presence of orthopedic hardware, valuable information can be obtained about possible infection, fracture, loosening, and osteolysis.

V. **Ultrasonography** may be used to evaluate soft tissue masses and characterize them as either cystic or solid. Popliteal cysts can easily be detected. Tendons are more echogenic than muscle and can be evaluated for continuity and the presence of inflammation. Tenosynovitis can be detected as fluid in the tendon sheath. Ultrasonography has been used in the shoulder for evaluation of the rotator cuff tendons. Complete and partial tears and tendinopathy can be diagnosed. Tendons in most other parts of the body can be evaluated in a similar manner. Plantar fasciitis can be diagnosed by evaluating the thickness and appearance of the plantar fascia. Calcific tendinitis can be detected as focal areas of high echogenicity. Injection of soft tissue ganglia, calcific deposits, tendon sheaths, and interdigital neuromas can be performed under ultrasonographic guidance (Fig. 7-5). Foreign bodies in the soft tissue can be localized. Ultrasonography is used for the evaluation of developmental dysplasia of the hip in infants to determine the position of the nonossified femoral head with respect to the acetabulum.

ARTHROCENTESIS, INTRA-ARTICULAR INJECTION, AND SYNOVIAL FLUID ANALYSIS

Jessica R. Berman, Theodore R. Fields, and Richard Stern

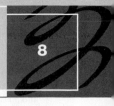

8

■ KEY POINTS

■ Aspiration of a joint should always be performed on an initial evaluation or whenever a diagnosis is in doubt or in the case of monoarticular arthritis when infection must be excluded.

■ The fluid aspirated should always be analyzed for cell count, Gram stain, culture, and the presence of crystals at a minimum.

■ A known diagnosis of rheumatoid arthritis, gout or pseudogout does not exclude infection especially when one joint is disproportionately affected.

I. **Arthrocentesis,** or aspiration of fluid from a joint, is a safe and relatively easy procedure that plays both diagnostic and therapeutic roles in the management of arthritis. It should be included in the initial evaluation of every patient with a joint effusion, especially those with monarthritis.

II. **Synovial fluid analysis** following aspiration may help in differentiating a primary inflammatory process such as rheumatoid arthritis (RA) from a noninflammatory process such as osteoarthritis. It can provide a specific diagnosis in crystalline arthritis.

   A. Diagnostic indications
   1. As part of an initial evaluation.
   2. To rule out infection or hemorrhage.
   3. To rule out crystalline disease.

   B. Therapeutic indications
   1. Drainage of an effusion to relieve pain and restore range of motion.
   2. Instillation of medication (e.g., steroids and viscosupplementation).
   3. Drainage of a septic joint.
   4. Drainage of a hemarthrosis.

   C. Absolute contraindications. Infection in overlying skin or surrounding soft tissue.

   D. Relative contraindications. Coagulation disorder, especially if severe.

III. **Intra-articular injection** is primarily used to deliver intra-articular corticosteroids to treat inflamed joints (a similar technique is employed for injection of inflamed soft-tissues such as bursae or tendons). Contraindications are the same as for arthrocentesis. Corticosteroids should not be injected into a joint until infection has been excluded. In general, joints should not be injected more than three to four times per year. Injection of corticosteroids directly into a tendon or tendon insertion can sometimes result in tendon rupture.

PREPARATION FOR ASPIRATION/INJECTION

I. **MATERIALS FOR ASEPTIC SKIN PREPARATION**
   A. Sterile gloves.
   B. Iodine solution.
   C. Alcohol solution.
   D. Sterile gauze pads.

II. **MATERIALS FOR LOCAL ANESTHESIA**
   A. One percent lidocaine for skin, subcutaneous tissues, and joint structures.
   B. Ethyl chloride spray for skin.

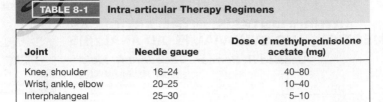

TABLE 8-1	Intra-articular Therapy Regimens	
Joint	Needle gauge	Dose of methylprednisolone acetate (mg)
Knee, shoulder	16–24	40–80
Wrist, ankle, elbow	20–25	10–40
Interphalangeal	25–30	5–10

III. **NEEDLES.** Sterile 18- to 25-gauge needles, depending on the size of the joint. Inflamed joint fluids may be thick and may require a large-bore needle for removal. Sterile 30-gauge needles may be used for local anesthetic instillation, and for injection into small joints such as the proximal interphalangeal (PIP) joints and when no fluid aspiration is anticipated.

IV. **SYRINGES.** The size varies from 1 to 50 mL depending on the joint and amount of effusion.

V. **TUBES FOR SYNOVIAL FLUID ANALYSIS**
   A. Hematology tube for cell count and differential.
   B. Sterile tubes for Gram stain, cultures, and smears.
   C. Heparinized tube for crystal analysis. Powdered anticoagulant may interfere with crystal identification.
   D. Cytology bottle (if neoplasm is suspected).

VI. **INTRA-ARTICULAR MEDICATIONS.** At the Hospital for Special Surgery, methylprednisolone acetate (Depomedrol), a long-acting, insoluble corticosteroid preparation is used. The dose varies with the size of the joint. Betamethasone (Celestone) may be used when the goal is avoidance of a joint flare reaction and a shorter 2- to 4-week duration of action is acceptable (e.g., with attacks of crystal disease). Doses and appropriate needle sizes are summarized in Table 8-1.

 JOINT-SPECIFIC TECHNIQUES

The most important maneuver before aspirating a joint is to locate the appropriate landmark. This can best be done by making a skin impression with the round end of an unopened pen point or pen mark. Local anesthesia of the overlying skin and subcutaneous tissues is recommended. As a general rule, if it is important to obtain fluid for diagnostic purposes, a larger needle should be used (so as to avoid the need for reaspiration if the fluid is too thick to be aspirated by a small needle).

I. **SHOULDER.** The shoulder can be entered either anteriorly or posteriorly.
   A. **Anterior approach** (Fig. 8-1). With the patient's hand on the lap and with the shoulder muscles relaxed, the glenohumeral joint can be palpated by placing the fingers between the **coracoid process** and the humeral head. As the shoulder is internally rotated, the humeral head can be felt turning inward and the joint space can be felt as a groove just lateral to the coracoid process. When the skin over this area is anesthetized, a 20- or 22-gauge needle can be inserted lateral to the coracoid (the thoracoacromial artery lies medial to the coracoid). The needle is directed dorsally and medially into the joint space. The needle should be directed slightly superiorly to avoid the neurovascular bundle.
   B. **Posterior approach** (Fig. 8-2). The posterior aspect of the shoulder joint is identified with the patient's arm internally rotated maximally. This position is achieved by placing the patient's ipsilateral hand on the opposite shoulder. The humeral head can then be palpated by placing a finger posteriorly along the **acromion** while the shoulder is rotated. A 20- or 22-gauge needle is inserted approximately 1 cm inferior to the **posterior tip of the acromion** and directed anteriorly and medially.

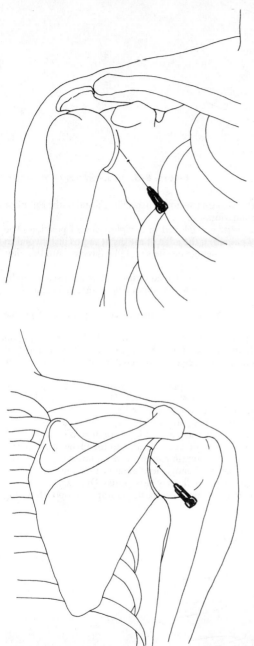

Figure 8-1. Arthrocentesis of the shoulder—anterior approach.

Figure 8-2. Arthrocentesis of the shoulder—posterior approach.

II.   **ELBOW.** The **elbow joint** (Fig. 8-3) can be identified by placing the patient's relaxed arm on the lap. With the palm facing the patient, the elbow is flexed to a 45-degree angle. By placing the finger on the **lateral epicondyle,** the shallow depression distal to it can be noted, which represents the elbow joint. A 22-gauge needle is introduced perpendicular to the joint.

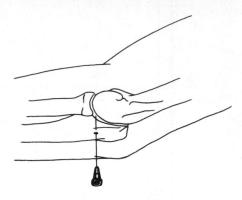

Figure 8-3. Arthrocentesis of the elbow.

III. **Wrist** (Fig. 8-4) aspiration is performed on the dorsal aspect just distal to the radius or ulna as indicated by clinical examination.

A. Radial entry. The hand and wrist are relaxed in a slightly flexed position. The joint space can be located by palpating the edge of the distal radius just medial to the **thumb extensor tendon.** A 22-gauge needle should be directed into the joint from the dorsal aspect.

B. Ulnar entry. The wrist is kept in the same relaxed position. The joint space can be identified by palpating just distal to the **distal ulna**. The 22-gauge needle is directed in a volar and radial direction.

IV. **ANKLE.** For both approaches (Fig. 8-5), the foot is first placed at about a 45-degree angle of plantar flexion.

A. Medial approach. A 22-gauge needle is placed approximately 1 cc proximal and lateral to the distal end of the **medial malleolus**. The flexor hallucis longus tendon is just lateral to this point. The needle is directed 45 degrees posteriorly, slightly upward, and laterally.

B. Lateral approach. A 22-gauge needle is placed approximately 1/2 cc proximal and medial to the distal end of the **lateral malleolus**. The needle should be directed 45 degrees posteriorly, slightly upward, and medially.

V. **KNEE.** The knee (Fig. 8-6) is the easiest joint to enter. It may be entered either medially or laterally. The patient should be supine with the knee comfortably extended. A 19- to 22-gauge needle is introduced in a direction parallel to the plane of the posterior surface of the patella in a medial position (in patients with a known coagulopathy or in those taking anticoagulant drugs, a 25-gauge needle can be used). In the presence of thick exudative effusions, a larger bore needle may be required. Drainage of the knee suprapatellar bursa can be facilitated by compressing the suprapatellar pouch during

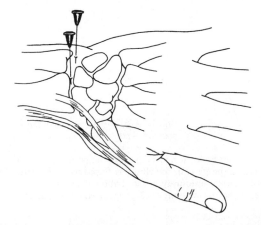

Figure 8-4. Arthrocentesis of the wrist—medial and lateral approaches.

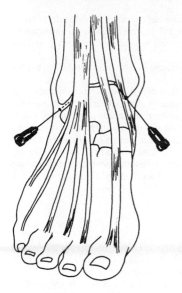

Figure 8-5. Arthrocentesis of the ankle—medial and lateral approaches.

aspiration. With large knee effusions, the distended suprapatellar pouch can be aspirated directly from either the medial or lateral aspect of the quadriceps muscle mass.

VI. **Small joints of the hands and feet** may be difficult to enter. Occasionally the effusion bulges and facilitates aspiration. Often, a corticosteroid injection can be given just adjacent to the joint rather than within it; this may result in an equivalent clinical response.

   A. **The metacarpophalangeal (MCP) joint** can easily be palpated on its dorsolateral aspect with the finger slightly flexed and relaxed. The joint is entered on the dorsolateral aspect with a 22- to 25-gauge needle. Because this is a ball (distal metacarpal) and cup (first phalanx) joint, the needle should not be directed at a 90-degree angle but rather distally at about a 60-degree angle.

   B. **The PIP joint** margin is barely palpable but may be felt on its dorsal aspect just distal to the skin crease. The joint is entered from the dorsal aspect with a 25- to 30-gauge needle that is directed slightly distally.

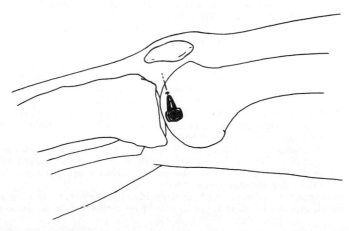

Figure 8-6. Arthrocentesis of the knee—medial approach.

    C. The distal interphalangeal (DIP) joint is extremely small and difficult to enter. The technique is the same as for aspirating the PIP joint. If there is no suspicion of infection, a 30-gauge needle may be the least uncomfortable for the patient and the easiest for joint entry.

    D. The metatarsophalangeal (MTP) joint is aspirated in a fashion similar to that for the MCP joint.

VII. OTHER JOINTS. There are external landmarks that can direct aspiration and injection of the hip joint, but success in this venture requires some experience. Because the hip joint lies deep within the pelvis, aspiration can be more readily performed under fluoroscopic or ultrasonographic guidance. Ultrasonography, in particular, enables direct visualization, accurately defines the presence and size of an effusion, and allows for successful and safe aspiration to be performed if the need arises. The injection of corticosteroids for treatment can also be carried out with greater precision in administration. The spinal and sacroiliac joints often demand fluoroscopic or CT guidance to carry out these procedures.

COMPLICATIONS

I. **"POSTINJECTION FLARE."** Long-acting intra-articular steroid preparations like methylprednisolone acetate may induce a crystal synovitis 24 hours after the injection. Application of ice at the onset of a postinjection flare may be helpful.

II. **BRUISING.** The needle itself may traumatize the joint, especially if the joint is small; for this reason, the patient should be warned of possible short-term aggravation of symptoms in the injected joint and receive appropriate instructions regarding analgesia.

III. **Skin Atrophy** can sometimes occur if corticosteroids are injected close to the undersurface of the skin.

IV. **TENDON RUPTURE.** Injection of corticosteroids directly into a tendon or tendon insertion can cause tendon rupture. If a tendon injection is desired, ultrasound-guided injections directly into the paratenon (not the tendon proper) may be both effective and safe. Ultrasonography-guided injections, for example, into the retrocalcaneal bursa, can minimize the risk of injection into the Achilles tendon.

SYNOVIAL FLUID ANALYSIS

Fluid analysis is an extremely useful diagnostic tool in the evaluation of rheumatic diseases. It should be included in the initial evaluation of most arthritic conditions that generate effusions. It can yield a specific diagnosis in infectious and crystal-induced arthritis and can be helpful in categorization, definition, and the diagnosis of other arthritides.

I. **SYNOVIAL FLUID STUDIES (TABLE 8-2)**

    A. Gross examination can be helpful in establishing the nature of a joint fluid. After air bubbles are allowed to clear, a heparinized specimen is examined for the following:

        1. Color. Normal synovial fluid is straw colored. Inflammatory fluids range from yellow to greenish yellow. Bloody fluid to a certain degree occurs in patients with coagulation disorders, trauma, neoplasms, and tuberculous arthritis and in patients receiving anticoagulant therapy.

        2. Clarity. Normal synovial fluids are clear enough for print to be read through them. As inflammation increases from mild to marked, the fluid becomes first translucent and then opalescent.

        3. Viscosity. Synovial fluid viscosity is tested by allowing a drop of fluid to fall from the needle tip. Normal synovial fluids are quite viscous, and a "string" of fluid will form. Because viscosity is decreased in inflammatory synovial fluids, no string sign is seen.

    B. Cell count. A cell count for both white blood cells (WBC), including a differential, and red blood cells (RBC) should be performed. Inflammatory fluids

TABLE 8-2 Synovial Fluid Analysis

Classification	Condition	Color	Clarity	Viscosity	WBC/mm³	NTP (%)	Crystals	Glucose (% serum)	Complement	Culture/smear
Normal	Normal	Yellow	Translucent	High	<200	<25	0	Same	Normal	0
Group 1 (non inflammatory)	Osteoarthritis	Yellow	Transparent	High	<2,000	<25	0	Same	Normal	0
	Trauma									
Group 2 (inflammatory)	SLE	Pink or red	Transparent	High	<2,000	<25	0	Same	Normal	0
		Yellow	Translucent	Slightly decreased	0–9,000	<25	0	Same	Normal	0
	Acute rheumatic fever	Yellow	Translucent	Slightly decreased	0–60,000	25–50	0	Same	Normal	0
	Pseudogout	Yellow or white	Translucent or opaque	Low	50–75,000	90	+	Same	Normal	0
	Gout	Yellow or white	Translucent or opaque	Low	100–160,000	90	+	Same	Normal	0
	Rheumatoid arthritis	Yellow or purulent	Translucent or opaque	Low	3,000–50,000	50–75	0	75–100	Normal or low	0
Group 3 (purulent)	Tuberculosis	Purulent	Opaque	Low	2,500–100,000	50	0	50–75	Normal or low	+
	Bacterial arthritis	Purulent	Opaque	Low	50,000–300,000[a]	>90	0	<50	Normal or low	+[b]

[a] Can be lower earlier in infection.
[b] Often negative in gonococcal arthritis.
NTP, neutrophils; SLE, systematic lupus erythematosus; WBC, white blood cells.

generally have WBC counts above 1,000, whereas noninflammatory fluids have WBC counts under 1,000. It must be noted that the ratio of RBC/WBC is approximately 750/1. This can be important in hemorrhagic fluids that are inflammatory or infected. The WBC differential can be useful diagnostically, with greater than 50% polymorphonuclear neutrophil (PMN) cells a common finding in inflammatory effusions and greater than 90% PMN cells commonly seen with infection.

  C. Crystal examination can be performed using polarized microscopy of a specimen of heparinized fluid (see Chapters 43 and 44). Urate crystals parallel to the polarizer axis appear yellow, and urate crystals perpendicular to the polarizer axis appear blue. The opposite is true for the calcium pyrophosphate crystals of pseudogout. Urate crystals are needle-shaped and calcium pyrophosphate crystals are rhomboid. It must be kept in mind that the finding of crystals does not rule out the possibility of an infection.

  D. Microbiologic studies

    1. Stains should include both Gram stain method and acid-fast method if infection is suspected or the fluid appears turbid or cloudy.

    2. Cultures should include routine bacterial studies. Fungal and mycobacterial cultures are ordered if clinically indicated. Some fastidious or slower growing organisms may need to be watched for growth for up to 4 weeks. Synovial fluids raising suspicion of gonococcal or *Borrelia burgdorferi* infection may be specifically sent for polymerase chain reaction (PCR) analysis if the diagnosis is in question.

  E. Biochemical studies

    1. Glucose. Determination of synovial fluid glucose, when interpreted with a simultaneous serum value, is helpful in diagnosing infectious arthritis. In bacterial infection or tuberculosis, the synovial fluid glucose level will be less than half the level in the serum. Occasionally, low values may be seen in RA.

    2. Protein determination does not provide additional useful information and should not be routinely ordered.

    3. Complement may be decreased in RA, but the test is rarely helpful for diagnosis because synovial fluid complement is usually normal in early RA.

II.   **DIAGNOSIS BY FLUID GROUP.** Synovial fluid can be divided into three groups based on the degree of inflammation (see Table 8-2).

  A. Group 1 fluids are clear and transparent and have few white cells on cell count. They include normal, osteoarthritic, and systemic lupus erythematosus (SLE) joint fluids.

  B. Group 2 fluids generally have a higher WBC count and are not as reactive as group 1 fluids; they appear translucent. This group includes fluids from most noninfectious, inflammatory arthritic conditions, such as gout, pseudogout, psoriatic arthritis, reactive arthritis and RA. Leukemia or lymphoma occasionally presents in this category, but the differential count reveals more than 90% mononuclear cells.

  C. Group 3 fluids are opalescent or purulent. Group 3 fluids include those from bacterial infections and tuberculosis (although joint fluid from gonococcal arthritis can be either group 2 or group 3). Group 3 fluids typically have 50,000 to 300,000 WBC/mm^3; these are mostly neutrophils. Occasionally, the synovial fluid from a patient with an inflammatory arthritic condition such as RA or gout may have as many as 50,000 to 75,000 white cells/mm^3 and appears opalescent or even purulent. As Table 8-1 shows, there is considerable overlap between the various arthritic diseases; this table is meant to serve as a guideline rather than provide a rigid set of criteria.

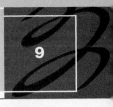

MEASURING CLINICAL OUTCOMES IN RHEUMATIC DISEASE

Melanie J. Harrison and Lisa A. Mandl

9

■ KEY POINTS

■ Understanding the purpose, design, proper application, and clinical meaning of outcomes instruments is necessary for correct interpretation of the medical literature.

■ The heterogeneity of the rheumatic disease often requires disease-specific assessment using validated instruments designed to detect clinically relevant outcomes that are unique to each condition.

■ Generic outcomes instruments are useful to compare different rheumatic disease populations with one another or with nonrheumatic disease populations with respect to common clinical manifestations, such as pain, disability, and general health.

■ Many different clinical outcomes are often assessed whether alone (e.g., tender joint count and pain) or as a composite [e.g., disease activity score (DAS)] in order to capture the overall effect of rheumatic diseases.

■ Clinical outcomes instruments are constantly changing to keep pace with the growing knowledge of the clinical manifestations and underlying pathophysiology of rheumatic diseases.

 any instruments have been developed to assess clinical outcomes. Some are designed for use in specific diseases, whereas others are applicable to more generalized populations; all instruments are intended to help make measurable assessments of the patients' physical and psychosocial status. Outcomes instruments are used routinely in rheumatic disease studies.

It is important to understand what these tools measure, in what settings they can be applied, and how their results are interpreted.

GENERAL CONCEPTS OF OUTCOMES MEASUREMENT

I. **Clinical outcomes instruments are essential for clinical research** and are useful for the evaluation of the status or change in status of an individual in the clinical setting. Instruments objectify what we see clinically, standardize measurement, and allow for comparison. However, reducing complex clinical information to statistically manageable data may result in oversimplification and loss of important detail.

   A. **Data reduction.** Outcomes analysis requires packaging of data qualitatively or quantitatively. **Qualitative** outcomes categorize individuals. For example, classification criteria classify subjects as with or without disease and American College of Rheumatology (ACR) response criteria classify patients as improved or not improved. **Quantitative** outcomes are expressed as scores and usually have a neutral or normal value for comparison.

   B. **Standardization.** Explicit procedures for distributing, administering, and scoring instruments are necessary to minimize error. Specific parameters to define each variable/outcome are needed to ensure that all evaluations are made in the same way; this is called **operationalization.**

C. Reliability. The precision of a measure can be described as its consistency, reproducibility, or reliability. It is divided into external and internal consistency.

    1. External consistency. Results are reproducible and have limited variability when the same measure is performed by the same assessor or on the same patient on different occasions (intraobserver) or different assessors simultaneously (interobserver).

    2. Internal consistency. Responses to items within an instrument that measure the same attribute are similar.

D. Validity. Instruments should accurately represent and measure what they purport to measure.

    1. Content validity. Is the instrument logical and meaningful, that is, does it make intuitive sense?

    2. Construct validity. Does the instrument examine the theoretical concepts and appropriately evaluate the relation between specific variables that are believed to explain the phenomenon being studied?

    3. Criterion validity. Do the results of the instrument correlate with an external measure of the true value, for example, a "gold standard"?

E. Responsiveness. Instruments that are used at two points in time to assess patient status over time should be sensitive to change; the results should vary consistently with the status of the patient (i.e., if the patient improves clinically, the change in outcome measurement should reflect improvement; if the patient's condition does not change, neither should the measurement).

F. Objectivity. The influence of individual interpretation by the patient or the assessor should be limited.

G. Feasibility. Instruments and their measurements must be practical and not cumbersome to use, easily understood by those administering and responding to them, patient-friendly, and scored without difficulty.

 ## CLASSIFICATION CRITERIA

There is no single definitive diagnostic test for most rheumatic diseases because many of these conditions are frustratingly heterogeneous. Classification criteria have been developed to allow accurate categorization of patients for clinical research studies.

I.   **Classification criteria are imperfect.** Sensitivity and specificity are maximized, but each is less than 100%. These criteria undergo revisions periodically as knowledge of these diseases grows.

II.   **Classification criteria are often used as the basis for subject selection for studies of specific diseases.** However, they are also used in epidemiologic surveys as the outcome measure (e.g., incidence and prevalence studies).

III.   **Classification criteria are not intended to serve as a diagnostic tool.**

 ## FUNCTIONAL STATUS QUESTIONNAIRES

I.   **HEALTH ASSESSMENT QUESTIONNAIRE (HAQ).** The HAQ measures functional disability, that is, how well individuals manage activities in their daily lives. The HAQ was one of the first patient self-report instruments. Previously, outcomes measurement relied on physicians' assessment or laboratory data. Although originally developed to evaluate arthritic conditions, the HAQ is now considered a generic instrument.

    A. Content. Individual questions that comprise the HAQ disability index evaluate the patient's ability over the preceding 2 weeks to perform various activities that fall into eight component areas: hygiene, dressing and grooming, arising, eating, walking, reach, grip, and outdoor activities.

    B. Scoring. HAQ scores range from 0 to 3; higher scores indicate greater disability and a 0.22 point change indicates a clinically important difference. The commonly used two-page version includes two visual analogue scales (VAS), one for pain and one for global health, and the HAQ disability index. The VAS global health scale is a validated measure of health-related quality of life and correlates strongly with other quality of life measurement tools.

C. There are different versions of the HAQ. The multidimensional HAQ (MDHAQ) identifies patients who have important functional limitations, but do not register a high enough HAQ to score as "disabled." The modified HAQ (mHAQ) includes fewer original items and additional questions regarding patient satisfaction and self-perception of health and performance.

D. Why is the HAQ important? The HAQ prospectively captures the effect of chronic illness over time. HAQ scores have been shown to correlate with work disability, health services utilization, and mortality, among other clinically important outcomes, especially in rheumatoid arthritis (RA) population.

II. ARTHRITIS IMPACT MEASUREMENT SCALE (AIMS). The AIMS evaluates health-related quality of life in patients with arthritis.

A. Content. The AIMS 2 is a 78-item questionnaire which evaluates physical, social, and emotional well-being. It is self-administered and takes approximately 20 minutes to complete. There is also a validated shorter version of the AIMS, which consists of 28 questions and takes approximately 8 minutes to complete.

B. Scoring. Items are additive. Lower scores indicate better quality of life. Single items are grouped into five scales: general physical health, affect, symptoms, work role, and social interaction. The numeric totals for the scales vary based on the number of individual items contained within each scale.

OSTEOARTHRITIS MEASURES

I. Western Ontario McMaster Universities Osteoarthritis Index (WOMAC) measures important, potentially modifiable, clinical outcomes in hip and knee osteoarthritis (OA). It is recommended by the Osteoarthritis Research Society International for use in clinical trials of knee and hip OA.

A. Content. Patients' reported experiences with OA played a significant role in developing the WOMAC in order to ensure that questions were patient-centered and clinically relevant. The 24 items are grouped into three subscales: pain, stiffness, and physical function. The WOMAC has well-documented reliability, validity, and responsiveness.

B. Scoring. Scores can be presented as the mean within each subscale or as a total instrument score.

II. KNEE INJURY AND OSTEOARTHRITIS OUTCOME SCORE (KOOS). Although originally used in patients with a previous knee injury, the KOOS can be applied to any patient with knee OA. It is particularly appropriate for use in younger or more active patients whose activities are affected by knee pain, but whose loss of function is not severe enough to be identified by the WOMAC.

A. Content. There are five subscales: pain, other symptoms, functioning in daily living, functioning in sport and recreation, and knee-related quality of life. WOMAC scores can be calculated from the KOOS.

B. Scoring. Scales range from 0 to 100, with 100 indicating no symptoms and 0 indicating severe symptoms. The KOOS is self-administered and takes 10 minutes to complete.

RHEUMATOID ARTHRITIS MEASURES

I. AMERICAN COLLEGE OF RHEUMATOLOGY (ACR) 20, 50, AND 70 RESPONSE CRITERIA

A. Content. The ACR response criteria include (a) tender joint count, (b) swollen joint count, (c) a measure of disability (e.g., HAQ), (d) patient's global assessment, (e) physician's global assessment of disease activity, (f) patient's assessment of pain, and (g) an acute phase reactant, either the erythrocyte sedimentation rate (ESR) or C-reactive protein (CRP). This index has been validated and is used extensively in most RA clinical trials.

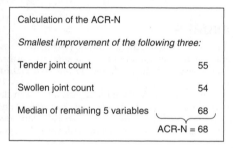

Components	Baseline	Follow-up	Percent Improvement	Calculation of the ACR 20
Tender joint count	20	9	55	Both joint counts MUST have improved by at least 20%
Swollen joint count	24	11	54	
Pain (VAS)	65	20	69	
Patient's global assessment (VAS)	89	50	44	Three of these five variables MUST have improved at least 20%
Physician's global assessment (VAS)	75	20	73	
Functional disability (HAQ)	2.5	1.8	28	
Acute phase reactant (ESR or CRP)	60	19	68	

Calculation of the ACR-N

Smallest improvement of the following three:

Tender joint count	55
Swollen joint count	54
Median of remaining 5 variables	68

ACR-N = 68

Figure 9-1. Example of American College of Rheumatalogy response criteria used to calculate in a patient with rheumatoid arthritis. (Patient illustrated here meets ACR 20 and ACR 50 response criteria, but not ACR 70 criteria.)
VAS, visual analogue scales; HAQ, health assessment questionnaire; ESR, erythrocyte sedimentation rate; CRP, C-reactive protein; ACR, American College of Rheumatology; RA, rheumatoid arthritis.

B. **Scoring.** Each component is measured at two points in time and the percentage change is calculated. An "ACR 20" (or improvement) is achieved if both the tender **and** swollen joint counts are at least 20% improved over baseline **and** if at least three of the five remaining component scores have also improved at least 20% (Fig. 9-1). ACR 50 and ACR 70 scores are similarly calculated.

C. **Limitations.** The means by which the ACR response criteria are calculated present several limitations to their use and interpretation.

1. **The ACR criteria do not evaluate a patient at a single point in time.** The criteria can only examine a change over a period of time and are therefore only useful in longitudinal assessments.

2. **ACR response criteria only classify patients with RA as improved or not improved.** They do not differentiate between deterioration in RA status and stable disease.

3. **Because these criteria depend on a positive change in RA status, they are best used in those with considerable room and potential for clinical improvement.** They are less useful in patients who have severely destroyed joints, have minimally active RA, or have stable disease because these patients are not likely to show clinically important positive change.

4. **They do not give a good qualitative sense of the patient's abilities.** Two patients who both improve 20% could each have a very different functional status. For example, a bedridden patient who improves 20% could have the same ACR 20 as a patient who can run 10 miles and then improves 20%; however, these patients are clearly not equivalent.

II. **The numeric ACR (ACR-N)** is a modification of the ACR response criteria and quantifies changes in patient status.

    A. **Content.** The ACR-N includes the same seven components as the ACR response criteria, as described in the preceding section.

    B. **Scoring.** A continuous variable summary measure that includes the lowest percentage change in (i) number of tender joints, (ii) number of swollen joints, and (iii) the median percentage improvement in (a) pain assessment, (b) physician global assessment, (c) patient global assessment, (d) physical function, and (e) acute phase reactant value.

    C. **The ACR-N is calculated for each patient over the course of a study at different points in time.** The area under the curve (AUC) is calculated for each patient; mean AUC can be compared between groups. Unlike the disease activity score (DAS) (in the subsequent text), the ACR-N AUC has yet to be validated and shown to correlate with relevant clinical outcomes, such as radiographic progression.

III. **DISEASE ACTIVITY SCORE.** The DAS can evaluate the status of a patient with RA at a single point in time.

    A. **Content.** The DAS requires a tender joint count, a swollen joint count, a patient global assessment of disease activity, and ESR; no follow-up is necessary for calculation. The DAS has been validated, is responsive to change, and has been found to correlate with functional disability and radiographic progression. The DAS 28 is the shorter version, evaluating only 28 joints.

    B. **Scoring.** The DAS is derived from a complex calculation:

$$DAS = 0.56 \times \sqrt{\text{(tender joint count)}} + 0.28 \times \sqrt{\text{(swollen joint count)}}$$
$$+ 0.70 \times \ln(ESR) + 0.014 \times \text{global assessment}.$$

    C. **Scores can be subtracted from one another to demonstrate change that is either positive or negative.** The DAS at different points in time can be used to calculate a DAS AUC. A DAS score less than 2.6 is considered remission. A patient whose DAS score decreases by greater than or equal to 1.6 over two points in time is considered to be clinically improved.

    D. **Limitation.** DAS scores are meaningless without familiarity with the scale.

SYSTEMIC LUPUS ERYTHEMATOSUS MEASURES

Systemic lupus erythematosus (SLE) is the prototypical autoimmune disease characterized by enormous within-patient and between-patient heterogeneity. This diversity results in considerable complexity and difficulty when attempting to measure the outcomes of groups of patients. SLE outcomes are usually measured in two dimensions: **activity** and **damage.**

I. **ACTIVITY.** Activity is the acute (or subacute) status of a patient that is presumed to be reversible. Activity is attributable to the underlying pathophysiology of SLE: immune-mediated inflammation. There are many instruments that measure SLE activity, each addressing a different methodologic issue. Three of the most common SLE activity instruments are described in the subsequent text. All have several versions, require trained administration, and have documented reliability and validity.

    A. **Systemic Lupus Erythematosus Disease Activity Index (SLEDAI)**

        1. **Content.** The SLEDAI includes 24 SLE manifestations (called descriptors) which are operationalized (called definitions). Data collection requires performance of a history, physical examination, and laboratory evaluation.

        2. **Scoring.** Each SLEDAI descriptor has been assigned a weighted score from 0 to 8, on the basis of its general clinical severity. Manifestations that have been present in the preceding 10 days are noted and summed to give a total activity score. Total SLEDAI scores range from 0 to 108.

B. Systemic Lupus Activity Measure (SLAM)

 1. Content. The SLAM consists of 33 clinical and laboratory manifestations of active SLE within nine organ systems. Each item is classified as active or inactive over the prior month and then expanded to evaluate its severity on the basis of categories of disability, destruction, and monitoring or treatment needs.

 2. Scoring. Each active manifestation is given a score based on category of severity and then summed. Summary scores express total activity and range from 0 to 84. The SLAM has excellent responsiveness.

C. British Isles Lupus Activity Group (BILAG). The BILAG was developed specifically for use in SLE clinical drug trials to determine change in disease activity within a particular organ system. Individual items are well operationalized; there is high inter-rater reliability and good responsiveness.

 1. Content. Manifestations within eight organ systems, including one for generalized manifestations (e.g., fever and weight loss), are evaluated for activity within the prior month. Each system is assigned a rating based on the physician's intention to treat a specific SLE condition within the system.

 2. Scoring. A modified version (1993) has five rating categories (scores 0 to 9): A—urgent, disease requiring greater than 20 mg prednisone or immunosuppression; B—less active than A, but requires symptomatic therapy; C—stable, mild disease; D—previously affected, but currently inactive; E—system never involved. The eight category scores are summed; total scores range from 0 to 72.

II. FLARE. Clinically important deterioration in SLE status constitutes flare.

A. Types of SLE flares. These changes may be qualitative (i.e., the development of new disease in a previously uninvolved organ) or quantitative (i.e., exacerbation of already existing organ dysfunction).

B. Measurement of flare. Ideally, the difference in scores on SLE activity instruments administered at two points in time should denote at least quantitative flare. However, as some organ disease may improve, and others deteriorate, use of the aforementioned instruments for this purpose is problematic.

III. DAMAGE. Damage is an assessment of the chronic, cumulative, physiological impact of SLE since its diagnosis. It is a measure of irreversible organ damage and dysfunction not related to active inflammation.

A. Assessment of damage does not require attributability to SLE itself. It may be the consequence of the disease and/or its treatment, primarily corticosteroids or cytotoxic medications; presumably, patients with more serious disease require more aggressive and longer duration of therapy, thereby exposing them to a greater risk of adverse events secondary to these treatments.

B. Measurement—The Systemic Lupus International Collaborating Clinics (SLICC)/American College of Rheumatology (ACR) Index.

 1. Content. The **SLICC/ACR Damage Index** includes clinical manifestations within 12 different organ systems. Items include cataracts, cerebrovascular accident(s), end-stage renal disease (regardless of dialysis or transplantation), pulmonary hypertension, avascular necrosis, chronic alopecia, premature gonadal failure, among others.

 2. Scoring. Clinical manifestations that are clinically ascertained and have been present for at least 6 months (repeat episodes must occur at least 6 months apart to be scored twice) are scored using a simple weighting system. The SLICC/ACR Damage Index is a reliable and valid measure of SLE-associated morbidity and higher scores have been associated with poor outcome.

 OTHER RHEUMATIC DISEASE-SPECIFIC MEASURES

The nuances of many rheumatic diseases make outcomes evaluation with generalized instruments insufficient. Several disease-specific instruments have been developed and validated. Examples include the **Bath Ankylosing Spondylitis Activity Index**, the **Fibromyalgia Impact Questionnaire**, the **Modified Rodnan Skin Score** for systemic sclerosis, and the **Birmingham Vasculitis Activity Score**.

RADIOGRAPHIC INSTRUMENTS

Two standardized methods for quantifying joint damage have commonly been used in RA studies. Both are validated measures that examine hand and foot films, evaluate erosions and joint space narrowing, and require trained raters. A third system for use in OA assessment is also described.

I. **SHARP/VAN DER HEIDJE SCORE.** Erosions and joint space narrowing are assessed separately, although scores are usually expressed as the total of both. Scores range from 0 to 448.

II. **LARSEN/SCOTT METHOD.** Global damage within each joint is assessed on a scale of 0 to 5 by comparing patient films with a set of standardized radiographs. Scores are primarily influenced by erosions and range from 0 to 200 when both hands and feet are evaluated.

III. **KELLGREN AND LAWRENCE SCORING SYSTEM.** Severity of OA is assessed on a five-point scale by comparing patient films to a set of standardized radiographs. The original version was limited by the simplistic view of OA as a stepwise progressive disease, lack of the clear meaning of different grades, and significant floor and ceiling effects of scoring. Modifications have partially addressed these issues.

 OTHER OUTCOME MEASURES

Rheumatic disease studies often include measurement of associated conditions that are common to these diseases, but not specific.

I. **GENERAL HEALTH AND HEALTH-RELATED QUALITY OF LIFE INSTRUMENTS**
   A. These instruments are useful for comparison of health status between different or unrelated disease groups (e.g., RA vs. SLE and RA vs. coronary artery disease).
   B. The short form **(SF)-36** is a self-report instrument designed for use as a generic measure of overall health status in population surveys and for health care policy decision-making. The 36 items measure eight dimensions, which are grouped into physical and mental health components; scores can be expressed for the dimensions or the components. It is often used as a proxy for health-related quality of life.

II. **COMORBIDITY.** The **Charlson Comorbidity Questionnaire** is a reliable and valid instrument that records specific common medical conditions other than the disease of primary interest. Each condition is assigned a weight, which is summed so that the burden of all disease can be quantified. It was designed to be used for medical record review, but has been modified for administration by trained personnel.

III. **PAIN.** Visual analog scales are often used to quantify pain. Several other self-report instruments are also available for use in qualifying and quantifying pain. The **McGill Pain Scale** is among the most commonly employed. This valid and reliable instrument uses 78 different words to describe three dimensions of pain (sensory, affective, and evaluative), and provides overall scores of pain intensity or scores for individual domains.

IV. **DEPRESSION.** Physiologic and reactive depressive symptoms are common to many rheumatic diseases and are often measured as confounders of outcome in clinical studies.
   A. Among the many different validated self-report scales assessing depression are three, brief (20-item) self-administered instruments: the **Beck Depression Inventory,** the **Center for Epidemiological Studies-Depression (CES-D),** and the **Geriatric Depression Scale.** None are diagnostic of clinical depression.
   B. As depression is often manifested by somatic signs, such as decreased energy and increased fatigue, all these measures are limited in that many items query these particular symptoms which may be due to rheumatic disease and not the psychological state of the patient.

V. **FATIGUE.** Although very common and debilitating, fatigue is one of the most abstract and difficult rheumatic disease manifestations to operationalize. Many validated instruments have been used to assess fatigue in various rheumatic disease studies.
   A. **Fatigue severity index** (a modified version of the Fatigue Severity Scale) provides an overall assessment of general fatigue.

   B. Multidimensional fatigue inventory (MFI) and the multidimensional assessment of fatigue (MAF) measure various dimensions of fatigue independently including general fatigue, physical fatigue, reduced motivation, reduced activity, and mental fatigue.

   C. Piper fatigue scale describes the temporal, intensity, affective, and sensory domains of fatigue in 41 items using 10 cm VAS.

VI. Self-efficacy is the belief in one's ability to perform a task effectively. The **Arthritis Self-Efficacy Scale** is a 20-item, validated, self-report instrument with subscales for physical functioning, pain management, and ability to control symptoms of arthritis. A modified 8-item instrument has also been validated. The total score is the average of responses using a 10-point numerical rating scale.

VII. LEARNED HELPLESSNESS. The current version of the **Rheumatology Attitudes Index (RAI)** is a brief, 5-item, self-administered Likert scale response questionnaire. It was developed from a longer version of the RAI and the **Arthritis Helplessness Instrument.** It is a validated measure of learned helplessness, common to many chronic diseases, and has been incorporated into the MDHAQ.

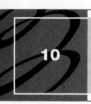

10 ETHICAL AND LEGAL CONSIDERATIONS
C. Ronald MacKenzie and Allan Gibofsky

 thics and the law are related because each field is concerned with norms of conduct. While ethics examines what behaviors might be considered desirable and articulates the ideals and virtues to which one should aspire, the law deals with standards of conduct and the consequences of failing to live up to them.

ETHICS

Ethics has been described as a "generic term for various ways of understanding and examining moral life." Drawing from the scholarship of multiple disciplines, the ethics of medical practice has, over the years, developed into a field that focuses on the problems and dilemmas that confront health care professionals and their patients and those that arise in the setting of caring for the sick. It is considered a "normative" discipline which sets out to answer such questions as "what ought to be done" in a given clinical circumstance. Although this describes the domain of "clinical ethics," the influence of ethics as a scholarly endeavor has come to play a much broader role in modern medicine. In addition to its more public form, familiar to health care professionals through such activities as hospital ethics committees, the field of ethics also plays an important role in defining professional norms and codes of conduct (professional ethics), helps define appropriate practices and standards for health care organizations (organizational ethics), and has an important role in providing an ethical and moral framework to guide the practice of clinical research (research ethics).

I. CLINICAL ETHICS (PATIENT AS THE FOCUS)

   A. The **practice of clinical ethics** deals with the common, everyday ethical challenges that arise in the practice of medicine. Developed and spurred on by the unrelenting pace of technologic advance over the last 40 years, it has largely been a "case-driven" field of inquiry, its moral foundations based on the concept of patient rights and guided by a broader set of principles or physician obligations that include:

1. **Beneficence.** To benefit patients in order to further their welfare and interests.
2. **Respect for autonomy.** To protect and defend the informed choices of capable patients.
3. **Nonmaleficence.** To prevent harm, or if risks of harm must be taken, to minimize those risks.
4. **Justice.** An obligation relevant to fairness of access to health care and its rationing.

B. On a more **individual** basis in clinical care, additional responsibilities are required of the physician and health care provider. These include such obligations as:

1. Respect for the patient's privacy and the preservation of confidentiality.
2. Open and honest communication concerning the patient's condition (diagnosis, treatment, and prognosis).
3. Ascertaining the patient's capacity for a shared decision-making process.
4. Insuring a valid process of informed consent.

   Failure of the clinician in any of these obligations constitutes a fundamental infringement of the patient's right to ethical health care delivery.

C. In the modern era of medicine, the medical ethicist and the Ethics Consultation Service are the **public face of medical ethics at large health care institutions,** specifically hospitals. The services provided by such individuals or entities are an important resource to all health care professionals as they provide a number of useful services including:

1. Providing specific case consultation.
2. Assisting in the development of institutional policies having to do with ethical issues arising in patient care.
3. Educating health care professionals, patients, and their families.
4. Participating in ethics-related research, which ultimately may inform practices of prevention for the future.

D. In practice, clinical ethics remains a case-based activity and those involved with medical ethics in a clinical environment draw on and apply a broadly founded base of bioethical theory to situations arising in the care of patients. Yet despite its theoretical and philosophical foundations, it nonetheless remains a very practical, problem-centered activity that draws widely on the expertise of those who work in the health care system. The composition of hospital ethics committees underscore this diversity, usually being composed of physicians and nurses, social workers, and psychologists, having legal representation, as well as the clergy, pastoral care, and the lay public. This sharing of authority is not only vital to the deliberative process but necessary for its perceived fairness.

II. **PROFESSIONAL ETHICS (PRACTITIONER AS THE FOCUS)**

A. Rather than the patient, the area of **professional ethics** is centered directly on the professional and the focus of this ethical domain is the maintenance of the integrity of the individual clinician within the profession at large. Rather than rights or principles, the bedrock foundation of professional ethics is generally articulated in its professional "codes" which are seen as the guiding beacons for the behavior of the practitioner. Such codes consist of advice and direction concerning the proper manner of responding to the problems that arise in clinical practice and they define certain fundamental character traits of the "professional" practitioner. Relevant examples of important professional codes of medicine include the Hippocratic Oath, as well as the Codes of Ethics of the American Medical Association, the American College of Rheumatology and the American Association of Orthopedic Surgeons, all of which are available on the websites of these organizations.

B. **Professionalism** in clinical care is based on the Hippocratic tradition and relates to the role of the physician as healer, fully focused on and committed to the patient. It implies a set of priorities and good conduct in a number of arenas:

1. **Competence** is based on good clinical skills, knowledge of the medical literature, and the capacity to apply it effectively in the correct clinical context.

2. **Engagement.** Includes the capacity to communicate effectively, and manage the clinical transaction in an empathetic collaborative fashion with the patient.
3. **Reliability.** Implies timely access to the physician and through him/her, the health care system.
4. **Dignity.** Refers to the interaction with and treatment of the patient in a respectful, dignified manner.
5. **Agency.** A concept that implies patient advocacy and a commitment to the patient's priorities.
6. **Focus on illness and disease.** An awareness of the distinction between disease, a biological event versus illness, a human experience characterized by symptoms, fears, and so on.
7. **Concern for quality.** The valid application of clinical procedures and clinical care.

C. Professional ethics concentrates on clinicians as **moral agents** whose primary obligation can be summed by the question: **What kind of person should I be to fulfill my professional obligation?** Professional ethics therefore perceives an ethical problem as a deviation from accepted professional norms.
D. Professionalism has also been discussed in the context of a given profession's **social contract** with society. This construct subsumes quality of care considerations, the problem of access to medical care, cost considerations, and the impact of health policy on the socially disadvantaged. Particularly relevant to the fields of rheumatology and orthopedics are the reports concerning race-based inequalities in joint replacement surgery and the differential survival rates amongst patients with systemic lupus erythematosus (SLE) based on socioeconomic class, education, and racial background. Further, the evolving interest in "early arthritis" and clinics devoted to early diagnosis and treatment of rheumatic disease coupled with the advent of highly effective but expensive, biologically based therapies raise concern about the access to such care for the more disadvantaged amongst us.

III. **ORGANIZATIONAL ETHICS (HEALTH CARE SYSTEM AS THE FOCUS)**
A. Health care organizations differ in important ways from patients as well as health care professionals. Recognition of this stimulated an entire field of ethical inquiry and has evolved to guide these large, corporate entities known as health care systems or organizations as they attempt to balance the often competing interests and priorities of the organization with those of its many stakeholders (employees, health care professionals, and patients). Groups such as the American Medical Association and the Joint Commission on Accreditation of Healthcare Organizations (JCAHO) have made important contributions to this area of ethical inquiry.
B. The development of standards that guide organizational decision making almost by definition will remain evolutionary, reacting to, and requiring modification as the health care system itself evolves. Certain principles or priorities have been suggested to guide the process and include:
1. **Priority of health care** establishes patient care to be central and superseding all other considerations such as profit.
2. **Priority of professional expertise** in decision making with respect to clinical matters (diagnosis, prognosis, and treatment).
3. **Priorities relating to** public health, unmet health care needs, advocacy for social reform in health care, acknowledging the relationship between the organization and its employees, acknowledging the necessity for organizational solvency and survival, and recognizing an organization's obligation to the community.

IV. **RESEARCH ETHICS (RESEARCH AS THE FOCUS)**
A. While producing great societal benefit, scientific research at the same time has raised many difficult questions. As a consequence of the abuses of human subjects participating in research experiments, professional organizations, and national agencies have been developed to monitor and oversee the conduct of scientific research. One important early National Commission (1979) articulated a set of guiding principles of research ethics in a document titled the *Ethical Principles and*

Guidelines for the Protection of Human Subjects Research commonly referred to as the *Belmont Report.* Since the publication of this report, these ethical principles have provided the foundation for subsequent federal guidelines. The basic principles outlined in the *Belmont Report* are as follows:

1. **Respect for persons.** This concept comprises two ethical convictions: that individuals are autonomous agents and should be treated as such, and that persons with diminished autonomy should receive increased protection. Federal regulation goes further and defines certain types of individuals as "vulnerable." These include those who are incarcerated (prisoners), children, individuals with impaired mental capacity, and pregnant women.

2. **Beneficence.** This category subsumes the concept of **"do no harm"** and that of maximizing benefits while reducing risks.

3. **Justice.** Implying fairness in distribution, specifically fairness in the selection of research subjects.

B. The application of these principles to the conduct of research requires additional responsibilities including:

1. Informed consent (discussed later).
2. Assessment of risk versus benefit.
3. Fair selection of subjects for participation in research.

C. Federal agencies (1991) adopted a "common rule" or set of regulations, which govern scientific research, and established three mechanisms of protection for research subjects, which include:

1. Review of research by a committee known as the **Institutional Review Board (IRB).**
2. Requirement for **informed consent** of the research subject.
3. Institutional assurance of compliance.

D. **Valid informed consent occurs only** when all of the following five elements occur:

1. **Disclosure** of relevant information that a reasonable person would need in order to make an informed decision.
2. **Competence** of the patient or surrogate receiving the information.
3. **Understanding** of the information by the patient or surrogate, in a language or utilizing those terms most appropriate for that individual (e.g., in their primary language and recognizing their educational level).
4. **Voluntary** evaluation of all factors by the patient or surrogate, free of influence or subtle coercion (e.g., "If you don't do what I recommend, I will be unable to be your physician after this point").
5. **Decision by the patient** or surrogate and not by the physician (e.g., "This is what I would do").

V. **CONFLICT OF INTEREST.** Conflict of interest considerations have become an important part of the landscape of modern clinical medicine and research. Such practices as the provision of industry-generated honoraria for the participation in sponsored symposia and speaking engagements, as well as the provision of gifts, honoraria, and the payment of other expenses to physicians have all come under close scrutiny.

A. In the **arena of clinical research,** the partnership between academic medicine and industry has been increasingly recognized as an ethically uneasy one, fraught with conflict for the clinical investigators and the institutions where they work. Conflicts of interest may arise as a consequence of a number of forces and present in various forms. Financial conflicts of interest are the most obvious but there are others including conflicts of commitment (to the performance of the investigation), the desire for professional success, advancement, and even fame, or simply conflict arising from such motivations as the satisfaction of one's altruism or curiosity.

B. **Disclosure** statements are now mandated in most academic medical centers, particularly in the research environment. Although disclosure is not a panacea for the problem, it is an important first step in the development of a set of guiding principles for dealing with this important challenge.

THE LAW

I. **INFORMED CONSENT.** Informed consent is the process whereby the physician provides information about the risks, benefits, and alternatives to recommended therapy or a procedure, as well as the risks and benefits of the alternatives (one of which is to have no therapy or procedure at all). It also has an important application in patient participation in clinical research. In each of these contexts, it is important to recognize that informed consent is a **process,** not simply a piece of paper. Although the paper is evidence that the process has occurred, it is not a substitute for it.

II. **AUTONOMY.** Sometimes in clinical medicine, ethics and the law may conflict, as for example, when a physician unwittingly violates a patient's right of autonomy in an effort to provide a therapeutic benefit. On the one hand, the physician is seeking to provide a "good" and certainly to "do no harm"; on the other hand, violation of the right of autonomy may result in criminal, administrative, and civil liability. A physician is required to obtain consent from a patient (or the patient's surrogate) for virtually **everything** he or she wishes to provide, even those therapies and/or procedures that may be beneficial to a clinical outcome or even life-saving. (There are specific exceptions for noninvasive activities, e.g., making the bed and taking vital signs.) Failure to obtain informed consent, no matter how pure the motivation, is viewed as an "unconsented touching," which the law defines as battery. Battery is not only a criminal act but also a violation of a state's code of professional conduct, subjecting the individual to administrative sanctions.

III. **DUTY.** A physician owes a duty of care to a patient. If this duty is breached (either by commission or omission), and the breach results in damage or injury to the patient, the physician may also be subject to civil liability under established principles of **tort law** (i.e., medical malpractice). If the elements of **duty, breach** of that duty, proof of **causation** and a justification for **damages** are proven, that patient may recover both economic loss (e.g., lost earnings and cost of subsequent treatment) and noneconomic loss (e.g., "pain and suffering").

IV. **HEALTH CARE DELIVERY.** Yet other problems, both ethical and legal, may arise for physicians in the context of the various cost-containment initiatives that have affected the delivery of health care recently. As a result, the diagnostic procedure or medication recommended by the physician must be "approved" for the patient's insurance provider to provide payment. The financial imperative to contain costs in health care sometimes conflicts with the physician's ethical responsibility to utilize his or her best judgment to recommend procedures or medications in the best interest of the patient. One trend is clear, however: If a physician complies without protest with the limitations imposed by a third-party payor and an adverse event occurs, the physician will not be able to "blame" the third-party payor or insurance carrier for what happened to the patient. Increasingly, courts are taking the position that insurance companies make payment decisions and physicians make medical decisions.

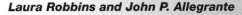

PATIENT EDUCATION

Laura Robbins and John P. Allegrante

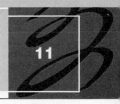

11

A t a time of groundbreaking medical advances in the diagnosis and treatment of arthritis and musculoskeletal diseases, patient education has become an essential component in providing comprehensive care and in achieving positive clinical outcomes. These advances, coupled with novel education delivery systems such as the Internet, have created consumer demand for information from patients, their families, and the general public. This is converging at a time when research and systematic evaluation have demonstrated that patient education can have an effect on pain, functional ability, and psychological status. Moreover, patient education for management of arthritis and related diseases includes not only providing information and knowledge, but also utilizing a variety of strategies to support healthy beliefs, behaviors, and skills to cope with the daily stresses and challenges that arthritis presents. This framework has led to the continued emphasis on demonstrating the efficacy of programs, the mechanism by which they work and for whom they will work, and the application of processes and programs that are designed to reach a broad base of patient populations.

 ## WHAT IS PATIENT EDUCATION?

Patient education has been defined as planned learning experiences designed to help individuals make voluntary adaptation of behaviors or beliefs conducive to health. The concept of "voluntary adaptation" is the key to successful patient education programs and relates to issues of motivation and compliance. There are three major components to effective education programs. First, education programs should have well-defined and measurable goals and learning objectives targeted toward specific groups of individuals with similar forms of arthritis. Second, they should be "user friendly," taking into account cultural beliefs and attitudes about the etiology and treatments of diseases and their impact on behavioral change. Third, patient education programs should be directed toward identifiable, achievable, and measurable outcomes. Patient education should be a process designed and tailored to help patients adopt, maintain, and prevent relapse of disease-relevant self-management behaviors. The key psychological construct underlying these components is fostering patient self-efficacy to help a person gain confidence in performing a particular disease-relevant self-management behavior and in overcoming barriers to the conduct of that behavior.

 ## WHAT MAKES PATIENT EDUCATION PROGRAMS SUCCESSFUL?

Patient education programs must have well-defined goals and objectives to be successful. Some authorities have emphasized that patient education goals are similar to those of traditional medical care: to improve function, relieve pain, enhance psychological well-being, maintain satisfactory social interaction and employment, and control disease activity. It has been demonstrated that the additional aims of patient education are to maintain or improve health and to slow down the deterioration. Most well-designed goals of patient education programs are provider-initiated and based on careful diagnostic assessment of the

TABLE 11-1 Goals of Patient Education Programs
• Understand disease and treatment(s) • Control or relieve pain and other symptoms • Enable psychosocial well-being • Control or alter disease activity and its consequences • Prevent or minimize disability • Decrease inappropriate use of health services • Increase use of appropriate health services and care systems • Increase/foster independence • Enhance functional health status • Enhance social functioning • Improve communication skills
From Robbins L. Patient Education. In: Klippel J, Weyand C, Wortman R, eds. *Primer on the Rheumatic Diseases*. 12th ed. Atlanta, GA: National Arthritis Foundation, 2001, with permission.

patient's educational needs. Other programs are designed based on mutual goals agreed upon by the patient and the health care provider. This design often utilizes assessment methods such as focus groups to understand what knowledge patients have about their disease, what their beliefs and attitudes are about their disease, what information and behavioral skills or supports they need to learn so as to feel empowered and be able to manage their arthritis or related illness. Table 11-1 summarizes the broad goals as they relate to effective patient education programs.

EDUCATION MODALITIES

A challenge to health educators is the fact that different individuals learn differently, making it difficult to develop educational programs meeting every individual's needs. It is a well-established principle of learning theory that people learn in different ways based on their education level, beliefs, and acquired patterns of behaviors. Moreover, language differences and literacy levels must be considered in designing effective patient education programs. In order to develop an effective patient education program, there must first be a thorough understanding of the patient population. Then, one must decide the optimal channels through which one can reach the patients. Rheumatology patient education programs are based upon a multitude of methods from formal, didactic education sessions led by a health professional, to information groups that are facilitated by patients who have a specific rheumatic disease. Table 11-2 summarizes the various patient education programs that are available.

In recent years, patient education programs have grown to keep pace with new technology. As more individuals use the Internet, the opportunities for patient education programs are becoming unlimited. Programs already exist that can be accessed by patients from their homes and have similar effects on health status as the more traditional face-to-face program formats. Maisiak's arthritis information telephone line also allows patients to access information via telephone (Maisiak et al. User evaluation of an arthritis information telephone service. *AC&R* 1989;2:75–79). Horton's Lupus Line, a peer-counseling telephone service, and its Spanish counterpart Charla de Lupus and the Asian version, Lantern, have been designed after assessing the patients' cultural as well as physical needs (Horton et al. Users evaluate LupusLine, a telephone peer-counseling service. *AC&R* 1997;10: 257–263). Building on interventions such as these, home-to-home education programs utilizing emerging technologies and tailored messages, are an untapped source for new programs targeted at specific patient populations.

TABLE 11-2	Education Program Modalities

- Hospital-based programs: presurgical, discharge planning, outpatient
- Community lectures, symposia
- Family education programs
- Peer education programs
- Social support programs
- Self-management programs
- Self-help groups
- Telephone-based programs
- Web-based, Internet programs

EDUCATION STRATEGIES

- Assess what the patient and his/her family members understand about the medical condition, diagnosis, and treatment options.
- Emphasize the importance of accurate information and questions.
- Encourage patients to take notes during the clinical visit and to write down or record instructions.
- Ask patients to repeat the information back to you so that you can clarify any misunderstanding.
- Repeat and reinforce the information at each office visit.
- Have patients set feasible short-term goals for behavior change that are challenging, yet manageable, and which can be reinforced with predetermined rewards.
- Encourage patients to use strategies, such as checklists and diaries, informing them that these are common ways to record and document their progress toward achieving their goals.
- Prepare written instructions and tip sheets for patients about medication and other complex aspects of a therapeutic regimen, in advance of the clinical visit; make these available in the clinic or office waiting areas.
- Call patients a day or two following an office visit to get a feedback, and to clarify and reinforce instructions.
- Ask the patients whether they would feel comfortable if a family or other significant member is included when presenting instructions to patients; have the family member take notes.
- Utilize a variety of audiovisual aids when teaching patients, including printed materials such as diagrams, tip sheets, pamphlets, newsletters, and videotape or DVD presentations, especially when explaining surgical procedures.
- Provide language translations, culturally relevant materials, and large-typesize versions of instructions to patients with special needs.
- Discuss with patients their expectations about the treatment and the significance they attach to alternative or competing treatment options.
- Assess each patient's level of self-efficacy when it comes to complying with medication or performing other prescribed disease-relevant self-management behaviors.

RESOURCES ON PATIENT EDUCATION

There is a plethora of resources available to individuals seeking information directly or through structured programs. Disease-specific organizations such as the Lupus Foundation, the Scleroderma Society, and the Fibromyalgia Association offer programs for patients and their families. Many of these organizations have national offices with regional or statewide local chapters. Hospitals and major academic centers also offer in-patient education programs, while some offer community-based education programs for a broader population of patients. The National Arthritis Action Plan has created collaborations with the Centers for Disease Control, resulting in statewide education programs for patients with arthritis.

The following are broad-based organizations that offer a variety of written or Web-based public and patient education programs, as well as education programs for health professionals on how to design and evaluate effective patient education programs.

A. Arthritis Foundation, www.arthritis.org.
B. American College of Rheumatology (ACR) and the Association of Rheumatology Health Professionals (a division of ACR composed of nurses, physical and occupational therapists, psychologists, social workers, and health educators), www.rheumatology.org.
C. American Academy of Orthopedic Surgeons, www.aaos.org.
D. National Institute for Arthritis and Musculoskeletal and Skin Diseases, www.niams.gov.
E. Centers for Disease Control and Prevention, www.cdc.gov/needphp.

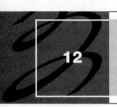

PSYCHOSOCIAL ASPECTS OF THE RHEUMATIC DISEASES
Sharon Danoff-Burg and Tracey A. Revenson

*T*his chapter addresses psychological and social issues that many patients face in the course of living with rheumatic diseases. Most patients are mentally healthy at the time their illness is diagnosed, but they may experience psychological distress throughout the course of their illness. At the same time, many patients report finding benefits in their illness, including an increased sense of spirituality and purpose of life, awareness of deepened interpersonal relationships, and an overall increased appreciation for life.

Living with rheumatic disease involves facing a number of psychosocial stresses and challenges. Depending on the type and severity of the illness, persons with rheumatic disease may need to cope on a daily basis with pain, stiffness, fatigue, and physical activity restrictions, as well as issues related to identity, body image, and even mortality. Many of these adaptive challenges require help from others. Therefore, patients with rheumatic disease need an available and satisfying network of interpersonal relations which they can count on, for both emotional sustenance and more practical help during periods of pain and disability.

Although, from a medical point of view, the rheumatic diseases may differ in regard to presentation and treatment, they have a number of psychosocial coping tasks in common. These include the following:

- Pain.
- Disability and loss of role functioning (as well as anxiety over anticipated losses).
- Increased risk for depression.
- Ongoing and often frustrating interactions with the health care system.
- The need to adhere to a prescribed and often changing treatment regimen.
- Changes in lifestyle and in appearance.
- Changes in interpersonal relationships.
- The need to tolerate uncertainty.
- In some, the possibility of death.

As symptoms, disease course, and prognosis are unpredictable and may change over time, the salience of these coping tasks changes as well. However, the need to tolerate uncertainty is an ever-present issue, one that can be both frustrating and frightening.

PSYCHOSOCIAL EFFECTS OF RHEUMATIC DISEASE

I. **DEPRESSION.** Most individuals with rheumatic disease do **not** experience clinical depression, although a significant minority do. At the same time, individuals with rheumatic disease are more likely to experience depression than are individuals without any serious chronic illnesses. If depression does occur, it can increase the pain and disability associated with rheumatic disease.

Patients with depression may feel unsupported by others. In some cases, this perceived lack of support reflects reality, as many individuals find it difficult to spend time with someone who is depressed.

Although depression is often linked to pain, the loss of the ability to perform valued roles and activities (because of pain, inflammation, fatigue, or disability) is a greater risk factor for developing depressive symptoms. Patients' interpretations of the **meaning of their limitations** and role changes may be more salient than their actual disease status.

Women with rheumatic disease are at greater risk for depression than are men. Within the US population, a clinical diagnosis of depression reveals a prevalence that is about twice as much among women than among men. Health practitioners need to be especially alert for depression in women so that both the depression **and** the rheumatic disease are treated.

If depression is overlooked, declines in functioning caused by depression can be attributed mistakenly to the rheumatic disease and result in overtreatment or unwarranted changes in the medical regimen. Complicating the clinical picture, some medications such as steroids may trigger or worsen depression.

It is important that health care professionals monitor their patients for depressive symptoms and, when necessary, ensure that they receive appropriate mental health treatment, rather than assume that depression is a "normal" and anticipated part of rheumatic disease.

II. **LIFESTYLE CHANGES.** Living with a rheumatic disease not only magnifies the stresses of everyday life but also creates additional ones. Most lifestyle changes are a direct or indirect result of frequent episodes of pain and disability. Most patients report a decrease in social, recreational, and leisure activities at one time or another. Some of these changes have great psychological significance for the patient, but may seem trivial to others. These include problems of engaging in activities that previously might have been taken for granted and as easily performable, such as household chores or getting around one's community easily. These "smaller" problems should not be dismissed offhand, as they accumulate over time and may lead to psychological distress.

A. **Changes in paid and unpaid work.** Rheumatoid arthritis (RA) has a profound effect on employment status, with many individuals unable to maintain their jobs as the disability worsens. This may exacerbate financial concerns. "Forced" retirement, medical leave, or the need to change careers in midlife because of physical limitations can increase psychological distress.

Rheumatic disease may interfere with the ability to perform valued activities at home, such as taking care of children. Particularly for women, loss of the caregiver role may lead to a decline in feelings of self-worth. Patients should be reassured that decreases in activity levels are normal, as is frustration with these changes. Patients should be encouraged to find new ways to perform tasks (perhaps with the aid of assistive devices), explore new leisure activities, and redefine roles at home and work.

B. **Changes in marital and intimate relationships.** Communication, day-to-day life, and sexual satisfaction seem to be the areas of intimate relationships that are most disrupted by rheumatic disease. The degree of disability is a major determinant of the extent to which relationships are affected. Partners may feel frustrated about a reduction in shared pleasurable activities, helpless in response to seeing their partner in pain, or fearful regarding the future of the relationship.

Contrary to common belief, positive effects of the illness on interpersonal relationships are as likely to be experienced as negative ones, although they are seldom reported to physicians. Commonly perceived benefits include an appreciation of support received from loved ones and increased empathy or compassion.

C. **Sexuality.** Persons with rheumatic diseases may be vulnerable to sexual problems because of illness symptoms, side effects of some medications, or emotional distress. However, studies comparing patients with rheumatic disease to healthy persons have found no differences in sexual satisfaction. Patients do report declines in sexual satisfaction with time, but this may be a consequence of aging as much as of pain. Sexual dissatisfaction is greater for those with more severe disease or greater functional disability. In one study, some spouses reported not having sex for fear that they would hurt their partners. However, another study found that some women perceived that their illness resulted in positive effects on their sexuality.

Although avoidance of sex because of embarrassment about joint deformities or steroid-induced changes in appearance has been emphasized in the clinical literature, another reason for reduced interest in sex may be exhaustion or anger created by role changes or added household demands resulting from the illness. This can be addressed by fostering communication between partners.

D. **Social life.** Relations with friends are at greater risk of being lost than those with the family. Reduced mobility and increased pain make social relations outside the home difficult to maintain; more than half of the patients with RA report that they visit other people less often because of their disease. In some cases, social isolation may arise because the patient seeks to avoid the stigma and embarrassment associated with the condition.

Changes in the quantity and quality of close relationships are common. In the years following diagnosis or with initiation of a new treatment, family and friends may be quite helpful. With the passage of time, however, friends and family may tire of providing help, and patients may interpret this as withdrawal from them or as criticism of how they are coping with the disease. This may occur at a time when patients are becoming less able to care for themselves and actually need more help.

E. **Effect on family members.** Spouses or live-in partners play a dual and sometimes conflicting role: They serve as the primary provider of support to the patient but, at the same time, they experience stress because of the illness. Partners often experience anxiety, communication difficulties, and problems at work, but they typically do not manifest clinical levels of psychopathology. Spouses report the greatest illness intrusion in the areas of social and leisure activities, family activities, and sex.

Frequent episodes of pain, increasing disability, an unpredictable course of the illness, and financial pressures brought on by the illness may add up to affect the partner's ability to be supportive over the long haul. The societal pressures embodied in marriage vows ("In sickness and in health 'till death do us part") may create feelings of resentment, anger, and guilt. If the patient is depressed, it can be difficult to empathize or help. With advancing age, many spouses have health problems themselves, which can make tending to the patient's physical and emotional needs more difficult.

Having a child with juvenile idiopathic arthritis (JIA) creates many new stressors and coping tasks, similar to those experienced by adults but handled differently in terms of the child's cognitive abilities and life context (e.g., school, team sports, and dating). Nonadherence to treatment can create family conflict, and healthy siblings may vie for attention. Many families, however, report being pulled closer together in coping with the illness.

III. **FACTORS PROMOTING PSYCHOLOGICAL ADAPTATION TO RHEUMATIC DISEASE**

A. **A sense of personal control over the illness.** The extent to which patients maintain a **sense of control** over their illness appears to have a significant impact on their adjustment. Perception of personal control over treatment is related to a positive mood, and perceived control over pain is related to reports of less pain. Similarly, perceived **helplessness** has been linked with pain, disability, and early mortality in patients with RA.

B. Coping. Coping efforts can be directed toward dealing with the stressful situation itself, managing psychological distress aroused by the situation, or maintaining interpersonal relationships. Most stressful situations evoke all three modes of coping. At the time of diagnosis, patients may need to minimize the seriousness of their situation, lest they be overwhelmed by emotions and are not able to act. Over a period, the patient is able to acknowledge emotions and deal with the situation more actively, such as by seeking the relevant information before accepting a treatment decision. However, some patients may try to "normalize" or pass as healthy, by performing activities that are not advisable.

The effectiveness of coping depends on many factors (see the subsequent text), and coping efforts should not be judged *a priori* as adaptive or maladaptive.

C. Effectiveness of coping. The coping strategies of actively seeking information about the illness, seeking support from others, and trying to view one's situation in a more positive light have been associated with better psychological functioning. Coping strategies that involve wishful thinking, fantasizing, self-blame, avoidance, and denial are associated with poorer psychological functioning. However, reports of emotion-focused coping strategies such as self-blame may reflect levels of psychological distress rather than actual coping efforts.

How effective a particular coping strategy is depends on many factors, including aspects of the patient's life context (e.g., age, interpersonal relationships, and financial stressors) as well as the medical condition. The degree of personal control that patients believe they have over their illness and treatment, and whether they believe their coping efforts will be effective, have been shown to influence psychological outcomes.

A particular coping strategy might result in positive well-being in some situations and psychological distress in another situation. For example, strategies to reduce tension, such as drinking or sleeping may make patients feel better temporarily but diminish their overall physical health status.

A person's coping efforts may not be effective if they conflict with the coping styles of family members. For example, expressing anger to a spouse may reduce a patient's tension but increase the spouse's tension, which may in turn lead to reduced support. Patients may also feel depressed if family members criticize their coping efforts.

Families of children with JIA that cope in a unified fashion and keep channels of communication open fare better than do families in which the coping styles of individual members conflict. However, dissimilar coping styles between spouses do not automatically result in psychological distress, as sometimes they may be complementary.

D. Social support. Social support refers to interpersonal exchanges that provide information, emotional reassurance, material assistance, and a sense of continued self-esteem. Family, friends, and health professionals are all important sources of support.

Patients who receive support from friends and family exhibit greater self-esteem, psychological adjustment, and life satisfaction; cope more effectively; and are less depressed. Family support can serve as an adjunct to professional treatment. Support from family members has been shown to enhance the effects of psychological treatment and help patients maintain the initial treatment gains.

Social support provides coping assistance. It provides feedback and new information, helps patients achieve a new understanding of their problems, increases their motivation to take positive action, and reduces emotional stress. It reinforces the performance of adaptive health behaviors and treatment recommendations, which lead to greater overall health and control of disease.

Social support can have a positive or negative effect. Even well-intentioned support from close friends and family may backfire if patients do not want the help or comfort that is offered.

Common types of unhelpful support are making light of the severity of an illness or the patient's pain; making pessimistic comments about the patient's ability level or health status; criticizing the patient's coping efforts; pitying the patient; and offering help when it is not wanted. For example, some patients resent offers of help because such offers interfere with their self-image as a healthy person and usurp valued social roles.

For patients to benefit from social support, the type of support offered must fit in with what the patient needs at that time. Unwanted or unhelpful support leads to negative affective states, diminished self-esteem, loss of autonomy, and decreased psychological well-being. New tensions within a relationship may emerge. Patients who receive little positive support but receive a lot of unhelpful support from their friends and family are at a greater risk for depression.

Social support can also be helpful for the patients' family members. Spouses of patients, who receive support outside the marital relationship, are able to be more supportive to their partner with rheumatic disease. Support may alleviate some of the family burden of providing care and also provide a safe outlet for expressing negative feelings.

E. Adherence to treatment. Treatment efficacy depends on the patient's understanding and effort toward carrying out therapeutic recommendations. Adherence to the appropriate use of prescribed medication ranges from 30% to 78% for patients with rheumatic disease. Rates of nonadherence to exercise regimens are equivalent to or are higher than those of oral medication. Both patients and physicians overestimate adherence, possibly because direct and specific questions regarding adherence are rarely asked during a medical visit.

Risk factors for nonadherence are numerous. Some are lodged within the person and others relate to the treatment or the patient–provider relationship. Patient characteristics may include age, social class, beliefs about treatment efficacy, and cultural concepts about disease. Characteristics of the treatment regimen that influence adherence include duration, complexity, number of changes, and side effects.

Characteristics derived from the patient's social context include support or criticism from friends and family, and encouragement and interest from persons in the health care setting. Because physicians have more kinds of power than do allied health professionals, patients are more likely to listen to physicians. Patient–physician communication may be the single most important variable affecting adherence and satisfaction with medical care. Poor patient–physician communication is a result of the time constraints at most medical visits, impersonal health care environments, and inequity in power and status residing with the patient–physician encounter.

Perceptions of a physician's caring, warmth, sensitivity, concern, friendliness, interest, and respect also affect adherence to treatment regimens. Satisfaction with care increases when the physician addresses the patient's concerns before the end of the visit. Unfortunately, some physicians do not elicit or discuss psychosocial concerns because they believe such concerns to be irrelevant, time-consuming, or outside their field of expertise.

F. Increasing adherence

   1. Treatment partnership. Make patients partners in their treatment. Talk about models of disease progression and treatment goals so that patients can share those goals. It is important for patients and physicians to share the same "cognitive models" of the disease and its treatment.

   2. Describe the treatment rationale. Help the patient understand why treatment is necessary, and what the short- and long-term goals of treatment are (e.g., functional improvement, decreased pain, and decreased inflammation). The expected time course for improvement should be made explicit.

   3. Set achievable goals. Set short-term goals that can be accomplished by the next visit.

   4. Explain and clarify. Present information clearly. Create a situation in which patients feel comfortable asking for clarification if they do not understand something. Identify and dispel any false beliefs about treatment (e.g., that medication loses its efficacy over time, that medication should be used only when symptoms are present or when pain is unbearable).

5. **Describe possible adverse effects.** Warn patients of any of the anticipated side effects and provide methods to minimize them.

6. **Simplify treatment regimens.** This can be done by adopting regimens, such as prescribing, if appropriate, daily medication in one dose instead of by multiple administration, or by recommending exercises that can fit into the patient's daily schedule. This is likely to enhance self-efficacy beliefs and promote treatment adherence.

   Identify potential and real difficulties with adherence. Before the end of the visit, make a plan, incorporating the patient's input, to overcome any difficulties by the next visit.

   Provide written treatment information. As the physician's handwriting is often illegible, have handouts prepared in advance to cover the most common situations. The Arthritis Foundation also can provide material.

7. **Respect the patient.** Respect the patients' use of holistic remedies as long as they do not interfere with the treatment. They may help and, at a minimum, may increase a patient's sense of control and well-being. Never threaten a patient. Statements such as, "You're killing yourself by not taking your medications," may jeopardize the patient's satisfaction with medical care and trust in the physician.

8. **Medication reviews.** Patients should be asked periodically to review their medication dosage and schedule with the physician, even in the absence of changes. Such reviews may uncover unintentional nonadherence resulting from simple misunderstanding. This and other behavioral technologies, such as putting tracking caps on pill bottles, may increase adherence by reinforcing its importance. Make clear that the purpose of such monitoring is to help patients with difficulties in adhering to a medication schedule, not to punish or humiliate them.

   Forgetful persons should be taught to leave themselves notes in prominent places or elicit the aid of a family member. Pill containers that separate administrations by day and time and programmable watches with beepers have been used successfully as reminders. If manual dexterity is severely limited, be sure that patients obtain medication bottles with easy-open caps.

9. **Family participation.** Depending on family members to remind patients to take medication or do exercises does not work consistently. In some instances, it can be of extreme help whereas in others it creates feelings of social control being imposed. This issue often arises in early adolescence for patients with JIA, when parents are transferring responsibility for taking medications to the patient or during a session of passive exercises for their child.

10. **Appreciate costs.** Be attentive to patients' concerns about out-of-pocket expenses. Explain the short- and long-term benefits of each medication. Suggest that the patient calculate the cost per day. Prescribe a generic drug, if possible, or contact the patient's insurance company if necessary. Many pharmaceutical companies have programs to make medications available to patients who need but cannot afford them.

11. **Fit treatment into the patient's life.** For increasing adherence to exercise regimens, ask the physical therapist if the exercises can be made more congruent with the patient's daily schedule or with other physical activities.

IV. **INFLUENCE OF GENDER.** Gender is an important factor when psychosocial aspects of rheumatic disease are considered, because many patients are women. Gender differences have been discussed in several places within this chapter. Although few studies have examined psychological differences between male and female patients in terms of their adjustment to rheumatic disease, it is important to acknowledge that there are areas in which gender differences are **not** apparent and also to note those areas where evidence of important gender differences does exist.

A. Reporting symptoms. When men and women are compared, women report more symptoms than men do. However, when differences between men and women regarding disease severity (e.g., joint appearance) and sociodemographic characteristics (e.g., age and income) are taken into account, women report fewer symptoms than do men. Women do not overreport symptoms and, in fact, report RA symptoms more conservatively than men do, given comparable disease severity.

B. Impact on work. Rheumatic disease may have an even more severe effect on employment for women than for men. The economic impact of women's work disability is probably underestimated because their nurturant, teaching, and housekeeping work in the paid labor market is economically undervalued. Furthermore, the economic value of work that women do at home without pay is undervalued even more. Women with RA, who have more homemaker responsibilities, are less likely to be disabled than women with fewer responsibilities (even after disease severity and functional status are equalized statistically). In fact, having more homemaker responsibilities may enhance a sense of self-worth and social functioning.

C. Effects on treatment. Some recent research suggests that gender may affect the nature and quality of treatment across a variety of medical conditions. However, there is currently little information on whether specific procedures, drugs, or treatment strategies differ for female and male patients with rheumatic disorders.

Any disparity may result from a number of factors. Physicians may base treatment outcomes on differential expectations of treatment success for men and women or may have stereotyped expectations about male and female patients. For example, female patients with fibromyalgia often report first that they were told at first that their symptoms were imagined or psychological in origin. One study found that women undergo major orthopedic surgery at a more advanced stage in their disease and that this gender difference could not be explained by other medical variables such as disease severity. A possible explanation is that women wait longer for surgery because of their caregiving responsibilities toward their families.

V. PSYCHOLOGICAL INTERVENTIONS. In addition to biomedical treatment, participation in psychological interventions can contribute to decreases in physical symptoms and improvement in quality of life. A wide variety of psychological and educational interventions for individuals with rheumatic disease have been developed. The overall aim of these interventions is to minimize the impact of rheumatic disease on patients' physical, psychological, and social functioning.

Most psychological interventions are multimodal and typically include one or more of the following components: provision of general information about rheumatic disease; instruction in self-management and coping skills; sharing of concerns; cognitive restructuring; behavioral techniques, such as goal setting; relaxation training; and hypnosis or biofeedback to facilitate pain control. Families occasionally participate in psychological interventions, which may augment the benefits of individual treatment.

A. Cognitive-behavioral therapy (CBT) is a type of psychological intervention in which patients work with a psychotherapist to learn specific skills, such as relaxation techniques, coping skills, goal setting, and activity pacing. CBT can occur within group or individual settings. Randomized, controlled studies of individuals with rheumatic disease who participated in CBT interventions have found positive effects (e.g., decreased pain, fatigue, and disability, and fewer depressive symptoms) at the end of treatment, which sometimes are sustained through subsequent follow-up assessments. More work is needed on how to integrate relapse prevention strategies into treatment so that long-term gains can be achieved.

B. The Arthritis Self-Help Course (ASHC), offered through local chapters of the Arthritis Foundation, is a structured group education program led by trained lay persons with arthritis or fibromyalgia. Reported benefits of the program include increased knowledge and self-care behaviors and decreased pain, depressive symptoms, and medical visits. The ASHC teaches basic self-management skills, such as development of individualized exercise regimens and pain management strategies.

Recent revisions of the ASHC emphasize the enhancement of patients' self-efficacy to manage their arthritis or fibromyalgia.

Mutual help or support group discussions provide avenues for discussing problems and arriving at coping solutions. They also reassure members that they are not alone. Individuals who are coping well with their illness may serve as strong role models. Such interventions also may build patients' social skills, such as assertiveness.

VI. PRACTICE GUIDELINES

   A. Increasing the psychological well-being of your patients

   1. Be on the lookout for symptoms of depression, so that effective mental health treatment can be provided immediately.

   2. Serve as a source of information concerning mental health before patients ask. Have information available about community resources, psychological counseling services within the hospital, and support groups or patient education programs available through the local chapter of the Arthritis Foundation. Patients may also be directed to reputable websites with current information. This resource sharing is best presented early in the illness. A brief list of resources can be found at the end of this chapter. It may be advantageous to have a printed list to hand to patients.

   3. Offer emotional support. Physicians can offer emotional support during medical visits with little effort, by asking patients about the stresses in their lives and simply listening. This not only increases patient satisfaction but also provides clues as to the onset of depression in the patient.

   4. Actively involve family members in the patient's care. On the most basic level, patients with stronger support systems are more adherent to treatment. Involve family members in treatment from the beginning, not merely during a medical crisis. Family members need to understand the nature and severity of the patient's illness and details regarding treatment if they are to be helpful. For example, giving information to family members about such things as what to expect when flares occur or the potential side effects of medication may minimize problems.

   Encourage family members to join in discussions during medical visits. Encourage family members to reinforce patients' coping efforts and to learn to offer help that does not undermine patients' self-esteem. Strengthen communication skills among family members. Many of the unintended negative consequences of helping result from faulty communication or misinterpretation of the patient's need for support. Ask about how the illness affects intimate relationships or daily family life.

   Encourage patients and family members to build support networks outside the family. Emphasize to patients and family members the benefits of having additional individuals available to provide help and emotional support. Suggest that they start with individuals in existing networks, such as groups involved in neighborhood activities, local churches or synagogues, and the workplace. Encourage families to join support groups or use telephone help lines.

   Social networks must be built up and strengthened in the early stages of the illness so that they are available during crises. This advice may be especially important for men, for whom their spouse is often the primary or sole source of support. Men tend to have fewer close ties and are less likely to seek support from them. Encourage male patients and male spouses to attend support groups and "open up," although it might be difficult. Alternatively, individuals who are unwilling to share personal information with others might benefit from writing privately about their deepest thoughts and feelings; in some studies this technique has been shown to improve the health status of patients with rheumatic disease.

   In supporting your patient, it is worthwhile to attend to family members' difficulties. Only about one-third of patients and partners seek any kind of help from mental health professionals or participate in support groups. Although the practitioner may feel responsible only for the patient's physical health, the psychological well-being of family members may directly or indirectly affect the patient's response to treatment.

B. Improving communication with patients and their families. The manner in which physicians inform patients about their illness plays an important role in how patients form beliefs about the implications of their illness, their views of treatment, and their impressions of health care professionals. It has been linked in numerous studies to patients' satisfaction with their physician and treatment and their adherence to prescribed treatment.

1. **Assess the disease knowledge of patients with newly diagnosed rheumatic disease.** Dispel any false beliefs, such as that the patient "brought on" the disease or that there is no treatment.

2. **Ensure understanding of treatment.** Ensure that the patient understands the basic details of treatment by giving instructions that are explicit, clear, and unambiguous. This may not be as obvious as it sounds, as it has been documented that many patients do not even know the names of their medications.

3. **Optimize communication of information.** Try not to give too much or too little information. Individuals can remember only 7 ± 2 bits of information at a time, and this number is probably reduced by the anxiety of being in a physician's office.

4. **Emphasize basic issues.** Go over basic issues slowly and clearly and provide any information necessary for making decisions about treatments. Do not be evasive, but do not overwhelm the patient with information either.

5. **Avoid jargon.** Work hard not to use medical jargon without defining terms.

6. **Assess feedback** by asking patients at the end of the visit to paraphrase the instructions that they have been given.

7. **Repeat and utilize information.** Summarize the most important information again at the end of the visit. Provide a written handout from your office and consider supplementing it with pamphlets from the Arthritis Foundation.

8. **Encourage questions.** Encourage patients to write down their questions before arriving for their appointments; by doing this, they will not have to worry about remembering everything during the visit.

C. Increasing satisfaction with care

1. **Optimize the physician–patient relationship.** Enough cannot be said about the importance of a good physician–patient relationship. What makes for a good relationship varies from patient to patient. Clearly, trust, communication, and empathy are essential. A patient's preference for casual versus formal styles of interaction may be influenced by the patient's age, ethnicity, and gender.

2. **Determine the patient's decision-making style.** Some patients find it important to be involved in a major way in any decision-making process; others want little or no part in it. It may take several visits to peg the patient's style. This may vary with age, ethnicity, and socioeconomic background and may change with time.

3. **Minimize waiting time and listen to the patient's responses to questions.** Minimize waiting time for medical visits. Length of perceived waiting time is inversely correlated with satisfaction and treatment adherence. Some physicians have receptionists call patients several hours in advance, if they are running extremely late, offering the opportunity to make a new appointment within the week.

   Always treat a patient, as you would wish you or your family members to be treated. Apologize for long delays, and do not rush the visit to make up time. Both satisfaction with care and adherence to treatment increase if patients **feel** that they have been given adequate time with the physician; perceived time spent with the physician does not always correlate with real time.

Asking patients if there are any issues of importance that were not covered or whether they have questions, yields considerable benefits. Address all the psychosocial concerns a patient voices, even ones that may seem to be of little importance.

VII. RESOURCES
A. For the health care professional
Arthritis Care and Research. This bimonthly, peer-reviewed journal of the Association of Rheumatology Health Professionals presents the best research on non-medical aspects of arthritis and musculoskeletal disease. It is published by the American College of Rheumatology.

DeVellis BM, Revenson TA, Blalock S. Rheumatic disease and women's health. In: Gallant SJ, Keita GP, Royak-Schaler R, eds. *Health care for women: psychological, social, and behavioral influences*. Washington, DC: American Psychological Association, 1997:333–347.

Keefe FJ, Smith SJ, Buffington ALH, et al. Recent advances and future directions in the biopsychosocial assessment and treatment of arthritis. *J Consult Clin Psych* 2002;70:640–655.

Newman S, Fitzpatrick R, Revenson TA, et al. *Understanding rheumatoid arthritis*. London: Routledge, 1996.

Seawell AH, Danoff-Burg S. Psychosocial research on systemic lupus erythematosus. a literature review. *Lupus* 2004;13:891–899.

B. For the patient
Arthritis Today. This health magazine, written for individuals with rheumatic disease and those who care for them, features articles on many of the issues discussed in this chapter. It is published bimonthly by the Arthritis Foundation.

Arthritis Self-Help Course (ASHC) is offered through local chapters of the Arthritis Foundation. Support groups are also offered through local chapters of the Lupus Foundation of America.

Lorig K, Fries JF, Gecht MR. *The arthritis helpbook: a tested self-management program for coping with arthritis and fibromyalgia*. 5th ed. New York: HarperCollins, 2000.

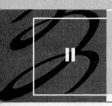

The Stat Rheumatology and Orthopedic Consultation: Your Guide to Acute Care

II

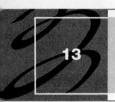

ACUTE MANAGEMENT OF MUSCULOSKELETAL AND AUTOIMMUNE DISEASES

13

Arthur M. F. Yee and Edward Su

 his chapter is meant to be your curbside consultation with a rheumatologist. Once you have rapidly narrowed down the diagnostic possibilities, you can go to the chapters that focus specifically on that problem, to be guided further in your diagnostic and therapeutic options.

THE PAINFUL, SWOLLEN JOINT (NONTRAUMATIC)

The acute onset of a painful joint with an effusion, in the absence of trauma, indicates the presence of an inflammatory or infectious intra-articular pathology. It is important to elicit the cause of the effusion in order to treat it effectively. Some joints that may commonly have effusions are the knee, hip, elbow, ankle, wrist, and shoulder.

The presence of fever elevates the problem to a possible infectious arthritis and emergency status.

I. DIFFERENTIAL DIAGNOSIS
   A. Nongonococcal septic arthritis.
   B. Gonococcal septic arthritis.
   C. Crystalline-related arthritis (gout, pseudogout).
   D. Inflammatory synovitis [rheumatoid arthritis (RA), systemic lupus erythematosus (SLE), psoriatic arthritis, reactive arthritis (ReA), colitic arthritis].
   E. Hemarthrosis due to hemophilia or anticoagulation.
   F. Osteoarthritis.

II. KEY DIAGNOSTIC QUESTIONS
   A. Does the patient have any systemic signs or symptoms suggestive of infection? Fevers, chills, or night sweats may indicate a septic arthritis with bacteremia. Possible risk factors for infection should be investigated, such as skin lesions, immunosuppressive therapy, comorbid disease such as diabetes, prior joint damage, and iatrogenic sources such as cortisone injections or surgery.

B. **Does the patient have a history of gout or pseudogout [calcium pyrophosphate disease (CPPD)]?** Although gouty flares typically localize to the great toe, crystalline deposition in the larger articular joints may lead to acute, symptomatic effusions. A history of podagra may suggest an inflammatory effusion due to crystalline arthropathy.

C. **Does the patient have a recent history of overuse of the joint?** Although the patient may not recall a traumatic incident, joints with underlying arthritis may develop an effusion after minimal overuse. For example, a previously asymptomatic arthritic knee may develop an effusion overnight after a tennis match.

D. **Does the patient have any signs or symptoms of a gonococcal infection; is the patient in the at-risk population?** A history of dysuria or urethral discharge may suggest a gonorrheal infection; patients younger than 30 are at greatest risk.

E. **Is there a history of inflammatory arthritis?** RA, SLE, and spondyloarthropathies may periodically flare and cause joint effusions.

F. **Is there a history of hemophilic arthropathy?** Typically, there is a target joint that may experience bleeding despite periodic infusion of clotting factors. Patients on anticoagulants are at risk of bleeding with less than severe trauma.

III. **PHYSICAL EXAMINATION**

A. Some joints are more accessible to palpation than others; the knee and elbow lend themselves to direct palpation of an effusion, whereas the hip does not. An assessment of the amount of fluid can be performed by milking (i.e., pushing or shifting) the fluid from one area of the joint to another. Joint effusions are subjectively graded as 1+ (small), 2+ (moderate), and 3+ (large). A septic arthritis will usually have a large, 3+ effusion.

B. Inspection and palpation of the joint may reveal warmth and tenderness. A palpable warmth in the joint indicates either an inflammatory or septic arthritis; a degenerative joint with a reactive effusion will not be noticeably warmer than the surrounding skin. Generally, a septic joint will be diffusely tender to palpation, whereas a reactive effusion due to osteoarthritis will not. Hemarthrosis can be warm due to the pyrogenic effect of the blood.

C. The joint is typically held in such a way as to maximize volume. The knee and hip are held in slight flexion so as to decrease painful capsular stretch. Weight-bearing joints may have pain with ambulation. Intra-articular pain is present with both active and passive range of motion. The range of motion may be limited due to the effusion. A degenerative joint with effusion will have the sensation of limitation at the extremes of motion whereas a patient with a septic effusion may guard against examination, holding the joint rigidly to avoid motion.

IV. **INVESTIGATIONS**

A. **White blood cell (WBC) with differential.** A septic arthritis with transient bacteremia may lead to an elevation of the WBC with a left shift. It must be emphasized that a normal WBC does not rule out the possibility of septic arthritis.

B. **Erythrocyte sedimentation rate (ESR) and C-reactive protein (CRP).** These nonspecific acute phase reactants will be elevated in inflammatory and septic arthritis. An ESR greater than 25 mm suggests an inflammatory etiology. The higher the ESR and CRP, especially when associated with fever, the greater the likelihood of infection.

C. Radiologic studies may demonstrate asymmetric narrowing of the articular surfaces in degenerative disease or symmetric narrowing in inflammatory arthritis. Chondrocalcinosis, or deposition of calcium in the articular cartilage or fibrocartilage, is strongly suggestive of CPPD. However, 20% of elderly patients have such deposits and never have an episode of joint inflammation.

D. **Joint aspiration** (see Chapter 8). This is the most important of all the laboratory investigations. A joint aspirate should be analyzed for its gross and microscopic appearance, and for microbiologic evaluation. The gross appearance of a reactive, noninflammatory effusion is typically of clear, yellowish, synovial fluid. An inflammatory effusion may be turbid, owing to the relative increase in cellularity. A septic arthritis will range from turbid to grossly purulent.

E. A cell count with differential of the aspirated fluid should be obtained. A WBC greater than 1,000/mm^3 is suggestive of an inflammatory effusion; if WBC is greater than 50,000/mm^3, presence of a septic arthritis is of prime concern. Additionally, the differential will reveal a relative neutrophilia, with polymorphonuclear neutrophils (PMNs) greater than 80% of the cells. Microscopic analysis should focus upon the identification of bacteria on Gram staining; also, for the presence of crystals within the PMNs. A diagnosis of gout is made by the presence of negatively birefringent, needle-shaped crystals; CPPD is confirmed by visualizing positively birefringent, rhomboid-shaped crystals in PMNs.

F. It must be kept in mind that infectious arthritis can "strip" gout and/or pseudo-gout crystals off the wall of a joint. So, the finding of crystals does not provide assurance that an infection does not exist. The higher the fever and the peripheral white count, the greater is the concern about infection.

G. Microbiologic analysis should also be done when there is a suspected infectious etiology. A sample of fluid for aerobic and anaerobic cultures may reveal bacterial growth in 48 to 72 hours if septic arthritis is present. Although white cell counts generally can be a guide to the likely diagnosis, infectious arthritis can **only** be defined by Gram stain and culture.

V. **TREATMENT**

A. Once infection has been ruled out, one can choose from among the many therapeutic options, guided by the cause and comorbidities.

B. An inflammatory effusion may respond to a short course of oral anti-inflammatory medication. The patient should also avoid inciting further synovitis, by resting the joint. A gently compressive ace bandage may help prevent reaccumulation of the effusion. If the synovitis is severe or recurrent, intra-articular steroid injections can be quite helpful.

C. If uric acid crystals are identified within the synovial fluid, then gout is the presumptive diagnosis. Patients may be treated with indomethacin or alternative anti-inflammatory medication. Institution of allopurinol may help prevent future recurrences, but should never be started in the presence of active joint inflammation and without colchicine coverage.

D. A clear, reactive effusion in the presence of pre-existing degenerative joint disease may be managed by drainage of the fluid. Patients will usually get symptomatic relief with the initial aspiration of fluid. A gently compressive bandage and avoidance of additional overuse will help prevent recurrence. Intra-articular steroid injections can be quite helpful.

E. A septic arthritis, supported by a "septic clinical picture" or a WBC greater than 50,000/mm^3 in the synovial fluid and a definitive diagnosis by a positive Gram stain and positive microbiologic cultures, requires emergency attention. Time is of the essence because articular cartilage is immediately at risk of permanent damage (see Chapter 46).

F. The main thrust of treatment, along with optimal antibiotic coverage, is joint drainage. Studies have shown that, in most situations, similar results are obtained from both surgery and daily or twice daily closed needle drainage. However, in the face of persistently positive synovial fluid cultures despite the use of specific antibiotics, lack of clinical improvement, hip infections, or the presence of an aggressive organism such as *Staphylococcus aureus* or gram-negative rods, orthopedic consultation is appropriate and arthroscopic surgery is indicated and quite effective in improving the short- and long-term outcome.

G. If the patient is medically stable for surgery, and the above poor prognostic signs exist, a surgical consultation should be obtained from an orthopedic surgeon. Irrigation and debridement of the joint should be performed expeditiously to prevent the destruction of articular cartilage and the onset of osteomyelitis. The irrigation and debridement of the joint may be performed arthroscopically or open, along with continued administration of intravenous antibiotics.

H. A joint effusion caused by gonococcal infection will typically respond to appropriate antimicrobial medication and will not require surgical intervention. Daily aspirations of the joint effusion can help symptomatically by removing inflammatory mediators.

THE PAINFUL, SWOLLEN JOINT (TRAUMATIC)

Trauma to a joint, such as twisting injuries, forced motion, and direct impact, can lead to intra-articular swelling. Although many of these injuries will need imaging studies to diagnose the pathology, the initial management should be focused upon preventing further damage to the joint. Here we will focus mostly on the knee, hip, and shoulder, which are the most commonly traumatized joints. However, what is said here will likely apply to other joints as well.

I. DIFFERENTIAL DIAGNOSIS

    A. Fractures (e.g., tibial plateau fractures and tibial eminence avulsions).

    B. Ligamentous rupture (e.g., anterior cruciate ligament or posterior cruciate ligament tears of the knee).

    C. Ligamentous sprain (e.g., medial collateral or lateral collateral ligament sprain).

    D. Fibrocartilage tear (e.g., labral tear of the hip or shoulder; meniscal tears of the knee).

    E. Articular contusion.

II. KEY DIAGNOSTIC QUESTIONS

    A. How did the injury occur? A detailed description of the injury mechanism can give clues to the diagnosis. For example, a blow to the side of the knee suggests an injury to the medial collateral ligament, and possibly an anterior cruciate ligament tear. Hyperflexion of the hip can cause a labral tear.

    B. Did the patient hear or feel a crack or a pop at the time of injury? Often complete ligamentous ruptures are associated with a distinct sensation of a "pop."

    C. Was the patient able to bear weight after the injury? The inability to comfortably bear weight suggests the possibility of a fracture in the hip or tibial plateau.

    D. Does the patient feel any clicking within the joint? Mechanical symptoms such as clicking suggest a fibrocartilage tear. Knee meniscal tears can cause clicking when doing pivoting-type activity or with hyperflexion.

    E. Has the patient experienced joint locking? True locking of a joint, defined as the inability to actively move the joint for a certain period of time, indicates that there is something interposed between the articular surfaces, such as a loose body. Patients can usually shake the joint or passively move it to unlock the joint.

III. PHYSICAL EXAMINATION

    A. The joint should be palpated for any obvious tenderness, which may indicate areas of contusion, sprains, or occult fractures. The ligament examination should not only check for the competency of the ligaments, but also whether or not pain is elicited. Pain, without any compromise of ligamentous competency, indicates a sprain; pain and failure of ligamentous competency indicates a rupture.

    B. Motion should be assessed as to whether certain joint positions elicit pain. Rotatory motions of the knee that cause pain may indicate a meniscal tear; pain with hyperflexion and adduction of the hip may indicate a labral tear.

IV. INVESTIGATIONS

    A. Joint aspiration may provide additional information about the type of injury. A hemarthrosis with fat droplets indicates a fracture of bone. The fracture may be a periarticular fracture or an avulsion fracture of ligamentous attachments.

    B. X-ray analysis in two planes can help identify periarticular fractures.

    C. Magnetic resonance imaging (MRI) is the best imaging modality to look at the soft tissues inside and surrounding the joint.

V. TREATMENT

    A. Immediate management includes RICE: rest, ice, compression, and elevation. This algorithm should be followed for at least 48 to 72 hours.

    B. Joint aspiration may provide symptomatic relief, but is not necessary. Fluid will usually reaccumulate despite attempts to keep it down.

    C. Splinting may take the stresses off the injured area. Many traumatic injuries of the knee are managed with a hinged knee brace (knee immobilizer), which alleviates stresses on the collateral and cruciate ligaments.

D. A sling may help relieve the stresses on the elbow and shoulder by supporting the weight of the arm against gravity.

E. If the patient has pain with ambulation, protected weight bearing may help unload the stresses upon that joint. A cane, crutches, or a walker can be used depending on the age of the patient and the amount of pain.

F. If a sprain is diagnosed, once the acute swelling has subsided, a physical therapy program can help regain range of motion.

G. In the case of a hemarthrosis, the inability to bear weight, ligamentous laxity, or swelling that does not improve, referral to an orthopedic surgeon is indicated to determine whether or not surgery is required.

H. A short course of nonsteroidal anti-inflammatory drugs (NSAIDs) is helpful to treat pain and inflammation.

I. Orthopedic consultation is appropriate in setting a likely fracture or significant joint or ligamentous damage.

THE INABILITY TO WALK DUE TO PAIN

The inability to walk due to pain implies a serious mechanical problem in the load-bearing joints or axial skeleton. Diagnosis will require additional imaging studies, but a careful physical examination can localize the problem, allowing the physician to narrow the differential and prevent further damage.

I. DIFFERENTIAL DIAGNOSIS
 A. Hip fracture/occult hip fracture.
 B. Stress fracture of the femoral neck.
 C. Stress fracture of the tibial shaft or plateau.
 D. Insufficiency fracture of the sacrum with or without a pubic ramus fracture.
 E. Compression fracture of the thoracolumbar spine.
 F. Exacerbation of existing osteoarthritis.
 G. Exacerbation of RA or other systemic inflammatory disorders.
 H. Femoral head collapse in the setting of osteonecrosis.
 I. Acute lumbosacral sprain with or without radiculopathy.
 J. Vascular occlusion.

II. KEY DIAGNOSTIC QUESTIONS
 A. Over what time period has this condition evolved? An insidious onset suggests a gradual mechanical failure brought on by repetitive activity (a stress fracture). An acute onset preceded by a traumatic event suggests a fracture.
 B. Has the patient adopted any new activity recently? An increase in the activity level of the patient beyond the body's ability to adapt can lead to a stress fracture. An example is marathon training leading to stress fractures in the metatarsals, tibial shaft, or femoral neck.
 C. Is there a history of osteoporosis? Osteoporotic bone can succumb to relatively minor loads; a vertebral body compression fracture can occur with lifting of grocery bags or with a cough.
 D. Is there a history of hip osteoarthritis? With pre-existing osteoporosis and degenerative joint disease of the hip, subchondral fractures of the femoral head may occur, leading to rapidly progressive osteoarthritis, and difficulty in bearing weight. RA or other inflammatory disorders rarely lead to total inability to walk. If that is the case or if walking ability is severely limited, either a very severe joint disease with superimposed secondary osteoarthritis or a superimposed infection, fracture, and mechanical joint problem must be considered.
 E. Is there a history of steroid use, alcohol abuse or diseases such as sickle cell disease or Gaucher's disease that could lead to osteonecrosis? Does the patient have systemic lupus, with or without a history of steroid therapy?
 F. Is there a history of back pain, sciatica, or spinal stenosis?
 G. Does the patient have a history of vascular disease such as angina, myocardial infarction, or peripheral vascular disease with claudication?

III. PHYSICAL EXAMINATION

A. The patient should be observed while attempting to walk. A decreased stance phase with a shortened stride length is the definition of an antalgic gait due to joint pain. Asking the patient to localize the pain while ambulating will help the physician focus on the correct area.

B. All weight-bearing joints (tarsal, ankle, knee, hips, and sacroiliac) should be inspected for tenderness, swelling, and range of motion. Point tenderness over a bone may indicate a stress fracture. Active straight leg raising in the supine position increases joint reactive forces across the hip. Pain while straight leg raising is a localizing finding suggesting hip pathology such as an occult fracture. Internal rotation of the hip is the most sensitive position to bring out hip pathology, be it fracture or arthritis.

C. The spine, including the sacrum, should be palpated over the spinous processes and paraspinal musculature. Point tenderness over the spinous processes may suggest a compression fracture, whereas tenderness in the paraspinal musculature may indicate a sprain. A careful neurovascular examination is a requisite to evaluate neurologic deficit caused by compression fractures.

D. Because the back can be the origin of pain that "presents" all along the sciatic nerve distribution in the lower extremity, examination of the back is important as is a neurologic examination that includes testing of reflexes and muscle strength.

E. Vascular occlusion can lead to severe leg pains and therefore an examination of leg pulses is mandatory.

IV. INVESTIGATIONS

A. Plain radiographs are quite helpful in defining the presence of joint damage due to RA or osteoarthritis. A fracture can be missed either because the reactive bone changes may not occur for 1 to 2 weeks, or the patient could be osteopenic and the fracture line may not be obvious. Osteonecrosis may not be seen at all with this imaging technique and requires assessment with a bone scan or MRI.

B. Radiographs in two planes can help identify whether or not a fracture is the cause. A chronic stress fracture may appear as sclerosis, but often radiographs are unrevealing.

C. Nuclear medicine studies, such as a Technetium 99 three-phase bone scan, will demonstrate areas of increased bone turnover. A bone scan is helpful especially when the physical examination was not able to localize the problem. The caveat is that an occult fracture occurring after trauma will not show up on the bone scan until 48 hours have elapsed. A sacral insufficiency fracture will show up as an "H pattern" on the bone scan.

D. Computed tomography (CT) scan of the region of interest can demonstrate occult fractures of the hip, tibial shaft, and tibial plateau. Three-dimensional reconstructions may be necessary to visualize the fracture lines.

E. MRI of the region of interest can similarly evaluate for occult and stress fractures. MRI has the added benefit of imaging bone edema patterns and avoiding the use of ionizing radiation.

V. TREATMENT

A. The affected area should immediately be protected from weight bearing by the use of crutches or a walker, depending upon the age and physical condition of the patient.

B. Stress fractures of all types, especially if the trauma that led to it was minimal (this is called a fragility fracture), should stimulate an evaluation for osteopenia/osteoporosis and possible treatment for it. This includes a dual energy x-ray absorptiometry (DEXA) and a search for the cause (see Chapter 53).

C. If an occult fracture or stress fracture of the femoral neck is diagnosed, an orthopedic surgeon should be consulted as to whether operative fixation is advisable. Depending upon the location of the stress fracture on the compression or tension side of the femoral neck, the patient may be treated with a protracted course of protected weight bearing, or with operative fixation.

D. Stress fractures of the tibia may be treated with a period of rest and re-evaluation in 4 to 6 weeks.

E. A stress fracture in the foot should be treated with a hard-soled shoe, which distributes weight more evenly, and a period of rest. A repeat examination should be performed at 4 to 6 weeks to monitor improvement.

F. The acute pain related to sacral insufficiency, vertebral or pubic fractures can improve over 6 to 8 weeks, but such fractures may also require a protracted course of protected weight bearing for as long as 6 to 9 months.

G. A vertebral compression fracture that causes severe and persistent pain or neurologic deficit should be assessed by a spine surgeon to decide if a brace, kyphoplasty/vertebroplasty or surgery is indicated.

H. Anti-inflammatory medications may be used to help with symptomatic relief; generally, narcotic analgesics may be necessary if the patient is unable to regain full weight bearing.

 "MY BACK HURTS AND I CANNOT MOVE"

Back pain is the most common musculoskeletal complaint, and is estimated to affect 60% to 80% of individuals at some point in their lives. It can be difficult to ascertain the exact cause of an acute episode of pain that limits mobility, as most occurrences are self-limited and will resolve with rest, time, and symptomatic treatment. However, it is the physician's responsibility to ensure that there is no persistent, underlying condition that may require intervention.

I. DIFFERENTIAL DIAGNOSIS

A. Herniated nucleus pulposus.

B. Lumbosacral sprain.

C. Mechanical back pain (e.g., spondylolisthesis and degenerative disc disease).

D. Vertebral compression fracture.

E. Osteomyelitis of the spine.

F. Epidural abscess.

G. Neoplasm of the spine.

II. KEY DIAGNOSTIC QUESTIONS

A. Has there been any loss of bowel or bladder control? Loss of function of the bowel or bladder sphincters may indicate cauda equina syndrome, which is a compression of the inferior portion of the spinal cord. Cauda equina syndrome is a surgical emergency and requires immediate decompression.

B. Was there a history of back pain prior to this acute event? A history of lower back pain preceding this acute event may indicate previous disc annulus degeneration that has now acutely herniated.

C. Is there anything temporally related to the onset of pain? Many patients can cite a specific traumatic incident, episode of heavy lifting, or rotational/torsional overuse. Such a history suggests the possibility of a herniated disc, exacerbation of facet arthropathy, or lumbosacral sprain. A history of heavy lifting in a patient with osteoporosis can indicate a compression fracture of the thoracolumbar spine.

D. Does the patient have a history of repetitive hyperextension, such as gymnastics or diving? Hyperextension of the lumbar spine may cause a fracture of the lumbar spine pars interarticularis, allowing one vertebra to shift forward on another (spondylolisthesis).

E. Is the pain worse at night? Pain that increases at night raises the possibility of a tumor in the spine, either a primary or metastatic lesion. Some possible primary neoplasms of the spinal column include eosinophilic granuloma, aneurysmal bone cysts, giant cell tumors, and chordomas. Metastatic lesions involving the vertebral elements include multiple myeloma, and breast, lung, renal, and prostate malignancies. Rarely, severe mechanical or degenerative back disease can give pain both during the day and night, but this is uncommon.

F. Are there any systemic signs of infection, or history of any other recent infections? A history of fevers, chills, or night sweats heightens the possibility of an infectious process. Urinary tract infections, or respiratory infections may cause seeding of the lumbar vertebrae, which may not be symptomatic until 8 weeks after the initial event. Risk factors for vertebral osteomyelitis include diabetes mellitus, immunocompromised patients, intravenous drug users, and elderly, debilitated patients. A patient who has a history of travel to a tuberculosis endemic area raises the possibility of Pott's disease (tuberculous spondylitis).

G. Spondyloarthropathies such as ankylosing spondylitis cause early morning stiffness that gets better as the day goes on. This is different from mechanical back disease that is generally better in the morning after rest and worsens with activity. Rarely, however, does inflammatory back disease lead to an inability to move. If this occurs in that setting it could be due to the other problems listed in the preceding text, because these patients are not immune from them, are generally osteoporotic, and can fracture with minimal trauma.

III. PHYSICAL EXAMINATION
    A. Vital signs including temperature.
    B. The patient should be observed while ambulating, if possible. Although the problem may be in the midline of the spine, it is common that the patient feels pain primarily on one side of the body. The entire spine should be palpated for point tenderness, which could indicate a compression fracture or vertebral osteomyelitis. Forward bending and hyperextension should also be assessed; limitations of these motions may indicate involvement of the facet joint complex.
    C. The examination of a patient with back pain and limited mobility must include a complete neurologic evaluation to assess for radiculopathy or myelopathy. Passive straight leg raising places tension on the lower lumbar nerve roots, and pain elicited by this maneuver indicates a compressive lesion. Motor strength, sensation, and deep tendon reflexes must be checked to ensure symmetry. If cauda equina syndrome is suspected, perineal sensation and anal sphincter tone must be assessed.

IV. INVESTIGATIONS
    A. Complete blood count and differential count to assess for leukocytosis due to infection. ESR and CRP can be important diagnostic branch point tests which, when elevated, could reflect the presence of an infection, tumor, or inflammatory back disease.
    B. Radiographs of the spine should include anteroposterior, lateral, and oblique views. X-rays may provide some indication of the level of spinal involvement, as well as indicate if there are degenerative changes, neoplastic involvement, or fracture.
    C. The presence of severe back pain and fever should raise suspicion for an epidural abscess. An MRI should be performed on an emergency basis to assess this medical emergency.
    D. If symptoms persist without resolution with a conservative approach, cross-sectional imaging may be required to identify the pathology. MRI has the advantage of visualization in the axial, coronal, and sagittal planes without ionizing radiation or use of contrast material. However, a CT myelogram may be preferable when attempting to identify bony pathology.
    E. A bone scan can identify areas of increased bone activity in the spine, which can indicate a neoplastic, degenerative, or traumatic process. It is imperative to note that a negative bone scan does not rule out the possibility of multiple myeloma.

V. TREATMENT
    A. The initial management of acute back pain is purely symptomatic, as the cause may remain unclear. Patients often feel less pain when lying on a firm surface. A period of rest for 2 to 3 days (limited walking, no lifting, and avoidance of torsional activity) is recommended.
    B. NSAIDs, narcotic analgesics, and muscle relaxants may be effective in combination to help the patient through the acute period.
    C. If paraspinal spasm is a component of the pain, heating pads may help the muscles relax.
    D. Limited use of a lumbar corset can provide relief of pain in the acute period.
    E. Once the pain has begun to subside, a program of lumbar paraspinal muscle stretching and strengthening can help prevent exacerbation or recurrence. Abdominal stretching and strengthening is equally important in helping with support of the axial skeleton.

F. If there are any radicular symptoms, cross-sectional imaging is recommended to identify the cause of compression. A spine specialist can provide input as to whether epidural steroid injections or surgical decompression is indicated.

G. If symptoms of cauda equina syndrome or vertebral osteomyelitis are present, immediate surgical consultation is needed.

H. If symptoms of epidural abscess are present, immediate MRI is needed and, if abnormal, surgical consultation is mandatory.

I. If fever is associated with back pain of this level of severity, the diagnostic algorithm and treatment plan must change, with a new focus upon possible infection or tumor.

 THE "RED HOT" JOINT

Acute pain, swelling, redness, and warmth within and about a single joint. This is an uncommon clinical entity in rheumatology and is due to infection until proven otherwise.

I.   DIFFERENTIAL DIAGNOSIS

    A. Infectious arthritis.

    B. Crystal-related synovitis.

    C. Flare of an underlying systemic, inflammatory disorder such as RA, ReA, psoriatic arthritis, or colitic arthropathy.

II. KEY DIAGNOSTIC QUESTIONS

    A. Is this an intra- or extra-articular process or both? Inflammation within the joint space should be differentiated from that within the surrounding soft tissue. Intra-articular inflammation such as that with septic arthritis, gout, or pseudogout is painful with passive and active movement, and in any direction in which the joint is moved; extra-articular inflammation generally allows more passive range of motion. If the inflammatory reaction is circumferential such as in cellulitis, this dictum may not hold true. A tendinitis will be exacerbated by stretching or by resisted contraction of the associated muscle. A superficial bursitis (e.g., olecranon bursitis) or cellulitis will generally limit motion at the extremes (i.e., full flexion or full extension) of the arc of the involved joint.

    B. Which joint is involved? A septic joint is the most important and emergent condition to consider, with the knee and the hip the most commonly affected areas. However, any joint may become infected, particularly in the chronically ill or immunosuppressed, in patients with prosthetic joints or fixation devices, in patients with portals of entry for infection (e.g., foot ulcers and indwelling catheters) or with known foci of infection (e.g., endocarditis), or intravenous drug abusers. Particular care should be taken not to overlook a disproportionately inflamed (i.e., infected) joint in a patient with a chronic arthropathy such as RA. A migratory arthritis in a sexually active or young adult should raise the suspicion of gonococcal arthritis, especially if supported by the presence of skin lesions, tenosynovitis, urethritis or cervicitis and recent sexual contact. Although monarthritis of the first metatarsophalangeal (MTP) joint is stereotypical of gout, any joint may be involved, particularly the small joints of the hands and feet and the ankles. Pseudogout commonly involves the wrists and knees. Low-grade fevers and leukocytosis can occur in crystalline diseases, but the higher their levels are the less likely is a diagnosis of crystal-induced disease. Concurrent infection with the presence of crystals of gout or pseudogout is not rare and it seems to be related to joint crystals stripping off due to the infectious process.

    C. Are there associated clinical symptoms or signs? High-grade fevers, chills, and rigors suggest infection, but may not be prominent in many cases, and may be masked by the anti-inflammatory, analgesic or oral antibiotic regimen the patient has earlier been started on. A toxic, septic state is often not associated with disseminated gonococcemia. Peripheral signs of endocarditis (e.g., Osler's nodes and Janeway lesions) indicate that the joint disease may be an embolic manifestation of the infection. All potential sources of bacteremia (e.g., pneumonia, cellulitis, and urinary tract infection) should be sought.

D. Does the patient have a past history of an inflammatory joint disease such as RA? A red hot joint, and out of proportion to all other RA joints, is infection until proven otherwise. This is especially true in a patient whose disease is quiescent due to immunosuppressant drugs.

III. **INVESTIGATIONS**

   A. Joint aspiration is mandatory in order to define the cause of an uncommonly severe, acute inflammatory synovitis, be it related to infection or a flare of an underlying inflammatory joint disorder such as RA, gout, or pseudogout.

   B. Acute septic arthritis is a true emergency and must not be missed, and so arthrocentesis and synovial fluid analysis is mandatory. Fluid should be examined by a Gram stain and sent for cultures and sensitivities. A positive Gram stain should be considered diagnostic of infection, whereas a negative Gram stain is not sufficient evidence to exclude infection. Examination for intracellular crystals diagnostic of gout or pseudogout under polarizing light microscopy is also indicated and should be done promptly, within hours of receiving the specimen if possible, to ensure sensitivity. Synovial cell counts greater than 50,000/mm^3 increases the suspicion of infection, but it must be appreciated that in patients who are neutropenic, synovial cell counts may be much lower.

   C. If gonococcal arthritis is included in the list of differential diagnosis, then swabs of the pharynx, urethra, and rectum should be ordered for microbiologic testing.

   D. A mild peripheral leukocytosis and fever can be seen with crystalline arthritis, but higher levels of both (WBC >15,000/mm^3; temperature >38.5°C) are associated with an increased likelihood of infection.

IV. **TREATMENT**

   A. Empiric intravenous antibiotics and daily or twice daily **joint aspirations** are appropriate management if the clinical suspicion for septic arthritis is high, even while the results of microbiologic tests are pending. Surgical consultation may also be indicated for possible debridement, especially if joint effusions persist or remain positive for microbial growth, when deep joints such as the shoulder or hip are involved or if virulent organisms are found, such as gram-negative rods or *S. aureus*.

   B. Crystalline arthropathies respond readily to anti-inflammatory agents, intra-articular or systemic corticosteroids, colchicine, or parenteral corticotrophin [adrenocorticotrophic hormone (ACTH)].

   C. In the rare situation that such a red hot joint is related to a flare of RA, ReA, psoriatic arthritis, or colitic arthritis without infection, once cultures are negative and infection is definitively ruled out, local injection of steroids into the inflamed joint will be helpful.

 SEVERE JOINT PAINS AND FEVER

A patient presenting with fever indicates a systemic inflammatory process; joint pain may reflect direct involvement of the disease or an indirect "reactive" process.

I. **DIFFERENTIAL DIAGNOSIS**

   A. Infection
   1. Infectious arthritis.
   2. Superimposed on an already established systemic inflammatory disorder such as RA or SLE.

   B. Flare of an established systemic inflammatory disorder
   1. SLE.
   2. Inflammatory bowel disease (IBD).
   3. ReA.

   C. New-onset systemic inflammatory disorder
   1. SLE.
   2. Adult-onset Still's disease.
   3. ReA.
   4. IBD.
   5. Sarcoidosis.

     6. Vasculitides.
       a. Polyarteritis nodosa.
       b. Wegener's granulomatosis.
       c. Henoch-Schönlein purpura.
       d. Churg-Strauss vasculitis.
       e. Polymyalgia rheumatica (PMR)/giant cell arteritis (GCA).
     7. Allergic reaction.

II. **KEY DIAGNOSTIC QUESTIONS**

   A. **What is the duration of onset?** Acute fever and joint pain most typically describe a pyogenic infectious arthritis or a crystal-induced arthritis. A more insidious presentation is suggestive of an immune/inflammatory disorder such as SLE, adult-onset Still's disease, ReA, IBD, sarcoidosis, or adverse drug reaction. Occult or atypical infections such as bacterial endocarditis, mycobacterial or fungal disease can also present more slowly. RA should not be considered a febrile disease, unless prior flares have been associated with fever. However, fever in a patient with RA should always be considered a red flag and infection must be ruled out.

   B. **What is the distribution of joint symptoms?** Involvement of a single joint increases the likelihood of an infectious etiology although rarely it can be polyarticular, especially in disseminated gonococcemia or in immunosuppressed hosts. Crystalline arthritis also usually presents as a monarthritis, but can be polyarticular at times. Oligoarthritis (<four or fewer joints inflamed) is commonly seen in spondyloarthropathies such as psoriatic arthritis, ReA, or colitic arthritis. They tend to involve large, lower extremity joints in an asymmetric fashion. As more and more joints are involved, the likelihood of direct joint infection diminishes, and the likelihood of an immune/inflammatory condition increases. Bilateral arthritis and periarthritis of the ankles are highly suggestive of the Löfgren's variant of sarcoidosis, especially when accompanied by bilateral hilar adenopathy and erythema nodosum. Symmetric polyarthritis is characteristic of SLE, Still's disease, and viral infections.

   C. **Are there extra-articular findings?** Associated dermatologic signs can be pathognomonic as for SLE, Still's disease, acute rheumatic fever (ARF), endocarditis, and tophaceous gout. Erythema nodosum should suggest Löfgren's syndrome or IBD; SLE and sarcoidosis, in particular, are associated with many types of rashes. Prominent pulmonary complaints should be sought to assess for sarcoidosis, whereas gastrointestinal manifestations are present in IBD; the vasculitides have tell-tale signs such as mononeuritis multiplex with foot drop in polyarteritis nodosa; asthma, and eosinophilia with Churg-Strauss; sinus, lung, and kidney disease with Wegener's granulomatosis; palpable purpura, abdominal pain, and rash with Henoch-Schönlein purpura; and PMR, headache, visual symptoms, and elevated ESR in PMR/GCA. A thorough review of systems is essential to establish a complete clinical picture. It must be remembered that for many of the chronic diseases, new manifestations may appear over an expanded period of time, and ongoing vigilance is necessary until a firm diagnosis is made.

III. **INVESTIGATIONS**

   A. Septic arthritis must not be missed, and so arthrocentesis and synovial fluid analysis is essential if this diagnosis is a consideration. Fluid should be examined by Gram stain and sent for culture and sensitivity. If clinically appropriate, mycobacterial and fungal studies should also be done. Examination for crystals under polarizing light microscopy is also indicated and should be done promptly, within hours if possible, to avoid crystal deterioration. If gonococcal arthritis is in the differential diagnosis, then swabs of the pharynx, urethra, and rectum should be ordered for microbiologic testing.

   B. Serologic testing may be helpful if conditions such as SLE (e.g., antinuclear antibodies), ARF (antistreptolysin O antibodies), cytoplasmic-antineutrophil cytoplasmic antibodies (c-ANCA) in Wegener's granulomatosis, perinuclear-antineutrophil cytoplasmic antibodies (p-ANCA) in Churg-Strauss vasculitis are possible.

   C. Radiologic testing is often unrevealing during the initial onset of disease. One exception is pseudogout in which chondrocalcinosis (that had been previously asymptomatic) may be seen. However, baseline x-rays of septic joints may be helpful to follow the course of illness, and x-rays of the joints in more chronic presentations can offer some clues as to etiology (e.g., bony involvement in sarcoidosis).

D. Chest radiograph may demonstrate infiltrates or nodules in Wegener's granulomatosis or Churg-Strauss vasculitis; and bilateral hilar adenopathy is characteristic of sarcoidosis.

IV. Treatment. Empiric intravenous antibiotics are appropriate if the clinical suspicion for septic arthritis is high, while the results of microbiologic tests are completed. Otherwise, therapy is directed toward the underlying condition.

 LUPUS AND FEVER

Fever in a patient with known SLE raises the question of whether the patient is having an exacerbation (flare) of the illness, an acute infection, or both.

I. KEY DIAGNOSTIC QUESTIONS

A. Are there localizing signs or symptoms indicative of infection? Any part of the history or physical examination suggesting a potential focus of infection should be thoroughly investigated (e.g., meningeal symptoms, respiratory complaints, diarrhea, skin ulcers). Immunosuppressive therapies, leukopenia, hypocomplementemia, nephrosis/nephritis, functional asplenism, and other factors render the patient with SLE susceptible to infections by any type of organism, notably encapsulated bacteria and opportunistic organisms. Atypical presentations by common pathogens (e.g., pneumococcal peritonitis) and infections with atypical organisms (e.g., *Pneumocystis carinii*) should always be considered. Some patients with lupus are infection-prone and have a history of many such infections. However, a patient who has previously been free of infections and yet treated with steroids or immunosuppressive agents is always prone to be infected for the first time.

B. Are there signs or symptoms suggestive of lupus flare? SLE exacerbations are often anamnestic; that is, they often recall the presentations of past flares, although new manifestations may add-on to past patterns. Stereotypical rashes, mucosal ulcers, symmetric polyarthritis, and other manifestations, which are more suggestive of SLE than of infection, should be sought.

C. Is there a concurrent lupus flare and an acute infection? Patients with active SLE are more prone to infection, and infections may trigger lupus flares. Fever due to SLE is generally quite responsive to low-to-moderate doses of systemic steroids, and so if there is no obvious infection, a trial of low-dose steroids can be started. If the patient remains febrile, the likelihood of superimposed infection is greater.

II. INVESTIGATIONS

A. Leukopenia and thrombocytopenia point to an exacerbation of SLE, although leukocytosis and thrombocytosis suggest infection. It should be emphasized that a normal WBC or platelet count may be relatively elevated in the patient with lupus who may normally have low counts at baseline. Also, steroids at any dose will cause an elevated WBC count; therefore, such a finding may actually be related to the medication that could be predisposing the patient to an infection.

B. All fluids and specimen that raise the suspicion of infection should be subjected to microbial staining, culture and sensitivity tests. Appropriate imaging studies (e.g., chest radiograph) should be performed, as guided by the clinical picture.

C. Hypocomplementemia may suggest a lupus flare. Conversely, marked CRP elevations have been thought to indicate infection. However, such serologic tests should be used to support clinical suspicions but should never supersede clinical judgment.

III. TREATMENT

A. Both infection and SLE can be potentially life-threatening, and so if the patient appears severely ill, concomitant empiric broad-spectrum antibiotics and systemic corticosteroids are appropriate.

B. Stress doses of adrenocorticoids are appropriate in ill patients already receiving systemic corticosteroid therapy for SLE, even if an infectious etiology for fever is clearly identified.

C. Certain antibiotics, notably sulfonamides, have been thought to trigger lupus flares in some patients and should be avoided, if at all possible, so as not to confound the clinical picture. However, if they are needed in the setting of *P. carinii* infection, they should be used and rarely cause problems.

AN ELDERLY PATIENT WITH A SEVERE HEADACHE

In the case of an elderly patient with an acute or subacute headache of quality or severity that is atypical for the patient, infectious, inflammatory, neurologic, and vascular etiologies should be strongly considered.

I. **DIFFERENTIAL DIAGNOSIS**
   A. Meningitis.
      1. Septic.
      2. Aseptic.
         a. Viral.
         b. Medications such as NSAIDs.
   B. Cerebrovascular accident (CVA).
      1. Because of atherosclerotic disease or an embolus.
      2. Because of an underlying systemic disorder such as SLE or one of the vasculitides.
         a. CVA.
         b. Bleeding due to coagulopathy.
         c. Antiphospholipid syndrome.
         d. Vasculitic occlusion of an intracerebral vessel.
   C. Intracranial hemorrhage.
      1. Subarachnoid hemorrhage.
      2. Subdural hematoma.
   D. GCA.
   E. Herpes zoster or simplex.

II. **KEY CLINICAL FINDINGS**
   A. **Meningitis.** Fever, photophobia, meningeal signs, and mental status changes.
   B. **CVA.** Cognitive changes, aphasia, and focal neurologic symptoms and signs.
   C. **Intracranial hemorrhage.** History or physical evidence of head trauma, especially in a patient on anticoagulant therapy; an acute "worst headache of my life" warrants evaluation for a subarachnoid hemorrhage.
   D. **Subdural hematoma.** Recent onset of increasingly severe headache in a patient on anticoagulation or with thrombocytopenia and with a recent history of head trauma.
   E. **GCA.** Constitutional symptoms, fever, PMR, scalp tenderness, tender temporal arteries, diminished temporal artery pulses, facial or tongue pain, jaw claudication, and, most importantly, loss of visual acuity or amaurosis fugax.
   F. **Herpes zoster.** Generally unilateral and typical vesicular rash, although occasionally a rash cannot be definitively appreciated. Herpes simplex should be considered in an immunosuppressed patient with an encephalitic picture with cognitive changes, headache, and fever.

III. **INVESTIGATIONS**
   A. **Meningitis.** Leukocytosis in the cerebrospinal fluid.
   B. **CVA.** Neuroradiologic imaging.
   C. **Intracranial hemorrhage.** Neuroradiologic imaging (subarachnoid hemorrhage and subdural hematoma), evidence of hemorrhage in cerebrospinal fluid (subarachnoid hemorrhage).
   D. **GCA.** Laboratory evidence of inflammation (e.g., elevated ESR, elevated plasma CRP levels, anemia of chronic disease); temporal artery biopsy (preferable but not necessary to initiate therapy).
   E. **Herpes zoster.** Tzanck's test (not absolutely necessary if herpetic lesions are characteristic). Neuroradiologic imaging for herpes simplex encephalitis with a focus on the temporal lobes.

IV. **TREATMENT**
   A. **Meningitis.** If a bacterial etiology is suspected, intravenous antibiotics with a good central nervous system penetration are necessary. If aseptic meningitis is suspected, supportive care and discontinuation of suspected causes for the condition (e.g., medication) are appropriate.

B. CVA. If the cause is thrombotic, then anticoagulation is indicated. If the cause is hemorrhagic, then a neurosurgical consultation may be warranted.

C. Intracranial hemorrhage. A neurosurgical or vascular surgical consultation may be warranted.

D. GCA. If the clinical suspicion is high, empiric systemic corticosteroid therapy should be administered immediately, even without pathologic data. This is especially true if ophthalmologic involvement is suspected.

E. Herpes zoster. Antiviral agents. If the eyes are threatened, ophthalmologic consultation and intravenous therapy are indicated.

F. If the problem is due to SLE or one of the vasculitides, immunosuppression is likely to be required.

 THE GOUT THAT DOES NOT GO AWAY

A patient with presumptive gout whose symptoms, despite appropriate therapy for acute gouty attacks, are incompletely responsive, progressive, or frequently recurrent.

I.   KEY DIAGNOSTIC QUESTIONS

  A. Is the diagnosis of gout correct? Although a definitive diagnosis of gout can be made by the identification of uric acid crystals within neutrophils found in synovial fluid, patients are very often diagnosed clinically and therefore may actually have alternative diagnoses. An acute extremely inflammatory monarthritis should raise the suspicion of bacterial infection. A more indolent, yet persistent, inflammatory monarthritis may represent an atypical infection (e.g., mycobacterial or fungal) or an early inflammatory arthropathy such as a spondyloarthropathy. Oligoarthritis involving large lower extremity joints in an asymmetric pattern more strongly point to conditions such as a spondyloarthropathy; symmetrical polyarthritis points toward RA. It must be noted that not all joint inflammation that involves the first MTP joint is gout. Pseudopodagra can be caused by psoriatic arthritis, ReA, or even the early stirrings of RA. Rarely is the first MTP arthritis caused by infection.

  B. Are there comorbid conditions whose symptoms overlap with gout? Even when gouty arthritis has been established by synovial fluid analysis, comorbid conditions such as concurrent infection or structural damage to the joint (e.g., degenerative arthritis, tophi or gouty erosions) may account for persistent symptoms. The presence of a tophus in or near a joint can lead to persistent or recurring inflammation despite what appears to be optimal anti-inflammatory therapy for the gout.

  C. Is chronic therapy for gout a more optimal therapeutic tactic than intermittent therapy? In cases of gout where acute flares are increasingly difficult to control or occurring with increased frequency, therapeutic approaches aimed at prevention and prophylaxis may be more appropriate.

II.   INVESTIGATIONS

  A. Synovial fluid analysis can help confirm the diagnosis of gout (e.g., intracellular uric acid crystals) and also identify a concurrent infection (e.g., positive microbial stains or cultures). A leukocyte count greater than 50,000 cells/mm^3 is highly suggestive of a septic arthritis. If synovial fluid analysis is unrevealing, synovial biopsy specimen are more sensitive in identifying uric acid crystals and infectious causes (particularly atypical organisms), but require surgical intervention for sampling.

  B. Radiologic studies may show characteristic findings that may be more consistent with gout, spondyloarthropathies, RA, infection, or osteoarthritis.

III.   TREATMENT

  A. Appropriate therapy for any identified alternative or concomitant conditions should be instituted (e.g., antibiotics for infections; disease-modifying antirheumatic drugs for inflammatory arthropathies).

  B. Acute gouty flares normally respond readily to NSAIDs, systemic corticosteroids or intra-articular corticosteroids. Oral colchicine and parenteral corticotrophin are second-line options. However, since acute flares are generally self-limiting and pose no threat to life or vital organs, pure pain management with brief courses of low potency narcotics should not be discounted as suitable measures.

C. Chronic therapy for gout should include appropriate dietary modifications to reduce purine intake and avoidance (if possible) of medications that contribute to hyperuricemia. Colchicine, allopurinol or uricosuric therapies are available agents for the prevention of gouty flares. Surgical debridement is occasionally required to remove tophi that are symptomatic or threaten adjacent structures such as tendons and ligaments. Hypouricemic agents are usually required after surgical intervention to prevent regrowth of tophi.

 # A FEVER OF UNKNOWN ORIGIN

A fever of unknown origin (FUO) is an unexplained febrile illness with temperatures higher than 38.3°C for more than 3 weeks despite three outpatient evaluations or 3 days of investigation in the hospital. [Nosocomial FUO, neutropenic FUO, and FUO associated with human immunodeficiency virus (HIV) are classified separately and addressed differently than classic FUO and are not included in this discussion.]

I. DIFFERENTIAL DIAGNOSIS
   A. Infections of all types.
   B. Malignancy.
   C. Autoimmune disorder or vasculitides.
   D. Systemic granulomatous disorders such as Crohn's disease or sarcoidosis.
   E. Allergic disorders/drug reactions.

II. KEY DIAGNOSTIC QUESTIONS
   A. Are there any historical features, localizing symptoms, or clinical signs to direct inquiry? It is a truism that the etiology of an FUO is not obvious, and so a thorough clinical history, review of systems, and physical examination are essential at the outset to most efficiently arrive at a correct diagnosis. Any complaint, no matter how seemingly trivial, should be taken seriously. Drug or toxin exposures, recent travel, family medical history, psychiatric history, and other historical elements need to be assessed fully. Even a simple element such as the age of the patient can help to narrow the diagnostic process (e.g., advanced age should raise a suspicion of GCA). Often a "fresh look" is needed, preferably by someone who is not biased by the prior negative workup.
   B. Is there evidence of, or a predisposition to infection? In general, excluding an infectious etiology is the first priority. In recent studies, one-fifth to one-fourth of FUOs eventually has been determined to be caused by infections. Occult infections such as intra-abdominal abscesses, osteomyelitis or endocarditis; infections of indwelling foreign objects such as joint prostheses or fixation devices; and insidious and slow-growing pathogens such as mycobacteria or fungi, all need to be considered. Recent instrumentation or invasive procedures should be considered possible portals of entry for infectious agents.
   C. Is there evidence of an occult malignancy? Though this is as likely the result of better diagnostic techniques, malignancies now account for less than 10% of FUOs. The most common malignancies that cause fever are Hodgkin's disease, non-Hodgkin's lymphomas, leukemias, renal-cell carcinoma, and hepatoma.
   D. Is there evidence of an inflammatory disorder? Noninfectious immune-mediated and inflammatory disorders account for approximately one-third of FUOs. Vasculitides (notably GCA), adult-onset Still's disease, and granulomatous diseases (e.g., sarcoidosis, Crohn's disease, and granulomatous hepatitis) are consistently represented in case series of FUOs.

III. INVESTIGATIONS
   A. Documentation of fever in a controlled setting is essential. In one series, more than a third of FUO cases were either factitious or without evidence of actual fever.
   B. Reassessment of the prior records is mandatory because something may have been missed. Also, as the disease evolves, history and clinical findings that may not have

seemed important early on may furnish an important clue to the diagnosis at the time you see the patient.

C. The clinical picture should be the basis to direct laboratory testing, but initial studies should include complete blood count, biochemical profile, ESR, and CRP. Blood and body fluid specimen should be cultured to ensure growth of slow-growing bacteria, mycobacteria, and fungi. Serum specimen stored at initial evaluation may be helpful for future examination as clinically indicated, to assess for acute and convalescent antibody titers.

D. CT scans and MRI of the chest, abdomen, and pelvis are helpful to uncover abscesses or occult malignancies. Radionuclide scanning (e.g., gallium or indium) and positron-emission tomography (PET) can identify focal areas of inflammation and increased metabolic activity.

E. The accumulated clinical, laboratory, and radiologic data should dictate the requirement for biopsy of tissue, but bone marrow, liver, and (in the elderly) temporal artery biopsies are routinely obtained when other studies are not helpful.

F. Ophthalmologic examination is a helpful hint, which gives a unique view into the body condition and specifically the nervous system. Many systemic inflammatory and infectious disorders have an effect upon the eye that cannot be appreciated by a simple external eye examination. Persistent bacteremias arising from the gall bladder, blood vessels, and heart valves must be looked for. A fresh look by a rheumatologist and oncologist can be helpful because, once infection has been ruled out, those specialists, working together, can rule out many occult disorders that may not be apparent.

IV. TREATMENT

A. In general, therapy should be withheld until a putative diagnosis is better established. Empiric antibiotics may be appropriate if the patient is clinically unstable, but every effort should be made to have samples collected for microbiologic cultures before initiation of antibiotics.

B. Nonessential medications that are deemed to be possible causes of fever should be discontinued. Phenothiazines, which can cause the neuroleptic malignant syndrome, are notable causes of high fevers. For essential medications (e.g., antibiotics), alternatives should be considered.

C. Until a diagnosis is made, ongoing investigation and continued observation for new or changing clinical findings are mandatory.

 A PATIENT TOO WEAK TO STAND

Patients unable to bear their own weight due to muscle weakness.

I. DIFFERENTIAL DIAGNOSIS

A. Myopathy can be due to one or more of the following.

  1. Polymyositis, dermatomyositis or inclusion of body myositis.

  2. Myositis due to other systemic inflammatory disorders.

   a. SLE.

   b. Mixed connective tissue disease (MCTD).

   c. Vasculitis.

   d. Scleroderma.

  3. Metabolic.

   a. Hypothyroidism.

   b. Hypokalemia.

  4. Drug induced.

   a. Statins.

   b. Steroids.

   c. HIV medications.

  5. Infectious.

   a. Viral.

   b. Bacterial.

   c. Protozoan.

  6. Inherited.

B. Neurologic disorders
  1. Multiple sclerosis.
  2. Guillain-Barre syndrome.
  3. Amyotrophic lateral sclerosis.
II. KEY DIAGNOSTIC QUESTIONS
  A. Is the inability to stand truly due to muscle weakness? The proximal musculature of the lower extremities, notably the hip and knee extensors, provide the strength necessary for standing. However, subjective weakness may occur in diverse medical and psychiatric conditions such as anemia, depression, chronic infections, and malignancies. Functional weakness may occur with painful lower limb arthropathies.
  B. What is the distribution of weakness? Asymmetric weakness may suggest a unifocal neuropathic process such as a nerve root injury. Symmetric proximal weakness may suggest inflammatory diseases (e.g., polymyositis, dermatomyositis, SLE, MCTD, and sarcoidosis), endocrinopathies (e.g., thyroid, adrenal, or parathyroid dysfunction), drug toxicities (e.g., "statins," corticosteroids, colchicine, zidovudine, ethanol), or inherited myopathies. Involvement of proximal and distal musculature may suggest inherited myopathies, inclusion body myositis, Guillain-Barre syndrome, or electrolyte abnormalities.
  C. What is the evolutionary pattern of weakness? Rapid onset of weakness often points to electrolyte abnormalities or toxic disorders. Ascending weakness over hours to days suggests Guillain-Barre syndrome. Subacute or slowly progressive proximal weakness is characteristic of polymyositis, dermatomyositis, drug effects, and endocrinopathies.
  D. Are there extramuscular manifestations? Characteristic skin findings may be diagnostic for dermatomyositis, SLE, MCTD, or sarcoidosis. Inflammatory myopathies may be associated with dysphagia or pulmonary symptoms. Cushingoid features should raise the suspicion of excessive corticosteroid use or adrenal hyperfunction. Central nervous system disease or cardiomyopathy can be seen in mitochondrial myopathies.
III. INVESTIGATIONS
  A. General screening laboratory tests (e.g., complete blood count, basic biochemical profile that includes potassium, phosphorus, calcium, and magnesium), serum muscle enzyme tests (e.g., aldolase, creatine kinase, lactate dehydrogenase, aspartate, and alanine aminotransferases), and thyroid function tests should be routinely assessed. The clinical picture may indicate more specific tests.
  B. A full neurologic examination. Electromyography and nerve conduction studies can confirm the presence of and localize a neuromuscular lesion. They may also help to assess the evolution of the disease.
  C. Formal muscle strength testing such as torque analysis can quantify the degree of weakness as well as document effectiveness of therapy.
  D. MRI and ultrasonography can identify evidence of muscle inflammation and possible sites for muscle biopsy.
  E. Muscle biopsy often offers definitive diagnosis of a myopathic process, but identification of specific metabolic defects may require histochemical or biochemical techniques available only at specialized tertiary care centers.
IV. TREATMENT
  A. Electrolyte (sodium, potassium, calcium, magnesium, and phosphate) and endocrine abnormalities should be corrected, and the etiology of these abnormalities addressed.
  B. Many immune-mediated myopathies (e.g., dermatomyositis, polymyositis, and sarcoidosis) will respond rapidly to systemic corticosteroids.
  C. Myopathic drugs and toxins should be discontinued.
  D. Physical therapy is appropriate for all types of myopathic disorders.

Clinical Presentations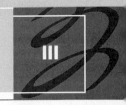

III

MONARTHRITIS/POLYARTHRITIS: DIFFERENTIAL DIAGNOSIS
Stephen Ray Mitchell and John F. Beary, III

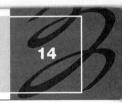

14

■ KEY POINTS

- ■ The number of joints involved and the time course of their involvement enable the physician to classify joint problems and to construct the appropriate differential diagnosis.
- ■ "Chronic" refers to joint symptoms that persist beyond 2 months. Oligoarthritis refers to the involvement of 2 to 4 joints, and polyarthritis is defined as the involvement of more than four joints.
- ■ Acute monarthritis can be due to infection, and septic arthritis is a rheumatologic emergency.
- ■ Gout is a classic example of acute monarthritis, but approximately 25% of gout cases present as polyarthritis, mainly in the lower extremity.
- ■ Rheumatoid arthritis (RA) is the classic example of chronic polyarthritis, but it is important to carefully confirm the diagnosis, as one occasionally encounters a patient with gout who has hand deformities that look like RA and has a relatively normal uric acid. Such a patient may even receive disease-modifying antirheumatic drugs (DMARDs) for a time, which are stopped when it is discovered that it is actually gouty tophi that are involved in the destructive hand lesions.
- ■ The importance of identifying the pauciarticular pattern in children with juvenile idiopathic arthritis (JIA) is that it is an important clue to seek, identify, and treat iridocyclitis, which is asymptomatic but can destroy the sight of children.

 ## INTRODUCTION

I. **The number of joints and the time course during which a joint disorder develops guide the approach to differential diagnosis.** Acute and severe monarthritis, especially one that presents along with fever, may represent septic arthritis, which is a rheumatologic emergency. The promptness of the diagnosis and treatment of a potentially septic process is likely to profoundly alter the outcome.

II. **Alternatively, a single abnormal inflamed joint that persists beyond 2 months presents a different diagnostic challenge,** with infection being a much less likely

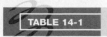

TABLE 14-1	Differential Diagnosis of Monarthritis by Presentation	

Monarthritis	Common	Less common
Acute	Bacterial arthritis Gout (CPPD) Spondyloarthropathies Reactive arthritis Psoriatic arthritis Inflammatory bowel disease JIA Hemarthrosis Trauma Anticoagulant therapy	Leukemia Rheumatoid arthritis Sarcoid arthritis Hemarthrosis Coagulopathy Dialysis/apatite crystals Osteochondromatosis PVNS
Chronic	Osteoarthritis Spondyloarthropathies Lyme disease (recurring)	Fungal arthritis Tuberculous arthritis Bacterial arthritis Monarticular RA CPPD Sarcoid arthritis PVNS Osteochondromatosis

CPPD, calcium pyrophosphate dihydrate; JIA, juvenile idiopathic arthritis; PVNS, pigmented villonodular synovitis; RA, rheumatoid arthritis.

disease process. In each case, one must view the overall clinical presentation, including factors such as extra-articular visceral involvement, constitutional signs and symptoms, severity of illness, limitation of function, potential foci of infection, skin lesions, hyperuricemia, and history of trauma or bleeding disorders.

III. **Often, an aggressive initial approach is indicated,** including joint aspiration with synovial fluid analysis and occasionally, in more refractory or unexplained situations, referral for synovial biopsy or arthroscopy. Therapy will vary significantly depending on the presumptive diagnosis. Specific therapy for each disease is discussed in later chapters. Tables 14-1 and 14-2 summarize the diagnostic approach to this group of disorders.

ACUTE MONARTHRITIS

I. **Infectious arthritis** has an abrupt onset and a marked systemic inflammatory response. Because prompt therapy is required to prevent irretrievable joint damage, it is important to diagnose bacterial infection promptly. One may be deceived, however, in a partially treated patient on oral antibiotics or in an immunosuppressed patient in whom the inflammatory response is dampened by steroid therapy. A prudent approach includes careful examination for associated infectious foci and clinical clues (e.g., cutaneous pustules with neisserial infection), prompt joint aspiration and synovial fluid analysis, synovial fluid culture and Gram stain, and empiric antibiotics (depending on age and epidemiology). A viral process is typically polyarticular and may be accompanied by rash or other viral signs and symptoms. Lyme arthritis, caused by a Borrelia spirochete in endemic areas, can present acutely in recurring episodes of knee monarthritis; but more often it presents early in the course of the disease as migratory polyarthralgias, is associated with a characteristic rash or tick bite, and has a less "toxic" presentation (see Chapter 47).

II. **CRYSTAL-INDUCED DISEASE**

 A. **Gout** classically presents as "podagra" with the abrupt and intense onset of pain and inflammation in the first metatarsophalangeal joint; it often affects the midfoot and ankle, but can involve any joint or bursa. Typically, a man in his fifties with

TABLE 14-2	Differential Diagnosis of Polyarthritis by Presentation	
Polyarthritis	**Common**	**Less common**
Acute		
Migratory	*Neisseria* infection	Viral
	Acute rheumatic fever	
	Lyme disease (early)	
Nonmigratory	Rheumatoid arthritis	Hematologic disorders
	Serum sickness	Polyarticular gout
	Systemic lupus	
	Polyarticular JIA	
Chronic		
	Rheumatoid arthritis	Sarcoid arthritis
	Polyarticular JIA	CTD and overlap syndromes
	Systemic lupus	Spondyloarthropathy
	Polyarticular gout	
	Oligoarticular OA	

CTD, connective tissue disease; JIA, juvenile idiopathic arthritis; OA, osteoarthritis.

hypertension, obesity, diabetes, and coronary artery disease presents with monarthritis of the lower extremity. However, approximately 25% present with polyarticular synovitis. Between episodes, the joints return to normal unless chronic disease develops. A careful check for tophi on the ears, elbows, hands, or feet is required. At a younger age of onset of gout, one must think of lymphoma or other disorders associated with rapid cell turnover. The finding of negatively birefringent, needle-shaped crystals within the white blood cells in the synovial fluid is diagnostic. Note that gout can coexist with pseudogout, and both can coexist with infection (see Chapter 43).

 B. Calcium pyrophosphate dihydrate (CPPD) deposition disease (pseudogout) is an acute or subacute process in the elderly with involvement of large or small joints (including the second and third metacarpophalangeal joints). Chondrocalcinosis can often be defined radiographically in the knee, symphysis pubis, or triangular cartilage of the wrist. Crystals found within synovial fluid white blood cells are rhomboid-shaped and positively birefringent. In those patients who present at a younger age, other diagnostically important, treatable medical conditions, such as hemochromatosis or hyperparathyroidism must be considered (see Chapter 44).

III. Hemarthrosis is defined through the aspiration of bloody joint fluid.

 A. Trauma usually is associated with a relevant history of injury. A layer of fat (from the bone marrow) seen on top of bloody fluid implies intra-articular fracture even in the presence of negative radiographs.

 B. Internal derangement. Meniscal tears involving avascular portions of knee fibrocartilage may not be bloody but can cause intermittent locking, giving way, and a positive MacMurray's maneuver (a painful click produced by extending the knee when the foot is internally or externally rotated). Instability of the collateral and cruciate ligaments is also a clue to this condition (see Chapter 24).

 C. Nontraumatic hemarthrosis may be seen in the setting of anticoagulation, after the use of heparin during dialysis, or with benign neoplasms such as pigmented villonodular synovitis, synovial osteochondromatosis, or hemangioma of the synovium. Diagnosis of the latter three disorders is confirmed with synovial biopsy, arthroscopy, or magnetic resonance imaging (MRI).

IV. PERIARTICULAR SYNDROMES. Any of the tissues surrounding the joint can be involved in an inflammatory or traumatic process. A careful musculoskeletal examination can distinguish between tendinitis, bursitis, overuse syndromes, and surrounding cellulitis. Erythema nodosum is often seen with drug reaction, inflammatory bowel disease, or acute sarcoidosis. It often causes a periarthritis about the ankles and can result in an associated joint effusion. Osteomyelitis or neoplasia should be considered with focal bone pain. Severe nighttime periarticular pain in a child is uncommon with juvenile arthritis and should always suggest leukemia.

V. NONINFECTIOUS INFLAMMATORY CONDITIONS

    A. Spondyloarthropathies. Because of the highly inflammatory, monarticular nature of some episodes of joint inflammation associated with reactive arthritis (ReA) or psoriatic arthritis, the clinical presentation may be indistinguishable from that of infection. The diagnosis may be supported by the presence of characteristic extra-articular features, such as a psoriasiform rash, eye inflammation, or urethritis. A history of low-back symptoms or tenderness over the sacroiliac joints suggests the diagnosis of spondyloarthritis and is an indication for radiographic study of the sacroiliac joints (see Chapter 39).

    B. Juvenile idiopathic arthritis (JIA). The child who presents with monarthritis, often subacute in character, and a negative infectious workup may well have **pauciarticular** (fewer than four joints) JIA (see Chapter 36). **Transient synovitis of the hip** characteristically presents as a monarthritis of the hip in a child following a viral illness. The child is nontoxic in appearance and has a culture-negative joint effusion. This self-limited disorder is felt to be mediated by a virus or immune complexes and responds to bed rest and anti-inflammatory medications.

VI. MONARTICULAR PRESENTATION OF A POLYARTICULAR DISEASE. Although rheumatoid arthritis (RA) characteristically evolves into a symmetric polyarthritis, some patients present, at the onset of the disorder, with a monarticular synovitis. Attacks of "palindromic rheumatism" resemble gout. These are intense inflammatory episodes that involve a single joint and periarticular tissues. The attacks typically last for days at a time, returning to normal between episodes. Later, the more typical, polyarticular pattern of RA may emerge (see Chapter 29).

CHRONIC MONARTHRITIS

Involvement of a single joint, which persists beyond 2 months, represents a somewhat different group of diseases. Clearly, the persistence of joint inflammation of a mild to moderate level, unassociated with fever, chills, or sweats, turns the differential diagnosis away from infection and toward more chronic joint disorders. Some conditions will resolve; others will progress to a polyarticular presentation. The finding of other involved joints alters the diagnosis significantly, in that the presence of oligoarthritis makes infection and neoplasia much less likely.

I. INFECTIOUS CONDITIONS

    A. Pyogenic bacterial infections. Most untreated pyogenic bacterial infections present in an acute fashion because of their virulence. These processes rarely persist in a chronic fashion unless they are partially treated.

    B. Bacterial osteomyelitis. There is the rare occurrence of bacterial osteomyelitis with an organism that is a low-virulence bacterial pathogen.

    C. Fungal infection in an immunocompromised host, or following penetration of a splinter or plant thorn, may develop subacutely and persist in a single joint.

    D. Lyme arthritis commonly persists from months to years after the primary infection as a recurring, inflammatory monarthritis, most commonly in the knee. Among children in endemic areas, it is as common for the child to have Lyme disease as it is to have JIA.

    E. Tuberculous (TB) arthritis usually presents subacutely as an inflammatory process in a single joint. Often, but not always, there is evidence of prior mycobacterial disease in the lung, a clinical history of travel to or residence in an endemic area for TB, and the patient demonstrates a positive skin test reaction to tuberculin. In contrast to a bacterial process, tuberculous arthritis may arise from a subchondral focus of osteomyelitis and often leads to bony erosions with the absence of joint space narrowing.

II. NONINFECTIOUS INFLAMMATORY DISORDERS

    A. Spondyloarthropathies may be the most common causes of chronic inflammatory monarthritis. Important clinical clues include a family history; the presence of low-back or buttock pain with morning stiffness reflecting spinal involvement or inflammation of the sacroiliac joints; extra-articular features such as pitting of the nails or a scaling skin rash (psoriasis); characteristic skin lesions such as keratoderma blennorrhagicum of the plantar feet or penile circinate balanitis associated with urethritis and conjunctivitis (ReA); a history consistent with inflammatory bowel disease (ulcerative colitis or Crohn's disease); or a history of uveitis.

B. **RA** can present as chronic monarthritis and requires additional months of observation before the typical symmetric joint distribution in the hands and feet develop.

C. **Pauciarticular JIA** is often monarticular. The joint involvement may be much less impressive than the **potentially devastating, asymptomatic chronic iridocyclitis** that can occur in patients with antinuclear antibodies. Older children in the 9 to 11 year age group, who present with pauciarticular disease in the lower extremities, will often develop spondyloarthropathy.

D. **Sarcoid arthropathy** can present as a monarthritis, and the associated erythema nodosum and hilar adenopathy (Löfgren's syndrome) will often suggest the diagnosis. More typically, there will be oligoarthritic involvement, with a prominent periarthritis about the ankles.

III. NONINFLAMMATORY CONDITIONS

A. **Osteoarthritis (OA)** is called osteoarthrosis in Europe to emphasize the low if not absent state of clinically obvious inflammation in this disease. OA usually is of insidious onset, involving the distal and proximal interphalangeal joints of the hands and the weight-bearing joints, in an asymmetrical fashion. It is less common, in the absence of trauma, in the wrist, ankle, elbow, or shoulder. Patients present with pain or brief morning stiffness in one or more hand joints or in a single weight-bearing joint. Symptoms may occur at the end of the day or following activity. Studies reveal normal laboratory data, a noninflammatory joint fluid, and a radiograph that may show asymmetric joint space narrowing, subchondral sclerosis, or osteophyte (spur) formation. The presence of chondrocalcinosis on radiographs may account for symptoms in joints uncommonly involved in OA, such as the wrist or second or third metacarpophalangeal joints.

B. **Internal derangement of the knee.** If untreated, this problem can lead to recurrent effusion, pain, and premature OA.

C. **Avascular necrosis of bone.** Avascular necrosis of bone (also called **osteonecrosis**) is associated with monarticular pain and decreased range of motion in hips, knees, ankles, or shoulders resulting from ischemic necrosis of bone and the underlying bone marrow. Although half of the patients have no obvious cause, this condition is associated with steroid use, systemic lupus erythematosus (SLE) (with or without a history of corticosteroid therapy), alcoholism, hemoglobinopathies, and Gaucher's disease. Avascular necrosis of bone may involve multiple sites, and some of them remain asymptomatic and are defined only radiologically. Typical radiographic changes are subchondral crescent-shaped, lucent areas (the "crescent" sign) within the femoral head. This may be followed by bone remodeling and collapse if weight bearing is not interrupted. In the chronic phase, secondary degenerative changes may occur. If the findings on plain films are normal, an early diagnosis can be made by a nuclear bone scan or MRI (see Chapter 52).

D. **Neoplasia.** As noted in the preceding section, the most common benign joint neoplasms are synovial chondromatosis and pigmented villonodular synovitis. The best preoperative diagnostic test is an MRI study, which will reveal radiolucent cartilaginous or iron-laden synovial lesions.

 ACUTE POLYARTHRITIS

The involvement of two to four joints (oligoarthritis) or more than four joints (polyarthritis) raises the possibility of several diseases listed in Table 14-2. The study of the pattern in which the arthritis develops often serves as a diagnostic aid.

I. **INFECTIOUS CONDITIONS.** When an acutely painful, warm, swollen joint develops, then returns to normal, even as synovitis occurs in another joint, the patient is categorized as having **migratory polyarthritis.** This group of disorders includes important, treatable diseases for which prompt diagnosis is crucial.

A. Bacterial infection. The young adult with migratory polyarthritis, often associated with tenosynovitis and cutaneous pustular lesions, may have a bacterial process such as **disseminated neisserial infection.** Most commonly seen with *Neisseria gonorrhoeae,* the same syndrome can occur with *Neisseria meningitidis.* The skin lesions in both conditions contain fluid that can show gram-negative diplococci. Both require prompt treatment with parenteral antibiotics. Most pyogenic bacteria produce a monarthritis, as does the late presentation of gonococcal arthritis. Polyarticular bacterial arthritis is unusual except in the immunocompromised host (see Chapter 46).

B. Reactive (or postinfectious) arthritis

   1. Acute rheumatic fever should be strongly considered in the young patient with migratory polyarthritis. A search for serologic evidence of a recent streptococcal infection with a rising antistreptolysin O (ASO) titer or a positive Strep Exoenzyme Screen test will support this diagnosis. Although the Jones's criteria are helpful in making the diagnosis, acute rheumatic fever may occur in the absence of carditis, rash, or chorea. The arthritis associated with acute rheumatic fever typically is exquisitely painful, sometimes out of proportion to any effusion or synovitis, and is usually abrupt in onset and associated with an elevated sedimentation rate (see Chapter 49).

   2. ReA can also cause an acute, reactive polyarthritis following dysentery or urethral infection. The arthritis is often more explosive and usually more sustained than in acute rheumatic fever. Patients may or may not demonstrate the characteristic Reiter's triad of arthritis, urethritis, and conjunctivitis.

C. Spirochetal infection. *Borrelia burgdorferi* infection during the primary, early stage of **Lyme disease** can lead to migratory polyarthralgias associated with low-grade fever and symptoms typical of viral infection. Late Lyme disease assumes a more oligoarthritic pattern that waxes and wanes. The diagnosis is supported by the clinical presentation, the presence of an erythema chronicum migrans rash, a history of being in an endemic area of Lyme disease and of tick bite and positive serologic testing.

D. Viral infection. Classically, viral arthritis is polyarticular and may, at times, be migratory. The prodromal, preicteric phase of hepatitis B can present classically with rash and arthritis. Other viruses known to produce a polyarticular presentation are rubella virus (including after vaccination), mumps virus, Epstein-Barr virus (infectious mononucleosis), and parvovirus B19. Parvovirus causes fifth disease or erythema infectiosum, a febrile exanthema in children. It can mimic acute rheumatic fever with a migratory polyarthritis or can produce an RA-like, seronegative (and even at times seropositive) self-limited polyarthritis in adults and some children.

E. Miscellaneous infections. Infections with *Rickettsiae,* fungi, or parasites can lead to polyarticular disease, but are less common.

II. NONINFECTIOUS INFLAMMATORY CONDITIONS

A. Rheumatoid arthritis. Although usually insidious in onset, RA can present with an acute polyarthritis. Early on, these patients may be seronegative for rheumatoid factor, but may have fatigue, anemia, and thrombocytosis. Fever is not commonly seen in RA.

B. Polyarticular JIA may present differently in subsets of children.

   1. The younger child has a **seronegative oligoarthritis** that is often **insidious in onset.** Serum will be positive for antinuclear antibodies in approximately 25%. A potentially destructive, and often asymptomatic iridocyclitis is seen in this group of children.

   2. Another group of children may present with **systemic-onset JIA,** with persistent, high-spiking fevers, a transient salmon-colored truncal rash, hepatosplenomegaly, lymphadenopathy, and polyarticular or oligoarticular joint complaints that develop later.

   3. The preadolescent girl, in contrast, may present with rheumatoid factor positivity, nodules, and an erosive polyarticular joint disease similar to adult RA (see Chapter 36).

C. SLE is a classic immune complex disorder that characteristically presents with an RA-like polyarthritis of the small joints of the hands and feet. Marked proliferative synovitis speaks against a diagnosis of SLE. **Erosive disease is rare in lupus, but the presence of reversible deformity is not.** Other clinical features, such as serositis, fever, skin rash, and renal disease, commonly provide clues to the diagnosis. Laboratory abnormalities can include the presence of serum antinuclear antibodies, anemia, and thrombocytopenia (see Chapter 30).

D. **Other connective tissue diseases (CTDs)** include a spectrum of disorders that produce inflammatory disease of muscles, soft tissues, small blood vessels, and viscera. The initial presentation may include polyarthritis, but more diagnostic features often evolve, including Raynaud's phenomenon with digital infarcts, skin thickening, dysphagia, and pulmonary fibrosis suggestive of scleroderma; proximal myopathy and skin rash characteristic of polymyositis/dermatomyositis; and the overlap features seen in mixed CTD (see Chapters 32 and 34).

E. **Spondyloarthropathies.** This group of diseases is characterized by presence of the class I histocompatibility antigen HLA-B27; axial arthritis, including spondylitis and sacroiliitis; and inflammatory disease of the eye, skin, and ligamentous and tendinous insertions (enthesopathy). The joint pattern is usually oligoarthritic and asymmetric, with involvement of large joints of the lower extremity. Rheumatoid factor and antinuclear antibodies are not found in the serum of these patients. The specific diagnosis is usually defined by the associated clinical features: psoriatic arthritis by the presence of psoriasis, Reiter's syndrome by the concomitant conjunctivitis and urethritis, and enteropathic arthritis by the presence of ulcerative colitis or Crohn's disease.

1. **Ankylosing spondylitis** has perhaps the least association with peripheral joint involvement of the group, with involvement of hip and shoulder arthritis in 25%; it usually presents insidiously with symptoms in the axial spine (see Chapter 39).

2. **Reactive arthritis** typically has a markedly acute presentation of polyarthritis. The triad of conjunctivitis, urethritis, and asymmetric oligoarthritis may not always occur simultaneously, and limited disease has been recognized. Disease onset often follows dysentery or urethritis caused by a number of pathogens, including *Salmonella* and *Shigella*, and *Chlamydia*, respectively. Extra-articular features that are most helpful in diagnosis include circinate balanitis (a psoriasiform rash encircling the glans penis) or a hyperkeratotic rash on the feet (keratoderma blennorrhagicum) (see Chapter 42).

3. **Psoriatic arthritis** can present as asymmetric oligoarticular arthritis of large and small joints, with the tell-tale involvement of the distal interphalangeal joints of the hands; it can also present as a symmetric polyarthritis indistinguishable from RA. Dactylitis, psoriasis, and nail dystrophy are clinical features used to distinguish psoriatic arthritis from RA. Enthesopathy (inflammation of ligamentous or tendon insertions) and joint inflammation cause the classic "sausage digit" or dactylitis that enlarges the joints and soft tissues of the toes or fingers. Nail involvement, often simple pitting, may be present in 60% of patients with arthritis and psoriasis and is found in only 5% of those with psoriasis alone (see Chapter 41).

4. **Enteropathic arthritis** usually presents as an asymmetric polyarthritis of the lower extremities, which can predate known inflammatory bowel disease by months to years. It is typically nonerosive, and the peripheral joint inflammation usually responds to therapy for the underlying bowel disease. The axial arthritis may not respond as well. Clues to the diagnosis include abdominal pain, abnormal bowel movements, erythema nodosum, or pyoderma gangrenosum associated with a spondylitic presentation.

F. **Crystal-induced disease**

1. **Gout** can present as polyarticular disease in the setting of long-established tophi. In men, there generally will be a history of previous, typical, acute monarticular or oligoarticular attacks; however, in postmenopausal women on thiazides, there is a well-described presentation of diffuse tophaceous, polyarticular disease without previous episodic disease. Virtually every joint can be involved, and significant fever and leukocytosis can be present. Diagnostic clues include palpable tophi in the olecranon bursa or along the pinna of the ear, and characteristic erosions with overhanging edges on radiographs of the hands or feet. Characteristic negatively birefringent crystals in the synovial fluid white blood cells and polyarticular or tophaceous disease make a septic process much less likely, but

gout and joint sepsis can coexist. Similarly, gout and pseudogout crystals can be found in the same inflamed joint (see Chapter 43).

2. **CPPD deposition disease.** The presentations of CPPD deposition disease include (a) acute monarticular pseudogout, (b) atypical OA involving the second and third metacarpophalangeal joints, (c) Charcot jointlike knee disease, and (d) polyarticular disease in the hands and wrists that can mimic RA. Clues include radiographic evidence of chondrocalcinosis of the triangular cartilage of the wrist, the symphysis pubis, or the knees, and the identification of typical, weakly positive birefringent rhomboid crystals in synovial fluid white blood cells. As previously discussed, it is important to exclude associated treatable medical illnesses such as hyperparathyroidism and hemochromatosis (see Chapter 44).

G. Serum sickness presents as an acute, sometimes migratory polyarthritis that develops 10 to 14 days after antigen exposure stimulates the formation of immune complexes. The antigen can be antibiotics or other drugs, or biologics such as horse or human antisera. The clinical response is fever, polyarthritis, pruritus, and a rash. The rash is often urticarial and sometimes petechial. Adenopathy and occasionally renal disease may occur. Laboratory assessment reveals mild leukocytosis, normal or mild elevation of the sedimentation rate, rare eosinophilia, and decreased serum complement. The heterophil reaction may be positive, and circulating immune complexes can be detected.

H. Sarcoidosis presents as a periarthritis or polyarthritis associated with hilar adenopathy, erythema nodosum, and fever (Löfgren's syndrome). A similar disorder can occur without adenopathy and can be due to infections (streptococci, TB), inflammatory bowel disease, and drug reactions to nonsteroidal anti-inflammatory drugs (NSAIDs), sulfa drugs, and birth control pills.

I. Vasculitis
1. **Small-vessel involvement.** Polyarthritis may be seen in types of vasculitis in which **small vessels** are inflamed. This includes the leukocytoclastic angiitis of **Henoch-Schönlein purpura.** Typically, dependent and at times confluent areas of nonthrombocytopenic purpura are present from the feet to the waistline in association with inflammatory arthritis of the ankles and knees.
2. **Medium-sized vessel involvement.** An inflammatory arthritis may also be present when medium-sized vessel involvement leads to systemic necrotizing vasculitides such as polyarteritis nodosa.
3. In children, **Kawasaki's disease** is characterized by a febrile exanthem associated with adenopathy, mucositis, ocular changes, and devastating coronary arteritis. This disorder, the most common vasculitis of childhood, causes an inflammatory polyarthritis in one-third of patients (see Chapter 36).

J. Hematologic disorders. Polyarthritis may be the presenting or early manifestation of leukemia, lymphoma, or sickle cell disease. Diagnostic clues are periarticular pain, bone pain, and nocturnal pain, as well as an associated known hematologic disorder. In children who present with these symptoms, a bone marrow aspirate is indicated, even in the presence of a normal peripheral blood smear.

 CHRONIC POLYARTHRITIS

This arthritis pattern is defined by involvement of four or more joints and persists longer than 2 months.

I. RHEUMATOID ARTHRITIS. The arthritis is usually an **additive** (joints do not return to normal between episodes), **symmetric polyarthritis** of the small joints of the hands and feet. Larger joints of the upper and lower extremities and neck are also commonly involved. Rheumatoid factor may not be present in the serum early in the disease. However, eventually 80% of patients are positive for rheumatoid factor. Extra-articular manifestations include constitutional features such as weight loss and fatigue, subcutaneous nodules, and anemia, but not fever (see Chapter 29).

II. SYSTEMIC LUPUS ERYTHEMATOSUS. Approximately 70% of patients will present with joint complaints. The arthropathy is usually an RA-like polyarthritis that is nonerosive. The diagnosis of SLE is based on the multisystem clinical presentation and is supported by the finding of serum antinuclear antibodies.

III. **OTHER CONNECTIVE TISSUE DISEASES AND OVERLAP SYNDROMES**
  A. **Scleroderma** (progressive systemic sclerosis) often produces arthralgias and morning stiffness, but signs of joint inflammation are uncommon. The diagnosis of scleroderma is based on a history of the Raynaud's phenomenon, and a multisystem illness involving the lungs, kidneys, and gastrointestinal tract, with its characteristic skin findings and tendon rubs.
  B. **Polymyositis.** Arthralgias may be reported in about one-third of patients with polymyositis, but joint problems are not a major aspect of this disease.
  C. **Overlap syndrome** is a term that recognizes that CTDs such as RA, SLE, scleroderma, and polymyositis have overlapping clinical and serologic features.
IV. **SPONDYLOARTHROPATHIES.** In patients with psoriatic arthritis, ReA, or ankylosing spondylitis, a chronic phase commonly develops. Characteristic features include sacroiliitis, asymmetric oligoarthritis or polyarthritis of the lower extremities, and spondylitis. Even ReA, with its typical episodic flares of activity, becomes chronic in approximately 75% of patients.
V. **CRYSTAL-INDUCED DISEASE.** As acute gouty attacks become more frequent, the joints may no longer return to normal. Patients begin to experience constant symptoms, including morning stiffness. Radiographs of patients with untreated chronic tophaceous gout can sometimes demonstrate joint changes similar to those of RA; such abnormalities may also be seen with the symmetric, polyarticular variant of CPPD deposition disease.
VI. **OSTEOARTHRITIS.** Despite the lack of systemic features, OA in some individuals can be diffuse in distribution, mildly inflammatory, and associated with significant, even if slowly progressive, deformity and disability. The joint distribution typically involves the first carpometacarpal joint of the thumb; first metatarsophalangeal joint; distal and proximal interphalangeal joints of the hands, hips, and knees; and the cervical and lumbar spine (see Chapter 51).

MUSCLE PAIN AND WEAKNESS
Lawrence J. Kagen

15

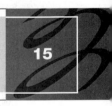

■ KEY POINTS

■ Consider the etiology of muscle pain and weakness in several categories.

■ Important diagnostic considerations should include the following: Is the presentation myopathic? Is the nervous system (central or peripheral) involved? Are there vascular factors to be considered? What medications and genetic, hormonal, or metabolic factors may play a role?

■ Laboratory testing (e.g., levels of enzymes, myoglobin, and creatinuria) is a useful indicator of the severity of myopathy.

■ Electromyography (EMG) is useful in distinguishing neurogenic from myopathic etiologies.

■ Magnetic resonance imaging (MRI) and ultrasonography are helpful in diagnosis, in selection of site for possible biopsy, and in determination of the extent and activity of the disease.

■ Muscle biopsy generally places the diagnosis of myopathy on its most secure footing.

*S*ymptoms of muscle pain (myalgia) and weakness are commonly encountered in clinical medicine. The history to evaluate these problems in affected patients should include not only the site(s), duration, character, and functional limitations but also the family background, medications taken, and other possible comorbid conditions.

ETIOPATHOGENESIS

I. **Myalgia and weakness can be considered under several etiologic categories**
   A. **Myopathies.** These disorders usually are manifested in proximal musculature and present initially with pain and weakness. Atrophy is generally a late finding. The causes of myopathies are many but an abbreviated list would include:
   1. **Inflammatory disorders.** Dermatomyositis, polymyositis, inclusion body myositis, other connective tissue disorders, especially scleroderma, and Sjögren's syndrome. Systemic lupus erythematosus (SLE), rheumatoid arthritis (RA), and sarcoidosis may also have myositis as a feature.
   2. **Endocrinopathies.** Many endocrine disorders affect muscles and their function (see Chapter 55). The most commonly encountered are thyroid diseases and diabetes.
   3. **Electrolyte disturbances.** Particularly those involving calcium, magnesium, sodium, and potassium.
   4. **Medications and toxins.** Such as the statin agents, penicillamine, and alcohol. Cocaine use may also lead to myopathy.
   5. **Genetic diseases.** The muscular dystrophies, particularly facioscapular humeral dystrophy, and the distal myopathies in adults should be considered in this category.
   6. **Metabolic disorders.** Genetic abnormalities of carbohydrate and lipid metabolism can produce pain and exercise intolerance.
   B. **Neurologic disorders**
   1. **Upper motor neuron diseases.** Diseases of the brain such as hemorrhage, infarction, infection, or neoplasm may be the cause of weakness and loss of function. Generally, the severity of involvement, its anatomical location, reflex abnormalities, sensory disturbances, and impaired cerebral function will alert the examiner to abnormalities in this area.
   2. **Spinal nerve root disorders.** Spinal stenosis causes muscle aching and heaviness, generally of the lower extremities, on exertion and may mimic symptoms of vascular ischemia.
   3. **Lower motor neuron disorders.** The presence of atrophic, flaccid musculature, with cramps, fasciculations, and loss of deep tendon reflexes characterizes these disorders.
   4. **Peripheral neuropathies.** Neuropathies of this type usually are associated with sensory loss. Weakness, if present, often begins in distal musculature. Atrophy and loss of deep tendon reflexes occur.
   5. **Myoneural junction disorders.** Myasthenic syndromes may appear similar to myopathies in many aspects. Ocular or facial involvement and marked fatigue are important characteristics.
   C. **Other disorders producing muscle symptoms**
   1. **Vascular.** Ischemia due to arterial disease may cause severe muscle pain, especially with exertion, generally of distal musculature.
   2. **Polymyalgia rheumatica.** This disorder, usually seen in elderly patients, is characterized by severe, often disabling, muscle and joint pain, stiffness, and soreness in the proximal regions that are particularly worse in the morning. Giant cell arteritis may be associated with this disorder.
   3. **Fibromyalgia.** This is a disorder of uncertain etiology characterized by muscle pain, fatigue, tenderness, and other manifestations often occurring in the presence of psychological stress.
   The reader should be aware that the above listing is presented as an initial step to organize an evaluation of the patient's symptoms. It is not intended to be a complete list of neurologic and myopathic disorders or their manifestations.
   It also should be kept in mind that more than one etiologic process may be present in a given circumstance. For example, coexistent hypothyroidism can worsen the muscle disease associated with polymyositis.

PREVALENCE

Information on the frequency of these disorders will be found under the appropriate chapter headings.

CLINICAL MANIFESTATIONS

I. **Weakness is a major problem** for patients with myopathy. In most cases, proximal musculature is primarily affected.
    A. **For the upper extremities,** tasks such as lifting objects, brushing teeth, using a hairdryer, hanging up clothing, or putting objects into cabinets or refrigerators will be difficult. Distal musculature used for fine manipulation (such as writing) will often be preserved in early stages but may be affected in severe and/or chronic disorders.
        Inclusion body myositis and myotonic dystrophy, however, are two examples of myopathies that demonstrate distal weakness early in the course.
    B. **With regard to the lower extremities,** difficulty in arising from a low seat or couch, crouching, climbing stairs, getting in and out of automobiles or buses, or lifting the legs to put on trousers, shoes, or socks can occur.
    C. **Muscles of the trunk** may also be affected. Rising from bed may require a lateral rolling maneuver while swinging the legs downward and pressing against the bed with the arms.
    D. **Respiratory muscle involvement** may be present and might be subtle in manifestation. Dyspnea can occur, although weakness of skeletal musculature may curtail activity and reduce the expression of this symptom. However, dyspnea can be seen early in inflammatory myopathies, both as a consequence of respiratory muscle involvement and the presence of associated interstitial pulmonary disease.
        Dyspnea is also noted in patients with acid maltase deficiency and carnitine deficiency.
    E. **Facial weakness is uncommon** in patients with myopathy but does occur in facioscapulohumeral dystrophy and myotonic dystrophy. Eyelid ptosis is a feature of myasthenia gravis and the Kearns-Sayres type of mitochondrial myopathy. Palatal weakness is uncommon in myopathies but dysphagia and change in phonation can occur in patients with inflammatory myopathy.
II. **Myalgia** or muscle pain can be a presenting complaint in a number of disorders. It may be an early feature of inflammatory muscle disease, infection-related myositis such as trichinosis or viral illnesses, or ischemic muscle disease in diabetes. Myalgia is a cardinal feature in polymyalgia rheumatica and fibromyalgia.
    A. **Stiffness** and pain may characterize a number of the connective tissue disorders. Myotonic dystrophy may present with stiffness and cramps. Painful sustained involuntary contractions occur in lower motor neuron disorders and pain on exertion can be noted in the metabolic myopathies of glycogen and lipid metabolism as well as in the mitochondrial myopathies.
    B. **Cramping pains** on exertion also occur in the myopathy associated with ingestion of lipid lowering agents.
    C. **Claudication** syndromes related to ischemia or spinal stenosis also produce muscle aching on exertion. An outline of causes of myalgia is shown in Table 15-1.
III. **Physical examination is essential** in documenting and assessing the nature and the degree of involvement because loss of strength is a central feature of most myopathies, especially in the context of the history of loss of function in relation to activities of daily living. However, pain, fatigue, and malaise can interfere with the patient's effort and complicate the examiner's physical assessment.
    A. Even so, objective information on function and strength obtained at each evaluation will facilitate the physician's task of discerning the course of illness and its response to therapeutic measures.

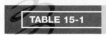

TABLE 15-1	Myalgia: Etiologic Considerations

1 Inflammatory-dermatomyositis, polymyositis, inclusion body myositis, and connective tissue disorders
2 Vascular–arterial ischemia
3 Neurogenic–spinal stenosis, lower motor neuron disorders
4 Infections—localized or systemic (e.g., bacterial, viral, and parasitic)
5 Medications and toxins
6 Electrolyte disorders (especially Na^+, K^+, Mg^{2+}, Ca^{2+})
7 Endocrinopathies (e.g., hypothyroidism)
8 Metabolic and genetic disorders (e.g., of lipid and carbohydrate metabolism)
9 Others (e.g., fibromyalgia and polymyalgia rheumatica)

B. A commonly used grading scheme for muscle strength is shown in Table 15-2. It is possible to increase the resolution of differences in strength in this scheme by the addition of the sign (+) or (−) for intermediate performance between grades.

DIAGNOSTIC INVESTIGATIONS

I. LABORATORY TESTS

A. Muscle enzymes.
These proteins leak from the muscle cell during the course of myopathy and are detected in increased amounts in serum.

1. **Creatine kinase (CK)** activity has proven to be a useful guide to muscle disorders and their severity. CK is present in the highest concentration in muscular and nervous systems. This enzyme catalyzes the interconversion of adenosine triphosphate (ATP) and creatine phosphate, controlling the flow of high-energy phosphate within the cell. During injury or inflammation, rapid rises in blood CK concentration occur earlier and in higher concentrations than those of the other commonly tested enzymes.

2. **Aspartate aminotransferase (AST) and alanine aminotransferase (ALT)** are both found in many tissues of the body including muscle tissues. In patients with a myopathy, serum AST is more frequently elevated than ALT.

3. **Lactate dehydrogenase (LDH),** which catalyzes the interconversion of pyruvate and lactate, and **aldolase,** which catalyzes the splitting of fructose phosphate into two fragments, are both widely distributed in body tissues. Aldolase A is a major form in skeletal muscle. The activities of both these enzymes are increased in serum in the course of myopathy and their concentration may remain elevated for a longer period than that of CK.

TABLE 15-2	Muscle Strength Testing

Grade	Muscle strength
0	No contraction detectable
1	Contraction observed—no motion produced
2	Motion produced but not enough to overcome gravity
3	Can only overcome gravity
4	Can overcome moderate resistance
5	Can overcome considerable manual resistance

B. Myoglobin is the heme-containing, oxygen-binding protein of both skeletal and cardiac muscles. Elevations in serum content of myoglobin have greater specificity for muscle than do those of the enzymes. Levels of myoglobinemia can be used as an indicator of the severity and course of myopathy.

In severe states of muscle damage (rhabdomyolysis), marked myoglobinemia may lead to myoglobinuria after renal clearance, which may be associated with a risk of renal failure in the presence of increased concentration of myoglobin.

C. Creatinuria can occur not only in active myopathies but also in any condition leading to muscle atrophy. This is due to two factors: Creatine uptake from the circulation by the muscle cell (to be used to store energy as creatine phosphate) is decreased and its retention within the muscle is diminished. Both circumstances lead to an increased level of creatine being delivered to the kidney for excretion.

II. OTHER DIAGNOSTIC TESTS

A. Electromyography (EMG) and nerve conduction. These techniques can be useful in distinguishing neurogenic from myogenic causes of muscle pain and weakness.

B. Imaging techniques. Magnetic resonance imaging (MRI) and ultrasonography can not only provide diagnostic information but can also help in selecting sites for biopsy and in defining extent or activity of disease and response to treatment.

C. Muscle biopsy. Histologic, and in some cases biochemical, assessment of affected muscle tissues can be an extremely valuable guide to diagnosis. Actively inflamed, but not end-stage atrophic, muscle is generally most suitable for sampling.

 DIFFERENTIAL DIAGNOSIS

Areas to be considered are briefly mentioned in the preceding text.

 TREATMENT AND PROGNOSIS

See chapters referring to specific disorders (especially Chapter 32).

RASH AND ARTHRITIS

Henry Lee, Rachelle Scott, and Animesh A. Sinha

16

■ KEY POINTS

■ Mucocutaneous lesions are an important clinical feature of a number of conditions presenting with arthritis, ranging from infectious to autoimmune etiologies.

■ Detailed cutaneous examination, including an examination of nail folds, genitalia, and oral mucosa, may aid in the proper diagnosis.

■ Description of mucocutaneous lesions should include the color, shape, and morphology of the primary lesion, the pattern in which the lesion occurs, and its distribution.

■ Biopsy of the lesion may aid in proper diagnosis. Immunofluorescent (IF) studies and tissue culture should be analyzed in appropriate cases.

INTRODUCTION

I. The differential diagnosis and approach to arthritis and rash are complex. Cutaneous lesions may provide insights into the underlying disease and diagnosis.

II. Mucocutaneous lesions may precede other systemic symptoms and may herald the onset of a multisystemic disease process. The diagnosis of several rheumatologic conditions relies on dermatologic manifestations as part of the diagnostic criteria, reinforcing the importance of a thorough cutaneous examination. In Table 16-1, we discuss some of the basic terminology of the morphology and the description of cutaneous lesions. In Table 16-2, we categorize the diseases that commonly present with both arthritis and rash according to their etiologies. This chapter follows the organization set in Table 16-2.

III. Although many of the diseases are protean and overlap in their presentations, in Table 16-3 we outline a basic guide to some of the primary lesions that may aid the physician in arriving at the proper diagnosis. The goal of this chapter is to provide the physician with diagnostic information about specific cutaneous findings in each disorder and to offer insights to these multisystemic conditions through the perspective of a dermatologist.

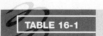 **TABLE 16-1**   **Fundamental Dermatologic Descriptive Terminology**

Term	Definition
Macule	A flat area of color change that is nonpalpable, <1 cm in diameter
Patch	A large macule >1 cm in diameter
Papule	A solid elevation, palpable with no visible fluid, <1 cm in diameter
Plaque	A large papule >1 cm in diameter
Nodule	A palpable, solid, round, or ellipsoidal lesion; depth of lesion and/or palpability may differentiate it from papule
Wheal	An evanescent, edematous, and flat-topped elevation of various sizes; no surface change, as the epidermis is unaffected
Vesicle	A circumscribed elevation that, unlike papules, contains fluid, <1 cm in diameter
Bulla	A large vesicle >1 cm in diameter
Pustule	An elevation similar to vesicles that contains purulent material (composed of leukocytes, ±cellular debris, ±bacteria)
Scale	An accumulation of stratum corneum; can vary in color and texture
Crust	Dried serum, pus, or blood resulting in hardened debris ±epithelial cells, ±bacterial debris
Excoriation	An abrasion produced by mechanical means
Fissure	A linear cleft through the epidermis with variable involvement of dermis
Erosion	Loss of all or portion of epidermis; if only epidermis is involved, there is no scar
Ulcer	An excavation that has lost its epidermis and some of its dermis. Will form scars with healing (dermis involvement)
Telangiectasia	Dilated, small vascular lesion that blanches with pressure
Atrophy	Thinning of skin that may affect any level of skin; loss of skin surface texture and structures ±translucency
Petechia	An intradermal hemorrhage that is nonpalpable <3 mm in diameter
Purpura	A large petechia that is >3mm in diameter
Poikiloderma	Triad of atrophy, telangiectasia, and pigmentary change (hyper- or hypopigmented)
Alopecia	Loss of hair; usually categorized as scarring vs. nonscarring

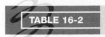

TABLE 16-2	Diseases that Manifest with Both Cutaneous and Joint Complaints

1. Spondyloarthropathy
   a. Reactive arthritis
   b. Psoriatic arthritis
   c. Inflammatory bowel disease
2. Lupus erythematosus
3. Dermatomyositis/polymyositis
4. Systemic scleroderma–mixed connective tissue disorder
5. Sjögren's syndrome
6. Rheumatoid arthritis
7. Juvenile idiopathic arthritis
8. Vasculitis
   a. Small-sized vessel vasculitis (e.g., LCV, HSP, mixed cryoglobulinemia, and UV)
   b. Medium-sized vessel vasculitis (e.g., PAN)
   c. ANCA-positive vasculitides (e.g., WG, CS, and MPA)
9. Behçet's disease
10. Sarcoidosis
11. Multicentric reticulohistiocytosis
12. Relapsing polychondritis
13. Acne fulminans
14. Sweet's syndrome
15. Pyodermic gangrenosum
16. Erythema nodosum
17. Infections
    a. Viral (e.g., parvovirus B19, rubella, varicella-zoster, and hepatitis B/C)
    b. Bacterial (e.g., disseminated gonorrhea infection, acute meningococcemia, syphilis, Lyme disease, and mycobacterium)
    c. Fungal (e.g., sporotrichosis, candida, histoplasmosis, coccidioidomycosis, and cryptococcosis)
    d. Rheumatic fever–postinfectious condition

ANCA, antineutrophil cytoplasmic antibodies; CS, Churg-Strauss; HSP, Henoch-Schönlein purpura; LCV, leukocytoclastic vasculitis; MPA, microscopic polyangiitis; PAN, polyarteritis nodosa; UV, urticarial vasculitis; WG, Wegener's granulomatosis.

DISEASE STATES

I. **Spondyloarthropathies** (see Chapter 39) refer to a family of disorders that share a predilection for spinal and sacroiliac joint inflammation and enthesitis. Mucocutaneous findings are prominent in three of these disorders.

A. **Reactive arthritis** (see Chapter 42) was originally described as a triad of arthritis, conjunctivitis, and nongonococcal urethritis. Many have expanded this triad to a tetrad to include mucocutaneous lesions.

1. **Balanitis circinata** are moist superficial ulcers on the glans or corona of the penis and may coalesce to give a circinate appearance. They are reported to occur in approximately 36% of patients. Erosion, erythema, and asymptomatic superficial ulcers may be seen in the mouth and pharynx.

2. **Keratoderma blennorrhagica** are hyperkeratotic papules and plaques usually found on the palms and soles. These lesions begin as clear vesicles on an erythematous base and cannot be clinically differentiated from pustular psoriasis. The less specific findings of psoriasiform dermatitis and erythroderma can be found in a subset of patients.

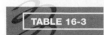

| TABLE 16-3 | Characteristic Cutaneous Morphologies of Selected Conditions Presenting with Arthritis and Skin Findings |

Erythematous papules/plaques	Ulcers
Psoriasis	Reactive arthritis
SCLE	Behçet's disease
DLE	Pyoderma gangrenosum
Gottron's papules	Vasculitis
Sarcoid-lupus pernio	Sarcoidosis
Secondary syphillis	**Nodules**
Sweet's syndrome "relief of mountain range"	Erythema nodosum
	Lupus profundus
Lyme-ECM	Rheumatic fever nodules
Secondary syphilis	Vasculitis
Disseminated gonorrhea infection	Sarcoidosis
Erythematous-violaceous patches	**Hyperkeratotic palms/soles**
ACLE (i.e., malar rash)	Reactive arthritis/Reiter's (keratoderma blennorrhagica)
DM-heliotrope rash (more violaceous)	Palmoplantar psoriasis
DM–shawl sign	
Parvovirus–slapped cheek	**Palpable purpura**
Lyme-ECM	Vasculitis (i.e., LCV)
Rheumatic fever–erythema marginatum	**Erythematous macules**
Annular plaques	JIA—generalized erythematous macules
SCLE	Rubella
DLE	
Sarcoid	**Calcinosis cutis**
Psoriasis	DM
	Scleroderma

Please note that this is a simplified categorization. Many of the above entities may present in a number of manifestations.
ACLE, acute cutaneous lupus erythematosus; DLE, discoid lupus erythematosus; DM, dermatomyositis; ECM, erythema chronicum migrans; JIA, juvenile idiopathic arthritis; LCV, leukocytoclastic vasculitis; SCLE, subacute cutaneous lupus erythematosus.

3. Nail changes include erythema of the nail fold, subungual hyperkeratotic deposits, onychodystrophy (abnormal growth of nails), and a yellowish discoloration of the nails.
4. **Treatment of simple mucocutaneous lesions.** Topical corticosteroids and topical keratolytics (i.e., 20% salicylic ointment) if necessary.

B. **Psoriatic arthritis** (see Chapter 41) is broadly defined as an inflammatory arthritis associated with the cutaneous findings of psoriasis. These patients are often rheumatoid factor (RF) negative. The arthritis exhibits a more limited involvement of the spine, when compared to other types of spondyloarthropathy, and exhibits more peripheral involvement of the joints.
   1. Cutaneous lesions usually precede arthritic complaints.
   2. Classic **psoriasis vulgaris** cutaneous lesions are described as well-demarcated erythematous plaques with nonadherent scale that are commonly found on elbows, knees, scalp, and lumbosacral region.
   3. **Inverse psoriasis** localizes to intertriginous area (usually no scale).
   4. **Guttate psoriasis** presents as small teardrop-shaped psoriatic lesions.
   5. **Pustular psoriasis** presents as sterile pustules that may coalesce to form "lakes of pus." It may be accompanied by fever and leukocytosis.
   6. **Palmoplantar psoriasis** presents as pustules on soles and palms that progress to scaly, erythematous patches/plaques.
   7. **Erythroderma** presents as thickened, erythematous, and scaly skin.

8. **Nail changes** can be associated with any form of psoriasis. These changes are seen in 80% of psoriatic arthritis and only 30% of pure cutaneous psoriasis. Nail findings include "**oil spots**" (yellow–brown spots), **nail pits, onycholysis,** and **onychodystrophy.**
9. **Auspitz sign** is the removal of scale, which leads to punctate blood drop.
10. **Köbner phenomenon** is the appearance of new lesions at sites of trauma.
11. Medications that may cause a flare include β-blockers, lithium, and chloroquine. Withdrawal of systemic steroids may cause a flare.
12. Topical treatments for rash include topical corticosteroids and vitamin D_3 analogs (i.e., calcipotriol). They are often used together.
13. Systemic treatments include psoralen plus ultraviolet A (UVA), narrow band ultraviolet B (UVB), retinoids, methotrexate, cyclosporine, and biologic agents (i.e., etanercept, infliximab, adalimumab, efalizumab, and alefacept). The use of systemic steroid leads to transient improvement but patients may experience withdrawal flare.

C. **Inflammatory bowel disease (IBD)–related spondyloarthropathy** (see Chapter 40)
1. **Erythema nodosum (EN)** occurs in approximately 7% or less of patients with ulcerative colitis.
2. **Pyoderma gangrenosum** (see section **XII** of this chapter) occurs in approximately 1% of patients with Crohn's disease and approximately 5% of patients with ulcerative colitis.
3. Patients may also exhibit aphthous ulcers and nutritional deficiencies.

II. **SYSTEMIC LUPUS ERYTHEMATOSUS (SLE)** (see Chapter 30).
A. **Acute cutaneous lupus erythematosus (ACLE)** includes malar rash but can occur elsewhere on the body. **Malar** or "butterfly" rash presents as an erythema that covers the cheeks and nose (may extend onto forehead and chin). Lesions are often exacerbated by sunlight (see Table 16-4A for a differential diagnosis).
B. **Subacute cutaneous lupus erythematosus (SCLE)** lesions are papulosquamous or annular plaques. The papulosquamous plaques are confluent and discrete erythematous papules and plaques with scales. The annular plaques often coalesce into larger plaques, forming polycyclic shapes. The borders remain erythematous but the central areas exhibit subtle hypopigmentation and telangiectasia. These lesions are nonscarring and predominantly affect white women (see Table 16-4B for a differential diagnosis).
1. High frequency of anti-Ro antibodies is observed in patients with SCLE (approximately 70% of patients).
2. Approximately 50% of patients meet the SLE criteria but only 10% will develop severe disease.
C. **Chronic cutaneous lupus erythematosus (CCLE)** lesions include a variety of lesions, of which discoid lupus is the most prevalent.
D. **Discoid lupus erythematosus (DLE)** lesions are well-demarcated erythematous plaques with scale. As lesions mature, they may develop central atrophy. Keratinous plugging of hair follicles can be seen as tiny spikes across the lesion. Lesions are often found on the face, scalp, neck, and ears. Lesions may cause scarring. Approximately 5% of patients will go on to develop SLE (see Table 16-4C for a differential diagnosis).

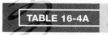

TABLE 16-4A	Differential Diagnosis of the Malar Rash of Acute Cutaneous Lupus Erythematosus

Dermatomyositis
Parvovirus
Photoallergic/phototoxic reaction
Seborrheic dermatitis
Acne rosacea
Polymorphous light eruption

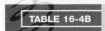

| TABLE 16-4B | Differential Diagnosis of Subacute Cutaneous Lupus Erythematosus |

Psoriasis
Dermatomyositis
Nummular eczema
Polymorphous light eruption
Contact dermatitis
Dermatophyte infection (i.e., Tinea corporis)
Cutaneous T-cell lymphoma

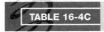

| TABLE 16-4C | Differential Diagnosis of Discoid Lupus Erythematosus, Facial Erythematous Plaque |

Condition	Significant cutaneous findings
Discoid lupus	Erythematous to violaceous well-demarcated plaque with follicular plugging May develop central atrophy
Dermatomyositis-heliotrope rash	Violaceous, on eyelids, and no follicular plugging seen
Sarcoid-lupus pernio	Violaceous, smooth, and shiny small nodule, plaque on nose/cheek/ear
Seborrheic dermatitis	Erythema typically involving the nasolabial fold, eyebrows, ears, and/or hairline; often has characteristic "greasy," yellow scale
Acne rosacea	Erythematous papules/plaques, pustules, often with telangiectasias
Polymorphous light eruption	Papule/edematous, indurated plaque without follicular plugging, usually occurs in spring 1–4 d after sun exposure
Chronic contact dermatitis	Ill-defined erythematous edematous plaque with scale, no follicular plugging, no atrophy
Tinea facei	Erythematous plaque with slight scale and indistinct borders, no follicular plugging, no central atrophy; potassium hydroxide smear shows dermatophyte
Lupus vulgaris (tuberculosis)	Typically, single plaque composed of grouped red–brown papule with adherent scales; may lead to ulceration; no follicular plugging

E. **Lupus profundus** lesions are deep subcutaneous nodules.
F. **Lupus tumidus** lesions include dermal mucin deposition, which leads to indurated, edematous erythematous plaques.
G. **Hypertrophic discoid lupus** lesions are verrucous and hyperkeratotic DLE.
H. **Chilblain lupus** lesions include erythematous to violaceous patches/plaques elicited by cold temperatures. These lesions are usually found on distal acral sites, elbows, and nose.
I. **Raynaud's phenomenon** is seen in up to 30% of cases (see Chapter 17).
J. **Periungual telangiectasias** develop on the fingers. This finding also commonly occurs in scleroderma and dermatomyositis (DM).
K. Two forms of **alopecia** are seen in LE. The first form, scarring alopecia secondary to DLE, is irreversible. The second form is a diffuse or patchy, nonscarring reversible alopecia.
L. **Vasculitis.** Any of the manifestations discussed in section **VIII.B.1** of this chapter may develop as a result of vasculitis.
M. **Lupus band test (LBT)** demonstrates immunoglobulin (Ig) and complement deposition at the dermal–epidermal junction by direct immunofluorescent (IF) staining. Positive LBT response may suggest lupus. Clinically normal skin of patients

with DLE exhibit a negative LBT response. Among patients with SLE and normal sun-protected skin, 50% have a positive LBT response, whereas among those patients with SLE and normal sun-exposed skin, 80% have a positive LBT response.

N. Treatment
1. Potent topical steroids have the risk of atrophy.
2. Antimalarials are the most popular initial systemic agents. **Hydroxychloroquine** 6 to 6.5 mg/kg/day to a maximum 400 mg/day is the recommended dosage. Quinacrine 100 mg/day may be added to the regimen if no improvement is observed in 2 to 3 months. Chloroquine can be used to replace hydroxychloroquine if there is no improvement. After achieving control, hydroxychloroquine should be decreased to 200 mg/day as maintenance dose.

III. DERMATOMYOSITIS (DM) (see Chapter 32)
   A. Cutaneous lesions of this disease are seen in 30% to 40% of adult patients and in approximately 95% of pediatric patients. Cutaneous lesions often predate musculoskeletal findings.
   B. Gottron's papules are pathognomonic of DM. They are violaceous, flat-topped papules that usually appear on the extensor aspects of the interphalangeal joints.
   C. Gottron's sign includes confluent, scaly erythematous patches on the dorsal surface of the digits and the extensor surfaces of the upper extremities.
   D. Heliotrope rash is a violaceous discoloration of the upper eyelid. It is often accompanied by edema.
   E. Diffuse erythematous patches located in a **"shawl-like"** distribution, involving the back, shoulder, and a V-shaped distribution of the anterior chest.
   F. Calcinosis cutis of skin, fascia, and muscle may occur, especially in children.
   G. Other findings include Raynaud's phenomenon and ulcerations or leukoplakia of mucous membranes.
   H. It may be difficult to distinguish DM from SLE. DM lesions preferentially involve dorsal interphalangeal joints, whereas SLE lesions usually spare them. Gottron's sign, heliotrope rash, and "shawl sign" support a diagnosis of DM.
   I. There is no relation between extent of cutaneous lesions and severity of myositis.
   J. Treatment. The therapeutic modalities are similar to SLE treatment options. Antimalarials have similarly been used to treat DM skin disease but the results have not been as promising. Systemic corticosteroids are the mainstay of therapy.

IV. SYSTEMIC SCLERODERMA (see Chapter 34). Scleroderma covers a wide spectrum of clinical entities, encompassing systemic sclerosis (including diffuse scleroderma and CREST syndrome) and localized scleroderma. The systemic form can involve the skin and can manifest musculoskeletal pathology and is discussed here; localized scleroderma is not discussed.
   A. The classic cutaneous finding is that of skin thickening, which usually begins specifically on the fingers/hands as erythema and swelling. The skin is taut or "bound down" and shiny. Hair growth is sparse and there is a loss of superficial skin landmarks. **Sclerodactyly** describes the above findings applied to the digits.
   B. The above skin changes may result in joint contractures primarily over small joints. Hand contractures may develop, which result in a "claw hand" deformity. Ulcerations may also occur.
   C. Development of "masklike" or expressionless facies is typical. There may be perioral furrowing. Patients develop limited oral opening. The nose may become pinched and "beaklike."
   D. "Neck sign" is ridging and tightening of the skin on extending the head.
   E. Telangiectasias (often matlike) occur in 50% of patients with diffuse sclerosis and can appear on the face, tongue, mucous membranes, gastrointestinal (GI) tract, and extremities.
   F. Calcinosis cutis occurs in approximately one-third of limited scleroderma and 10% of diffuse disease.
   G. Pterygium inversum unguis (distal portion of the nail bed remains adherent to ventral surface of nail plate) is seen in scleroderma and lupus. Approximately 80% of patients display dilated nail fold capillaries forming "giant" loops.
   H. Raynaud's phenomenon (see Chapter 17).

    I. Pigment abnormalities seen as either hypo- or hyperpigmented patches may occur. Hypopigmented patches that retain perifollicular pigment, resembling repigmenting vitiligo, have been described. Alopecia and anhidrosis may also be observed in affected areas.

    J. The extent of skin involvement correlates with internal organ disease and survival.

    K. CREST syndrome consists of calcinosis, Raynaud's phenomenon, esophageal dysfunction, sclerodactyly, and telangiectasia.

    L. Mixed connective tissue disease (MCTD) presents as an overlap between SLE, scleroderma, and DM. The condition is marked by high titers of anti-U1RNP antibodies. Raynaud's phenomenon and swollen hands are prominent features. Patients may have other skin changes associated with classic SLE.

    M. Arthritis. Early in the disease, many patients complain of arthralgias, which primarily involve both distal and proximal extremities. Joint inflammation and effusions are rare. Joint contractions and fibrosis of tendons does occur.

    N. Treatment

        1. Localized sclerotic skin. Case reports show that UVA, topical corticosteroids, topical calcipotriene, low-dose methotrexate, and D-penicillamine may increase skin softening or reduction in the involved area.

        2. Pruritus is managed with emollients and antihistamines. Topical steroids are rarely helpful.

        3. Telangiectasias are covered with cosmetic products or treated with laser therapy.

        4. There are no treatment guidelines for calcinosis cutis. Case reports show that diltiazem, but not verapamil, may improve the condition.

        5. Double-blinded studies have shown that both nifedipine and losartan reduce the number of Raynaud's attacks and perhaps the severity of the attacks.

V. **Sjögren's syndrome** (see Chapter 33) is an autoimmune multisystemic inflammatory disorder characterized by dryness of mucous membranes.

    A. The hallmark cutaneous finding is xerosis of skin and dry mucous membranes (e.g., oral, eyes, and vagina).

    B. Approximately 30% of primary patients with Sjögren's syndrome develop cutaneous vasculitis, of whom approximately 85% present with palpable purpura.

    C. Rare annular erythematous lesions are seen primarily in Japanese patients.

    D. There are documented cases of a cutaneous lupus and Sjögren's syndrome overlap. These patients typically present with SCLE lesions and are anti-Ro positive.

    E. Treatment options are primarily symptomatic.

        1. Symptomatic relief can be obtained with emollients and humidifier.

        2. Cutaneous vasculitis should prompt systemic evaluation.

        3. Infliximab failed to show statistical improvement in a recent randomized, double-blinded, placebo trial.

VI. **RHEUMATOID ARTHRITIS (RA)** (see Chapter 29). Rheumatoid nodules occur in up to 20% to 35% of patients with RA, most of whom are RF positive. The lesions are firm, nontender, flesh-colored papules or nodules, most frequently located subcutaneously. They are mobile and commonly affect pressure points (i.e., extensor surface of the forearms and the olecranon bursal region). They are not pathognomonic for RA and are found in other connective tissue disorders. They may ulcerate, may drain, and get infected. Small, painful nodules can occur on the fingers, and may be caused by methotrexate therapy.

    A. Vasculitic lesions are found on the digits. They present as nail infarcts, red or purpuric macules or papules that can progress to painful subcutaneous nodules or ulcers 2 to 3 mm in size. Leukocytoclastic vasculitis (LCV) with palpable purpura can occur in patients with severe, uncontrolled RA (see section **VIII.A.1**).

    B. Neutrophilic dermatoses including Sweet's syndrome, pyoderma gangrenosum, and rheumatoid neutrophilic dermatosis (RND) are rarely seen. RND is a chronic, erythematous urticarialike papule or plaque that occurs in patients with severe RA. RND is nontender and may develop into ulcers.

    C. Treatment. Optimal RA control may decrease the size and number of nodules. Interestingly, they tend to increase in number and size on treatment with methotrexate and decrease on treatment with anti-tumour necrosis factor (anti-TNF) medications.

VII. JUVENILE IDIOPATHIC ARTHRITIS (JIA) (see Chapter 36)
  A. Of the various forms of JIA, cutaneous findings only play a consistent role in those with systemic-onset disease.
  B. The characteristic lesions are erythematous to pink macules that typically erupt on the trunk. The macules vary in diameter from 3 to 10 mm. They may have paler centers. The rash is evanescent and is associated with the high-spiking fevers of JIA.
  C. Rheumatoid nodules are rarely found in these younger patients but may occur in those with the RA-like polyarticular disease that occurs in older children.
VIII. Vasculitis (see Chapter 37) disorders encompass a spectrum of clinical entities that share a destructive inflammation of blood vessel walls. Classification based on the size of affected vessels help distinguish the separate entities and account for clinical trends.
  A. Vasculitides that affect predominantly small vessels
    1. LCV of the postcapillary venules classically exhibits 3- to 10-mm palpable purpuric lesions found on dependent areas (i.e., lower extremities). Individual lesions tend to last approximately 1 to 2 weeks. Lesions are symmetrically distributed. Lesions begin as macules or urticarial papules that become purpuric and may progress to form hemorrhagic vesicles, bullae, nodules, or superficial ulcers.
      a. Common etiologies of LCV include medications [i.e., nonsteroidal anti-inflammatory drugs (NSAIDs), β-lactams, macrolides, sulfonamides, quinolones, β blockers, thiazides, anticonvulsants, allopurinol, and propylthiouracil], connective tissue disorders such as SLE, infections [i.e., cytomegalovirus (CMV), hepatitis B and C, human immunodeficiency virus (HIV), and *Streptococcus*] and malignancy (particularly hematologic).
      b. Treatment consists of treating the underlying etiology and symptomatic relief, such as leg elevation and nonsteroidal anti-inflammatory use. Steroids may be employed if there is evidence of extracutaneous involvement.
    2. Henoch-Schönlein purpura (HSP) is characterized by palpable purpura (on dependent areas) due to LCV, arthralgias, GI symptoms, and renal involvement. HSP occurs primarily in children following an upper respiratory infection. IF staining of early lesions reveals mainly IgA and complement deposition in the walls of vessels. The treatment involves treating the underlying etiology. Corticosteroids are utilized in severe cases with extracutaneous involvement. Dapsone and colchicine have been utilized in the treatment of active cutaneous disease.
    3. Mixed cryoglobulinemia presents with hepatosplenomegaly, lymphadenopathy, renal disease, and the cutaneous lesions of LCV. Mixed cryoglobulinemia, positive RF, and hypocomplementemia define this disease. There is a strong association with hepatitis C. IF staining of early lesions reveals Ig and complement deposition in the walls of affected vessels.
      The primary therapy is to avoid the cold in case of diseases that are precipitated by cold temperatures. In cases associated with hepatitis C, treatment should be directed at the viral infection, which may include pegylated interferon-α (IFN-α) and ribavirin. Severe cases have been treated with corticosteroids, cyclophosphamide, and plasmapheresis.
    4. Urticarial vasculitis presents with urticarialike lesions. These lesions tend to be smaller than urticarial lesions, ranging from 0.5 to 5 cm in diameter. Urticarial vasculitis lesions persist greater than 24 hours and often resolve with postinflammatory hyperpigmentation. Lesions are painful. Angioedema, dermal ulceration, livedo reticularis, and Raynaud's phenomenon may also be seen.
      a. When applicable, treatment of urticarial vasculitis should begin with treatment of the underlying disease process.
      b. Colchicine, NSAIDs, H1 and H2 blockers, and doxepin have not been effective in the treatment of hypocomplementemic urticarial vasculitis, although anecdotal reports state that these medications are effective in the treatment of urticarial vasculitis.
      c. Prednisone 30 to 60 mg/day has been shown to improve the urticarial vasculitis in most patients.
      d. Dapsone or hydroxychloroquine has been used successfully as an additional treatment in some patients.

B. **Vasculitides that affect predominantly medium-sized vessels**
   1. **Polyarteritis nodosa (PAN).** The cutaneous findings may include infarction, ulceration, and distal acral gangrene. Subcutaneous nodules (smaller than 10 mm) may be present. Smaller cutaneous vessels are not typically involved, and consequently, purpura is not as frequent as it is in the small vessel vasculitides. However, ruptured aneurysm(s) can occur and may present as extensive ecchymoses. Patients with PAN may also develop LCV.
   Immune deposits are present in tissue lesions and in blood in this disorder. Antineutrophil cytoplasmic antibodies (ANCA) are typically negative.
   2. **ANCA-positive vasculitides** (affect predominantly small to medium-sized vessels).
      a. **Wegener's granulomatosis (WG)** involves the kidney and upper respiratory tract. Forty percent to 50% of patients have skin findings, including palpable purpura, ulcers, necrotic papules, and subcutaneous nodules. Saddle nose deformities and gingival hyperplasia with petechia are rare findings but are suggestive of WG. The presence of cutaneous lesions may mirror systemic activity or at the least is a marker for potential systemic involvement.
      b. **Churg-Strauss (CS) syndrome** exhibits bronchial asthma, peripheral eosinophilia, and systemic vasculitis. Two-thirds of patients exhibit skin findings, including palpable purpura due to LCV, a maculopapular erythematous rash, hemorrhagic lesions, and/or cutaneous or subcutaneous nodules.
      c. **Microscopic polyangiitis (MPA)** involves the skin in 30% to 40% of patients. It typically exhibits palpable purpura and splinter hemorrhages. Cutaneous ulcers found on the lower extremities have also been reported.
C. **Vasculitides that affect predominately large vessels.** Cutaneous manifestations are not part of large vessel vasculitides (i.e., Takayasu's and giant cell arteritis) but LCV occurs rarely.
IX. **Behçet's disease** (see Chapter 37) was originally described as a triad of iritis and recurrent oral and genital ulcerations.
   A. Oral ulcers are often indistinguishable from common aphthous ulcers or "canker sores." They typically begin as small areas of macular erythema that develop into superficial gray ulcers. They most commonly arise on the buccal mucosa, gingival lips, and tongue.
   B. Genital lesions resemble the oral aphthae but have a greater propensity for scarring. In men, ulcers commonly arise on the penis or scrotum; in women they frequently occur on the vulva.
   C. Diagnostic criteria for Behçet's disease also include the nonspecific findings of erythema nodosum, pseudofolliculitis, papulopustular lesions, acneiform nodules, and positive pathergy test (cutaneous papulopustular lesions after cutaneous trauma).
   D. Treatment options include intralesional or topical potent steroids, tetracycline swish and swallows, topical anesthetics, dapsone, and colchicine. There are case reports of successful use of methotrexate, prednisone, thalidomide, IFN-α agents, and TNF-α antagonists.
X. **Sarcoidosis** (see Chapter 58) is a multisystemic disease characterized by noncaseating granulomas that can potentially affect any organ system.
   A. Cutaneous manifestations occur in 20% to 35% of patients and in some instances may precede all other symptoms. There does not seem to be any correlation between the extent of cutaneous lesions and extent of systemic disease.
   B. All the cutaneous manifestations discussed in the subsequent text, except erythema nodosum, exhibit sarcoid granulomas on biopsy. Diascopy (application of pressure using a clear lens or glass slide) of erythematous lesions may reveal yellow–brown nodules or **"apple jelly"** nodules.
   C. **Papular sarcoid** has a predilection for the face, eyelids, neck, and shoulders. Lesions range in color from translucent to reddish brown to violaceous. Papules are indurated and exhibit little epidermal change.
   D. **Annular plaques** with atrophic centers are described in Table 16-3. Plaques are usually violaceous and translucent. Telangiectatic vessels may be seen.

E. Violaceous, yellowish brown, reddish brown scaly macules and patches may also be seen in sarcoidosis. Lesions may develop atrophy and may mimic DLE, psoriasis, or even cutaneous T-cell lymphoma.

F. **Lupus pernio** is characterized by chronic indurated papules or plaques that involve the head and neck, with an increased predilection for the nose, cheeks, forehead, and ears. Lesions are typically violaceous, smooth, and shiny. When they occur on the fingers and toes, they may produce bulbous and sausage-shaped digits. They may be present in the setting of severe lung fibrosis.

G. **Subcutaneous sarcoidosis** presents as 1- to 3-cm deep nodules whose overlying epidermis may be violaceous.

H. **Hypopigmented sarcoidosis** presents as a hypopigmented macule or patch. The centers of these lesions often have a dermal palpable component.

I. **Ulcerative sarcoidosis** favors the lower extremities.

J. **Scar sarcoid** may arise in a pre-existing scar. Lesions resemble keloids.

K. **Morphea sarcoidosis** is rare. The associated dermal fibrosis resembles localized scleroderma, or morphea.

L. **Icthyosiform sarcoidosis** presents with fine scaling, usually on distal extremities.

M. Alopecia may occur either as a scarring process secondary to cutaneous lesions extending onto the scalp or rarely as a nonscarring alopecia that resembles alopecia areata. The latter form may be either permanent or reversible. Biopsy of either type of lesion reveals the characteristic dermal granulomas.

N. **EN** (see section **XIII**) is not specific for sarcoidosis. **Löfgren's syndrome** refers to presence of EN, bilateral hilar lymphadenopathy, polyarthralgia, periarthritis about the ankles, and/or anterior uveitis. EN associated with sarcoidosis may indicate a more benign course of disease.

O. Treatment of choice for systemic sarcoidosis is systemic corticosteroids. At times, antimalarial drugs and immunosuppressants are needed.

XI. **Sweet's syndrome** (acute febrile neutrophilic dermatosis) presents with fever, neutrophilia (usually ranging from 10 to 20,000 cells/mm^3), and cutaneous lesions.

A. It is estimated that approximately 50% of cases are associated with underlying disease, including malignancy (most commonly hematopoietic), bacterial infection (upper respiratory and GI tract, implicating *Streptococcus* and *Yersinia*), viral infection (CMV, hepatitis, and HIV), drugs [granulocyte-colony stimulating factor (G-CSF), lithium, furosemide, minocycline, hydralazine, sulfonamides, and oral contraceptives], connective tissue disorders, pregnancy, and IBD.

B. The primary skin lesion is a sharply demarcated, tender, erythematous to violaceous papule or plaque. There is marked inflammatory edema that may create a vesicular appearance. The papules may coalesce, forming the impression of a **"relief of mountain range."**

C. **Treatment.** The standard therapy is a systemic steroid taper, often starting with oral prednisone 40 to 60 mg/day, which is tapered to 10 mg over 4 to 6 weeks. Some patients require 2 to 3 months of treatment. Other agents include potassium iodide, colchicine, indomethacin, cyclosporine, and dapsone.

XII. **Pyodermic gangrenosum (PG)** is an idiopathic neutrophilic dermatosis in which 50% to 70% of cases are associated with an underlying systemic disorder, including IBD, hematologic diseases (including monoclonal gammopathy, leukemia, and lymphomas), and connective tissue disorders (including RA and SLE).

A. PG classically presents as an ulcer with a raised inflammatory, dusky border often described as **"undermined."** The base of the ulcer is often covered with necrotic material. Lesions generally begin as deep-seated tender nodules or superficial hemorrhagic pustules and typically occur on the lower extremities and trunk. A rim of erythema often surrounds the rapidly advancing border of a PG ulcer.

B. The diagnosis of PG often relies on ruling out other ulcer etiologies. Although a biopsy of PG is not diagnostic, an elliptical biopsy of the ulcer edge should be sent for histologic evaluation and culture.

C. **Treatment.** Therapy focuses on treating the underlying systemic disease. However, it should be noted that PG lesions might not follow the course of its associated systemic condition.

D. Topical therapies include intralesional and topical steroids, topical tacrolimus, sodium cromoglycate, topical 5-aminosalicylic acid, and nitrogen mustard.

E. Systemic steroids are generally the first-line agents among systemic therapies. Prednisone is usually started at 60 to 80 mg orally daily, but this dosage may be increased to 100 to 120 mg if there is no response after 10 days. Other agents include dapsone, clofazimine, thalidomide, rifampin, tetracycline, and vancomycin and mezlocillin. There are case reports of treatment success with cyclosporine, azathioprine, mycophenolate mofetil, cyclophosphamide, chlorambucil, and methotrexate.

XIII. **EN** is a reactive dermatosis due to a septal panniculitis associated with an underlying condition in approximately 50% of cases. Etiologies include infection [*Streptococcus*, tuberculosis, Epstein-Barr virus (EBV), HIV, and deep fungal infection], drug (oral contraceptives, sulfa drugs, and minocycline), malignancy (lymphomas and leukemias), and systemic conditions (sarcoidosis, IBD, Behçet's disease, and pregnancy).

A. EN classically presents as tender erythematous subcutaneous nodules usually limited to the extensor surfaces of the lower extremities. As EN lesions mature, they become more macular and undergo color changes associated with skin bruising. Lesions tend to resolve spontaneously within a few weeks without ulcerating or scarring.

B. Treatment focuses on the underlying etiology. In most cases, only symptomatic relief (i.e., NSAIDs, cool compresses, elevation of lower extremities, and bed rest) is needed. Potassium iodide, oral prednisone, and colchicine have all been used in refractory cases.

XIV. **Infectious diseases** affect both the skin and joints. Selected viral and bacterial etiologies are discussed here. Fungal infections and mycobacterial infections are rare causes of rash and arthritis and will not be discussed here.

A. **Parvovirus B19** classically presents with a **"slapped-cheek"** rash that spreads to the trunk and extremities, where it manifests in a reticulated pattern. This eruption begins a few days to a week after prodromal symptoms and fades after a few days. Adults may present without cutaneous findings or with just a reticulated rash on the extremities and trunk.

B. **Rubella.** The rash often begins as discrete pink macules and papules on the face, spreading to involve the trunk and extremities. Lesions may become confluent or present in a morbilliform or scarlatiniform pattern. Forchheimer's spots, pinpoint pink macules, and petechiae on the soft palate can be seen. The rash resolves in 2 to 3 days. Tender lymphadenopathy may occur concurrent with the skin findings.

C. **Varicella virus** associated exanthems often begin on the scalp or trunk before extending to the extremities. Individual lesions are erythematous macules that develop into less than 5 mm vesicles surrounded by erythema. Vesicles develop into pustular and crusted papules within 3 to 4 days. Lesions at different stages of development that are simultaneously present on the same patient are the hallmark.

   1. **Treatment.** Children should be treated with antipruritic lotion and oral antihistamines. Salicylates should not be used because of the risk of Reye's syndrome.

   2. Varicella runs a benign course in most immunocompetent patients. Randomized-controlled trial of acyclovir showed that early treatment with oral acyclovir reduced healing time and duration of symptoms.

   3. For severe disease or severely immunocompromised patients, acyclovir 10 mg/kg intravenously every 8 hours is given for 7 days. For mild disease, treatment is with acyclovir 800 mg orally five times daily for 7 to 10 days.

D. **Herpes zoster** begins as burning pain or pruritus in the affected dermatome a few days before the development of the rash. The rash is characterized by grouped vesicles on an erythematous base and is usually present in one dermatome. Immunocompromised patients may present with disseminated zoster.

   1. **Treatment.** Among immunocompetent patients, one may choose to treat only symptomatically or administer acyclovir 800 mg orally five times daily.

   2. If the patient is severely immunocompromised, the disease may be treated with acyclovir 10 mg/kg intravenously every 8 hours for 7 to 10 days.

E. **Disseminated gonorrhea infection (DGI)** presents with four to 50 discrete erythematous papules or petechiae found on the extremities. Lesions quickly progress to painful pustules that may become necrotic. Lesions are reportedly less common if there is arthritic involvement. The diagnosis of DGI can be confirmed by positive cultures of the skin, blood, pharynx, urethra, cervix, and rectum. Synovial cultures are positive only 40% of the time. Recommended initial treatment is ceftriaxone 1 gm intramuscular or intravenously every 24 hours.

F. Acute meningococcemia may present with skin lesions in nearly half of patients. Classically, lesions are small petechiae with a "smudged" appearance and a pale gray vesicular center. Some develop into bullae and may even become necrotic. Lesions can present on the extremities and the trunk. The treatment regimen is usually penicillin G, 4 million units intravenously every 4 hours, continued for 7 days after the patient becomes afebrile.

G. Syphilis can rarely cause arthritic symptoms in congenital, secondary, or tertiary syphilis.

1. Congenital lesions may present as **condyloma lata** (moist and smooth verrucous plaques) or mucous patches.

2. Secondary syphilis is referred to as the **"great imitator,"** indicating its wide range of clinical presentation. Typical findings are **copper-colored** maculopapular lesions on the trunk and, characteristically, the **palms and soles.** Other findings may include annular plaques on the face, condyloma lata, patchy alopecia, mucous patches, and a papulosquamous reaction that may resemble pityriasis rosea.

3. Tertiary syphilis may present as nodules, noduloulcerative lesions, and gummas in the skin.

4. Diagnosis can be made by a positive venereal disease research laboratory (VDRL) or rapid plasma reagin (RPR) that is confirmed with specific treponemal tests. Dark-field microscopy may also allow for diagnosis by demonstrating the presence of treponemal spirochetes.

5. Treatment of early syphilis (primary or secondary) in immunocompetent patients is 2.4 million IU of benzathine penicillin G intramuscular for one dose (some recommend a second dose 1 week later). The HIV status of the patient should be checked and sexual partners should be evaluated and treated. Serologies should be monitored and followed to assess the efficacy of treatment.

H. Lyme disease (see Chapter 47) has the following three distinct cutaneous manifestations that include **erythema chronicum migrans (ECM),** borrelial lymphocytoma, and acrodermatitis chronica atrophicans (ACA).

1. ECM appears days to weeks after a tick bite. The lesion begins as a small red macule or papule usually at the actual site of the bite. As the lesion enlarges, the central area clears, creating a target-appearing patch/plaque. The initial lesion generally spontaneously resolves but may last months, stretching to over a meter in size. This lesion is thought to be pathognomonic of Lyme disease.

2. Borrelial lymphocytoma is a solitary bluish red papule to nodule that arises at a median of 30 to 45 days. It appears later and lasts longer than ECM. Like ECM, it resolves spontaneously. This lesion has been predominantly reported in Europe.

3. ACA begins as a bluish-red edematous plaque that commonly occurs on the distal dorsal extremities. The edema and color slowly subside and the atrophy gradually becomes more prominent. The skin becomes thin, atrophic, and may develop a violaceous hue. These lesions do not spontaneously resolve.

4. Treatment options for ECM and borrelial lymphocytoma include a 10- to 21-day course of oral doxycycline 100 mg twice daily, tetracycline 250 to 500 mg orally four times daily, or amoxicillin 500 to 1,000 mg orally three times daily. ACA may be treated with a 14- to 30-day course of ceftriaxone 2 g intravenously, doxycycline 100 mg orally twice daily, or amoxicillin 500 to 1,000 mg orally three times daily.

XV. RHEUMATIC FEVER (see Chapter 49). Three types of skin lesions are observed in rheumatic fever. They are listed in decreasing order of frequency. The first two of these findings are part of the Jones's major criteria for the diagnosis of rheumatic fever.

A. Subcutaneous nodules are firm, nontender mobile nodules smaller than 2 cm in size. The lesions are typically found over the bony prominences of the elbows, knuckles, ankles, and occiput. The nodules usually last less than 2 weeks.

B. Erythema marginatum is characterized by rapidly enlarging ringed lesions that are asymptomatic. They begin as erythematous macules or papules. While enlarging, their centers begin to clear. These lesions may last a few hours to days.

C. Erythema papulatum rarely occurs. It consists of asymptomatic macules or papules that are 3 to 4 mm in diameter, which appear in crops and have a predilection for the flexor surfaces of the large joints of the extremities.

D. Treatment with penicillin should be started and maintained for at least 10 days in adequate doses for eradication of *Streptococcus* pharyngitis.

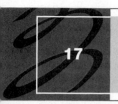

RAYNAUD'S PHENOMENON
Kyriakos A. Kirou

17

■ KEY POINTS

■ Raynaud's phenomenon (RP) is characterized by episodic vasospasm and occlusion of the digital arteries in response to cold and emotional stress. This manifests as the sequential change of digital skin color from pallor to cyanosis and then to rubor, but often not all three color changes are observed.

■ Primary RP (PRP) is symmetric and occurs in the absence of any known specific RP-associated disorder, peripheral pulse abnormalities, digital pitting/ulceration/gangrene, abnormal nailfold capillaries, and positive antinuclear antibody (ANA) test or a high erythrocyte sedimentation rate (ESR).

■ PRP is common in the general population, occurs in young women, has a familial predisposition, and carries an excellent prognosis.

■ Possible secondary RP (SRP) consists of those patients with some isolated laboratory or clinical abnormality that do not fulfill the diagnostic criteria for any specific RP-associated disorder. Most of them are patients who are ANA positive and those who have a relatively low progression rate (10% to 30%) to a connective tissue disorder.

■ SRP in the context of systemic sclerosis (SSc) is characterized by a structural micro- (and sometimes macro-) vasculopathy, which often leads to severe digital ischemia.

■ The management of RP includes general measures of protection from cold exposure and trauma, avoidance of drugs that promote vasospasm, and use of vasodilatory medications with a calcium channel blocker as the usual first choice.

■ Refractory SRP due to SSc will often respond to prostaglandin infusions but may require digital sympathectomy, microsurgical revascularization, or amputations.

*R*aynaud's phenomenon (RP) is characterized by episodic vasospasm and occlusion of the digital arteries, resulting in a well-demarcated ischemic blanching of the involved digits. This may be followed sequentially by cyanosis and rubor. Tingling may occur during the reactive hyperemia phase (rubor).

I. **Exposure to cold or emotional stress** is the typical inducer of RP. The duration of an attack may vary from several minutes to hours (usually 10 to 30 minutes). Upper extremities are most frequently involved, but 40% of patients have symptoms in their lower extremities.

II. **Primary RP (PRP)** is the RP that occurs in otherwise healthy individuals while **secondary RP (SRP)** is observed in association with other disorders.
   A. Proposed criteria for diagnosing PRP include the following:
      1. Appearance of symptoms with exposure to cold or emotional upset.
      2. Bilateral symmetric involvement of hands.

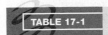

| TABLE 17-1 | Characteristics of Primary and Secondary RP |

Primary	Secondary
Women	Women (i.e., SSc or SLE) or men (i.e., HAVS and Buerger's disease)
Onset often in teens or 20s (<40)	Onset in 3rd and 4th decade (i.e., SSc) or even later (i.e., atherosclerosis)
Familial aggregation	Familial and nonfamilial, depending on the cause
Digital ischemia is episodic (vasospasm in response to cold or emotional stress)	Digital ischemia is episodic but can also occur at rest because of structural vascular abnormalities (i.e., SSc and vasculitis)
Symmetric	Symmetric (i.e., SSc) or asymmetric (i.e., atherosclerotic artery occlusion)
Normal pulse	Pulse can be absent or diminished
No significant tissue ischemic changes	Digital pitting, fingertip ulcerations, and gangrene may occur
Absence of an underlying RP-associated disorder	Underlying SSc, MCTD, SLE, vasculitis, etc.
Serologic tests for ANA and RF are negative and ESR is low	Positive ANA (i.e., SLE and SSc) or RF (SS, RA, and MC); high ESR (i.e., vasculitis and multiple myeloma)
Normal nailfold capillaroscopy	Abnormal nailfold capillaries (i.e., SSc, DM, and SLE)

ANA, antinuclear antibodies; DM, dermatomyositis; ESR, erythrocyte sedimentation rate; HAVS, hand–arm vibration syndrome; MC, mixed cryoglobulinemia; MCTD, mixed connective tissue disease; RA, rheumatoid arthritis; RF, rheumatoid factor; SLE, systemic lupus erythematosus; SS, Sjögren's syndrome; SSc, systemic sclerosis.

   3. Normal pulse.
   4. Absence of digital gangrene, or if present, only superficial.
   5. Absence of an underlying disorder commonly associated with the symptom complex.
   6. Symptoms present for longer than 2 years without the appearance of an underlying cause.
   B. In 1992, a stricter definition of PRP was developed that excluded all patients with evidence of digital pitting, ulcerations, or gangrene; abnormal nailfold capillaries; a positive antinuclear antibody (ANA) test; or an abnormal erythrocyte sedimentation rate (ESR) upon presentation.
   C. The main characteristics of PRP and SRP are summarized in Table 17-1.

ETIOPATHOGENESIS

I.   **PRP** is caused by vasospasm of the digital arteries and cutaneous arterioles. Its familial predisposition may be due to shared genetic or environmental factors.

II. **Vascular tone** is determined by the balance of vasoconstrictor and vasodilatory mediators that act on the vascular smooth muscle cells.
   A. Vasodilatory **neuromediators** from sensory (i.e., calcitonin gene-related peptide) and parasympathetic terminals (acetylcholine), as well as vasoconstrictor mediators from sympathetic fibers (i.e., norepinephrine), act on vascular smooth muscle cells to modulate vascular tone.
   B. **The endothelium** plays a central role in mediating the effects of several neurotransmitters (i.e., acetylcholine and neurokinin A), circulating factors (i.e., thrombin and histamine), as well as mechanical shear stress on smooth muscle cells, by producing relaxing (i.e., nitric oxide and prostacyclin or PGI$_2$) or constricting (i.e., endothelin-1) products.

C. **Exposure to cold** activates vasoconstriction of cutaneous blood vessels by amplifying the effect of norepinephrine on the α_2C-adrenoreceptors of the vascular smooth muscle cells.

D. The excessive vasoconstrictive response to cold in RP may be due to increased α_2C-adrenoreceptor sensitivity to cold. Other factors likely include a loss of vasodilatory sensory fibers or an overactivity of vasoconstrictive neuromediators. Interestingly, living in cold climates may predispose to PRP.

III. **The etiopathogenesis of SRP** varies according to the specific associated disorder (Table 17-2).

A. **In systemic sclerosis (SSc) or scleroderma,** the RP is due to a vasculopathy that mainly affects the cutaneous arterioles/capillaries and the proper digital arteries but often also larger vessels such as the ulnar artery and the superficial palmar arch.

1. **Endothelial cell damage** or dysfunction is a prominent and early characteristic of this vasculopathy. Reactive oxygen species (ROS) generated during the reperfusion injury from repeated ischemic attacks, as well as antiendothelial antibodies, have been implicated.

2. **Histologically, intimal hyperplasia and fibrosis** that may be accompanied by thrombosis occur. Adventitial fibrosis and telangiectasias of the vasa vasorum are also common and the former has been implicated in digital ischemia by virtue of external compression.

3. SRP due to mixed connective tissue disease (MCTD) and other scleroderma-overlap syndromes share the same pathogenesis.

B. **The SRP associated with systemic lupus erythematosus (SLE), rheumatoid arthritis (RA), Sjögren's syndrome, and polymyositis (PM)** is usually benign and vasospastic in nature. However, when caused by vasculitis or thrombosis in the context of the antiphospholipid syndrome, it can lead to tissue damage and gangrene.

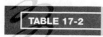

TABLE 17-2	Causes of Secondary Raynaud's Phenomenon

Connective tissue diseases
- Systemic sclerosis
- Mixed connective tissue disease
- Polymyositis and dermatomyositis
- Systemic lupus erythematosus
- Sjögren's syndrome
- Rheumatoid arthritis

Systemic vasculitis
- Polyarteritis nodosa
- Takayasu's arteritis
- Giant cell arteritis
- Wegener's granulomatosis
- Microscopic polyangiitis

Traumatic vasospastic/occupational
- Hand–arm vibration syndrome
- After frostbites

Occlusive/structural arterial diseases
- Atherosclerosis
- Atheroemboli
- Hypothenar hammer syndrome
- Thrombangiitis obliterans (Buerger's disease)

Nerve compression
- Thoracic outlet syndrome
- Carpal tunnel syndrome

Hematologic disease
- Cryoglobulinemia
- Cold agglutinin disease
- Polycythemia vera
- Waldenström's macroglobulinemia

Drugs and chemicals
- Ergot alkaloids
- Methysergide
- Vinyl chloride
- Chemotherapy agents (e.g., bleomycin, vinblastine, and cisplatin)
- β-Blockers
- Sympathomimetics
- Anticholinergics
- Cyclosporine A
- Interferon-α

Other disorders
- Hypothyroidism
- Complex regional pain syndrome type 1
- Paraneoplastic

C. **In systemic vasculitis,** the inflammatory occlusion of vessels usually leads to severe digital ischemia and gangrene.

D. **The hand–arm vibration syndrome (HAVS) or vibration-induced white finger (VWF)** occurs in workers who use vibratory tools such as pneumatic hammers and chain saws.

E. **Occlusive arterial disease** can occur in advanced atherosclerosis (i.e., in patients with diabetes mellitus) with asymmetric involvement of medium-sized vessels, in thromboangiitis obliterans (Buerger's disease) where smoking plays a key pathogenetic role, and in thromboembolic disease due to proximal cardiovascular clotting, thrombophilia, or trauma (hypothenar hammer syndrome).

F. **Nerve compression.** Compression (i.e., by a cervical rib or a pectoralis minor tendon) of brachial plexus sympathetic fibers and the subclavian artery has been implicated in the RP of the thoracic outlet syndrome (TOS). A similar mechanism may explain the RP seen in patients with the carpal tunnel syndrome (CTS).

G. **Drugs and chemicals.** Ergot alkaloids have a direct vasoconstrictive action on blood vessels. Methysergide may cause intimal fibrosis. Exposure to vinyl chloride and bleomycin can cause a sclerodermalike illness with RP. β-Blockers, sympathomimetics, cocaine, cyclosporine, interferon-α, vinblastine, and cisplatin have been all implicated in the development of RP.

H. **Hematologic abnormalities.** RP has been reported in cryoglobulinemia, cold agglutinin disease, polycythemia, and macroglobulinemia. Blood hyperviscosity is the presumed mechanism.

I. **Malignancy** should be suspected in RP that progresses in an abrupt and rapid manner to severe digital ischemia.

J. **Other disorders** associated with RP include malignancy, complex regional pain syndrome (CRPS) type 1, and hypothyroidism.

 PREVALENCE

Population-based studies estimate the prevalence of PRP to be 3% to 16% among women and 1% to 6% among men, the highest noted in the coldest geographic regions assayed. PRP is much more common than SRP and usually presents in teenagers. The prevalence of SRP in SSc or scleroderma-overlap disorders is greater than 90%, whereas in other CTD it is approximately 20% to 30%. SRP usually occurs at older ages, often above 40 years, and a male preponderance can be seen according to the etiology.

 CLINICAL MANIFESTATIONS

I. **PRP** is characterized by brief episodes of digital ischemia upon exposure to cold or emotional stimuli.

A. A history of the classic triad of sequential digital pallor, cyanosis, and rubor is diagnostic. However, white alone, white and blue/purple, or white and red color changes are frequently seen.

B. Reduced digital blood flow can be triggered by either a whole-body cold exposure (through a sympathetic reflex mechanism), or local digital cooling.

II. **CLINICAL FEATURES SUGGESTIVE OF SRP ARE SHOWN IN TABLE 17-1.**

A. **Persistent digital ischemia independent of vasospastic episodes** indicate structural occlusive vascular lesions because it can be seen in scleroderma, and occlusive arterial disease (see the preceding text).

B. **The asymmetric involvement of hands and/or feet** should suggest atherosclerosis or thromboembolic disease.

C. **In SSc,** RP is often the presenting feature and it can be a major cause of morbidity. Cold-induced vasospasm in the heart (angina) and other internal organs has been noted in SSc and is called systemic or visceral RP.

D. **Occupational history of use of vibratory tools** will suggest SRP due to HAVS. RP in this condition is triggered by exposure to vibration as well as the cold and it often involves the nonexposed hand as well.

E. A detailed drug/toxic-exposure history should always be obtained. Medications could be the cause of or an aggravating factor for existing RP, such as when β-blockers are used in patients with RP in the setting of autoimmune disorders.

PHYSICAL EXAMINATION

I. Examination of patients with PRP between attacks is unrevealing. Nevertheless, the clinician should look for clues of an underlying disease.

II. **Asymmetric peripheral pulse** should raise suspicion of an occlusive arterial disease.

III. **Puffy hands, sclerodactyly, tendon friction rubs, and telangiectasias** are features of the sclerodermalike disorders. Presence of severe ischemic pain, in association with digital coolness and cyanosis, as well as digital pitting, ulcers, and gangrene, indicate a compromised, resting, digital blood flow that occurs with a fixed arterial obstruction.

IV. **The Allen test** should be done to exclude radial or ulnar artery involvement. Ulnar artery involvement is not uncommon in SSc and leads to worsened digital ischemia.

V. **Maneuvers to detect thoracic outlet compression or CTS** should be undertaken.

VI. **Nailfold capillaroscopy** can help in differentiating PRP from SRP. An early nailfold videocapillaroscopic pattern consisting of a few enlarged and giant capillaries, as well as hemorrhages, is very specific for SSc, although with some variation this finding can also be observed in dermatomyositis (DM), MCTD, and SLE. Later in the disease process of SSc, loss of capillaries, ramified capillaries, and vascular architectural disorganization are seen.

This examination can be done either with application of mineral oil on the nailfold and visualization of the capillaries by ophthalmoscopy or with direct visualization using a dermoscope.

DIAGNOSTIC INVESTIGATIONS

I. **LABORATORY TESTS**

A. **Laboratory investigations** are performed as dictated by the patient history and physical examination findings. Accordingly, they may include a complete blood count with differential blood count, serum electrolytes, glucose, and creatinine levels; urinalysis; liver function test; thyroid-stimulating hormone (TSH) level; ESR; ANA level; rheumatoid factor (RF) level; serum protein and immunoelectrophoresis; and cryoglobulin level.

B. In ANA–positive cases where the probability for SSc is higher, testing for the anticentromere and antitopoisomerase antibodies is indicated. For other diagnostic tests used in SSc, please refer to Chapter 34.

C. Antiphospholipid antibodies should be tested for when the clinical suspicion for spontaneous thromboembolic disease exists.

D. **Electromyograms or nerve conduction** studies should be performed when nerve compression is a possibility.

E. **Echocardiography** is indicated when cardiac emboli are suspected.

F. **Vascular laboratory studies** can assess disease at the microvascular, macrovascular, or at both levels. They are not necessary for the diagnosis of PRP, but they may help in the assessment of the several forms of SRP (i.e., in defining the extent and severity of arterial disease).

    1. **Doppler studies** of the palmar arch and proximal larger arteries are indicated when such involvement is suspected clinically (i.e., occlusive arterial disease).

    2. **Finger photoplethysmography (PPG) and finger systolic blood pressure** determination (i.e., by a pneumatic cuff around the proximal phalanx and a photoplethysmograph placed over the distal phalanx) performed in a warm ambient temperature to avoid vasoconstriction may prove very useful. Abnormal

PPG waveforms and brachial–finger pressure gradients of more than 20 mm Hg indicate fixed arterial obstruction somewhere in the vascular pathway supplying the terminal phalanx.

3. **Laser Doppler imaging** (LDI) and thermography are additional research techniques for the assessment of the microvascular integrity.

4. **Cold provocation tests** (in association with PPG, LDI, etc.) have been used in research studies but are not necessary for the diagnosis of RP.

II. **RADIOLOGIC STUDIES**

A. A chest and neck x-ray might reveal a bony cervical rib in the case of TOS.

B. **Angiography** (or magnetic resonance angiography) is necessary only when a proximal arterial embolic source is suspected; the proximal extent of vascular compromise needs to be defined or a microsurgical arterial reconstruction of the palmar arch is contemplated. If dye is to be injected into an artery, a sympathetic block should be done proximally to avoid reflex vasospasm.

 DIFFERENTIAL DIAGNOSIS

RP must be differentiated from processes characterized by persistent vasospastic ischemia. In the following disorders, vasoconstriction is probably limited to arterioles and not the digital arteries.

I. **Acrocyanosis,** like RP, is exacerbated by low temperatures and emotional stress. However, cyanosis is not confined to the digits but extends diffusely to the hands or feet. The idiopathic form is a benign disorder.

II. **Livedo reticularis,** characterized by a persistent purple or blue mottling of the skin, predominantly involves the extremities. It is usually a benign condition but can be a prominent feature of cutaneous vasculitis syndrome (livedo reticularis with ulceration or atrophie blanche), due to the antiphospholipid syndrome, or secondary to a systemic disorder such as systemic lupus.

 TREATMENT

I. **General measures** are adequate for patients with mild to moderate PRP but necessary for all RP. They include the following:

A. Avoidance of a cold environment and the use of warm clothing, mittens, or gloves with Thinsulate, and even electrically heated gloves.

B. Tobacco use should be discontinued. β-Blocker drugs, if used, should be appropriately substituted. The newer vasodilatory β-Blocker drugs may be better tolerated and potentially beneficial.

C. In cases of PRP, reassurance about the good prognosis of the disorder should be offered.

II. **Therapy for SRP** should be aimed at correction of the underlying disorder. For example, vasculitis will require corticosteroids and/or immunosuppressive therapy; antiphospholipid syndrome, other thrombophilic disorders, and thromboembolic events need appropriate anticoagulation therapy; Buerger's disease will usually respond to smoking cessation; severe involvement of large vessels (i.e., secondary to trauma, atherosclerosis, or vasculitis) will require vascular surgery.

III. **PHARMACOLOGIC THERAPY**

A. **For severe PRP or SRP,** pharmacologic therapy with vasodilators is often required in addition to the general measures. Goals for SRP include the reduction of frequency of attacks and prevention of digital ulcer formation.

B. **Calcium channel blockers** are the best-studied agents in RP and, therefore, often the first drug choice in managing vasospasm. They have been shown to have moderate effects in decreasing the frequency and severity of RP. However, if a significant occlusive component is present, as in advanced SSc, the benefit may be minimal. At times, a "steal phenomenon" can exist with worsening of the ischemia because blood flow may preferentially be directed to normal vessels and not to the abnormal ones. They might aggravate esophageal reflux or constipation and they should be avoided during pregnancy.

1. **Nifedipine** can decrease the number and severity of episodes of RP. Side effects are common and include headache, tachycardia, flushing, light-headedness, and edema. Initial dosage is 10 mg three times daily, with upward adjustment to the maximum tolerated dose. The slow-release preparations (30 or 60 mg/day) are thought to have fewer side effects.

2. **Amlodipine** in a dosage of 5 to 10 mg/day, and **diltiazem** (30 mg three or four times daily) may be used as well.

C. α-Blockers

1. **Prazosin,** an α-1 receptor blocker, has been found to be beneficial in PRP, but the clinical improvement may not be sustained with prolonged treatment. Syncope may occur with the first dose but can be prevented by giving the drug at bedtime and by limiting the dose to 1 mg. Subsequent doses are better tolerated. Most patients can be managed on 1 to 2 mg three times daily.

2. **A selective $α_2$C-adrenoreceptor** antagonist improved digital skin perfusion during recovery from cooling in a recent small study of patients with SSc. Further studies are needed to establish its usefulness in RP.

D. Nitrates. Topical 2% ointment and sustained-release transdermal glyceryl trinitrate patches can reduce the number and severity of attacks in both PRP and SRP, but their use is limited by the high incidence of headaches.

E. Prostaglandins, in addition to being potent vasodilators and platelet aggregation inhibitors, probably have additional biologic functions of longer-lasting benefits to microcirculation. Although beneficial when given intravenously, there is not yet sufficient evidence for the clinical usefulness of available oral prostaglandin preparations. They are mainly used at the early stages of severe digital ischemia in SSc. Side effects are common during infusion and include headaches, nausea, and jaw, thigh, or chest pains. They should be avoided in patients with coronary disease or strokes.

1. **Iloprost** is a chemically stable prostacyclin analog. Recent controlled studies have shown that iloprost intravenous infusions promote healing of digital ischemic ulcerations and may reduce the frequency and severity of RP attacks in patients with SSc. Improvement in microcirculation after intravenous infusion of iloprost at the rate of 0.5 to 2 ng/kg/minute for 6 hours/day for 5 days can last for 2 to 4 weeks and repeated monthly 1-day infusions may maintain these effects. It is currently not available in the United States.

2. **Epoprostenol or prostacyclin (PGI2)** has also been effective in RP secondary to SSc. It is currently approved for use in primary pulmonary hypertension where it is given continuously (via a portable infusion pump linked to a central vein) at a starting dosage of 2 ng/kg/minute.

3. **Alprostadil or prostaglandin E1 (PGE1)** requires a central intravenous line and has been given in infusions of 6 to 10 ng/kg/minute over a 72-hour period. It is available in the United States for maintaining the patency of the ductus arteriosus. More stable analogs of PGE_1 have also been used with success.

F. Angiotensin receptor blockers (ARB) and angiotensin converting enzyme inhibitors (ACEI). Losartan has been shown to be superior to nifedipine in one study. Notably, in SSc, ACEI (and less so the ARB) have a special role in the management of scleroderma renal crisis.

G. Antiplatelet agents such as 81 mg of aspirin have been advocated for use in RP with ulcer formation where some degree of thrombosis might have occurred. Heparin is reserved for more severe cases.

H. Pentoxifylline at dosages of 400 mg orally three times a day is a rheologic agent that has been advocated by some, but there is little supporting evidence for its use in RP.

I. Phosphodiesterase-5 inhibitors have been anecdotally used with success in refractory RP cases.

J. Ketanserin, an antagonist of the S2 serotonin receptors on vascular smooth muscle cells and platelets, may be effective in PRP and SRP. This medicine is no longer available in the United States.

K. Selective serotonin reuptake inhibitors (SSRI) have been used with success in RP in some studies. More data are needed to establish their role in RP.

L. The endothelin-antagonist (Bosentan) has been shown to prevent new digital ulcer formation in patients with SSc and may have a role in the management in RP of such patients.

M. Antioxidant drugs such as intravenous infusion of N-acetylcysteine are presumed to have a beneficial effect by ameliorating reactive oxidant species-induced damage.

N. Narcotic analgesics are often needed for severe ischemic pain.

IV. Surgery is indicated in refractory cases of RP with severe ischemia ("finger at risk") and nonhealing digital ulcers despite medical therapy.

   A. Cervical sympathectomy is not recommended for upper extremity RP because it does not offer long-term benefits and may have significant long-term adverse effects. However, peripheral or proximal sympathetic blocks may have a place in the acute management of severe digital ischemia (digit at imminent risk for tissue loss) in connective tissue disease and often will stabilize the condition sufficient enough to allow maintenance medical therapy. For lower extremity RP, lumbar sympathectomy is usually effective.

   B. Digital sympathectomy (adventitial stripping) can be digit saving, often with immediate restoration of blood flow. The technique, in experienced hands, is a relatively safe procedure and achieves not only interruption of the vessel sympathetic innervation but also a mechanical release of arterial constriction by the adventitial and periadventitial fibrosis ("decompression arteriolysis").

   C. Microsurgical revascularization can be effectively employed for occlusive lesions affecting the ulnar artery at the wrist and the superficial palmar arch, as may be seen in SSc.

   D. Amputations will occasionally be required for ulcers associated with distal phalanx osteomyelitis and/or distal interphalangeal (DIP) sepsis, or severe pain due to gangrene. However, autoamputation of mummified tissue is preferable because this procedure allows the maximum possible tissue salvage. The use of oral or parenteral antibiotics for active infections in the site of ischemic finger ulcers can avoid rapid tissue breakdown.

V. "THE FINGER AT RISK." At times, patients with limited scleroderma or CREST (calcinosis, Raynaud's phenomenon, esophageal dysfunction, sclerodactyly, and telangiectasis) syndrome will develop the rather sudden onset of severe pains in one finger, along with marked ischemia manifested by a totally white finger. This is an emergency because prolonged ischemia will likely result in tissue loss and secondary infection. The treatment regimen that is employed in this setting is the following:

   A. Avoidance of trauma and removal from a cold environment.

   B. Use of anticoagulants, usually aspirin, at times heparin, to avoid local clotting and a low flow state.

   C. Institution of vasodilator medications, as noted in the preceding text.

   D. Consultation with an anesthesiologist for an immediate sympathetic block either in the neck or in the hand. Often, this "breaks" the ischemic event. It should be noted that digital arteries may be totally encased by fibrous tissue in the vessel adventitia and no amount of sympathetic block can help.

   E. Consideration of adventitial stripping if ischemia persists, especially if a hand, vascular, or plastic surgeon who is skilled at this microsurgery is available.

   F. Adventitial stripping is usually quite effective but patients may still have some pain after the procedure. In this case, one should consider anticoagulation to avoid microthrombi due to the low flow state.

VI. Local care of existing ulcers with wet to dry dressings and antibiotic ointments is crucial to prevent local infectious complications.

PROGNOSIS

I. **PRP,** as diagnosed by using the more strict criteria (excluding those patients with digital pitting/ulcerations/gangrene, positive ANA, high ESR, and abnormal nailfold capillaries), has an excellent prognosis, and in only up to 10% of patients will PRP evolve into an autoimmune disorder.

II. **SRP**
   A. **Possible SRP** consists of those patients with RP who do not qualify as PRP with the strict definition and do not clearly fulfill the criteria for any of the secondary diagnoses. These patients often have an isolated positive ANA test or nonspecific nailfold capillary abnormalities. Their prognosis is also very good in that only 10% to 30% will develop a CTD.
   B. **The prognosis of SRP** depends on the underlying disease. Fixed-obstruction arterial lesions upon vascular laboratory evaluation (see laboratory studies in the preceding text) have been strongly correlated with digital ulcerations (50% of the patients) and amputations (10% to 20% of the patients).

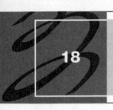

AUTOIMMUNE AND INFLAMMATORY OPHTHALMIC DISEASES

Sergio Schwartzman, C. Michael Samson, and Scott S. Weissman

■ KEY POINTS

■ There are multiple autoimmune diseases that can affect the eye with different implications. These can include idiopathic illnesses or the association of ophthalmic diseases with systemic autoimmune illnesses.

■ The systemic therapy for autoimmune ophthalmic illnesses frequently overlaps that used in systemic autoimmune illnesses.

■ It is important to exclude infectious and malignant (lymphoma) diseases when treating autoimmune eye diseases.

■ Close communication needs to be maintained between the ophthalmologist and the rheumatologist treating patients with autoimmune eye diseases.

INTRODUCTION

Autoimmune ophthalmic diseases comprise a heterogeneous group of illnesses that have different etiologies, clinical presentations, laboratory findings, and responses to therapy.

I. **The eye and its associated orbital structures may exhibit pathologic changes in patients afflicted with many systemic autoimmune illnesses**. In certain inflammatory joint diseases, such as rheumatoid arthritis (RA), there is a similarity in the pathologic processes occurring in the joints and in the eye. Inflammation in the conjunctiva and sclera seems to be somewhat analogous to that occurring in the synovium and cartilage, where uncontrolled and relentless immunologically mediated inflammation in either organ results in its destruction.

II. **Rheumatic illnesses in which ophthalmic involvement is most common are** the human leucocyte antigen-B27 (HLA-B27) associated diseases, RA, Sjögren's syndrome, systemic lupus erythematosus (SLE), juvenile idiopathic arthritis (JIA), Behçet's disease, and sarcoidosis.

III. **For the purposes of classifying the ocular manifestations of connective tissue diseases** (CTDs), it is convenient to conceptualize the eye anatomically as a structure consisting of three concentric spheres or coats: an outer collagen coat or scleral shell; a middle vascular coat, known as the uveal tract; and the inner coat or retinal layer. Each of the various CTDs shows a characteristic pattern involving one or more of these structures.

A. The outer collagen or corneoscleral layer becomes involved with RA, and a scleritis results.

B. The middle or uveal coat is more often involved with the spondyloarthropathies, such as ankylosing spondylitis (AS) or the oligoarticular juvenile arthritis, and iridocyclitis develops.

C. The inner, retinal layer is involved in SLE, so that a characteristic retinal vasculitis, retinopathy, or choroidopathy results.

IV. **The etiologies** of idiopathic uveitis, scleritis, and ophthalmic vasculitis are largely unknown. In all probability, the causes of these diseases differ and the findings of uveitis, scleritis, and vasculitis represent multiple disease processes. The ophthalmic manifestations of systemic autoimmune diseases are probably the consequence of the same mechanism that is responsible for the underlying systemic illness. It is, however, problematic to explain why all the patients with a given systemic illness do not develop ophthalmic involvement. This may be due to the requirement for a particular genetic profile and/or due to the need for specific exogenous exposures.

V. **When evaluating patients with autoimmune ophthalmic diseases,** it is critical to exclude infectious and malignant conditions that can affect the eye. These may span multiple etiologies including syphilis, tuberculosis, Lyme disease, rickettsia, viral infections, toxoplasmosis, histoplasmosis, and toxocariasis. Lymphoma may initially present as a form of uveitis.

VI. **It is critical that every patient with a rheumatic illness who develops ophthalmic involvement be evaluated by an ophthalmologist,** preferably one who has had experience with autoimmune illnesses, and a rheumatologist. Close communication should exist between these specialists in caring for patients with autoimmune diseases of the eye.

VII. **The workup for autoimmune ophthalmic illnesses** should be based primarily on the complete history and physical examination because the underlying illnesses dramatically vary. Although "laboratory screens" exist, we feel that the diagnostic workup of patients with autoimmune eye disease should be individualized and targeted. It is critical, however, to ensure that infectious and malignant illnesses be excluded. All patients who have inflammatory disease of the eye should have a full history and physical examination.

 IDIOPATHIC UVEITIS

In patients with uveitis, one needs to define the specific anatomic involvement of the uveal tract (ophthalmoscopy) and chronicity.

I. **ANATOMY**

A. Anterior uveitis. Involvement of the iris and/or the ciliary body with cells in the aqueous humor of the anterior chamber (Fig. 18-1).

B. Intermediate uveitis. Inflammation in the vitreous cavity.

C. Posterior uveitis. Choroid, retinal involvement, and/or optic neuritis.

D. Panuveitis. Involvement of anterior and posterior segments.

II. **CHRONICITY**

A. Acute uveitis. Less than 3 months.

B. Chronic uveitis. Greater than 3 months.

III. **SYMPTOMS AND OPHTHALMIC FINDINGS**

A. Anterior uveitis. Acute—pain, photophobia, and red eye. Ophthalmoscopy reveals cells in the anterior chamber. Chronic—similar to acute symptoms although less pronounced, however, with decreased visual acuity. Ophthalmoscopy may demonstrate anterior chamber cells, synechiae, band keratopathy, glaucoma, and cataract.

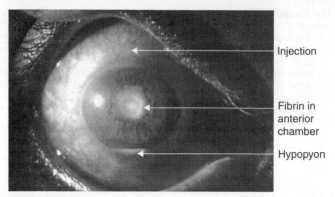

Injection

Fibrin in anterior chamber

Hypopyon

Figure 18-1. Anterior uveitis. (Courtesy of Biswas J, MD and Narayana K, MD, Chennai, India.)

B. **Intermediate uveitis.** Decreased visual acuity and floaters. Cells in the vitreous and "snowbanking" may be noted on ophthalmoscopy in cases of "pars planitis." Note the association of intermediate uveitis with multiple sclerosis.
C. **Posterior uveitis.** Decreased visual acuity and floaters, occasionally pain and photophobia. Ophthalmoscopy reveals cells in the vitreous, choroid, and retinal infiltrates, and vascular involvement.

IV. **DIFFERENTIAL DIAGNOSIS**
A. **Anterior uveitis**
1. HLA-B27 associated uveitis.
a. AS.
b. Reactive arthritis (ReA).
c. Psoriatic arthropathy.
d. Inflammatory bowel disease.
2. Whipple's disease.
3. Sarcoidosis.
4. Behçet's disease.
5. Fuchs' heterochromic iridocyclitis.
6. JIA.
7. Syphilis.
8. Lyme disease.
9. Tuberculosis.
10. Herpes simplex virus.
11. Herpes zoster virus.
12. Other infectious causes.
13. Postsurgical uveitis.
14. Tubular interstitial nephritis and uveitis syndrome.
B. **Intermediate uveitis**
1. Sarcoidosis.
2. Syphilis.
3. Lyme disease.
4. Multiple sclerosis.
5. Inflammatory bowel disease.
C. **Posterior uveitis**
1. Toxoplasma.
2. Cytomegalovirus (CMV) retinitis.
3. SLE.
4. Sarcoid.
5. EBV.
6. Toxocara.
7. Behçet's disease.

II. SIGNS AND SYMPTOMS. Acute anterior uveitis usually manifests with redness, pain, photophobia, and tearing, but the low-grade, chronic anterior uveitis of JIA may be asymptomatic, which makes it a particularly dangerous problem because extensive ocular disease may occur before the condition is recognized. There may be no correlation with joint inflammation. The most common sequela of anterior uveitis is the deposition of calcium beneath the corneal epithelium, causing band keratopathy. Band keratopathy is a nonspecific condition that develops after any longstanding inflammation. Chronic anterior uveitis also produces cataracts and secondary glaucoma. This chronic form of anterior uveitis can be unrelenting and have a progressive downhill course that may lead to significant vision loss. The treatment itself, which consists of topical or systemic corticosteroid therapy, can result in glaucoma and cataracts. New therapies have been studied and there are currently several publications on the use of anti-TNF agents in JIA-associated uveitis.

ANKYLOSING SPONDYLITIS

I. Anterior uveitis is so common in AS that it might be regarded as a clinical feature rather than a complication of the disease. It may be the presenting feature, antedating the joint symptoms by as much as 12 years or occurring when the disease is entirely quiescent. The anterior uveitis tends to affect one eye at a time and is generally fulminant at onset. In 20% of patients, it is the most disabling feature of the disease, because of both its severity and frequent recurrences.

II. In addition to anterior uveitis being found in a large number of patients with AS, spondylarthropathy is found in a significant percentage of patients presenting to an ophthalmologist with anterior uveitis. **Young men with anterior uveitis should be investigated** for signs and symptoms relating to AS. There is a striking association of this disease with the presence of the histocompatibility antigen HLA-B27, which is found in only 5% to 8% of controls, but in approximately 90% of the white patients with AS.

REACTIVE ARTHRITIS

I. The classic diagnostic triad of ReA includes nongonococcal urethritis, arthritis, and conjunctivitis (called Reiter's syndrome in the past).

II. The ocular findings may be the presenting feature of this disease, although they usually follow the other symptoms. Conjunctivitis, part of the classic triad, is the most common ocular manifestation of the disease. It is usually mild and presents with some burning and tearing. ReA and psoriatic arthropathy are the only conditions in which conjunctivitis is a complication. Anterior uveitis occurs in 8% to 40% of patients with this entity. It is more common with recurrent disease than in the initial stage of illness. ReA also shows an association with the HLA-B27 antigen.

ENTEROPATHIC ARTHROPATHY

Enteropathic arthropathy is the form of oligoarthritis associated with inflammatory bowel disease, including ulcerative colitis and Crohn's disease. Ocular findings associated with these entities involve mainly the uveal tract and manifest as an iridocyclitis. Scleritis has also been reported. The incidence of ocular findings in enteropathic arthropathy, however, is less than in the more common arthritis syndromes.

SYSTEMIC LUPUS ERYTHEMATOSUS

I. Unlike some of the other connective tissue disorders, SLE can involve almost every structure in the eye.

8. Syphilis.
9. Multiple sclerosis.
10. Herpes simplex.
11. Herpes zoster.
12. Vogt-Kayanagi-Harada syndrome.
13. Sympathetic ophthalmia.
14. White dot syndromes.

V. THERAPY

A. Anterior uveitis. Cycloplegic agents and topical steroids (e.g., prednisolone acetate 1% every 1 to 6 hours depending on severity). If disease is resistant, periocular steroids injections, systemic steroids (e.g., prednisone 1 mg/kg), or immunosuppressive agents (e.g., cyclosporine, azathioprine, mycophenolate mofetil, and methotrexate) can be used. Anti-tumor necrosis factor (anti-TNF) therapy has been demonstrated to be of benefit in patients who have uveitis resistant to immunosuppressive medications (although not approved for this indication). It is of interest that although the anti-TNF agents target the same cytokine, there appears to be a clear superiority of infliximab over etanercept.

B. Posterior uveitis and panuveitis. These illnesses tend to be resistant to therapy with topical corticosteroids and frequently require therapy with systemic steroids and immunosuppressive agents. Biological anti-TNF therapies may have their greatest benefit in this group of patients. Intravitreal sustained drug delivery systems that are either biodegradable or nonbiodegradable have also been employed.

IDIOPATHIC SCLERITIS

I. SYMPTOMS AND OPHTHALMIC FINDINGS. Severe eye pain is the most common complaint, with visual loss and photophobia also occurring. Inflammation of the scleral, episcleral, and conjunctival vessels occurs, resulting in a red, inflamed eye (Fig. 18-2). Particularly in chronic scleritis, the sclera may become thin with a consequent bluish appearance.

II. DIFFERENTIAL DIAGNOSIS. RA, Wegener's granulomatosis, relapsing polychondritis, AS, SLE, polyarteritis nodosa, Lyme disease, ReA, Behçet's disease, and sarcoidosis.

III. THERAPY. Nonsteroidal anti-inflammatory drugs (NSAIDs) (Indomethacin 25 mg four times a day), systemic corticosteroids (prednisone 1 mg/kg), and immunosuppressive therapy (cyclosporine, azathioprine, mycophenolate, and methotrexate). Cyclophosphamide has been used for the systemic vasculitides and in patients with scleromalacia perforans.

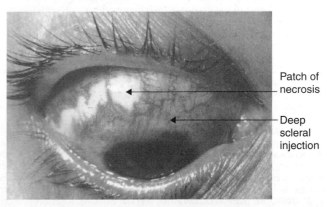
Patch of necrosis

Deep scleral injection

Figure 18-2. Scleritis. (Courtesy of Biswas J, MD and Narayana K, MD, Chennai, India.)

RHEUMATOID ARTHRITIS

The most characteristic and potentially serious ocular manifestations of RA are inflammation of the sclera, cornea, or both. The most common manifestation of RA is keratoconjunctivitis sicca. In the face of the new aggressive treatment paradigm employed for RA, all of these problems appear to be decreasing in frequency and severity.

I. **SCLERITIS.** The clinical spectrum of scleritis may range from a mild, localized, superficial episcleritis, to a dramatically painful, necrotizing scleritis with dire prognostic systemic implications. The various types of scleritis are probably different manifestations of a single pathologic process, which appears similar to that operating in the joints. An immune complex vasculitis in the sclera appears to be responsible for the inflammatory process. The specific clinical entity produced depends on the site, depth, and extent of the pathologic process.

   A. **The incidence of scleritis** in RA is approximately 5%; however, in patients who present to the ophthalmologist with scleritis, as many as one-third may have RA. Therefore, every patient with scleritis in an ophthalmology clinic should be evaluated for RA as well.

   B. **Prognosis for life and sight.** The prognostic significance of rheumatoid scleritis is conspicuously illustrated by a study in which 45% of patients with scleritis died within 5 years of being diagnosed, compared with 18% of a matched control sample of patients with RA without scleritis. In mild forms of scleral inflammation, such as local or generalized episcleritis, the swelling and inflammatory process is superficial, although painful, and it is usually easy to control with topical medications and resolves without serious sequelae. Deep scleritis, however, is one of the few severely painful eye problems; it has serious prognostic implications for sight and life, and requires systemic, often long-term treatment with one of several anti-inflammatory agents. In necrotizing scleritis, which is the most dramatic and destructive form of scleritis, a scleral vessel is suddenly occluded, causing an avascular patch (sequestrum) that eventually dissolves and exposes the underlying uveal tissue. Necrosis occurring slowly over time and without inflammation is called necrotizing scleritis without inflammation; it is referred to in older classic literature as scleromalacia perforans. Necrotizing scleritis represents the changes of the eye during the malignant phase of a systemic tissue disorder and usually occurs in patients in whom the disease has manifested into the advanced stages. It is also seen in polyarteritis nodosa, Wegener's granulomatosis, and SLE. Scleritis itself has serious ocular complications other than the production of a scleral defect; it can result in keratitis, cataracts, uveitis, and glaucoma.

   C. **Treatment.** Because of the depth and severity of the inflammatory process in scleritis, long-term (years) systemic anti-inflammatory agents are required. Those that have been reported to be effective include indomethacin, diflunisal, corticosteroids, azathioprine, cyclophosphamide, and cyclosporin A. In the most severe and sight-threatening cases, cyclophosphamide along with intravenous corticosteroids must be used. With the use of these two drugs, the clinician is in the unenviable position of balancing toxic treatments versus a destructive disease. There is preliminary data that anti-TNF therapies, particularly infliximab, may benefit patients with scleritis that is unresponsive to traditional immunosuppressive medications.

II. **CORNEAL COMPLICATIONS.** Corneal manifestations associated with RA are serious problems whose importance and occurrence are not generally appreciated. Corneal involvement may accompany inflammation of the adjacent sclera or may occur in the absence of any other ocular complications. One form is the development of peripheral ulcers or furrows at or near the limbus (limbal guttering), frequently occurring in the absence of significant inflammation. These ulcers may be nonprogressive or go on to cause marked thinning and perforation of the cornea. Central corneal ulcers and perforations can be seen in clinically quiet eyes. These patients are usually in an advanced stage of their disease and are often on maintenance doses of systemic corticosteroid drugs.

III. **SICCA SYNDROME (KERATOCONJUNCTIVITIS SICCA).** Keratoconjunctivitis sicca is one of the most common ocular manifestations of RA. It also occurs with several of the other CTDs and as an isolated entity. The syndrome as originally described by Sjögren consists of dry eye, dry mouth, and arthritis.

   A. **Signs and symptoms.** The most common symptom that patients complain of is a foreign-body sensation or a feeling of "something" (sand or lashes) in their eyes. The clinical spectrum of a patient with keratoconjunctivitis sicca may vary from symptoms only, with very few signs seen by the ophthalmologist, to mild signs consisting of punctate erosions on the inferior half of the cornea, with or without filaments that consist of a mixture of surface cells and mucus. There is one particularly devastating variation in which corneal infiltration and necrosis sometimes develop, leading to possible corneal perforation. Fortunately, this is quite rare.

   B. **Treatment**

      1. The first line of defense is replacement of tear volume through the use of artificial tears. This works best when combined with nightly eyelash lavage with baby shampoo to clean off accumulated debris that the compromised tear film cannot handle. Variable success has been reported with artificial tear inserts, such as Lacriserts.

      2. Another simple therapeutic intervention is the use of moist-chamber glasses. Clear plastic extends to the face, trapping any moisture produced and thereby decreasing evaporation.

      3. More severe cases require more aggressive treatments, all of which have inherent risks. Occlusion of the punctum can reduce the drainage of tears, but should only be used if less than 3 mm of wetting is noted on the Schirmer's test. Therapeutic soft contact lenses are extremely useful when foreign-body symptoms are so extensive that patients cannot keep their eyes open. This is also the case when filaments develop in a dry eye. The problem with contact lenses in patients with dry eyes is the possible development of corneal infections.

      4. Cyclosporin ophthalmic emulsion 0.05% (Restasis) has recently been approved for the treatment of keratoconjunctivitis sicca.

IV. **DIFFERENTIAL DIAGNOSIS OF "RED EYE."** These diagnostic possibilities hold for all the collagen diseases, but are presented in this section because RA is the most common underlying entity and is associated with the greatest number of possible causes of a red eye.

   A. **Scleritis,** either local or general. Pain is usually present.

   B. **Keratitis sicca** results in the eyes becoming irritated from lack of a normal tear volume to lubricate and protect the surface.

   C. **Conjunctivitis** occurs secondary to a tear volume deficit, which deprives the eye of its natural protection against infection.

   D. **Iridocyclitis** usually occurs acutely in spondyloarthropathies, with light sensitivity, a miotic pupil on the affected side, and a peripupillary red ring (ciliary flush). A more chronic iridocyclitis, with a white and quiet external appearance, is more typical of children with JIA.

   E. **Glaucoma,** secondary either to scleritis and inflammation of the trabecular meshwork or to corticosteroid therapy.

   F. **Herpetic keratitis,** complicating immunosuppressive drug regimens used to treat this group of patients.

JUVENILE IDIOPATHIC ARTHRITIS

JIA is sufficiently different in its ocular manifestations to warrant consideration as a separate entity. Adult RA most frequently affects the outer collagenous coat of the eye, producing scleritis, whereas in JIA, inflammation of the middle coat or uveitis is the classic ocular complication. The uveitis in JIA is characterized by an insidious inflammation of the anterior uveal tract (iridocyclitis). Scleral inflammation in JIA is rare.

I. The **incidence of uveitis** in JIA is approximately 10%, and uveitis is more common in women, antinuclear antibody positive, and with pauciarticular involvement. The uveitis usually develops after the arthritis, but may precede it by many years. Anterior uveitis is the most common.

II. It is critical to differentiate among the ocular manifestations of the disease itself, coincident antiphospholipid syndrome manifestations, and the ophthalmic toxicity of therapy targeting the systemic disease (glaucoma and cataracts).

   A. The most common **retinal findings** are cotton-wool spots sometimes termed cytoid bodies, retinal hemorrhages, and edema of the disc and surrounding retina. Similar changes can result from the associated hypertension seen in patients with SLE and nephritis. The findings associated with vasculitis are sometimes called lupus retinopathy.

   B. **Anterior segment involvement** may take the form of conjunctivitis, sicca syndrome, or scleritis. Ptosis and proptosis have been reported secondary to myositis of the extraocular muscles. Drug-induced SLE can also be associated with ocular manifestations.

 GIANT CELL ARTERITIS AND POLYMYALGIA RHEUMATICA

Giant cell arteritis (GCA), also known as temporal or cranial arteritis, can result in sudden, dramatic, and disastrous loss of vision. Polymyalgia rheumatica (PMR) is included in this section because a small percentage of patients with PMR have occult GCA and 50% of patients with GCA have PMR. The two disorders are parts of a single disease spectrum.

I. **GIANT CELL ARTERITIS.** Ocular manifestations may occur in 30% of patients and are among the most serious consequences of this illness. Ocular complications occur usually several weeks to months after the onset of systemic symptoms, but may also occur years later or develop first in the absence of systemic signs, a situation referred to as occult temporal arteritis. Inflammation of the ophthalmic, central retinal, or posterior ciliary arteries is responsible for the various ocular problems.

   A. The most frequent and disastrous problem is the sudden, irreversible **loss of vision** caused by inflammation either in the central retinal artery, which is the terminal branch of the ophthalmic artery, or in the posterior ciliary arteries, which supply the optic nerve; the latter situation can result in an ischemic optic neuritis. An altitudinal visual field deficit is characteristic of optic nerve inflammation in GCA.

   B. **Diplopia** also occurs from involvement of the posterior ciliary arteries, which supply the extraocular muscles.

   C. When several of the extraocular muscles are involved, the syndrome of **anterior segment necrosis** may occur, which essentially is ischemia of the front of the eye resulting in uveitis, iris necrosis, and scleritis.

   D. **Treatment,** which must be instituted rapidly, consists of systemic corticosteroids in doses sufficient to suppress the clinical and laboratory evidence (especially the erythrocyte sedimentation rate) of disease activity. Any visual symptoms must be treated aggressively, at times with prednisone doses more than 100 mg/day, or intravenously with 500 to 1,000 mg of methylprednisolone. In some cases, vision is lost despite massive doses of systemic anti-inflammatory medication. Unfortunately, bilateral blindness may occur in up to 25% of patients with giant cell arteritis. The purpose of treatment is prevention of further worsening in the condition. Improvement of visual acuity in an involved eye after commencing steroid therapy is only rarely noted.

 POLYARTERITIS NODOSA

I. **Ocular manifestations** can involve almost every tissue of the eye in this inflammatory disease affecting small and medium-sized arteries. The most common and serious manifestation is scleral keratitis, which is similar to that seen in RA, but usually more painful and sharply demarcated. Guttering of the peripheral cornea develops in the limbal region, which may spread circumferentially to form a ring. Bilateral involvement can be present. The process may extend centrally to involve much of the cornea, producing extensive scarring, vascularization, and perforation.

II. **Clinical syndromes** have been described in which polyarteritis nodosa is associated with specific eye and ear findings.

   A. In Cogan's syndrome, an interstitial keratitis (deep corneal haze and vascularization) is associated with audiovestibular disease, characterized by profound deafness, vertigo, and tinnitus.

   B. Other variations include an association of polyarteritis, scleritis, and otitis media. The retinopathy of polyarteritis includes retinal vasculitis and changes that are secondary to coexistent hypertension. A host of ocular signs and symptoms of polyarteritis reflect central nervous system complications.

 ## WEGENER'S GRANULOMATOSIS

Ocular and orbital complications are fairly common in Wegener's granulomatosis, the reported incidence being as high as 60%. If the orbit is involved by direct spread of the granuloma from the paranasal sinuses, the patient can have proptosis, limitation of movement of the globe, and a rapid destruction in vision from either involvement of the optic nerve or an exudative retinal detachment secondary to a posterior scleritis. Nasolacrimal duct obstruction may also be the presenting sign.

I. **Proptosis,** which is a common clinical feature and can be severe, results from invasion of the orbit, and later the sclera, by granulomatous tissue. The sclera becomes infiltrated, and the underlying collagen is attacked by granulation tissue. The histologic picture differs from that usually seen in scleral inflammatory disease in that the invasion is from the outside rather than from the foci within the sclera.

II. **Other types of scleritis** are also seen, in which intrascleral inflammation develops first. A particularly painful peripheral ulcerative keratitis, or necrotizing scleritis, may occur and be the presenting feature of the disease.

 ## BEHÇET'S DISEASE

I. Behçet's disease is an illness defined by recurrent oral and genital ulcers, relapsing iritis, and skin lesions. In addition, it can involve the musculoskeletal, gastrointestinal, vascular, renal, pulmonary, and central nervous systems. There is a genetic predisposition to this illness (HLA-B51 association) and it is predominantly found in countries bordering the Mediterranean and in Japan.

II. The ocular manifestations include anterior uveitis at times with hypopyon, posterior uveitis, panuveitis, and retinal vasculitis. The therapy for ophthalmic involvement includes topical cycloplegic agents and topical steroids. Periocular and subtenon steroid injections may provide benefit. Of the immunosuppressive agents, steroids, methotrexate, cyclophosphamide, cyclosporine, and chlorambucil are effective in some patients. Colchicine has been used to treat the systemic disease and may provide some benefit in patients with ophthalmic involvement. Interestingly, anti-TNF therapies, particularly infliximab, may prove particularly beneficial in treating ocular Behçet's disease.

 ## SARCOIDOSIS

I. The clinical presentation of ocular sarcoidosis varies and may include eye pain, red eye, photophobia, and decrease in vision. Occasionally, patients with sarcoidosis will have very prominent lacrimal glands. Granulomatous iritis with "mutton fat" precipitates is frequently noted by the ophthalmologist.

II. The therapy for uveitis should include cycloplegic agents and topical steroids. In patients unresponsive to local therapy, periocular steroids, systemic steroids, and immunosuppressive agents such as cyclosporine, mycophenolate, and methotrexate have been used. There are anecdotal reports on the use of anti-TNF agents in sarcoidosis.

POLYMYOSITIS AND DERMATOMYOSITIS

I. Polymyositis is an inflammatory disease of striated skeletal muscle. When a characteristic skin rash is present, the term dermatomyositis is used. The most common ocular finding, indeed one of the more characteristic findings of dermatomyositis, is lid discoloration. There is a lilac discoloration of the upper eyelids, often associated with periorbital edema. This violaceous discoloration, called heliotrope rash, is considered pathognomonic.

II. Other ocular findings have been reported, but none is specific. Extraocular muscle weakness is uncommon and may be caused by the myositis itself or by coexistent myasthenia gravis. In children with dermatomyositis, retinal vasculitis is a relatively common feature.

SCLERODERMA

The most common ocular manifestation of this chronic disease of connective tissue is involvement of the skin of the lids, which may have secondary effects on the cornea and conjunctiva. The eyelids lose their freedom of movement and become thin, smooth, and shiny. Tightness of the lids may result in only minimally decreased mobility or a marked restriction of lid movement. Lid restriction may in turn lead to a severe exposure keratitis, especially when it is combined with a hyposecretion of tears occasionally seen with this disease. Sicca syndrome is a significant feature of scleroderma, as it is with the other connective tissue syndromes.

NECK PAIN

James C. Farmer, David A. Bomback, and Thomas P. Sculco

19

■ KEY POINTS

- ■ Degenerative disease of the cervical spine, or cervical spondylosis, is an age-related process that affects many components of the cervical spinal column.

- ■ The spectrum of cervical spondylosis ranges from axial neck pain to radiculopathy to frank myelopathy.

- ■ Physical examination findings correlated with diagnostic imaging studies can aid in diagnostic evaluation.

- ■ Almost all patients with symptomatic cervical degenerative disease without neurologic involvement can be managed nonoperatively.

- ■ Surgery for patients with myelopathy is a reasonable option to prevent disease progression.

Neck pain is a common complaint and tends to occur with increasing frequency after the age of 30. Most episodes of neck pain are short-lived and tend to respond to nonoperative management.

The clinical manifestations of neck disorders range from midline posterior neck pain to the neurologic sequelae of cervical nerve root or spinal cord compression. Axial neck pain may radiate from the base of the skull down to the upper trapezius region. Cervical radiculopathy involves compression of a nerve root, with pain radiating down the arm in an anatomic distribution. Cervical myelopathy is characterized by dysfunction of the spinal cord. This may be caused by cord compression, vascular abnormalities, or a combination of both.

ETIOPATHOGENESIS

I.   **Degeneration of the intervertebral disc** can lead to pain referred to the neck, posterior skull, and/or upper shoulders. This occurs as a natural consequence of the normal aging process with a resulting decrease in the water content of the disc. Disc degeneration can be affected by many external factors including repetitive occupational mechanical strain, and a history of diving or heavy weight lifting. The structures affected within the neck include the intervertebral disc, zygapophyseal joint with associated facet capsules, ligaments, musculature, and the neural elements. Changes can be acute (e.g., traumatic), chronic, or acute on chronic.

II. **Acute herniation of the disc** material posteriorly may result in impingement of the nerve root and/or spinal cord. The distribution of pain in cervical radiculopathy often fits a dermatomal distribution characteristic for each particular nerve root. When cord compression occurs, the changes within the cord can be caused by acute compression by the disc material, as well as compression of the vascular supply to the cord.

III. **Cervical spondylosis** involves loss of disc space height. As a result of the degeneration within the disc and the decreased intervertebral height, altered spinal biomechanics ensue, with osteophytes forming along the area of the disc space as well as posteriorly along the facet joints. This can be associated with nerve root and spinal cord compression.

PREVALENCE

Prevalence of neck and referred shoulder/brachial pain has been reported to be 9%. In a series of 205 patients who presented with neck pain and were managed nonoperatively, 79% were noted to be asymptomatic or improved at a minimum follow-up of 10 years. Symptoms of 13% were unchanged, and only 8% had worsening of their symptoms. Radiographically, 25% of patients in their fifth decade have been shown to have degenerative changes in one or more discs. By the seventh decade, this number increases to over 75%.

CLINICAL MANIFESTATIONS

I.   **NECK PAIN**

  A. **Signs and symptoms.** Neck pain is a pain that is perceived by the patient as existing primarily within the axial portion of the spine. Pain may radiate to the base of the skull or to the midupper periscapular region. The pain may involve the posterior trapezius muscles or the posterior deltoids. The pain itself may be limited to a focal area or may involve a more global region. Night pain is common because the neck becomes a weight-bearing area. The longer the pain exists the more difficult it is for patients to localize it. Because the neck can be a prominent area of referred pain from thoracic organs such as the heart or aorta, the physician must be aware of the patient's comorbid medical issues.

  B. **Physical examination.** Examination of the patient with neck pain should include noting the position in which the neck is held. When there is severe neck spasm, the head may be flexed laterally to that side or even rotated. Muscle spasm can often be visualized and can be palpated posteriorly along the paraspinal musculature. Examination should include inspection of the symmetry of the paraspinal muscles as well as the trapezius and shoulder musculature. Any signs of atrophy must be noted. Strength and range of motion of the shoulder should be tested, as well as examination for focal tenderness within the shoulder (to help rule out the shoulder as a source of potential pain or to define coexistent shoulder disease).

  C. **Range of neck motion** should include flexion, extension, rotation, and lateral bending. Normal flexion demonstrates the ability to touch the chin to the chest. Normal neck extension allows the occiput to approach the prominent C7 spinous process. Rotation is normally 70 degrees bilaterally and lateral bending is

50 to 60 degrees bilaterally. Palpation for carotid artery pulses as well as for the presence or absence of supraclavicular adenopathy should be performed.

II. **CERVICAL RADICULOPATHY**

A. **Signs and symptoms.** Cervical radiculopathy implies pain traveling on the basis of an anatomic distribution to the shoulder or down the arm. Patients describe sharp pain and tingling or burning sensations in the involved area. There may be sensory or motor loss corresponding to the involved nerve root, and reflex activity may be diminished.

B. **Physical examination.** The shoulder abduction relief sign is characterized by having the patient place the palm of his hand flat onto the top of his skull; this causes symptomatic relief of the radicular pain. Spurling's test is performed by having the patient extend the neck and rotate and laterally bend the head toward the affected side; an axial compressive force is then applied to the top of the patient's head. The test is positive when the maneuver reproduces the patient's typical radicular arm pain.

C. **Herniation or degeneration of an intervertebral disc** may produce specific radicular patterns, depending on the level of involvement. Considerable overlap exists among the patterns outlined in the subsequent text. C5-6 and C6-7 are far more commonly involved than C7-T1 or C4-5.

1. **C5-6 (C6 nerve root affected).** Pain will radiate to the shoulder or lateral arm and dorsal forearm. Anesthesia and paresthesias may be present in the thumb and index finger. Weakness, if present, will involve the biceps and wrist extensors. The brachioradialis or biceps reflex is often decreased or absent.

2. **C6-7 (C7 nerve root affected).** The pain distribution is similar to that of a C7 radiculopathy. Anesthesia and paresthesias, when present, involve the index and long fingers. Weakness, if present, is noted in the triceps, wrist flexors, and finger extensors. The triceps reflex is often decreased or absent.

3. **C7-T1 (C8 nerve root affected).** Pain may occur along the medial aspect of the upper arm and forearm. Anesthesia and paresthesias involve the ring and small fingers. Weakness, if present, is noted in the finger flexors and intrinsic musculature of the hand. The triceps reflex may be reduced.

III. **CERVICAL MYELOPATHY**

A. **Signs and symptoms.** Cervical myelopathy alone (e.g., in the absence of radiculopathy) is painless. This is due to the fact that there is spinal cord compression only. The pain becomes apparent only when compression of the spinal cord is accompanied by compression of the nerve root (myeloradiculopathy). Symptoms associated with spinal cord compression include gait disturbances with balance difficulty, fine motor dysfunction in the hands, and motor weakness. Bowel and bladder dysfunction is found late in the progression of cervical myelopathy. Physical findings often include difficulty with tandem gait, dysdiadochokinesia, hyperreflexia, and various sensory and motor changes.

B. **Physical examination.** Hoffmann's reflex is often present, which is elicited by flicking the middle finger of the patient and observing forced finger and thumb interphalangeal joint flexion. There can be upgoing toes (e.g., a positive Babinski's reflex) as well as associated clonus at the ankles. Myelopathy-related hand abnormalities include atrophy of the thenar musculature and an inability to maintain the ring and small fingers in an extended and adducted position (e.g., finger escape sign). Lhermitte's sign involves flexion of the neck with an electric-shocklike sensation extending down the axial spine and/or extremities. In addition to the physical examination for neck pain, a thorough neurologic evaluation is necessary. This includes motor testing of all pertinent motor groups including the deltoid, biceps, triceps, wrist flexors/extensors, finger flexors/extensors, and the interossei. Additionally, lower extremity strength needs to be tested including hip flexors, knee extensors and flexors, hip abductors and adductors, ankle dorsiflexors and plantarflexors as well as the function of the extensor hallucis longus, and peroneals. Sensory examination should include light touch, pinprick, and vibration sense using a tuning fork. Reflex examination should include the biceps, triceps, and brachioradialis, quadriceps, and the Achilles tendon. Another abnormal finding is the inverted radial reflex, characterized by spontaneous finger flexion when the examiner attempts to elicit a brachioradialis reflex. Gait should be tested during normal gait as well as with toe to heel walking.

 DIAGNOSTIC EVALUATION

I. **LABORATORY STUDIES.** Laboratory studies should include routine blood workup; a complete blood count with differential, an erythrocyte sedimentation rate (ESR), and C-reactive protein (CRP). These results will most commonly be abnormal when an infectious or malignant process is involved.

II. **ELECTROPHYSIOLOGICAL TESTING.** An electromyogram (EMG) may be helpful in defining a specific anatomic level when nerve compression is present. Such a study may also be helpful in ruling out other neurologic disorders including peripheral neuropathy. At times, a double-crush syndrome may exist when cervical radiculopathy can coexist with carpal tunnel syndrome.

 IMAGING STUDIES

I. **PLAIN X-RAYS.** A plain x-ray series should include an anterior/posterior view, a lateral view, and oblique views. Degeneration can often be noted within the disc spaces and the facet joints. There are often osteophytes noted along the area of the disc space, and foraminal narrowing can be noted on oblique views. Clinical correlation with patient symptoms is often poor in those older than 40. Instability has been defined as greater than 3.5 mm of translation or 11 degrees of angulation between adjacent vertebral segments.

II. **MYELOGRAPHY.** Myelography can be used to help evaluate nerve root compression as well as compression of the spinal cord. Root compression is manifested by an extradural filling defect with obliteration of the nerve root sleeve. Flattening of the spinal cord can be appreciated on the lateral view. In cases of severe compression, there will be complete obstruction of flow of the myelogram dye. In most clinical situations, this test has given way to the magnetic resonance imaging (MRI) described in the subsequent text.

III. **COMPUTED TOMOGRAPHY.** Computed tomography (CT) is helpful in evaluating the degree of foraminal stenosis caused by bony osteophytes. In combination with myelography, it provides superior imaging compared to myelography alone. It permits the visualization of the specific levels (e.g., C6-7) and location (e.g., lateral recess and foraminal) of nerve root compression; filling defects allow for the determination of the extent of spinal cord compression. Measurement of the diameter of the spinal canal can be made to help define pre-existing stenosis. Individuals with an anteroposterior spinal canal diameter less than 13 mm are considered to have congenital cervical stenosis. In addition, patients with a cord-compression ratio (anteroposterior cord diameter divided by transverse cord diameter) less than 0.40 tend to have worse neurologic function.

IV. **MRI.** MRI is perhaps the primary imaging modality overall for cervical spine disorders. It provides excellent visualization of the spinal cord and soft tissues. Measurements of sagittal and axial canal diameters as well as cord-compression ratios can be calculated from an MRI.

 DIFFERENTIAL DIAGNOSIS

I. **Differential diagnoses** to consider with cervical disc disease are numerous. When a history of **trauma** is present, cervical sprain, traumatic injury to the brachial plexus, fracture, dislocation, or post-traumatic instability need to be considered.

II. **Inflammatory conditions** including rheumatoid arthritis and ankylosing spondylitis can also present with cervical pathology. An infectious process including discitis, osteomyelitis, or soft tissue abscess (especially in light of a clinical history that includes fever or chills) must be ruled out.

III. Tumors can be a cause of neck and upper extremity symptoms. These may include metastatic tumors, primary bone tumors, and tumors within the spinal cord. Additionally, tumors involving the upper lung (Pancoast's tumor) may cause symptoms consistent with a C8 radiculopathy and/or a Horner's syndrome. The presence of a history of weight loss, night pain, and present or past malignancy should increase the physician's sensitivity to the possibility of a malignant tumor.

IV. Shoulder disorders including rotator cuff disease, instability, and impingement may cause pain referred to the neck and can be confused with a C5 radiculopathy. More commonly, the neck refers pain to the shoulder and may actually be associated with the development of frank shoulder pathology.

V. Neurologic disorders such as the demyelinating disease, multiple sclerosis, as well as diseases involving the anterior horn cells must be considered in the differential diagnosis.

VI. Finally, many other conditions such as peripheral nerve entrapment syndromes, reflex sympathetic dystrophy, thoracic outlet syndrome, as well as coronary artery disease with angina pectoris may simulate radicular type symptoms. Pathology in the neck or shoulder may make those areas more likely sites to which visceral pain refers.

 TREATMENT

I. Conservative care is the primary treatment of patients with neck pain, with or without radicular symptoms. Lifestyle modifications should be instituted to avoid activities that tend to create or aggravate neck and arm symptoms.

   A. Typical activities to modify include athletic activities, sitting at a desk with neck flexion (e.g., reading and typing) for extended periods of time, and driving. An ergonomic assessment of the modern computerized office is often helpful in decreasing day-long stresses to the neck. A soft cervical collar can be used to limit motion and allow the spasm to settle down. The use of two or three pillows at night, in order to decrease reflux symptoms or breathing problems, exacerbate cervical spine problems and should be avoided. Therefore, use of a cervical pillow under the nape of the neck at night may help decrease spasms and pain, as it tends to optimize the position of the neck during sleep. Other modalities such as moist heat and light massage may prove beneficial.

   B. Use of medications including anti-inflammatory medications help decrease the amount of inflammation and provide pain relief. In cases of severe pain, mild narcotics may be useful. Muscle relaxants may also help decrease the amount of spasm and allow for more comfortable periods of rest. Short courses of steroids are sometimes needed to control the inflammatory process.

   C. Physical therapy is often useful in the treatment of neck and radicular arm pain, once the phase of severe pain and radicular problems resolve. Modalities including traction, ultrasound, or diathermy can give pain relief. Once the patient's symptoms have begun to decrease, an exercise regimen can be added taking note that this does not exacerbate the neck or arm pain symptoms. Active range of motion exercises along with some isometric exercises can help regain the strength of the neck.

II. Surgery is indicated in cases of significant radicular pain that has failed to respond to conservative treatment, or in the presence of significant neurologic deficits. Only a small percentage of patients with cervical spine problems eventually require surgery. However, if considered necessary, the surgical procedure is either an anterior cervical discectomy and fusion or a posterior laminoforaminotomy. For cases of myelopathy with significant disability, surgery can be a reasonable alternative. The goal of surgery with myelopathy is to prevent progression of the disease. Postoperatively, some patients show improvement from their preoperative neurologic status. For myelopathy, surgery consists of either multiple anterior cervical discectomies/corpectomies and fusion versus posterior procedures such as laminectomy alone, laminoplasty, or laminectomy and fusion. A small percentage of patients with significant multilevel disease or poor bone quality are good candidates for a combined anterior/posterior procedure. Surgery should be done emergently in the setting of an epidural abscess.

PROGNOSIS

I. **The prognosis for patients with axial neck pain** is, in general, good. In a follow-up of a series of 205 patients with neck pain and treated nonoperatively, 79% were noted to be either asymptomatic or improved at 10-year follow-up, 13% were noted to be unchanged, and 8% were felt to have worsening symptoms. Surgery for axial neck pain by itself is rarely indicated, except perhaps in the setting of instability.

II. **The prognosis for patients with cervical radiculopathy** is also, in general, favorable. A significant number of patients tend to respond to nonoperative measures and show significant improvement 2 to 3 months after the onset of symptoms. A series of 26 patients with cervical disc herniation and radiculopathy were managed nonoperatively with traction, medications, and education. A 1-year follow-up showed successful nonoperative management in 24 of the 26 patients. For patients who have persistent radicular symptoms despite 2 to 3 months of nonsurgical treatment, or who have significant weakness, surgery is a reasonable option. The prognosis for improvement with surgery is generally favorable. Most patients experience significant improvement in their radicular pain.

III. **Cervical myelopathy** with early myelopathy and no significant neurologic deficits can initially be followed in an outpatient setting. The prognosis for cervical myelopathy in general shows that a high percentage of these patients slowly deteriorate over time. The deterioration is often slow and occurs over years; a small percent of cases may display signs and symptoms of rapid progression. In patients with gross findings of myelopathy with significant cord compression and impairment, surgery is a reasonable option. The goal of surgery is to prevent deterioration and potentially promote improvement in their overall neurologic status. In a series of patients treated surgically for cervical myelopathy, 90% of patients had significant neurologic improvement and 80% had significant pain relief.

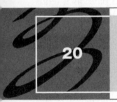

LOW BACK PAIN
20
H. Hallett Whitman, III, Daniel J. Clauw, and John F. Beary, III

■ KEY POINTS

■ Low back pain (LBP) is the second most common condition seen in primary care practice, and the most common problem seen by musculoskeletal specialists. It is essential that physicians be comfortable with the nuances of diagnosis and treatment of LBP.

■ Less common causes of LBP such as infection (fever and focal pain) and cancer (weight loss, unexplained pain, and oncologic risk factors) must not be overlooked. If the pain persists and is unexplained, then the case must be investigated further.

■ Magnetic resonance imaging (MRI) images have a 30% false-positive rate, and therefore must be used in a discriminating manner. Remember that most patients with acute LBP and without neurologic signs and symptoms will respond to conservative therapy, and need no diagnostic tests.

■ Prolonged bed rest is harmful. An extended period of inactivity is a risk factor for converting acute LBP into chronic LBP. Start an appropriate regimen of exercise as soon as possible to preserve strength and flexibility in the muscles that support the lumbar spine.

■ Sensitization of peripheral or central pain processing systems will explain some cases of chronic LBP that persist despite the correction of the anatomical factors. Therefore, the first 3 to 6 months of assessment and treatment of patients with LBP are critical with regard to preserving and optimizing function of the lumbar spine.

INTRODUCTION

I.   **Low back pain (LBP)** can affect up to 80% of the population at some point in their lives, making it second only to the common cold as an illness affecting the general population, and the fourth or fifth most common reason for a visit to the physician's office in the United States.

II. **Acute LBP** usually resolves spontaneously, but up to 10% progress to chronic LBP resulting in temporary or permanent disability. This results in a loss of more than 1,000 work days per 1,000 workers each year, costing more than $20 billion annually, and disabling several million individuals in the United States alone at any one time.

III. **Risk factors for the development of LBP** include heavy manual work, poor job satisfaction, exposure to vibration, cigarette smoking, and pregnancy. A sedentary lifestyle is also probably a cause.

IV. **Most patients with acute and chronic LBP have "idiopathic" LBP,** meaning that despite testing, no clear cause can be found for their pain.

V.   **Most patients who present with acute LBP in the absence of significant neurologic physical findings** need no diagnostic tests and will respond to conservative management.

VI. **Patients who do not respond to a conservative regimen** may need imaging studies, and rarely surgery.

ETIOPATHOGENESIS

Any of the components of the lumbosacral spine when combined with related conditions listed in the subsequent text may be responsible for LBP.

I.   **VERTEBRAL BODY** (fracture, osteoporosis, metastatic disease, sickle cell disease, and infection).

II.   **INTERVERTEBRAL DISC** (herniation and infection).

III. **JOINTS** (osteoarthritis and ankylosing spondylitis).
   A. Apophyseal joints.
   B. Sacroiliac joints.

IV.   **LIGAMENTS** (strain and rupture).
   A. Anterior and posterior longitudinal ligaments.
   B. Interspinous and supraspinous ligaments.
   C. Iliolumbar ligaments.
   D. Apophyseal ligaments.

V.   **NERVE ROOTS** (herniated nucleus pulposus and spinal stenosis).

VI.   **PARASPINAL MUSCULATURE** (strain and spasms).

VII. **PAIN FROM ADJACENT STRUCTURES** (referred pain).
   A. Kidney (pyelonephritis and perinephric abscess).
   B. Pelvic structures (pelvic inflammatory disease, ectopic pregnancy, endometriosis, and prostate disease).
   C. Vascular (aortic aneurysm and mesenteric thrombosis).
   D. Intestinal (diverticulitis).

VIII. **Pain amplification syndromes** where there is no identifiable abnormality of the peripheral tissue, but there is localized or widespread hyperalgesia (e.g., myofascial pain and regional forms of fibromyalgia).

PREVALENCE

Prevalence of LBP ranges from 38 to 93 per 1,000 population, with female sex, white ancestry, and increasing age being independent risk factors for increased incidence.

CLINICAL MANIFESTATIONS

I. **Clinical history** of the patient is of great importance in obtaining information regarding associated symptoms and establishing a pattern of pain. A thorough review of symptoms that would suggest a nonmechanical cause for LBP is required.

   A. **Fever or chills** would raise the possibility of an infectious process.

   B. **Weight loss, chronic cough, change in bowel habits,** or **night pain** may suggest malignancy.

   C. Similar pain or morning stiffness in different areas of the body would increase the suspicion of a more generalized rheumatic condition such as ankylosing spondylitis, psoriatic arthritis, or reactive arthritis (ReA).

   D. **If fatigue or sleep disturbance is present,** in the setting of a diffuse pain syndrome, the diagnosis of fibromyalgia should be considered.

   E. **Morning stiffness or back pain that improves with exercise** should prompt consideration of a spondyloarthropathy such as ankylosing spondylitis.

II. **PAIN.** The quality of pain, its distribution, and modulating factors are helpful in determining etiology.

   A. **Onset of pain**

      1. Sudden onset especially following trauma suggests injury.

      2. Indolent onset suggests a nonmechanical cause.

      3. Episodic or colicky pain suggests an intra-abdominal or pelvic source.

   B. **Localization of pain**

      1. Localized pain provides a focus for the diagnostic workup.

      2. Radicular pain, suggesting nerve root impingement.

      3. Pain that is not easily localized, migratory, or multifocal suggests fibromyalgia.

   C. **Modulating factors**

      1. Exercise-induced pain, especially on walking, suggests osteoarthritis or spinal stenosis, whereas pain that improves with exercise especially following morning stiffness suggests an inflammatory process, for example, a spondyloarthropathy.

      2. Valsalva maneuvers such as coughing, sneezing, or bowel movements that worsen pain suggest nerve root impingement.

III. **NEUROLOGIC SYMPTOMS.** The presence of neurologic symptoms should be specifically sought in patients with LBP. Their presence can not only help to delineate the site of the abnormality but also can prompt more rapid intervention.

   A. **Weakness, numbness, or paresthesias** in a dermatomal distribution suggests nerve root impingement (Table 20-1) (see also the dermatome figure in Appendix B).

      1. The most common cause of nerve root impingement in individuals between the ages of 20 and 50 years is a herniated nucleus pulposus.

      2. Radicular symptoms in individuals older than 60 are more likely to be secondary to spinal stenosis resulting from osteoarthritis.

   B. **Bowel or bladder dysfunction** suggests the presence of cauda equina syndrome and should prompt emergent investigation.

   C. **LBP in the presence of fever and neurologic symptoms** should trigger the mind to the possibility of an epidural abscess.

 PHYSICAL EXAMINATION

Specific abnormalities and provocative maneuvers designed to elicit pain associated with certain syndromes should be tested for in patients with LBP.

I. **PATIENT IN STANDING POSITION**

   A. Note the alignment of the spine looking for a pelvic tilt that may indicate a paravertebral spasm, for loss of normal lumbar lordosis that could indicate either spasm or ankylosis, and for evidence of structural scoliosis.

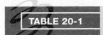

| **TABLE 20-1** | **Signs and Symptoms of Common Disc Lesions** |

Site	Pain	Sensory findings	Motor weakness	Reflexes
L3-4[a]	Anterolateral thigh, medial knee	Anterolateral thigh	Knee extensors	Patellar decreased
L4-5[b]	Posterior thigh, lateral calf, dorsum of foot, great toe	Posterolateral calf, dorsum of foot, web of great toe	Ankle dorsiflexors, extensor of great toe	No specific reflex change
L5-S1[c]	Buttock, posterior thigh, calf, heel, ball of foot, lateral toes	Buttock, posterior thigh, calf, lateral foot, or lateral two toes	Normal or weak plantar strength of ankle	Achilles decreased

[a]L3-4 disc affects the L4 nerve root.
[b]L4-5 disc affects the L5 nerve root.
[c]L5-S1 disc affects the S1 nerve root.

B. Evaluate gait, station, and posture.
C. Evaluate the patient's ability to flex, hyperextend, rotate, and tilt the spine.

II. PATIENT IN SUPINE POSITION
   A. Straight leg raising (SLR). Flex each leg at the hip with the knee extended and record the angle at which pain occurs and whether it radiates below the knee. A true positive SLR test is defined as radicular pain radiating below the knee, is a sensitive indicator of nerve root impingement, and should be confirmed by extending the knee while the patient is sitting, to eliminate malingering.
   B. A crossed SLR test (radicular pain contralateral to the leg being raised) is highly predictive of nerve root compromise.
   C. Evaluate hip and knee range of motion to eliminate these areas as a source of pain.
   D. Carry out thorough neurologic (see Table 20-1) and vascular examinations. The combination of neurologic examination and symptoms define a "root signature," allowing the physician to localize the source of the problem and potentially correlate it with the results of the imaging test.

III. PATIENT IN PRONE POSITION
   A. Look for evidence of sciatic notch tenderness, sometimes seen in sciatica.
   B. Results of the femoral stretch test (extending the hip) may be positive in L4 radiculopathy.
   C. Palpate bony structures, especially the vertebral structures, for localized tenderness, and examine for the presence of trigger points, not only in the low back but also in other areas of the body.

DIAGNOSTIC INVESTIGATIONS

I. **Laboratory tests** should be performed as indicated by the history and physical examination, age of the patient, and duration of symptoms.
   A. The erythrocyte sedimentation rate (ESR) and C-reactive protein reflect acute phase reactants and will usually be elevated in infection, inflammatory joint disease, and metastatic malignancies.
   B. Determinations of calcium, phosphorus, and alkaline phosphatase levels screen for metabolic bone diseases.
   C. Serum and urine protein immunoelectrophoresis should be performed if multiple myeloma is suspected because of the coexistence of back pain, elevated ESR, and anemia.

II. IMAGING STUDIES

A. **Imaging studies are not performed until the patient fails a trial of conservative therapy or unless neurologic or constitutional symptoms are present.**

1. **Plain films** should be taken as an **initial study** in the evaluation of LBP.

   a. Anteroposterior, lateral, and cone-down views of the lower two interspaces are standard procedure.

   b. Oblique views will identify subtle spondylosis and help to visualize the neural foramina, but are not routinely necessary.

   c. Flexion extension views may be obtained to document instability and range of motion.

2. **Bone scintigraphy** is useful as a screening study when malignancy (other than multiple myeloma), infection, or occult fracture, which are not visualized on plain films, are suspected.

3. **Magnetic resonance imaging (MRI)** has revolutionized the imaging of the lumbosacral spine and can visualize both bony and soft tissue structures well. MRI is now the imaging modality of choice for imaging intraspinal pathology. The principal problem with MRI is the high rate of false-positive results. Up to 30% of asymptomatic individuals will be shown to have significant abnormalities on MRI. Therefore, MRI-defined abnormalities need to be viewed in the context of the findings based on history and physical examination.

4. **Computed tomography (CT) scan.** When used without intradural contrast, CT scan is the modality of choice for delineating the bony structures of the spine (e.g., to detect spinal stenosis). With the addition of intrathecal metrizamide, the sensitivity for detecting neural involvement is enhanced. CT scan does not detect intraspinal pathology as well as MRI does, and false-positive results may also be present as in MRI.

5. **Myelography** outlines the dural theca and its contents after injection of a contrast media into the dural sac. This is a good study to delineate neural compression. It remains the study of choice when metal hardware is present or when arachnoiditis is suspected. Myelography is slowly falling from favor because of its invasiveness, side effects, and because of the improvement in imaging techniques with MRI and CT scan.

6. **Riskography** is performed by injecting dye into the disc space. If symptoms are reproduced during the procedure, it may be particularly helpful, especially if other imaging studies have been nondiagnostic.

B. Radiologic signs

1. **Degenerative disc disease.** Radiographic abnormalities correlate poorly with symptoms and they must be correlated with the patient's history and physical examination findings.

   a. Narrowing of the intervertebral disc.

   b. Vacuum phenomenon defined as radiolucency in the disc space.

   c. Traction osteophytes defined as anterior osteophytes on the lumbosacral spine indicative of spinal instability.

2. **Osteoarthritis**

   a. Osteophyte formation.

   b. Facet joint arthritis.

   c. Spinal stenosis.

   d. Acquired spondylolisthesis.

3. **Congenital and developmental defects**

   a. Spondylolysis refers to the dissolution or failure of the development of the neural arch, typically noted as a lucency in the "neck" of the "Scotty dog" noted on oblique spine radiographs (the "eye" of the Scotty dog is the pedicle, the "ear" is the superior articulation of that vertebral body, and the "neck" is the par interarticularis). Failure of the pars can lead to slippage (usually anteriorly) of one vertebral body over the other.

   b. Spondylolisthesis is slippage of one vertebral body on another. It can be a consequence of spondylolysis or an acquired condition.

   c. Transitional vertebrae, with lumbarization of S1 or sacralization of L5.

   d. Schmorl's nodes are defects in the vertebral end plates that allow vertical disc herniation.

   e. Scoliosis or kyphosis.

4. Spondyloarthopathies (ankylosing spondylitis, ReA, psoriatic arthritis, and arthritis associated with inflammatory bowel disease).

   a. Erosions or sclerosis of the sacroiliac joints are best seen in a Ferguson (sacroiliac) view of the pelvis, a special view that allows better visualization of the joint.

   b. Syndesmophytes. Calcification of the ligamentous structures leads to a bridging of the adjacent vertebral bodies.

5. Neoplasm

   a. Typically leads to destruction of the vertebral body.

   b. Loss of the outline of the pedicle on the anteroposterior films.

   c. Pathologic fracture.

6. Infection should be suspected when destruction of adjacent vertebral end plates is present or bony destruction is accompanied by constitutional symptoms.

7. Miscellaneous

   a. Osteoporosis. Loss in mineralization, compression fractures with characteristic anterior wedging, "fish mouth" appearance to the intervertebral spaces.

   b. Metabolic bone disease (i.e., osteomalacia, Paget's disease, or hyperparathyroidism).

   c. Sickle cell disease.

 DIFFERENTIAL DIAGNOSIS

I.   VERTEBRAL BODY DISEASES

   A. Fracture.

   B. Metabolic bone disease.

   C. Multiple myeloma.

   D. Metastatic cancer.

   E. Infection.

II.   INTERVERTEBRAL DISC DISEASES

   A. Herniation.

   B. Infection.

III.   JOINT DISEASE

   A. Apophyseal joint disease due to osteoarthritis.

   B. Sacroiliac joints.

IV.   LIGAMENTOUS DISEASE

   A. Anterior and posterior long ligaments.

   B. Interspinous and supraspinous ligaments.

   C. Iliolumbar ligaments.

   D. Apophyseal ligaments.

V.   NERVE ROOT IMPINGEMENT

   A. Herniated nucleus pulposus.

   B. Spinal stenosis.

   C. Neoplasm.

VI.   PARASPINAL MUSCULATURE

   A. Fibromyalgia.

   B. Myofascial (localized pain).

VII.   REFERRED PAIN

   A. Renal.

   B. Pelvic.

   C. Vascular.

   D. Gastrointestinal.

TREATMENT

I. **Because more than 90% of cases of LBP are self-limiting and resolve spontaneously,** any treatment algorithm must account for this and should avoid immediate laboratory or imaging studies unless constitutional symptoms, weakness, or neurologic dysfunction suggests that there is an urgent problem.

II. **ACUTE TREATMENT**

   A. **Rest versus activity.** Many longitudinal studies suggest that prolonged rest, and/or "fear" on the part of patients that activity will worsen their pain, are associated with a higher likelihood of the acute LBP becoming chronic. Patients should avoid extended periods of inactivity.

   B. **Spinal traction** has no direct benefit, but may help enforce bed rest if this is desirable for a very short period of time.

   C. **Pharmacologic treatment**

   1. **Pain control.** This is often brought about with the use of single or combination drug therapy with nonsteroidal anti-inflammatory drugs (NSAIDs), other classes of analgesics, and topical pain patches (i.e., Lidoderm 5%).

   2. **Muscle relaxants.** The mechanism of action of these drugs is not entirely clear, but they are helpful in some patients with acute LBP. Examples include cyclobenzaprine (Flexeril) 5 to 10 mg either as a single nighttime dose or up to a maximum of every 6 hours, methocarbamol (Robaxin) 750 to 1,500 mg up to every 6 hours, and chlorzoxazone (Parafon Forte) 500 to 750 mg up to every 6 hours. Benzodiazepines such as diazepam (Valium) may also be used for a limited period of time.

   D. **Physical measures**

   1. Moist heat. Heating pads, hot tubs, steam, and sauna baths.

   2. Massage, ultrasound.

   3. Bracing for any extended period of time may lead to muscle weakness.

III. **Failure of conservative treatment** as outlined at the end of 4 to 6 weeks is considered an indication to initiate a diagnostic workup and consider surgical intervention. The workup should include plain radiographs of the lumbosacral spine, and usually an MRI of the lumbosacral spine, as well as any other laboratory studies deemed necessary based on the patient's history and physical exam.

IV. **OTHER TREATMENT MODALITIES**

   A. Injection of myofascial trigger points with lidocaine alone or combined with corticosteroids if the patient exhibits only a few specific areas of tenderness.

   B. Facet or nerve block procedures can be both diagnostic and therapeutic, but require specific skills and experience.

   C. Transcutaneous electrical nerve stimulator (TENS).

   D. Physical therapy (see subsequent text).

V. **Invasive intervention** should be considered if there is a failure of conservative therapy and when there is a radiographically demonstrable anatomic lesion that could explain the pain, or when malignancy or infection cannot be excluded with noninvasive techniques.

   A. **Surgery should rarely be performed** before 2 months of conservative therapy, except in circumstances that require urgent intervention such as worsening neurologic deficit. However, a delay of more than 6 months may also be unwise because of a higher risk of the development of chronic pain.

   B. **Types of surgical intervention.** These operations usually are performed after conservative therapy has failed and intractable pain, other sensory findings, or motor weakness are present. Depending on the skill and experience of the surgeon, usually the least invasive operation has the best chance of success. For pure disc disease, artificial disc replacements are being developed and hold promise for less invasive surgery that does not disrupt the normal bony structures.

   1. **Laminectomy or hemilaminectomy.** Removal of all or part of the lamina while preserving the apophyseal joints or in the case of spinal stenosis trimming the joints to decompress the neural tissues.

2. **Laminotomy or hemilaminotomy.** An opening is created in the lamina without it being totally removed.
3. **Discectomy.** Removal of the nucleus pulposus by standard surgical approach or fiberoptic approach.
4. **Microdiskectomy.** Removal of a portion of the herniated nucleus pulposus under microscopic guidance with a fiberoptic scope.
5. **Spinal fusion.** The precise indications for this surgery are controversial; this is usually performed in combination with one of the above operations.

VI. **Chronic pain** may arise from a failure of conservative or more aggressive therapies, and these patients remain difficult to treat even in specialized settings. A subset of this group has fibromyalgia.

VII. **REHABILITATION AND EXERCISE.** Flexibility and strengthening exercise is frequently recommended for patients with LBP. Basic principles regarding rehabilitation in these patients should be followed, and physical therapists are very helpful in instructing patients in these programs.

A. **Postsurgical patients**
   1. Ambulation is encouraged early and prolonged sitting is avoided.
   2. Lifting should be avoided.

B. **Nonsurgical patients.** "Exercises" for LBP probably should not be initiated until the acute phase of recovery has been completed and the patient can move freely without pain, whereas resumption of normal "activities" should be encouraged as early as possible. In the beginning of an exercise program, patients should be instructed to begin with only three to five repetitions of each exercise and proceed slowly to increase the repetitions.
   1. **Pelvic tilt.** Buttocks are tightened, and the lumbar spine is flattened isometrically.
   2. **Modified sit-ups.** With the patient supine, knees bent, and arms at the side, the head and shoulders are lifted off the ground for 5 seconds.
   3. **Knee–chest stretch.** With the patient supine, knees bent, and arms at the side, each knee is brought to the chest one at a time and held with the arms for 5 seconds. Then the knee is extended and that leg is lowered to the ground slowly.
   4. **Wall exercise.** The patient leans against the wall with the feet approximately 1 foot from the wall, depending on the height of the patient. Knees are then bent to approximately 45 degrees or until the lumbar spine feels flat against the wall for a few seconds. The patient then returns to the upright position.

C. **Other suggestions**
   1. Weight reduction.
   2. Increase aerobic fitness with walking, swimming, or other low impact activities. Do stretching activities as a workup before aerobics.
   3. Lifestyle modifications such as proper lifting techniques (while lifting, the knees should be flexed and the back straight, and twisting while lifting should be avoided); use of a firm mattress to sleep on; and vocational training that may be of help.

PROGNOSIS

I. **In long-term follow-up,** most patients with LBP without a serious underlying disorder such as malignancy, herniated nucleus pulposus with spinal cord or nerve root compression, or significant spinal stenosis will do well with a short period of rest, a conservative exercise program (in some cases, supervised by a physical therapist) that emphasizes flexion and extension exercises, stretching regimens, and gradual aerobic conditioning and weight loss.

II. **Factors associated with a poor prognosis** include malignancy, fracture, multiple level spinal stenosis, or a herniated nucleus pulposus, or other conditions with spinal cord or nerve root impingement that is not corrected surgically in a timely manner.

III. **Patient characteristics that usually indicate the need for surgery** are sphincter and sexual dysfunction due to the compression of the conus medullaris or cauda equina and persistent radicular symptoms especially if associated with neurologic motor deficits that progress. The surgical procedure chosen is determined by the anatomic lesion that needs correction, and the training and skill of the surgeon called upon to do the surgery. Choosing a surgeon with extensive experience and good outcomes is an important role that medical consultants can fulfill on behalf of the patients with LBP.

IV.   Serious intraoperative or perioperative complications can occur during low back surgery if important neurologic structures are compromised due to surgical error, infection, or bleeding that causes pressure and subsequent damage to the spinal cord or nerve roots.

V.   Patients with LBP who have uncorrected pain for more than 3 to 6 months may have difficulty being totally free of pain even after the anatomic cause of their original pain is corrected. This may occur because of behavioral (e.g., fear of movement leading to inactivity and isolation) or neurobiologic (e.g., "sensitization" of peripheral or central pain processing systems) reasons, or misdiagnosis (e.g., pain coming from a different cause than that originally treated), or may be due to multiple causes.

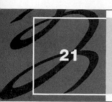

21 SHOULDER PAIN
Andrew D. Pearle and Russell F. Warren

■ KEY POINTS

■ The prevalence of shoulder pathologies varies with age, with instability and superior labral anterior posterior (SLAP) lesion common in the younger population, and impingement and rotator cuff disease more common in the older population.

■ A trial of conservative management including physical therapy, nonsteroidal anti-inflammatory drugs (NSAIDs), and subacromial injection are usually the initial management for shoulder impingement.

■ Rotator cuff tears are often associated with impingement syndrome and should be evaluated with careful examination as well as advanced imaging such as magnetic resonance imaging (MRI) or ultrasonography.

■ Adhesive capsulitis is characterized by stages that have distinct clinical manifestations and treatment strategies.

■ Acromioclavicular (AC) joint pain is diagnosed by physical examination, with attention to localized tenderness to palpation directly over the joint; radiographic findings support but do not establish the diagnosis.

■ Shoulder instability should be properly classified by its degree, frequency, etiology, and direction. Recurrent shoulder instability is more common in the younger, athletic population (<25 years old).

$\mathcal{T}$he diagnosis and treatment of problems of the shoulder region require an understanding of the anatomy and function of this joint.

I.   The three joints of the shoulder are the acromioclavicular (AC), sternoclavicular, and glenohumeral articulations, and the gliding planes consist of the scapulothoracic surface and the subacromial space. Elevation of the arm is produced by the combined rotation of the glenohumeral joint and of the scapula on the chest wall.

II.   The rotator cuff consists of four muscles, the supraspinatus, the infraspinatus, the teres minor, and the subscapularis. In addition to assisting in internal and external rotation, these muscles act to depress or "center" the humeral head during shoulder elevation. This centering action of the rotator cuff provides a fulcrum that allows the deltoid to elevate the arm rather than simply shrug the shoulder.

III. **The glenohumeral joint has the most mobile articulation in the body and is the most commonly dislocated diarthrodial joint.** Static shoulder restraints consist of the glenoid labrum, the articular anatomy, negative intra-articular pressure, joint fluid adhesion, and the capsuloligamentous structures. Dynamic shoulder stabilizers include the rotator cuff muscles, the biceps, and the periscapular muscles.

CLINICAL MANIFESTATIONS AND PHYSICAL EXAMINATION

Examination of the shoulder region includes observation, palpation, range of motion, strength testing, and special tests for specific pathologies. In addition, extrinsic sources of shoulder pain should always be considered, and evaluation of the cervical spine, entire upper extremity, and chest wall must be part of any shoulder examination.

I. **OBSERVATION**
  A. The **position of the shoulder** relative to the contralateral side should be noted. Asymmetry in the form of an elevated or depressed position of the shoulder may be related to scoliosis, congenital spinal or shoulder deformities, or simply athletic activity.
  B. **Swelling** about the shoulder may be secondary to inflammation of the joint, a bursa, or associated with rotator cuff tears.
  C. **Shoulder range of motion** should be assessed; it is essential to visualize shoulder motion from behind the patient to note the scapulohumeral rhythm.
  D. **Specific muscle atrophy** may indicate either rotator cuff tears or neurologic involvement.

II. **PALPATION**
  A. The **supraclavicular fossa** should be carefully palpated for masses as well as for tenderness of the brachial plexus, which is seen in the thoracic outlet syndrome.
  B. **Local tender spots** indicative of trigger points should be sought along the interscapular region and overlying musculature of the shoulder. If pressure is applied to these spots, radiation of pain into the upper arm may be observed.
  C. Specific sites of tenderness that should be carefully palpated include the **biceps tendon,** the **subdeltoid bursa,** the **rotator cuff,** the **AC joint,** and the **sternoclavicular joints.**

III. **MOTION**
  A. In examining the shoulder, one should observe the full range of **active** and **passive** motion, noting any discrepancy that may reflect a rotator cuff tear. Active elevation in the plane of the scapula may demonstrate altered scapulothoracic rhythm with a "shrug sign" if a rotator cuff tear is present.
  B. **Range of motion** examination should include **abduction** in the plane of the scapula, and **forward flexion. External rotation** of the humerus is noted with the arm at the side as well as with 90 degrees of abduction. **Internal rotation** is recorded by placing the hand behind the back and noting which spinous process the thumb will reach. It is also tested at 90 degrees of abduction.

IV. **STRENGTH TESTING**
  A. Strength testing includes evaluation of the shoulder **flexion** (anterior deltoid), **abduction** (middle deltoid), **adduction** (pectoralis major and latissimus dorsi), and **extension** (latissimus dorsi and posterior deltoid).
  B. **Rotator cuff strength** must be evaluated with every shoulder examination. The **supraspinatus muscle** is evaluated by applying downward pressure to the arm when it is abducted to 90 degrees in the scapular plane and in maximal internal rotation. Weakness of external rotation with the arm at the side is present with large rotator cuff tears involving the **infraspinatus** or with C5-6 nerve root problems. The lift-off test for **subscapularis** tears is performed by placing the back of the hand over L5 and pushing away from the back. Loss of strength is associated with subscapularis tears.

V. **SPECIAL TESTS**
  A. **The impingement sign** is positive in patients with rotator cuff inflammation or tears, and is noted by flexing the arm forward to the full overhead position. Pain is

present during the last 10 degrees of passive elevation. Passive abduction to the 90-degree position with internal rotation will similarly produce pain.

B. The impingement test is positive if a positive impingement sign is relieved with a subacromial lidocaine injection. A positive impingement test is indicative of impingement syndrome or a rotator cuff tear.

C. The cross-body adduction test consists of fully adducting the humerus across the chest. This test stresses the AC joint and will cause pain if degeneration of the AC joint is present.

D. The active compression test is performed with the arm straight and maximally pronated (thumb facing down) and the shoulder flexed to 90 degrees and adducted 15 degrees. Downward pressure is applied to the arm which places compression on the intra-articular portion of the long head of the biceps. Deep anterior pain and weakness with this test, which is relieved by performing the maneuver with the arm in supination is indicative of a **superior labral anterior posterior (SLAP) lesion.**

E. Instability of the glenohumeral joint is assessed by placing the patient in the supine position with maximal muscle relaxation. To evaluate **anterior instability,** the shoulder is placed in the abducted, externally rotated position and gentle pressure is applied in an anterior direction behind the humeral head. Instability is assessed by noting the degree of anterior humeral head translation. In addition, **apprehension** due to fear of dislocation with this maneuver is characteristic of anterior instability **(apprehension test). Posterior instability** is assessed with the shoulder adducted and internally rotated with pressure placed in the posterior direction; a click or a clear subluxation may be noted during this maneuver. In some patients, **inferior instability** is demonstrated by distracting the arms inferiorly to see if a sulcus forms **(sulcus sign)** distal to the acromion. This sign is frequently present in **multidirectional instability.**

VI. NEUROVASCULAR EXAMINATION

A. A complete neurologic examination should be performed. Weakness may be the result of intrinsic shoulder lesions, as in a cuff tear, or of nerve lesions of the brachial plexus or cervical roots.

B. The circulation of the arm and the hand must be carefully evaluated. Several tests are used for assessment of **thoracic outlet syndrome.**

   1. The **Adson's test** consists of palpating the radial pulse while the patient's head is turned to the involved side and a Valsalva maneuver is performed. A decrease in the pulse is suggestive, but not diagnostic, of thoracic outlet syndrome. A reduced radial pulse on testing should be compared with the pulse on the contralateral side.

   2. The **modified Adson's or Wright's test** is performed with the arm abducted and externally rotated, noting any decrease in the pulse.

   3. The **Roo's test** is performed with the patient's shoulders abducted and externally rotated; the patient is instructed to open and close the hands for 1 to 2 minutes in an attempt to reproduce the symptoms of thoracic outlet syndrome.

 IMAGING STUDIES

I. Standard radiographic views of the shoulder generally include anteroposterior views in neutral, internal, and external rotation. Because the scapula lies on the chest wall at approximately a 40-degree angle, radiographs should be taken at a right angle to the scapula and glenohumeral joint rather than to the chest.

II. Lateral and axillary radiographic views of the scapula are useful in identifying degenerative changes of the glenohumeral joint and calcification of the rotator cuff; they are particularly important in the evaluation of acute injuries to the shoulder.

III. Special radiographic views are used to assess for specific pathologic shoulder conditions.

A. The **supraspinatus outlet view** is a lateral view with a 10-degree caudal angle. This view is used to assess acromial shape (flat or curved or hooked) in impingement syndrome.

B. The **West Point view** is used to look for anterior inferior glenoid rim fractures **(bony Bankart's lesion)** seen with some cases of anterior instability. The x-ray is taken with the patient prone and the beam angled 25 degrees in the coronal and sagittal planes.

C. The **Stryker Notch view** is taken with the patient supine and with the hand placed on the head. The x-ray beam is directed anterior to posterior with a 10-degree cephalic tilt. This view is used in glenohumeral instability to assess for **Hill-Sachs's lesion** (impaction fractures on the posterior aspect of the humeral head).

IV. **Magnetic resonance imaging (MRI)** is particularly useful to evaluate for rotator cuff tears, labral pathology (Bankart's lesions and SLAP lesions), and cartilage lesions.

V. **Ultrasonography** is commonly used for rotator cuff lesions and calcific tendinitis.

 COMMON SHOULDER PROBLEMS

I. **OVERVIEW. The most common shoulder problems are** impingement syndrome, rotator cuff tears, calcific tendinitis, adhesive capsulitis, AC joint pain, thoracic outlet syndrome, and shoulder instability.

A. **Shoulder pain that is intrinsic in nature** is generally worse at night because of increased lying on the shoulder and the fact that it becomes a weight-bearing joint. Shoulder motion will generally aggravate the pain, particularly full elevation in the forward flexed position or abduction to 90 degrees. Specific problems of the shoulder region tend to occur at certain age intervals. From ages **20 to 30 years,** instability problems and SLAP lesions may present as a painful shoulder. From ages **40 to 50 years,** the impingement syndrome, calcific tendinitis, and adhesive capsulitis become more common. From ages **50 to 70 years,** the impingement syndrome may progress to a full-thickness rotator cuff tear. Degenerative lesions of the AC, sternoclavicular, and occasionally the glenohumeral joints become more frequent. Pain from metastatic disease should be considered.

B. **Extrinsic (referred) shoulder pain** must always be considered when examining the shoulder. Cervical spondylosis of C5-6 often results in a referred type of pain to the shoulder. If the radiculopathy includes weakness of shoulder abduction and external rotation, it may closely mimic a torn rotator cuff. Shoulder pain that originates in the cervical spine is usually increased by neck motion, particularly extension with rotation to the involved side. Multifactorial pain syndromes may be present; for example, in patients with cervical spondylosis and referred pain to the shoulder, limitation of shoulder motion secondary to adhesive capsulitis may also develop. Also, pain can be referred from diseases involving the heart, lung, or gall bladder.

II. **Impingement syndrome** generally develops during the fifth decade and may progress to a rotator cuff tear by the age of 55 years. The underlying pathology consists of degeneration of the tendons of the rotator cuff. As a result, the insufficient cuff fails to prevent superior migration of the humeral head during elevation. This results in pressure (or impingement) on the rotator cuff and increasing pressure on the bone. Spurs may develop within the coracoacromial ligament over time with cuff degeneration. In some patients, a hooked acromion will increase the pressure on the cuff.

A. **Clinical manifestations** include **pain** on performing overhead activities. The pain may increase during specific activities, such as throwing a ball and swimming. **Night pain** is particularly common. The **impingement sign** may be positive and the **impingement test** will relieve pain.

B. **Radiography** may show some sclerosis of the greater tuberosity or of the acromion. MRI may show a partial or complete cuff tear.

C. **Treatment** is based on an initial period of activity modifications, physical therapy, and anti-inflammatory medications. Surgery should be considered if the symptoms are recalcitrant to conservative interventions.

1. **Physical therapy** should focus on elimination of contractures about the shoulder region with a stretching program. A muscle-strengthening program of exercise must be established because shoulder pain often leads to weakness, particularly of the rotator cuff. In carrying out these exercises, the patient should avoid the pain-producing positions.

2. **Oral anti-inflammatory** agents may be helpful and a subacromial injection of 40 mg of methylprednisolone acetate (Depo-Medrol) is administered if the previous methods have failed. However, injections should be limited to one or two during a 3-month period.

3. After 3 to 6 months, if there is no improvement, **arthroscopy with subacromial decompression,** followed by physical therapy, may be of value.

III. **Rotator cuff tears** are usually due to impingement but may be associated with trauma, overuse, and instability. Based on a postmortem study, one-third of the patients who die after the age of 70 years have a rotator cuff tear. It is thought that during the **sixth or seventh decade,** rotator cuff degeneration develops as a result of decreased vascularity of the supraspinatus tendon. As the rotator cuff becomes attenuated as well as degenerative, partial tearing occurs that progresses to full-thickness tearing in some patients.

A. **Clinical manifestations** are **similar to impingement syndrome,** which usually coexists with the rotator cuff tear. This includes **pain on performing overhead activities, night pain,** and a positive **impingement sign.**

1. **Crepitation** of the subacromial space from an inflamed, thickened subacromial bursa may be present. **Biceps tendinitis** and **subacromial bursitis** may form during cuff degeneration.

2. **Atrophy of the infraspinatus and supraspinatus regions** may be present, particularly with large cuff tears. Rarely, nerve injury that exacerbates pain and muscle atrophy may coexist with a cuff tear.

3. When a small tear of the rotator cuff is present, shoulder motion may initially be normal, but as the tear increases, elevation will gradually be replaced by a shoulder-shrugging movement.

4. **Loss of external rotation** may develop; however, it is seen only in patients with large, extensive tears that involve both the supraspinatus and infraspinatus.

5. In patients with large tears of the rotator cuff, a **drop sign** will be positive. This sign is elicited by having the patient elevate the arm either actively or passively into the full overhead position, then lowering it in the plane of the scapula. At approximately the 90-degree position, marked weakness is noted, and the arm drops 30 to 40 degrees, often accompanied by pain.

B. **Shoulder radiographs** will demonstrate sclerosis of the acromion with a reversal of the normal convexity of the inferior surface of the acromion.

1. Occasionally, a **large spur** will develop at the anterior inferior edge of the acromion in the coracoacromial ligament. A supraspinatus outlet radiograph of the shoulder may demonstrate the spur, a curved acromion, or both.

2. If a cuff tear is suspected or if the patient does not respond to treatment, an **MRI** should be obtained, which will demonstrate cuff degeneration and a tear, if present. The size of the tear can be noted in addition to the degree of retraction and muscle atrophy.

C. **Treatment** algorithms are similar to that of impingement syndrome and include a trial of physical therapy and anti-inflammatory medications followed by surgery if necessary.

1. **Physical therapy** consisting of stretching and strengthening in the setting of **anti-inflammatory** agents may be beneficial.

2. **Injection** of the subacromial space on one or two occasions may be helpful in allowing the patient to restore shoulder function; a long and repeated course of injections, however, will lead to further degenerative changes of the rotator cuff.

3. **Surgical treatment** consists of **acromioplasty** and, if a significant tear is present, **rotator cuff repair.**

IV. **Calcific tendinitis** may be present in either an acute or chronic form. In the **acute** process, the patient notes the sudden occurrence of severe shoulder pain and will present to the doctor, holding the arm carefully at the side to avoid all shoulder movement. In the **chronic** situation, the calcific deposit becomes indurated within the rotator cuff and there may be a long history, often of multiple attacks of shoulder pain. Complaints will often mimic those of the impingement syndromes.

A. Clinical manifestations may include a distinct swelling overlying the humeral head, and gentle palpation may reveal a well-localized area of extreme tenderness. Movement of the shoulder may be resisted by pain.

B. Shoulder radiographs may show a fluffy calcific deposit within the rotator cuff tendons, most commonly of the supraspinatus. It should be noted that some patients aged 40 years or more have asymptomatic calcium deposits in the shoulder.

C. Treatment of the acute situation consists of injecting the deposit with 2 to 3 mL of 1% lidocaine and 40 mg of methylprednisolone acetate. After some local anesthesia is achieved, the deposit should be needled in an attempt to break it up, thus allowing the deposit to migrate into the subacromial bursae, where it will be absorbed. This procedure is typically done under ultrasonographic or fluoroscopic guidance. Occasionally, the calcific deposit will rupture spontaneously, with prompt resolution of the patient's pain.

1. Because pain may be temporarily increased following injection to the calcium deposit, ice should be applied to the shoulder for 20 to 30 minutes at periodic intervals during the subsequent 24 hours. In addition, anti-inflammatory medications should be used for 3 to 4 days.
2. When pain abates, full shoulder motion should be encouraged to avoid development of a contracture.
3. If pain persists or repeated attacks occur, operative removal of the calcium may be required.

V. Adhesive capsulitis (frozen shoulder), frequently seen during the fifth and sixth decades of life, may develop as a result of intrinsic shoulder pathology or occur secondary to extrinsic causes, particularly cervical spondylosis. A history of **diabetes** is frequently present. Often, no specific etiologic factor can be found.

A. The clinical course of adhesive capsulitis typically involves **four stages.**

1. **Stage I** is characterized by **pain,** particularly at night and at the extreme range of motion. There may be mild loss of external rotation. This stage typically lasts for 1 to 3 months and is associated with significant intra-articular synovitis.
2. **Stage II** is associated with **freezing** of the shoulder. There is pain with range of motion, pain at night and also while at rest, and characteristically, a loss of motion, particularly in **external rotation.** On occasion, extensive **loss of shoulder motion** will develop so slowly that the patient remains unaware of the magnitude of the problem. Conversely, the onset may be sudden and severe, with marked loss of glenohumeral motion and a restriction of abduction to the 90-degree range. This stage lasts for 3 to 9 months; intra-articular findings include synovitis and fibrosis.
3. **Stage III** is considered the **frozen** phase and may last 9 to 16 months. There is increased contracture, but decreased pain and synovitis.
4. **Stage IV** is the **thawing** phase. Patients typically improve clinically with gradual increase in range of motion. There is minimal pain during this stage.

B. Radiographic findings will often be negative in the early stage, but with time may show osteoporosis. **MRI findings** reveal synovitis in the early stages. In the later stages, findings include a loss of articular volume and a thickened capsule, particularly in the axillary recess.

C. Treatment is determined by the clinical stage of the adhesive capsulitis. In stage I or II, steroid injections into the joint and oral anti-inflammatory agents should be used as an adjuvant to aggressive physical therapy directed at maintaining or restoring motion. **Arthroscopic synovectomy and release** are indicated in the early stages if there is progressive loss of motion and is often used in stage III.

VI. AC JOINT. Pain secondary to pathology of the AC joint is frequently overlooked. The joint lies directly over the rotator cuff, and therefore any alterations of the inferior surface will result in inflammation of the supraspinatus tendon deep in this joint. **Degenerative lesions** of this joint may result in thickening and swelling and create an impingement syndrome.

A. Clinical manifestations include pain on performing overhead activity of the arm, often aggravated by adduction of the arm across the chest. Pain occurs at night and is often increased by lying on the shoulder. **Tenderness** is well-localized to the involved joint.

B. Radiographs demonstrate narrowing of the joint with sclerosis and marginal osteophytes. Specific views taken at a 15-degree cephalic tilt allow better visualization of the AC joint.

C. Therapy for the chronic situation consists of anti-inflammatory medication as well as intra-articular injections with lidocaine and steroids. The degree of relief obtained from these injections confirms the diagnosis.

  1. In the post-traumatic condition, muscle-strengthening exercises, particularly for the deltoid and trapezius, will result in improvement if significant degenerative changes are not present.

  2. In the chronic situation in which pain persists despite one or two injections, resection of the outer 2 cm of the clavicle may be warranted.

VII. Instability of the shoulder is an important cause of pain in the younger population. Often, the patient will state that the shoulder "comes out," although some patients will complain only of shoulder pain, particularly in the posterior humeral region. Shoulder instability is classified by the degree, frequency, etiology, and direction **(anterior, inferior, posterior, and multidirectional)** of instability. It is important to determine the etiology of instability **(traumatic vs. atraumatic)** to help direct management.

A. Clinical manifestations include recurrent dislocations or episodes of instability, particularly with athletic activities. Pain or instability with particular movements or positions may reveal the direction of instability. Patients with **anterior instability** report symptoms with the arm in an abducted and externally rotated position. **Posterior instability** often occurs with the arm flexed, internally rotated, and adducted. The patient may experience symptoms while pushing open a door or a heavy object. Patients with **inferior instability** often have pain while carrying heavy objects; they may also experience traction paresthesias. Patients with **multidirectional instability** often have no history of trauma or generalized ligamentous laxity, and may experience frequent, transient, and bilateral subluxation episodes as well as impingementlike symptoms.

B. Specific testing for shoulder instability should be performed (see Clinical Manifestations and Physical Examination, section **V.E.**), and any positions associated with apprehension should be noted.

C. Radiographic evaluation must initially be directed on confirming reduction of the joint and should include an **axillary view.** Special radiographic views (Stryker Notch and West Point views; see Imaging Studies, section **III.C.**) may provide corroboration of shoulder instability such as a bony Bankart's lesion (fracture of the anterior inferior glenoid) or a Hill-Sachs lesion (impaction fracture of the posterior humeral head).

D. MRI examination is an excellent means of evaluating the labrum and capsule for evidence of shoulder instability.

E. Treatment is tailored to the type of instability present. In those patients who have a traumatic dislocation, rotator cuff and shoulder strengthening exercises may be helpful. If symptoms persist despite this approach, surgical stabilization may be required. In patients with generalized ligamentous laxity and multidirectional instability, prolonged physical therapy is recommended prior to considering surgical intervention.

VIII. SLAP lesions are lesions of the superior labrum that destabilize the anchor of the long head of the biceps. These lesions typically occur in the younger population, particularly with overhead athletes. The lesions are often associated with other shoulder pathology including rotator cuff tears, instability, and chondral defects.

A. Symptoms include pain, the sensation of instability, and mechanical intra-articular complaints (e.g., catching and clicking).

B. Diagnosis is established by physical examination and MRI evaluation.

C. Treatment is usually surgical with debridement or repair of the lesion.

IX. ADDITIONAL SHOULDER CONDITIONS. Although the more common causes of shoulder pain have been discussed, a wide variety of conditions may affect the shoulder.

　A. The **thoracic outlet syndrome** with vascular or brachial plexus involvement may be the basis for extremity pain or fatigue.

　B. Any type of **arthropathy,** including rheumatoid arthritis, degenerative joint disease, and syndromes such as polymyalgia rheumatica, may be expressed as rheumatologic shoulder pain; however, in contrast to the conditions reviewed in this chapter, such problems are often part of more generalized rheumatologic syndromes.

　C. Osteonecrosis (avascular necrosis) commonly affects the humeral head and should be considered in the differential diagnosis of shoulder pain (see Chapter 52).

　D. The **shoulder–hand syndrome (reflex sympathetic dystrophy),** a poorly understood and uncommon basis for shoulder pain, is associated with diffuse swelling, pain, and vasomotor changes in the distal upper extremity. The problem occurs in elderly subjects and is sometimes related to myocardial infarction or other cardiopulmonary conditions. Unless an exercise program supported by the use of analgesics and anti-inflammatory drugs is vigorously instituted, **adhesive capsulitis** may be the outcome. If agents such as indomethacin (100 to 150 mg orally daily) do not control pain sufficiently to permit exercise, a short course of prednisone (25 mg orally daily for 3 to 4 days) may be instituted.

　E. A variety of **intrathoracic problems** (including coronary ischemia, pulmonary embolus, pleuritis, and pneumonitis) and **diaphragmatic irritation** from abdominal lesions should be considered in the differential diagnosis of pain referred to the shoulder region.

ELBOW PAIN
Robert N. Hotchkiss

22

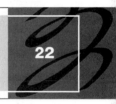

*T*he articular anatomy of the elbow is unique because it contains two independent axes of motion in the same synovial pouch. The ulnohumeral joint determines flexion and extension, and the radiocapitellar joint determines pronation and supination of the forearm. The axis of rotation moves very little throughout flexion and extension, making a nearly perfect hinge that is highly constrained. The normal range of motion is 0 to 140 degrees of flexion and extension, 80 degrees of pronation, and 90 degrees of supination.

　The elbow naturally deviates away from the body (the "carrying angle"), the extent of the deviation varying from person to person.

　The hemicircumferential articulation of the humerus and ulna combined with tension in the biceps–brachialis and triceps makes the elbow extremely stable. The radial head also contributes to stability by providing a wider base of support.

I.　LIGAMENTS

　A. Because of the natural valgus (away from the body) angulation at the elbow, valgus stress develops when a load is thrown or borne. The medial collateral ligament, specifically the anterior portion, is the most important stabilizer.

　B. On the lateral side, the radial collateral ligament helps stabilize the ulna and humerus. The annular ligament wraps around the radial head, securing the proximal radius to the proximal ulna while allowing rotation of the radius.

II.　MUSCLES

　A. Flexors. The biceps and brachialis combine to function as the most powerful muscles in the upper extremity. Because of the location of the long head of the biceps, proximal ruptures can occur. The distal biceps tendon can also rupture. Depending on the patient's needs of function and mobility, some of the ruptures should be surgically repaired.

B. Extensors. The triceps is less powerful than the combined flexors. Active extension is needed for throwing and is especially important for patients who use their arms while transferring from bed to wheelchair or while using crutches. The triceps is much less prone to injury or rupture than the biceps.

III. NERVES. The medial, ulnar, and radial nerves cross the elbow. The ulnar nerve is subcutaneous along the medial side and is palpable posterior to the medial epicondyle in the cubital tunnel. The radial nerve courses along the lateral side and is not palpable. The median nerve lies next to the brachial artery in the cubital fossa.

CLINICAL MANIFESTATIONS AND PHYSICAL EXAMINATION

I. ETIOLOGY. In the examination of a painful elbow, it is helpful to categorize patients according to the suspected etiology.

A. Acute pain after trauma is most likely to be associated with fracture or dislocation. Muscle tears of the biceps can also occur in middle-aged men. Acute pain on the medial or lateral sides of the elbow may be associated with sports such as golf or tennis because of an acute muscle tear. In the absence of a history of trauma, inflammation from gout, infection, rheumatoid arthritis (RA), or other rheumatic conditions should be investigated.

B. Chronic pain that develops slowly may be related to repetitive use; it is sometimes seen in assembly line workers and in golf or tennis players. RA can present as recurrent, warm effusions in the elbow or progressive, indolent loss of motion.

C. Episodic pain, characterized by sudden twinges and locking of the elbow, may be caused by loose cartilaginous fragments, commonly referred to as loose bodies.

II. Localization of pain by the patient is the single most important part of the examination. If the patient can specifically identify a reproducible location for the pain, the chances of diagnosis are greatly enhanced. Once the pain has been localized, or at least regionalized, the most common causes of pain in the given region can be investigated.

III. PALPATION

A. Point of maximal tenderness. Once the pain is localized by the patient, he/she should be examined for tenderness at that same location. It should be checked whether the application of direct pressure (gently applied) reproduces the discomfort. If pressure causes pain, local inflammation, from any of the sources listed in the subsequent text, should be suspected.

B. Synovitis and effusions. Proliferative synovium is usually associated with RA. Unlike effusions in the knee, effusions in the elbow are often difficult to notice. Effusions can sometimes be palpated just anterior or posterior to the radial head, where arthrocentesis is performed.

C. Crepitus. Grinding and popping in a joint as it moves through a range of motion can often indicate severe erosions of articular cartilage. Both flexion–extension and pronation–supination should be checked. The status of the radial head can be assessed by placing a thumb over the radiocapitellar joint during passive forearm rotation.

IV. RANGE OF MOTION

A. Flexion–extension. Flexion and extension should be recorded both actively and passively. With mild inflammation or minor trauma, loss of the range of extension is the first to be noted. It is helpful to compare active and passive extension in the affected joint against the range of motion on the other side.

B. Pronation–supination. Forearm rotation should also be measured and compared with that on the other side.

IMAGING AND OTHER DIAGNOSTIC TECHNIQUES

I. PLAIN RADIOGRAPHS. Plain radiographs of the elbow should include a true lateral and an anteroposterior film. The lateral film is the most difficult to obtain. If a flexion contracture exists, an anteroposterior film of the distal humerus and of the proximal forearm can be of help. A radiocapitellar view can sometimes be helpful in assessing the radiocapitellar joint. In the normal elbow, the head of the radius always points toward the capitellum in all views. If an effusion is present, the lateral view may demonstrate displacement of the anterior or posterior fat pad.

II. **Bone scans** can be useful in an attempt to localize or diagnose pain of unknown origin. A single-phase, "bone static" image may show uptake in a particular region and may lead to closer scrutiny.

III. **Computed tomography (CT)** scan of the elbow can be useful in fracture and reconstructive problems. It is important to review the clinical history with the radiologist and to describe the area of interest. The slice thickness for proper detail is usually 0.8 to 1 mm.

IV. **MAGNETIC RESONANCE IMAGING (MRI).** The effectiveness of MRI in detecting a variety of painful conditions has dramatically improved. The detail and resolution of images obtained with specialized surface coils permit visualization of ligament, cartilage, nerve, and muscle. The condition of cartilage, tendon ruptures, and ligament tears can now be assessed with great reliability using MRI.

V. **ARTHROCENTESIS.** As in all conditions of the joints, analysis of joint fluid may be valuable (see Chapter 8). Tapping the elbow requires knowledge of the surface anatomy to visualize effective needle placement. In addition to synovial fluid analysis, instillation of 1% lidocaine or 0.5% bupivacaine can be diagnostically helpful if the examiner is unsure whether the source of the pain is intra-articular or not.

 SPECIFIC PROBLEMS

I. **LATERAL ELBOW PAIN**
   A. Lateral epicondylitis
      1. Sports-related. "Tennis elbow" associated with racquet sports is common in amateurs and professionals. The onset can be rather acute or can build up slowly over months.
         a. The **diagnosis** is made by palpating the area of the lateral epicondyle with the elbow in near-full extension and by asking the patient to extend the wrist against resistance. This movement usually reproduces the pain.
         b. Proper racquet size and proper backhand technique can lessen the severity of pain. The **first line of treatment** is rest, a short course of anti-inflammatory medicine, and a wrist splint. Specialized braces or forearm bands that encircle the proximal forearm have also been used with some success, but on a case-by-case basis. It is also often helpful to speak to a "tennis pro" to assess other aspects of the game performance, such as foot speed and point of contact. These experts can also suggest changes in grip and racquet technique.
         c. The **second line of treatment** is local steroid injection in the area of greatest pain and symptom. The patient should be warned of possible skin depigmentation. It is mandatory for the patient to reduce the load on the elbow for at least 2 weeks after the injection by refraining from lifting in the "palm-down" or forearm-pronated position.
         d. If these measures fail, excision of the degenerative fascia with or without reattachment of the tendon origin can be helpful in decreasing pain and in restoring function. Recently, successful use of arthroscopic release without repair has also been reported. Surgery should be reserved for severe, recalcitrant cases. Consideration should also be given to a change in avocation (i.e., avoiding racquet sports).
      2. Cumulative trauma from work. Lateral elbow pain from repetitive labor is typically more resistant to treatment than is sports-related "tennis elbow." The onset can be insidious or can begin with a direct blow to the lateral elbow. The pain is usually more diffuse throughout the extensor muscle mass. The same conservative measures as those listed in section **I.A.1** should be tried. It is often difficult for the patient to return to work. Surgery in this cohort of patients is less successful.

B. Radial tunnel syndrome
  1. **Diagnosis.** Entrapment of the posterior interosseous nerve, a branch of the radial nerve at the elbow, is a diagnosis that can be difficult to make. These patients frequently are indistinguishable from those with lateral elbow pain caused by work trauma (see section **I.A.2**). Exquisite but dull pain over the anterior lateral elbow, distinct from the lateral epicondyle, may be present. Direct pressure over this same area should reproduce the symptoms. Weakness and pain during active extension of the middle finger can be present but is not necessarily diagnostic of this condition. Nerve conduction studies and electromyography have not been helpful in diagnosing this condition the way they are in carpal tunnel syndrome.
  2. **Treatment.** Surgical release of the radial and posterior interosseous nerves has been advocated for this condition, but consistent and effective treatment remains elusive.
C. Radial head fracture. Individuals who fall on an outstretched hand are at special risk for this fracture.
  1. The **diagnosis** is frequently missed because of inadequate radiography and examination. The symptoms may be a vague discomfort of the elbow, with little swelling. An ipsilateral fracture of the distal radius (Colles's fracture) may draw attention away from the elbow, and the radial head fracture goes unrecognized. Palpation of the radial head during gentle passive pronation and supination can be diagnostic, revealing exquisite tenderness or crepitation. Anteroposterior and lateral radiographs usually are diagnostic.
  2. **Treatment** depends on the degree of displacement and other features. Most nondisplaced fractures require no splinting and benefit from early active motion.
D. Bicipital tendinitis and distal biceps rupture. Distal bicipital tendinitis can occur and may presage a distal biceps rupture.
  1. **Diagnosis.** A patient who describes a tenderness and soreness along the distal biceps tendon following heavy lifting activity should be warned and the arm should be rested. An MRI may show tendon degeneration or partial tear near the insertion at the bicipital tuberosity of the radius. The biceps tendon can rupture at either end, but it is the distal end that can present as elbow pain or weakness. The rupture is usually seen in men aged 45 to 60 years, but it can also occur in younger weight lifters. Most patients feel a sudden snap or tearing in the elbow while lifting and notice a sudden bulge in the distal forearm with weakness of supination. Ecchymosis may or may not be evident. Given the appearance of the arm, the amount of discomfort can be surprisingly mild.
  2. **Treatment.** The decision to repair this rupture surgically must be individualized. If repair is contemplated, it is best accomplished within days of injury.

II. MEDIAL ELBOW PAIN
A. Medial epicondylitis. Inflammation of the medial side of the elbow is less common than inflammation of the lateral side. Overuse at work or **throwing sports** can initiate the process. As in lateral epicondylitis, there may be some tearing of the fibers of the muscle that originate from the medial side of the elbow.
  1. **Diagnosis.** Direct palpation over the medial epicondyle usually elicits pain. This tenderness can be accentuated by resisted active flexion of the wrist. The zone of tenderness in medial epicondylitis is usually less discrete than that on the lateral side. The cubital tunnel, through which the ulnar nerve passes, is posterior to the epicondyle, and the examiner should attempt to distinguish between medial epicondylitis and cubital tunnel syndrome. Entrapment of the ulnar nerve can occur in patients with medial epicondylitis (often in throwing athletes), but the two conditions are separable and should be distinguished.
  2. The **treatment** of medial epicondylitis is the same as that for the lateral side, but success is less predictable.
B. Cubital tunnel syndrome. Entrapment of the ulnar nerve at the elbow can occasionally begin as pain in the elbow. The symptoms of nerve entrapment, paresthesias, numbness, and weakness in the ulnar nerve distribution are associated with the local pain. If the ulnar nerve subluxates over the medial epicondyle during flexion

and extension, the pain can have quite an "electric" quality. It is useful to try to palpate the nerve during flexion and extension if subluxation is suspected. Tapping the ulnar nerve (Tinel's sign) may elicit paresthesia or dysesthesia in the distribution of the ulnar nerve. A full assessment of ulnar nerve function by motor and sensory examination is essential. Nerve conduction studies can be helpful in detecting a decreased rate of conduction across the elbow.

   C. Valgus strain. When a person falls on an outstretched hand, a sudden valgus loading or near dislocation can result. Tenderness along the medial side of the elbow, as well as swelling, is usually present. Fractures of the radial head or avulsions of the medial epicondyle must be looked for. The medial collateral ligaments are commonly found to calcify several months later. This usually causes no functional loss and does not require any treatment.

III. STIFFNESS AND CONTRACTURE OF THE ELBOW

   A. Post-traumatic. Stiffness of the elbow after trauma is quite common, and physical therapy is usually required to minimize it. The functional range of motion of the elbow is in an arc of approximately 30 to 130 degrees of flexion and is in the range of 50 to 150 degrees of pronation–supination. Each patient must be examined individually to determine whether treatment should be tried and the specific modality that is appropriate. Forced, sudden, and passive motion could be deleterious.

   B. Heterotopic bone formation. Loss of motion may also be caused by juxta-articular bone formation at the elbow. Patients who have experienced head trauma with neurospastic injury are especially prone to heterotopic bone formation and may require excision and contracture release. The precise mechanism for increased heterotopic bone formation after head injury is not understood.

IV. OLECRANON BURSITIS. Acute inflammation of the olecranon bursa is a common condition that can result from infection or an acute gouty attack. Distinguishing infection from nonseptic inflammatory conditions such as gout or RA is often impossible on clinical examination alone. The differentiation becomes especially difficult in the patient with diabetes with a history of gout. Both conditions demonstrate erythema, fluctuance, and generalized tenderness. Adenopathy may be more prominent in infection, but it is not always present. Traumatic bursitis can cause bursal swelling and even some warmth. Fluid analysis demonstrates bloody or xanthochromic fluid that gives negative culture results.

   A. Laboratory studies. Aspirating the bursal fluid for Gram stain, culture, crystal examination, and cell count is helpful, and findings can be diagnostic. Unfortunately, some patients are given antibiotics before specimens are taken, and the diagnosis remains elusive. The simultaneous use of anti-inflammatory agents and antibiotics, although not technically acceptable, may be prudent in some of these patients until the final culture results are available. Because *Staphylococcus aureus* is most commonly cultured, the patient must be started on dicloxacillin or a cephalosporin when the results of the culture are pending. In those patients with infection who do not respond to a 1- to 2-day course of oral antibiotics, intravenous therapy is indicated. Daily aspiration of the bursa is also mandatory.

   B. Treatment. Recurrent bouts of inflammatory olecranon bursitis can be treated with repeated aspirations. In noninfectious cases, treatment of the underlying systemic disorder or avoidance of local trauma are indicated. If the source of the bursitis is judged to be inflammatory, a single injection of corticosteroid followed by splinting of the elbow should be considered. Repeated injections should be avoided. If these nonoperative measures fail to reduce symptomatic pain and swelling, operative bursectomy should be considered.

V. OSTEOARTHRITIS. Primary symptomatic osteoarthritis is less common in the elbow than in the weight-bearing joints of the lower extremities and interphalangeal joints of the hands. Inflammatory arthritis of the elbow is more likely to be RA or a crystal-based arthropathy than a primary degenerative joint disease.

VI. RA. Rheumatoid involvement of the elbow usually begins with repeated effusions. Control of the effusions may require the use of systemic medications or intra-articular steroid injections. Depending on the severity of the disease, there is a gradual loss of motion as the joint surfaces become barren of articular cartilage. The loss of motion becomes more debilitating and self-care becomes more difficult when the adjacent joints become affected. Arthroscopic synovectomy can be helpful in the early stages in select patients. For patients with significant pain and joint destruction, total elbow replacement is often the best option.

VII. HEMOPHILIA. Recurrent hemarthrosis of the elbow may lead to a gradual loss of elbow function. In the early stages of recurrent hemarthrosis, a mild flexion contracture exists, with little chronic pain. Recurrent bleeding leads to destruction of the articular cartilage and a generalized arthropathy with pain and eventually to fibrosis of the joint.

    A. Medical management. In the early phases of bleeding, standard care includes factor VIII or IX infusions, with plasma levels being monitored. Initially, activity should be restricted to some extent, but when the acute bleed has resolved, motion exercises should be encouraged. Control of pain is always difficult.

    B. Surgery. Synovectomy of the elbow may be indicated for recurrent hemarthrosis unresponsive to medical management. For painful arthropathy, total elbow replacement offers improved function in select cases.

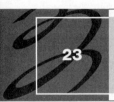

23   HIP PAIN
Thomas P. Sculco and Paul Lombardi

*A*n evaluation of hip pain begins with considering the multiple structure/function relationships that comprise the joint itself and the surrounding soft tissue structures. The **hip joint** comprises the proximal femur and acetabulum, articular surfaces, and synovium. The **periarticular soft tissues** comprise **bursae** (e.g., greater trochanteric, iliopsoas, and ischial), **tendons** (e.g., hip abductor, adductor, internal–external rotators, extensors, flexors, and hamstrings), and **acetabular labrum** which is the soft tissue rim surrounding the acetabulum.

    The clinician should also consider other structural abnormalities, such as inguinal and femoral herniae, and the possibility that the complaint of pain in the hip is actually referred from another location, for example, lower back, knee, and even visceral organs such as the gastrointestinal tract, prostate, ovary, and aorta.

 CLINICAL MANIFESTATIONS

The most important initial step while obtaining the patient's clinical history is to ask the patient to point to the area of "hip pain." Most will point to their back or their lateral thigh, not their groin. In general, hip pain is groin pain. Patients with true hip pain usually complain of limitation of hip motion, a painful limp, and pain in the groin on movement. Pain occurs less often at rest and rarely at night. Care while obtaining the patient's clinical history may reveal childhood hip disorders, such as Legg-Calvé-Perthes disease, slipped capital femoral epiphysis, developmental dysplasia of the hip, and septic arthritis. Concomitant disorders such as osteoarthritis, rheumatoid arthritis (RA), psoriatic arthritis or ankylosing spondylitis, malignancy, or low back pain may provide insight into the etiology of the hip pain. A history of alcohol or steroid use is pertinent in patients suspected of having osteonecrosis. Response to prior therapies, including physical therapy, anti-inflammatory medications, modification of activity, night pain, or use of assistive devices helps one to assess the severity of the pain. Accompanying fever, chills, weight loss, or fatigue, or a history of recent infection are important symptoms that could reflect an infected hip or metastatic lesion.

I. DURATION AND LOCATION OF PAIN

    A. Pain of short duration is usually post-traumatic or inflammatory.

    B. Pain that is chronic and progressive may indicate mechanical joint incongruity related to an underlying arthritis. The pain of osteoarthritis is usually alleviated by rest.

Constant hip pain, especially if severe and unresponsive to simple pain medications, is characteristic of an inflammatory/septic or neoplastic process. Synovitis due to RA or psoriatic arthritis tends to be worse in the morning; however, it may not go away completely during the day. It rarely causes night pain unless there is an associated infection or it has led to severe secondary osteoarthritis.

C. Groin pain that radiates to the buttock indicates hip joint dysfunction. Pain that is confined purely to the buttock or back, without affect on the groin, usually has its origin as a back pain. When patients say their hip hurts, they mostly point to the buttock. Lateral hip pain with radiation to the lateral thigh may be related to greater trochanteric bursitis or abductor tendinitis. Discomfort over the anterior superior iliac spine extending down the anterior thigh is associated with meralgia paresthetica (inflammation of the lateral femoral cutaneous nerve). Medial groin pain can be due to adductor tendinitis, sometimes associated with overuse or yoga positions, or a pubic ramus fracture. Hip pain can also be referred to the knee through the obturator nerve.

D. Buttock pain may be related to ischial tuberosity bursitis or spinal disorders, such as spinal stenosis, ruptured intervertebral disc, and instability.

II. RELATION OF PAIN TO ACTIVITY
  A. Pain from the hip joint and surrounding soft tissues is usually aggravated by weight bearing and relieved by rest.
  B. Patients will usually describe a specific position of the limb which exacerbates or relieves their symptoms.

III. DECREASED FUNCTION. Patients complain of a progressive decrease in the maximum distance they are able to walk and tolerance to exercise. Ability to perform activities of daily living is decreased. These decreases can be quantified with functional assessment scores such as Western Ontario McMaster Arthritis index (WOMAC), the Harris Hip Score, and Short Form-36 health survey questionnaire (SF-36) (see Chapter 9). A persistently severe hip pain that limits function and awakens a patient at night should stimulate consideration of an infection, a fracture, metastatic lesion, or very severe osteoarthritis.

 PHYSICAL EXAMINATION

I. GAIT. The patient is observed while entering the examination room, and the presence of a limp or an expression of pain is noted.
  A. Abductor lurch (Trendelenburg's gait). The patient shifts the center of gravity away from the affected limb during the stance phase of gait to unload the weakened abductors and to avoid pain.
  B. Coxalgic gait. The patient quickly unloads the painful leg while bearing weight. Decreased stance phase of gait and stride length on the affected side will be seen.
  C. Stiff hip gait. The patient will walk by rotating the pelvis and swinging the legs in a circular fashion.

II. PATIENT IN STANDING POSITION
  A. Measure unequal leg lengths by balancing the pelvis with calibrated blocks, if necessary. Note for fixed pelvic obliquity if present.
  B. Evaluate the spine for scoliosis or kyphosis.
  C. Trendelenburg's sign. While bearing weight with the leg on the affected side, the opposite side of the patient's pelvis will droop because the hip abductor, which normally elevates the pelvis, is weakened. This may take 30 to 45 seconds to become apparent.

III. PATIENT IN SUPINE POSITION
  A. Record active and passive range of motion bilaterally, and compare the values of the two sides.
    1. Note flexion, extension, abduction, adduction, and internal rotation and external rotation in both flexion and extension. Internal rotation is usually the most affected motion in most types of arthritis (osteoarthritis and RA) and this motion will commonly stimulate pain along with the limitation in range of motion.

   2. Snapping hip (coxa sultans) can be elicited with range of motion.
   3. Thomas's test for hip flexion contracture. Flex the contralateral knee and hip; extend the affected hip while keeping the lower back flat on the examination table. Note the amount of flexion present in the affected hip against the horizontal.
   4. Patrick's test for sacroiliac joint symptoms. While the patient is supine, place the affected side in a figure of 4 position with knee flexed and ankle on opposite knee. Apply pressure to the knee. A positive result exists if significant pain is present in the contralateral sacroiliac joint.
   5. Hip apprehension test for acetabular labrum pathology. Flex, adduct, and internally rotate the affected limb while observing for pain.
   B. Palpate the anterior hip capsule by applying pressure just inferior to the inguinal ligament over the femoral triangle, and evaluate the degree of tenderness. Assessment for adenopathy is important to rule out a systemic disease.
   C. Palpate the groin in supine and standing positions to rule out femoral or inguinal herniae.
   D. Measure thigh circumference bilaterally to assess muscle atrophy.
   E. Measure leg lengths with a tape measure, recording from umbilicus to medial malleolus and from anterior superior iliac spine to the medial malleolus. Note whether a fixed pelvic obliquity is present.
   F. Perform a complete neurovascular examination.
   G. Examine the knee and ankle. Patients with RA will often present with polyarticular involvement. Functional status often reflects the integral of the effects of back, hip, knee, and ankle disease.
IV. PATIENT LYING ON UNAFFECTED SIDE
   A. Palpate the greater trochanteric area for bursal tenderness.
   B. Assess abductor muscle power.
   C. Ober's test for iliotibial band tightness. With the patient in the lateral position, extend the affected hip and attempt adduction. If this cannot be achieved, the test result is positive.
V. PATIENT LYING PRONE
   A. Palpate the lumbosacral area to evaluate the low back as a potential source of pain.
   B. Evaluate hip extensor power.
   C. Palpate the sciatic notch for tenderness.
   D. **Ely's test for hamstring tightness.** With the patient prone, extend the knees until the buttocks are raised involuntarily. This indicates a positive result.

 LABORATORY STUDIES

I. A **complete blood cell count** with differential, measurements of erythrocyte sedimentation rate (ESR), or C-reactive protein are appropriate if the doctor believes that a systemic illness might be the cause of hip pain. Rarely, a hip aspiration should be performed if inflammatory joint disease and/or infection are suspected.
II. **Serum and urine immunoelectrophoreses** should be performed to rule out multiple myeloma in patients with bone pain in the setting of anemia and an elevated ESR.

 IMAGING STUDIES

I. **Radiographs** should include an anteroposterior view of the pelvis, and anteroposterior and lateral views of the affected hip. Lumbosacral films should be obtained if spinal pathology is present. Current films should be compared with prior ones, if available, to look for radiographic evidence of the progression of disease. In osteoarthritis, the patients' symptoms may often not correlate with the degree of radiographic involvement of the affected hip.
   A. Degenerative changes in the hip joint, with osteophytes, subchondral sclerosis, localized joint space narrowing, and cyst formation, are consistent with osteoarthritis.

B. Periarticular osteoporosis and global joint space narrowing is seen in RA. Osteophytes are not typically present unless the patient has had longstanding joint damage and has developed secondary osteoarthritis.

C. In cases of bone involvement by a neoplastic process, bone erosion of 50% can occur before being detected on radiographs.

II. Ultrasonography can define joint space narrowing, synovitis, and effusion and can optimally guide joint aspiration and steroid injections. Power Doppler can give a rough estimate of the amount of synovial inflammation.

III. Computed tomography (CT) scan may be used to visualize complex acetabular pathology, and to determine the degree of bone involvement in a neoplastic or fracture process.

IV. Magnetic resonance imaging (MRI) is the most sensitive tool for diagnosing occult hip fractures and osteonecrosis.

 DIFFERENTIAL DIAGNOSIS

I. HIP JOINT

A. Acetabulum and proximal femur

1. Fractures may occur in the femoral neck or intertrochanteric region. Fractures may also occur to the acetabulum after trauma. Stress fractures of the femoral neck or acetabulum, particularly in distance runners and patients with osteoporosis, may be seen. Pubic ramus fracture can lead to medial groin pain and tenderness. These can sometimes occur bilaterally along with sacral fractures in patients with osteoporosis.

2. Primary or metastatic tumors may infiltrate the femoral head and acetabulum, and pathologic fractures may occur. The most common tumors to metastasize to bone are breast, lung, prostate, kidney, and thyroid. The most common primary tumor of bone is multiple myeloma.

3. Osteonecrosis of the femoral head with or without collapse may produce severe hip pain, especially in alcoholics, patients taking steroid preparations, and steroid-treated patients with systemic lupus (see Chapter 52).

4. Transient regional osteoporosis can affect the hip and cause severe hip pain and dysfunction.

B. Articulating surfaces

1. Osteoarthritis, RA, ankylosing spondylitis, psoriatic arthritis, or septic arthritis may cause hyaline cartilage destruction with resultant hip joint incongruity and pain. The association of fever and hip pain must bring up the specter of an infected hip, which is a medical emergency.

2. Incongruity of the femoral head and subsequent arthritis can be seen in osteonecrosis with segmental collapse, or in the adult manifestations of pediatric hip disorders such as Legg-Calvé-Perthes disease, slipped capital femoral epiphysis, and developmental dysplasia of the hip.

C. Synovium

1. Synovitis of the hip joint may result from RA, spondyloarthropathies such as ankylosing spondylitis and psoriatic arthritis, and viral infections, especially in children who can present with transient synovitis of the hip and hemophilia.

2. Septic arthritis is most commonly caused by gram-positive organisms such as *Staphylococcus aureus* and streptococci and more rarely by gram-negative bacilli. In prosthetic joint infections, one must also consider *Staphylococcus epidermidis*. The patient who is most likely to develop this type of infection is the immunosuppressed individual with a history of prior hip joint damage. The common presentation is of severe pain of acute onset along with fever and chills. This is a medical emergency and demands optimal cultures, antibiotics, and often, hip drainage by needle or by surgical intervention (see Chapter 46).

3. Tuberculosis may lead to a proliferative synovitis and severe joint destruction on both sides of the joint. Hip aspiration, followed by acid-fast staining, rarely polymerase chain reaction, culture of the aspirate, and histologic assessment confirm the diagnosis. This problem is discussed in Chapter 46.

4. **Synovial chondromatosis** is a benign cartilage tumor of the synovium, which usually presents with pain and a decreased range of motion.

5. **Pigmented villonodular synovitis** is a benign but aggressive synovial proliferation in the hip joint, characterized histologically by hemosiderin-stained synovium and giant cells. This may lead to cyst formation in the femoral neck or joint destruction. The radiographic changes seen are present on both sides of the joint.

II. PERIARTICULAR SOFT TISSUES

A. Bursae

1. Greater trochanteric bursitis is common and produces acute pain over the lateral thigh, which usually radiates distally. Swelling and pain with weight bearing are often present, and a limp may result. Pain is present when the patient is lying on the affected side and will often awaken the patient from sleep.

2. Iliopsoas bursitis is uncommon. It may communicate with the hip joint in 15% of patients.

B. Tendons and fascia

1. **Hamstring, adductor, abductor, and rotator tendons** may become inflamed at their insertions into bone. Piriformis syndrome is diagnosed by the presence of pain in the sciatic notch on palpation and resisted external rotation.

2. The **fascia lata** is quite taut as it passes over the greater trochanter and may produce a snapping sensation and pain, particularly on hip flexion and adduction. Other causes of a "snapping hip" (coxa sultans) include a tight iliopsoas tendon and hypertrophic fovea.

C. Herniae

1. **Inguinal herniae,** if symptomatic, may produce severe groin pain and limitation of hip motion.

2. **Femoral herniae** with prolapse may produce severe groin pain and limping. However, pain is intermittent until incarceration occurs.

D. Referred pain

1. **Lumbosacral.** Osteoarthritis involving the lumbosacral apophyseal joints can produce buttock pain. Radicular pain from nerve root irritation may be manifested in the lateral thigh or groin. Disc herniations involving L1-2 and L2-3 may produce these symptoms. Pott's disease, a tuberculous infection of the intervertebral discs and vertebral bodies, may spread to the hip joint via the psoas muscle insertions along the anterior portion of the lumbar spine. At times, an injection of lidocaine and steroids into the hip joint via ultrasonographic guidance is needed to differentiate whether the "hip pain" arises from the hip itself or is referred from the back.

2. **Visceral origin**
   a. Renal colic can radiate to the groin. Ovarian or prostate disorders may mimic hip pathology.
   b. Vascular occlusive disease of the aorta can produce buttock pain; femoral vein phlebitis can present with thigh and groin pain.

 THERAPY

I. **Joint rest** may be accomplished by unloading the affected hip with various forms of external support. A **cane** should be held in the contralateral hand to assist weakened abductors and to unload the hip. Forearm crutches or axillary crutches can be used in more severe disease or bilateral involvement.

II. **COMPRESSES**
   A. If an acute inflammatory condition involves a tendon or bursa, ice compresses are useful.
   B. For chronic pain, moist heat improves local blood supply and relaxes spastic musculature.

III. **MEDICATIONS**
   A. **Anti-inflammatory medications** are useful for arthritic problems involving the hip joint. Nonsteroidal anti-inflammatory drugs (NSAIDs) can be helpful. These

medications may be contraindicated in patients taking anticoagulants or who have peptic ulcer or renal disease.

B. Analgesics may be used in conjunction with an anti-inflammatory drug.

C. Soft tissue injections. For bursitis or tendinitis, local injection with a corticosteroid such as 40 mg of methylprednisolone acetate (Depo-Medrol) and 3 to 5 mL of 1% lidocaine is effective. If no improvement occurs after one injection, two more weekly injections may be given or the injection can be performed under ultrasonographic guidance to ascertain optimal needle placement. For details of therapy for specific disease entities, see the appropriate chapters.

IV. EXERCISES

    A. Attempts should be made to maintain passive and active hip motion without aggravating the underlying pain.

    B. Gentle isometric exercises for the quadriceps and hamstrings and antigravity exercises as tolerated by the patient, for hip flexors, extensors, abductors, adductors, and rotators are recommended. See Chapter 61 for specific exercise prescriptions. Weight reduction is an important aspect of the treatment of hip disorders when we consider that hip mechanics is such that every pound of weight is perceived by the hip as being 5 lbs. The prognosis in many hip disorders is guarded if aggravating factors such as obesity are not addressed.

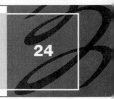

KNEE PAIN
Norman A. Johanson and Paul Pellicci

24

ANATOMY

I.   JOINTS. There are three articulations in the knee, referred to as compartments. They can be affected separately or together as part of a single process.

    A. Patellofemoral compartment.

    B. Medial tibiofemoral compartment.

    C. Lateral tibiofemoral compartment.

II. LIGAMENTS. The knee ligaments are specially designed to accommodate a wide range of motion and flexibility while providing essential stability for weight bearing.

    A. Medial collateral ligament.

    B. Lateral collateral ligament.

    C. Anterior cruciate ligament.

    D. Posterior cruciate ligament.

III. Menisci are crescent-shaped fibrocartilaginous structures that are peripherally situated in the medial and lateral tibiofemoral compartments. These structures are involved in the weight-bearing process and augment the stability of the knee.

IV. PERIARTICULAR STRUCTURES. Several musculotendinous structures pass across the knee to insert at or near the joint. Injury or inflammation of any of these structures can result in knee pain.

    A. Quadriceps mechanism (quadriceps tendon and patellar tendon).

    B. Pes anserine tendons (sartorius, gracilis, and semitendinosus).

    C. Semimembranosus.

    D. Biceps femoris.

    E. Iliotibial band.

    F. Popliteus.

    G. Gastrocnemius (medial and lateral heads).

CAUSES OF KNEE PAIN

I. **TRAUMA.** The mechanism of injury is important in formulating a differential diagnosis; however, components of several mechanisms may be present in a given injury.
    A. **Hyperextension** (anterior cruciate tear).
    B. **Varus** (lateral collateral ligament tear and anterior cruciate tear).
    C. **Valgus** (medial collateral ligament tear and anterior cruciate tear).
    D. **Torsion** (meniscal tears).
    E. **Axial impact on femur and posterior displacement of tibia (dashboard injury),** patellar fracture, posterior cruciate ligament tear, femoral shaft fracture, and fracture-dislocation of hip.
II. **SPONTANEOUS**
    A. **Inflammation** (synovitis and tendinitis).
    B. **Vascular disorder** (osteonecrosis and sickle cell crisis).
    C. **Degeneration** (meniscal tear and articular erosion).
    D. **Neoplasm** (primary or metastatic bone tumors near the knee; soft tissue tumors around the knee).
    E. **Referred pain** from hip or spine disorder.

 COMMON PRESENTING SYMPTOMS ASSOCIATED WITH KNEE PAIN

I. **Swelling**—enlargement of the knee with loss of normal contour.
II. **Locking or severe stiffness** (meniscal tear and chondromalacia patellae).
III. **Giving way or buckling** (anterior cruciate tear or patellofemoral disorder).
IV. **Clicking or crackling sound** in the knee (meniscal tear or chondromalacia patellae).
V. **Audible pop** at the time of knee injury (cruciate or meniscal tear).

 PHYSICAL EXAMINATION

I. **OBSERVATION**
    A. **Contour** of the knee.
    B. **Alignment** of the knee while the patient is standing (varus, valgus, flexed, or hyperextended).
    C. **Gait**
II. **PALPATION**
    A. **Effusion.** The presence of fluid in the knee may be demonstrated by sweeping the hand distally over the knee to empty the suprapatellar pouch. Medial and lateral bulging of the capsule can be felt and sometimes seen (as distinguished from synovial thickening).
    B. **Popliteal fullness** is suggestive of Baker's cyst.
    C. **Joint-line tenderness** exacerbated by tibial rotation (Steinmann's test) is suggestive of meniscal tear.
    D. **Tenderness on patellofemoral compression** with the knee slightly flexed is suggestive of chondromalacia patellae.
III. **Range of motion** (active and passive flexion and extension, fixed flexion deformities).
    A. Note presence of **patellofemoral crepitus** throughout the range of motion.
    B. **McMurray's test.** With the knee at first in full flexion, the tibia is rotated internally and externally while the knee is brought slowly into extension. A palpable jumping at the joint line sometimes accompanied by an audible click is suggestive of a meniscal tear.
IV. **STRENGTH**
    A. **Thigh circumferences** are measured and compared (10 cm above patella).
    B. **Quadriceps strength.** It must be noted whether an apparent weakness is secondary to pain, stiffness, or actual muscle dysfunction. Presence of any thigh atrophy is noted.
    C. **Hamstring** strength.

V. STABILITY

   A. Varus and valgus stability is best demonstrated by cradling the knee with one hand and, with the knee in extension, applying a medial or lateral knee stress. Any more than a jog of motion is suggestive of the laxity of the medial or lateral collateral ligament.

   B. The **anterior and posterior cruciate ligaments** are tested with the knee in flexion and in extension. While sitting by the patient's foot with the knee of the patient flexed to 90 degrees, the examiner applies anterior and posterior displacement force on the proximal tibia. A firm end point should be present in each direction (anterior drawer test). With the knee in extension, the tibia is lifted anteriorly on the femur (Lachman's test). Minimal excursion and a firm end point should be noted.

 DIAGNOSTIC INVESTIGATIONS

I. Radiography should be performed while the patient is in the standing position (anteroposterior and lateral views) to demonstrate joint space narrowing. Tangential patellar views (Merchant's views) are obtained to assess the patellofemoral compartment. A tunnel view is obtained to assess the contour of the intercondylar notch.

II. Screening blood tests such as complete blood cell count; erythrocyte sedimentation rate, rheumatoid factor, and biochemistry profile should be performed if systemic disease is suspected.

III. Aspiration of synovial fluid for analysis of cells and crystals is helpful in rheumatoid arthritis (RA), gout, and pseudogout. Culture and sensitivity are definitive in infectious arthritis.

IV. Arthrogram is helpful in confirming meniscal and cruciate tears and to demonstrate a popliteal cyst or nodular synovitis. This test has generally been supplanted by the magnetic resonance imaging (MRI).

V. Bone scan is helpful in demonstrating early osteonecrosis (increased or decreased uptake in subchondral bone) when radiographic findings are still normal or when there is a stress fracture present. It can also define the diffuse increased uptake in RA or medial uptake in osteoarthritis (OA).

VI. MRI has become the imaging procedure of choice for evaluating torn menisci and ligaments.

 TREATMENT

I. ACUTE PHASE

   A. Rest through decreased activity and weight bearing (crutches and cane if needed).

   B. Anti-inflammatory medications.

   C. Therapeutic aspiration of synovial fluid (or blood in traumatic effusion) often relieves pain. This can be supplemented by injection of a local anesthetic into the joint.

   D. Injection of a steroid preparation into the knee is recommended for older patients with arthritic changes on radiography or in patients with inflammatory joint disease in whom infection is not present.

II. CONVALESCENT PHASE

   A. Quadriceps and hamstring exercises are frequently used for many knee disorders. Straight leg raising without weights is helpful in patients with arthritis because it minimizes patellofemoral stress. Exercises with weights are more effective in rehabilitation after athletic injuries.

   B. Progressive activities (e.g., swimming and bicycle riding) preserve knee motion and strength without excessive impact loading.

   C. Braces are used according to the condition being treated (usually not effective in arthritis but beneficial in chondromalacia patellae and mild ligament injuries).

COMMON DISEASES ASSOCIATED WITH KNEE PAIN

I. **Chondromalacia patellae** is a spectrum of knee disorders resulting from excessive pressure on the patellar cartilage and the subsequent softening and fibrillation of the articular surface. Increased pressure may be caused by an abnormality of patellar tracking during knee motion. Associated conditions include femoral anteversion, external tibial torsion, valgus knee alignment, hypoplastic high-riding patella, or foot pronation. Excessive malalignment may cause subluxation or dislocation of the patella.

A. **History**
   1. **Anterior knee pain** is felt during climbing or descending stairs, sitting for long periods, or squatting.
   2. There may be a history of **direct trauma** to the patella (dashboard injury).
   3. Sports that may cause overloading of the patellofemoral joint (e.g., jogging, basketball, gymnastics, and dancing) are associated with chondromalacia.

B. **Physical examination**
   1. **Mild peripatellar swelling** may be present, but joint effusion is rare.
   2. **Crepitus of the patellofemoral joint** is usually palpable during range of motion. Full flexion may elicit an increase in pain.
   3. In cases of **patellar malalignment or recurrent subluxation/dislocation,** the patella may exhibit mediolateral hypermobility, and in case of lateral patellar displacement, the patella may elicit significant apprehension.

C. **Radiographic findings**
   1. **Tangential view** of the patella (Merchant's view) may demonstrate lateral displacement or tilt of the patella. Narrowing of the joint space is suggestive of patellofemoral arthritis.
   2. **Lateral view** of the knee may demonstrate a high-riding patella (patella alta), which has been associated with patellofemoral pain. Patella alta is defined as a ratio of the length of the patellar tendon to the length of the patella greater than 1.2:1.

D. **Differential diagnosis.** Chondromalacia patellae must be distinguished from **meniscal tears.** Meniscal tears are more frequently associated with a specific traumatic event and even more likely to result in a knee effusion, locking, and a reduction of range of knee motion. Meniscal tears may be ruled out by an arthrogram, MRI, or arthroscopic evaluation.

E. **Treatment**
   1. Those activities that exacerbate pain are temporarily discontinued.
   2. **Quadriceps muscle strengthening** is the most important objective. This is accomplished through quadriceps exercises in the range of 90 to 30 degrees or through straight leg raising.
   3. In some cases, **nonsteroidal anti-inflammatory drugs (NSAIDs)** are necessary to control acute pain in chondromalacia. Ibuprofen in a dosage of 600 mg four times daily may be effective.

II. **MENISCAL TEARS.** Traumatic tears of the medial and lateral menisci are common causes of knee pain, particularly in athletic individuals. The medial meniscus is by far the most frequently affected.

A. **History**
   1. A **twisting injury** is often the cause of a meniscal tear.
   2. **Swelling** of varying severity is often reported.
   3. Knee **stiffness, pain, and limitation of motion** are frequent complaints. A history of locking of the knee is less common.

B. **Physical examination**
   1. Swelling and knee effusion are frequently present.
   2. Tenderness is present along the medial or lateral joint line.
   3. Range of motion may be limited in extension and flexion, or the knee may be locked in one position.
   4. Result of the McMurray's test or Steinmann's test (tibial rotation) is often positive in case of meniscal tears.

C. Diagnostic studies
  1. **Radiographic findings** in the knee are usually normal except for the demonstration of a knee effusion.
  2. **Arthrography or MRI** will demonstrate meniscal tears in most cases.
  3. **Arthroscopy** is an important therapeutic modality for meniscal tears.
D. Differential diagnosis
  1. **Medial collateral ligament sprains** may produce medial joint line pain and tenderness with a limp and an effusion. Locking is not present. Arthrography finding is negative or demonstrates leakage of dye in the area of the ligament injury. MRI is diagnostic.
  2. **Acute chondromalacia patellae** may produce anteromedial pain. An effusion is rarely present, and locking is also very uncommon. Findings on arthrogram or MRI are negative.
  3. **A pes anserine bursitis** presents with pain and tenderness over the proximal medial tibia just below the joint line without effusion, limitation of motion, or locking. Direct tenderness is present over the bursa, and the arthrographic or MRI findings are negative.
  4. **Medial compartment tibiofemoral OA** may produce an effusion with medial joint line pain, tenderness, and a limp. Radiography demonstrates sclerosis and joint space narrowing in the medial aspect of the knee joint.
E. Treatment. In patients with a locked knee or recurrent symptoms from a torn medial meniscus, **surgical removal** is the treatment of choice. If the tear is longitudinal, simple excision of the injured segment may be performed. Arthroscopic techniques are the preferred method of treatment.

III. Tibial tubercle apophysitis (Osgood-Schlatter disease) occurs primarily in adolescents and presents as pain located at the insertion of the patellar tendon into the tibial tubercle. Some investigators believe the syndrome represents an injury to the apophysis that is similar to mild avulsion.
  A. Physical examination. There is localized pain on palpation of the tubercle.
  B. Radiography often shows a displaced ossicle of bone anterior to the tubercle within the tendinous insertion.
  C. Treatment. The pain usually disappears when the ossicle fuses with the underlying tibia. Until this time, the patient's activity level must be monitored. Depending on the severity of the pain, some or all athletic activity must be discontinued. A cylindric cast for 4 to 6 weeks may be necessary in resistant cases. Ibuprofen 600 mg three times daily or other NSAIDs may be used during the acute phase.

ANKLE AND FOOT PAIN
David S. Levine

25

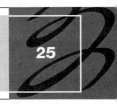

■ KEY POINTS

■ A sound understanding of foot and ankle anatomy is essential for establishing the cause of associated pathologies.

■ Understanding the "essential" nature of the mobile hindfoot and forefoot joints and the "nonessential," rigid nature of the midfoot joints is important.

■ With the exception of acute fractures, weight-bearing plain radiographs provide the most important information for the diagnosis and treatment of foot and ankle pathologies.

■ Understanding the contribution of the "tight" or shortened Achilles tendon in the pathogenesis of posterior tibial tendon insufficiency and plantar fasciitis is important.

■ Understanding the contribution of a "hypermobile" first ray in the presence of hallux valgus deformity, as well as the generation of second metatarsal overload conditions (metatarsalgia, hammertoes, and stress fracture of the second metatarsal, etc.), is important.

ANATOMY

I. The **joints** of the foot and ankle can be divided into two groups: **essential joints,** which have appreciable motion and are "required" for normal functioning of the foot, and **nonessential joints,** which have little appreciable motion and are largely responsible for providing stability.

A. Essential joints

1. The **ankle (tibiotalar) joint** maintains an axis through the malleoli such that dorsiflexion and external foot rotation are coupled. Similarly, plantar flexion and internal foot rotation are coupled motions. Surrounding ligamentous structures limit inversion or eversion through the ankle joint.

2. The **subtalar (talocalcaneal) joint** is responsible for hindfoot inversion and eversion. Motion occurs around an axis inclined 15 degrees lateral to the longitudinal axis of the foot. Along with the ankle joint, the subtalar joint forms a "universal joint," thereby enabling the hindfoot to accommodate to uneven surfaces.

3. The **talonavicular and calcaneocuboid (transverse tarsal) joints** function to link the mobile hindfoot to the immobile midfoot.

4. The **metatarsophalangeal (MTP) joints** of the forefoot have significant dorsiflexion and plantar flexion capability, which enables the center of gravity of the body to be propelled forward efficiently at the end of the gait cycle.

B. Nonessential joints such as the **navicular-cuneiform, intercuneiform,** and **tarsometatarsal** joints (collectively known as the "midfoot") have little motion because of stout ligamentous reinforcement. These joints serve to provide a rigid lever-arm during weight transfer from the hindfoot to the forefoot. Movement in this part of the foot is considered to be pathologic.

II. LIGAMENTS

A. The **deltoid ligament** is the prime stabilizer of the medial (inner) side of the ankle joint. It runs from the medial malleolus to the talus, calcaneus, and navicular. Its deep portion resists lateral translation of the talus within the ankle joint. The superficial portion blends with other capsular and ligamentous structures over the medial hindfoot.

B. The **lateral collateral ligaments** consist of the anterior and posterior talofibular ligaments and the calcaneofibular ligament. As a group, these ligaments are the prime stabilizers of the lateral (outer) side of the ankle joint. The anterior talofibular ligament is the most frequently injured ligament, especially during plantar flexion of the foot. With increasing energy of motion or when the foot is in a neutral position or in slight dorsiflexion, the calcaneofibular ligament may also be injured.

C. The **plantar talocalcaneonavicular (spring) ligament** has been increasingly noted to be important in supporting the head of the talus and in preventing loss of the medial longitudinal arch height.

D. The **plantar intertarsal (interosseous) ligaments** (the long and short plantar ligaments, as well as the many intertarsal ligaments, are often collectively referred to as the plantar intertarsal ligaments) stabilize the bones of the midfoot, thereby maintaining their static contribution to the medial longitudinal arch.

III. MUSCLES

■ Movement: dorsiflexion of the foot and ankle;
■ Muscles effecting that movement: tibialis anterior, extensor digitorum longus, extensor hallucis longus, and peroneus tertius.

■ Movement: plantar flexion of the foot and ankle;
■ Muscles effecting that movement: gastrocnemius and soleus.

■ Movement: hindfoot inversion;
■ Muscles effecting that movement: posterior tibialis and gastrocnemius.

- Movement: hindfoot eversion;
- Muscles effecting that movement: peroneus brevis and peroneus longus. The intrinsic muscles of the foot contribute to the bulk and padding of the sole, help maintain the architecture of the transverse and longitudinal arches, and influence the alignment of the toes. The toes are flexed and extended by their long and short flexors and extensors, respectively.

IV. FASCIA. The plantar fascia originates on the posteromedial tubercle of the calcaneus and inserts into the bases of the proximal phalanges via the plantar plate and flexor tendon sheaths. It maintains a static support of the longitudinal arch via a "windlass" mechanism (the windlass mechanism refers to the ability of the plantar fascia to elevate the longitudinal arch of the foot when the great toe is dorsiflexed). This mechanism is observed at the push-off phase of the gait pattern and supports the arch during this period of high force transmission.

V. The **blood supply** of the ankle and foot comes principally from the dorsalis pedis artery (an extension of the anterior tibialis artery), which is palpable between the first and second metatarsal bases on the dorsum of the foot, and the posterior tibialis artery, which is palpable about one finger's breadth posterior and inferior to the medial malleolus. Communicating branches from the peroneal artery provide an inconsistent anastomosis with the above-named arteries.

VI. Innervation of the foot and ankle is from the superficial and deep peroneal nerves, which supply the dorsum of the foot. The medial and lateral plantar nerves provide sensation to the plantar surface of the foot and innervate the intrinsic muscles. The sural nerve provides sensation to the outer border of the heel and the dorsolateral border of the foot. The saphenous nerve, a terminal branch of the femoral nerve, provides sensation to the medial border of the ankle and foot.

 HISTORY

I. PAIN
 - **A.** Exact localization of pain and radiation to other areas.
 - **B.** Aggravating and alleviating factors.
 - **C.** Associated findings.
 - **D.** Acute or insidious onset.
 - **E.** Traumatic or atraumatic.
 - **F.** Intensity.
 - **G.** Quality (radiating pain with an "electric" quality may be consistent with neuroma).

II. FOOTWEAR
 - **A.** Recent alterations in usual footwear (i.e., heel height) should be taken into account.
 - **B.** Attitude toward footwear influences expectations.
 - **C.** Barefoot activities can be associated with increased or decreased symptoms.

III. PAST MEDICAL HISTORY. Numerous conditions, including gout, rheumatoid arthritis (RA), neoplasm, peripheral vascular disease, diabetes mellitus, congenital deformity, and neurologic conditions, can contribute to foot or ankle dysfunction. Similarly, the altered gait pattern related to foot and ankle dysfunction can contribute to other musculoskeletal complaints, such as lower-back pain, hip pain, and medial knee pain. Similarly, musculoskeletal dysfunction and pain arising from those joints can alter the gait pattern and can have an impact upon the foot. Often, the ultimate disability is the integral of all of these factors. A deformity of the knee may be associated with a "compensatory" deformity of the foot.

IV. PAST SURGICAL HISTORY. Any prior history of surgical procedures on the foot and ankle should be thoroughly discussed.

 PHYSICAL EXAMINATION

I. Gait and alignment should be evaluated with the patient in shoes and barefoot.
 - **A.** At **heel-strike,** the hindfoot should assume a valgus attitude, allowing shock absorption through the flexible hindfoot. Weight is transferred forward during

foot-flat. At **heel-rise,** the hindfoot is inverted (by the tibialis posterior muscle). The transverse tarsal joint becomes rigid when the hindfoot is inverted, enabling the body weight to be transferred through the rigid midfoot to the MTP joints preparing for toe-off. The **swing phase** then completes the gait cycle.

B. An **antalgic gait** involves a shortened stance phase, which signifies a painful limb.

C. A **steppage gait** involves hip and knee flexion to clear the foot during swing phase in the setting of a "drop foot" (e.g., after a peroneal nerve palsy).

D. The **patient's standing position should be observed from behind.** Physiologic hind foot valgus (i.e., away from the midline) should be readily apparent. Excessive valgus (as in a flatfoot) or hindfoot varus (as in clubfoot sequelae or the cavovarus foot) should be noted.

E. Heel-rise should be associated with hindfoot inversion (a tibialis posterior function).

F. Total limb alignment should be evaluated from the hips to the toes.

G. Rotational deformities (i.e., intoeing) due to internal tibial torsion or excessive femoral anteversion are best evaluated with the patient in the prone position.

II. **Range of motion** should be compared with that of the contralateral extremity. Both active and passive range of motion should be evaluated.

A. **Ankle dorsiflexion** must be examined with the hindfoot in the neutral position. Dorsiflexion with the knee in extension versus flexion should be noted to differentiate between tendoachilles tightness and gastrocnemius tightness.

B. The **subtalar joint** is assessed by inverting and everting the heel while stabilizing the tibia.

C. **Forefoot inversion** (supination) and **eversion** (pronation), as well as **abduction** and **adduction,** are assessed by holding the heel in the cup of the examiner's hand to lock the subtalar joint in a neutral position and by noting the forefoot position.

D. **Active and passive motion of the MTP and interphalangeal joints**
  1. **Hammertoes** are lesser toe deformities having a fixed or flexible flexion–contracture of the proximal interphalangeal (PIP) joints.
  2. If MTP hyperextension coexists, the term **clawtoe** is used.
  3. A **mallet toe** exists when a fixed or flexible flexion contracture of the distal interphalangeal (DIP) joints of the lesser toes exists.
  4. **A cock-up toe** is a toe deformity in which there is a component of hyperextension at either the MTP joint or the PIP joint. It is a general term that is probably best replaced by the terms explained in the earlier points: hammertoe, mallet toe, or clawtoe.

III. **TENDERNESS.** The point of maximal tenderness is crucial in establishing a correct diagnosis. Systematic palpation of the foot to localize tenderness and evaluate bony and soft-tissue asymmetry is required to elicit these findings.

A. Tenderness over a prominent medial eminence of the hallux MTP joint is commonly seen in hallux valgus (bunions).

B. Tenderness over the lateral ankle ligaments is seen commonly after an inversion ankle sprain.

C. Tenderness over the MTP joint of the hallux may be seen in gout and osteoarthritis.

D. Metatarsalgia is signified by tenderness along the plantar surfaces of the metatarsal heads.

E. Medial hindfoot tenderness or posterolateral hindfoot tenderness is often associated with acute or chronic posterior tibial tendon insufficiency, respectively.

F. "Squeeze" tenderness of all of the forefoot MTP joints approximates them and augments the tenderness in the setting of inflammatory disorders such as RA and is an important early sign of active forefoot disease.

IV. **Swelling** may be nonspecific or the manifestation of a systemic disease (i.e., RA, congestive heart failure, or venous obstructive outflow disease).

A. **Dorsal forefoot** swelling along with pain on weight bearing suggests a metatarsal stress fracture.

B. Swelling anterior to the **distal fibula** following a "turned ankle" indicates an anterior talofibular ligament sprain.

C. Swelling distal to the **medial malleolus** along with inability to invert the heel is consistent with posterior tibial tendon insufficiency.

D. Swelling, especially when associated with pain and **erythema,** is consistent with musculoskeletal infection, or it may be seen in severe flares of inflammatory disease such as RA or gout.

E. Swelling that involves the tendons on the dorsal surface of the foot may represent tenosynovitis, an inflammation of tendon sheaths that can be seen in RA and infections such as gonococcemia.

V. **SKIN**

A. Callosities (keratoses) are areas of thickened skin that reflect areas of increased weight bearing. Calluses under the second and third metatarsal heads may represent lesser metatarsal overload secondary to a hypermobile first ray. This is common in advanced RA, where disease-related joint damage leads to misplacement of the metatarsal heads.

B. Corns. A hard corn (clavus durum) is frequently seen over the dorsolateral aspect of the PIP joint of the fifth toe where it contacts the shoe upper. A soft corn (clavus mollum), caused by moisture, is most frequently seen in the fourth web space.

C. Ulceration may be the consequence of shoe pressure on underlying bony prominences; altered protective sensation as in diabetic neuropathy and vasculitides; or systemic vascular insufficiency due to atherosclerosis.

VI. **Neurologic and vascular** examinations, including evaluation of sensation, motor function, reflexes, position sense, skin temperature, pulses, and capillary refill, should be performed carefully.

A. Charcot arthropathy may develop in patients with diabetes with peripheral neuropathy. The resulting destruction of normal midfoot architecture leads to deformity and ulceration. This can be so severe that it mimics osteomyelitis, a disorder that can also occur in patients with diabetes.

B. Skin breakdown resulting from vascular disease with arterial or venous insufficiency may be amenable to vascular bypass surgery to improve flow.

VII. **Footwear** should be examined. Insufficient insole support may contribute to posterior tibial tendinitis. The wear pattern of the sole of the shoe may provide insight into the overall alignment of the foot. A constrictive toe box may aggravate a hallux valgus or deformity of the lesser toes. Insole wear patterns can provide insight into points of high pressure during weight bearing.

 ADDITIONAL INVESTIGATIONS

I. **Blood testing** to evaluate the white cell count, erythrocyte sedimentation rate, and C-reactive protein level may support a diagnosis of infection or RA. Measurements of rheumatoid factor, anticyclic citrullinated peptide, and uric acid levels may be helpful in suspected cases of inflammatory arthropathies.

II. **Joint aspiration** in the presence of an effusion with culture, cell counts, and analysis of crystals should be performed to rule out a septic joint, RA, or a crystal-induced arthropathy such as gout or pseudogout.

III. **Radiographs** provide a confirmation of the suspected diagnosis after the history and physical examination have been performed. All radiography should be performed during weight bearing whenever possible.

A. The ankle series consists of anteroposterior, mortise (30-degree internal rotation), and lateral views of the ankle. The joint space, alignment, and distal tibia–fibula syndesmosis, as well as bony structures themselves, should be carefully evaluated. Contralateral radiographs are often useful for evaluating asymmetries.

1. Ankle fractures are usually readily apparent. The presence of a medial malleolar fracture without a concomitant lateral malleolar fracture necessitates a full-length radiograph of the fibula.

2. Osteochondral fractures of the talar dome are often not visible on films of initial injuries. Repeated films obtained when symptoms persist should be carefully scrutinized.

3. Chronic lateral ankle instability, seen after 20% of ankle sprains, may be further assessed with stress radiographs. Talar tilt (mortise) and anterior drawer (lateral) views must be compared with those of the contralateral, uninjured limb.

B. The **foot series** consists of weight-bearing anteroposterior and lateral radiographs. Joint spaces, bone density, alignment, and presence of deformity should be noted.

    1. Forefoot, midfoot, and hindfoot relations cannot be evaluated in the non-weight-bearing condition (i.e., flatfoot or cavus feet).

    2. An **oblique radiograph** may provide additional information about the midfoot bony architecture (e.g., Lisfranc's fracture-dislocation) and about a suspected tarsal coalition (calcaneonavicular).

    3. Broden's views (taken with the ankle in 30 degrees of internal rotation and in a neutral position, with varying degrees of tilt to the x-ray beam) provide information about the congruity of the posterior subtalar joint after calcaneal fractures.

    4. Canale's view (taken with the ankle in plantar flexion, the foot internally rotated 15 degrees, and the x-ray beam tilted 15 degrees cranially) profiles the talar neck after talus fractures.

    5. A sesamoid view of the forefoot demonstrates the sesamoid-first metatarsal articulation for arthrosis, fracture, and subluxation.

IV. **Computed tomography (CT)** scan provides high-resolution anatomic detail of the cortical and cancellous structures of the foot and ankle. Computer-assisted reconstruction can provide images in planes other than those actually imaged. Arthrosis of the tarsal bones, coalitions, and osteochondral lesions are seen clearly with this modality. In addition, the complex fracture patterns of the distal tibia, talus, calcaneus, and midfoot structures are well-delineated on CT scan, which offers improved preoperative planning and management.

V. **Magnetic resonance imaging (MRI)** provides exquisite anatomic detail of the soft tissue elements of the foot and ankle, such as the ankle ligaments (after suspected talofibular ligament tear), tendons (e.g., a diseased posterior tibial tendon), skin, and subcutaneous structures. In addition, the condition of the articular cartilage surfaces can be well-visualized on certain sequences. The extent of soft tissue involvement of a neoplastic lesion can also be more accurately assessed on MRI. Synovitis and tendosynovitis due to RA or spondyloarthropathies can be clearly defined.

VI. **Technetium 99m bone scans** provide information about the metabolic activity of the bones of the foot and ankle. Increased activity as seen diffusely in RA and locally in a stress fracture is visualized as a "hot spot." However, low specificity makes the differentiation of the multiple diagnostic possibilities difficult, without additional clinical information.

COMMON FOOT PROBLEMS

I. **Achilles tendinitis** is a common condition of the Achilles tendon that presents with pain either at or just proximal to its insertion into the calcaneal tuberosity. It is frequently caused by overuse related to athletic participation. Degenerative changes within the tendon itself may be the cause in older persons. Occasionally, inflammatory disorders (such as gout) or spondyloarthropathies (such as ankylosing spondylitis, psoriatic arthritis, colitic arthropathies, or reactive arthritis) may precipitate such a condition.

A. Physical Examination. The tendon itself may be thickened approximately by 2 to 3 cm proximal to the insertion. Local tenderness is frequently present. A palpable bony prominence may be noted at the calcaneal insertion. An overlying adventitial bursa may be present as well. Active ankle plantar flexion may reveal subtle weakness in comparison with the contralateral extremity. The Thompson's test (squeezing the calf) causes ankle plantar flexion, thereby ruling out a rupture of the tendon.

B. Radiography may demonstrate a soft tissue thickening at the level of the tendinopathy. Alternatively, a degenerative spur may be seen "growing" up into the tendon at its insertion.

C. The **treatment** of acute tendinitis involves reducing the associated inflammation. A brief period of rest in a walking boot or cast may result in significant resolution of symptoms. Anti-inflammatory medications, judicious use of cryotherapy, and gentle physiotherapy upon resumption of athletic activity are valuable adjuncts. Steroid injection can lead to tendon rupture and should be avoided. Particular attention should be paid to the gastrocnemius equinus contracture, which is frequently present in recalcitrant cases. Chronic tendinitis unresponsive to conservative measures will frequently benefit from surgical debridement of the diseased tendon with excision of a bony spur, if present. Augmentation with a flexor hallucis longus tendon transfer is particularly useful if considerable weakness exists in the degenerative condition or if insufficient tendon remains after debridement.

II. **Plantar heel pain** is one of the most common disorders seen by physicians who manage foot and ankle problems. Plantar fasciitis, an irritation of the plantar fascia at its origin on the posteromedial tubercle of the calcaneus, is the most common cause of plantar heel pain. Atrophy of the normal plantar fat pad may result in difficulty in walking because of plantar heel pain. Entrapment of branches of the posterior tibial nerve as they cross in close proximity to the heel may also result in plantar heel pain. Inflammatory arthropathies (i.e., psoriatic arthritis and reactive arthritis) frequently present with plantar heel pain, occasionally even before the systemic nature of these diseases is appreciated.

A. **Physical examination** may reveal tenderness at the origin of the plantar fascia. Dorsiflexion of the MTP joints may exacerbate the tenderness because this stretches the fascia. "Start-up" pain during the first step in the morning or after prolonged sitting is common. Gastrocnemius equinus contracture (continuous with the plantar fascia) is frequently present.

B. **Plain radiographs** are frequently normal. An incidental traction spur may be present at the origin of the flexor digitorum brevis muscle. This is rarely, however, the source of the discomfort.

C. **Treatment** should be directed at unloading the heel, with soft cushioning in the shoe, vigorous stretching of the plantar fascia–gastrocnemius complex, and administering nonsteroidal anti-inflammatory medications. Occasional night splinting is helpful in the persistent case. Patients should be counseled about the often prolonged nature of the disorder. In more than 95% of cases, symptoms will resolve within 12 months. In the presence of significant tendoachilles or gastrocnemius contracture, tendon release and lengthening are often curative.

III. **Pes planus (flatfoot) deformity and posterior tibial tendon insufficiency** have received considerable attention recently. A flat foot, in and of itself, is not pathologic. However, when associated with progressive pain and deformity, it warrants intervention. Static factors contributing to the integrity of the medial longitudinal arch include the plantar fascia, the spring ligament, and the capsular and ligamentous structures associated with the bones of the medial column of the foot. The dynamic factor most commonly associated with the maintenance of the medial arch is the posterior tibial muscle and its tendon. When overloaded (e.g., by a gastrocnemius equinus contracture and obesity), the posterior tibial tendon fails. The hindfoot remains in valgus. Eventually, the static supports of the longitudinal arch fail and a sag is noted in the midfoot. The foot assumes a pronated posture and exacerbates the hindfoot valgus, which increases the gastrocnemius contracture. Eventually, degenerative changes occur in the midfoot and hindfoot joints if the problem is left untreated.

A. **Physical examination** demonstrates a complex deformity with varying degrees of hindfoot valgus and midfoot pronation and abduction. Early in the course of the disorder, tenderness is noted along the posterior tibial tendon below the medial malleolus. However, in the advanced case, pain along the posterolateral hindfoot predominates because of calcaneofibular impingement. The "too many toes" sign may be viewed from behind with excessive hindfoot valgus. The inability to perform a single-limb heel-rise or to invert the heel may be noted. Clawtoes and a hallux valgus deformity may develop secondarily.

B. **Radiography** should always be performed while weight bearing. The lateral radiograph will often demonstrate a sag in the longitudinal arch of the foot and an increase in the talocalcaneal angle. The anteroposterior radiograph will similarly demonstrate an increase in the talocalcaneal angle and a loss of coverage of the talar head by the navicular. In longstanding cases, degenerative arthrosis may be noted in the hindfoot, particularly the subtalar joint.

C. Treatment depends on the stage of the disease.

1. **Stage 1** disease, marked by posterior tibial tendinitis (without deformity), is treated by immobilization of the foot to allow the posterior tibial tendinitis to resolve, followed by use of a supportive insole orthosis. Lengthening of a contracted tendoachilles complex, when present, is particularly helpful in arresting progression.

2. **Stage 2** disease, marked by tendon insufficiency and flexible pes planus deformity, is best treated surgically with tendoachilles lengthening, posterior tibial tendon augmentation, and medial column stabilization through arthrodesis of the nonessential joints of the midfoot or by lateral column lengthening via osteotomy.

3. **Stage 3** disease is characterized by either fixed pes planus deformity or degenerative arthrosis of one or more of the essential hindfoot joints (i.e., the subtalar joint). However, the resulting significant limitation of normal gait mechanics warrants early, aggressive intervention when the deformity is flexible and hindfoot arthrodesis can be avoided.

IV. **Metatarsalgia** represents a condition characterized by plantar pain under the weight-bearing surfaces of the metatarsal heads. Its many causes include hypermobility of the first ray with compensatory overload of the lesser metatarsals, clawtoes (in which the plantar fat pad is drawn distally to expose the plantar metatarsal heads), and a rigid cavovarus foot and tendoachilles–gastrocnemius equinus contracture. It may be prominent in RA.

A. Physical examination. Prominence of the metatarsal heads may be noted on palpation of the plantar forefoot. The plantar metatarsal fat pad may be displaced distally in the presence of hammertoe or clawtoe deformities. A hypermobile first ray with overload of the lesser toes will present with plantar keratoses beneath the second (and third) metatarsal heads. Gastrocnemius equinus contracture and clawtoes routinely coexist in this syndrome.

B. Radiography. Clawtoe deformities may be demonstrated on weight-bearing lateral radiographs. A forefoot cavus posture may be evident as well. Longer standing cases may result in dislocation of the MTP joints. The anteroposterior radiograph will demonstrate a long, hypertrophied second metatarsal in the hypermobile first-ray syndrome.

C. Treatment is directed at unloading the excessive plantar pressure beneath the metatarsal heads. Various nonoperative measures that are particularly helpful include placing a metatarsal pad just proximal to the metatarsal heads. Accommodative inserts can also provide unloading of the metatarsal heads. Surgical correction of lesser clawtoe deformities can replace the plantar fat pad beneath the metatarsal heads. Stabilization of the hypermobile first ray can redistribute plantar weight-bearing forces. Gastrocnemius equinus contracture can be relieved through tendoachilles or gastrocnemius tendon lengthening.

V. **Morton's neuroma** is the presence of pain in the web space between the third and fourth toes caused by irritation of the common plantar interdigital nerve at this location. Many etiologies are thought to contribute to this disorder, including constrictive shoes with a narrow toe box, forefoot overload with metatarsalgia, and gastrocnemius equinus contracture. Patients typically complain of a numbness or burning sensation radiating into the toes that is promptly relieved by removing the shoes and rubbing the feet.

A. Symptoms may be reproduced during compression of the metatarsal heads of the patient by the examiner (Mulder's click). A palpable mass may be appreciated in the appropriate web space.

B. Plain radiographs are routinely normal. MRI can be helpful when the diagnosis is not clear.

C. Treatment includes wearing appropriate shoes to accommodate the natural width of the forefoot. A metatarsal pad may serve to "splay" the metatarsal heads and provide symptom relief. In recalcitrant cases, local steroid injection or surgical excision is warranted.

VI. **Inversion ankle injuries (sprains)** are among the most common musculoskeletal injuries seen by the physician. One must recall that the talus is wider anteriorly than posteriorly, which renders it particularly susceptible to inversion injury in the plantar-flexed position. Approximately 20% of ankle sprains will progress to varying degrees of chronic ankle instability or pain.

A. **Physical examination** shortly following an inversion ankle injury reveals swelling located over the anterolateral aspect of the ankle joint. Ecchymosis may be present. Tenderness over the anterior talofibular ligament will be noted on palpation. Involuntary guarding and apprehension to attempted inversion maneuvers will be evident. Depending on the severity of the injury, weight bearing may not be possible. Additional findings on the medial portion of the ankle indicate a higher-energy injury. Manual stress testing with anterior drawer and talar tilt maneuvers, if tolerated, may reveal asymmetry in comparison to the uninjured extremity.

B. **Radiographs** should always be obtained to rule out a fracture of the fibula or medial malleolus. Small avulsion fractures of the distal fibula are frequently seen and require no specific treatment. As mentioned previously, anteroposterior and lateral stress radiographs comparing the injured and uninjured extremities may prove helpful in subtle cases.

C. **Treatment** initially is supportive. **R**est, **I**ce, **C**ompression, and **E**levation **(RICE)** and nonsteroidal anti-inflammatory medications are instituted until the patient is comfortable. Organized physical therapy to restore normal muscle strength and proprioception is essential for a good outcome. Weight bearing in a light-weight orthosis that controls inversion and eversion is particularly helpful. Normal activities can gradually be resumed when strength in the injured ankle is equal to that in the uninjured extremity. Chronic ankle instability is most often associated with premature return to athletic activities and early reinjury. Long-term use of a protective orthosis may provide symptomatic relief to those with chronic ankle instability. Surgical repair or reconstruction of the elongated lateral ankle ligaments is helpful in those cases in which nonoperative therapy has failed.

VII. **Hallux valgus** is a common condition that is likely caused by multiple factors. Tight and constrictive shoes, ligamentous laxity with muscle imbalance, and hereditary predisposition all contribute to a lateral deviation of the hallux on the first metatarsal. Hallux valgus may often be a part of a larger deformity—namely, the planovalgus foot with a pronated midfoot that gradually stretches the medial capsule of the hallux MTP joint into valgus.

A. **Physical examination** reveals a lateral deviation of the hallux phalanx, often with impingement of the lesser toes that causes an overlapping second-toe deformity (hammertoe). Prominence of the medial aspect of the hallux metatarsal head may cause local paresthesias or ulceration of the overlying soft tissues. Bursal swelling can occur and can become infected. Gastrocnemius equinus contracture and a hypermobile first ray are often present.

B. **Radiography** will demonstrate an increased hallux valgus angle and an increased intermetatarsal angle (metatarsus primus varus). Second metatarsal overload may be present. Lateral radiographs may reveal hammertoe deformities. Loss of medial column height (sag) may be noted as well.

C. **Treatment** should be based on the severity of the deformity and the degree of functional limitation and should be directed at the cause of the deformity. Nonoperative measures include accommodative shoes with a wide toe box and insole orthoses to support a flexible pes planus deformity associated with hallux valgus. Operative intervention, when nonoperative measures are not successful, should be directed at the restoration of soft tissue and osseous stability. Operative intervention is largely successful in appropriately selected patients.

VIII. **Hallux rigidus** is a painful condition characterized by a limitation of hallux dorsiflexion. It often coincides with degenerative arthrosis to varying degrees. Remote injuries to the hallux MTP joint may be recalled by the patient. Alternatively, an elevated first ray causes the hallux proximal phalanx to "jam" into the first metatarsal head rather than "glide" over it in a smooth arc.

A. **Physical examination** reveals restricted dorsiflexion at the hallux MTP joint. Prominent osteophytes may be readily palpable, especially over the dorsolateral aspect of the joint.

B. Radiography may reveal varying degrees of osteoarthrosis, from osteophyte formation to joint space narrowing. An elevated first ray may be noted on the lateral radiograph.

C. Treatment in which a steel rocker bar is used in the sole of a shoe to relieve motion at the MTP joint can be quite effective. Surgical intervention, including cheilectomy, is of limited short-term value. In intractable cases, arthrodesis of the MTP joint can be quite helpful.

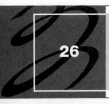

26 SPORTS INJURIES
Riley J. Williams and Thomas L. Wickiewicz

During the past decade, the importance of regular exercise in the maintenance of good health has been well-established. Consequently, with increasing attention now focused on personal fitness, the incidence of sports-related injuries has increased significantly. Both primary care physicians and specialists can expect to see a variety of athletic injuries. All clinicians should be able to recognize these conditions and administer appropriate care. A thorough history, physical examination, musculoskeletal imaging, and laboratory testing are all important in arriving at the proper diagnosis. A treatment plan is then developed for the injured athlete based on these objective findings.

 CERVICAL SPINE

Injuries to the cervical spine range from mild to severe. Certain athletic activities (football, diving, and gymnastics) are associated with an increased incidence of cervical spinal injury in comparison with other sports. Prompt recognition and treatment of individuals who suffer cervical spinal injuries may prevent the progression or severity of the associated neurologic injury.

I. **ANATOMY** (see Chapter 19).

II. **CLASSIFICATION OF CERVICAL SPINAL INJURIES.** Neck injuries can be classified according to neurologic sequelae or the type of force acting on the cervical spine at the time of injury.

A. **Cervical spinal injury with minimal, transient, or no neurologic symptoms**
   1. **Muscle strains.** Pain and neck stiffness with no neurologic findings and negative imaging studies. Usually resolve spontaneously.
   2. **Brachial plexus injuries ("stingers" or "burners").** Transient symptoms. See subsequent text.
   3. **Bony fracture, ligamentous injury, disc injury without neurologic involvement.**

B. **Cervical spinal injuries accompanied by incomplete or complete spinal cord syndromes.**

III. **CLASSIFICATION BY MECHANISM OF INJURY AND SYNDROME**

A. **Flexion without axial load or rotation.** These forces usually cause a compression fracture of the cancellous cervical vertebral body without tearing of the stabilizing ligamentous complex of the facet joints. Avulsion fractures of the transverse processes can also occur. These are stable fractures that are usually not associated with neurologic loss.

B. **Flexion with rotation.** These forces place high loads on the facet joint capsules and the posterior interspinous ligaments. Unevenly applied forces can cause unilateral facet dislocation resulting from facet capsular rupture. Larger loads can lead to bilateral facet dislocations with associated anterior subluxation of the vertebral bodies and fractures of the facets, laminae, or vertebral bodies. Neurologic trauma associated with these injuries is quite variable, ranging from no injury to complete spinal cord injury.

C. Axial compression. This type of load usually results when the head strikes a hard object, as when a swimmer dives into shallow water. With the forward flexion of the head, the cervical lordosis decreases such that the spinal column is essentially straight. The resultant force is transmitted to the cervical spine and can cause vertebral body fracture with retropulsion of bony elements into the spinal canal. Neurologic loss, including quadriplegia or complete motor paralysis secondary to anterior spinal cord syndrome, is commonly associated with this pattern of injury.

D. Extension. Extension forces that exceed the normal range of motion of the cervical spinal facet joints can lead to fracture of these elements or an avulsion of the superior margin of the vertebral body. Neurologic loss is variable. Occasionally, the spinal cord impingement occurs between the lamina posteriorly and a disc anteriorly. A complete spinal cord injury or a central cord syndrome can result.

IV. SPINAL CORD SYNDROMES

A. Central. Extension forces; injury affects upper extremities more than lower extremities; motor and sensory loss; fair prognosis; most common type.

B. Anterior. Flexion–compression; incomplete motor and sensory loss; poor prognosis.

C. Brown-Séquard's. Results from penetrating trauma; ipsilateral loss of motor function; contralateral pain and loss of temperature sensation; best prognosis of all spinal cord syndromes.

D. Complete. Spinal canal disruption and canal compression; no function below site of injury; poor prognosis.

E. Single root. Avulsion or compression (disc); symptoms related to level; good prognosis.

V. PHYSICAL EXAMINATION. In suspected cervical spinal injuries, a brief screening examination should be administered to assess the magnitude of the injury at the scene of the accident.

A. Observation. The position of the head and neck at impact should be noted to categorize the mechanism of injury.

B. History

1. In the on-site evaluation after cervical spinal injury, the examiner must first apply the ABCs of resuscitation. When unconsciousness follows neck injury, basic life-support measures should be applied. (Note: Hyperextension of the neck should be avoided during these efforts.)

2. If the patient is awake and alert, a history is taken to establish whether consciousness was lost at any point during or following the injury (amnesia for the event to be checked).

3. The location and quality of any pain (neck, arms, shoulders, hands, back, or legs) is noted.

4. Numbness patterns must be defined. In the event of complaints of numbness, the clinician must define whether the pattern is global (all extremities) or partial (upper vs. lower extremities) and whether it was transient or is persistent.

C. Motion. If the patient is not amnesic for the event, did not lose consciousness, and has no self-reported neurologic loss, the clinician can then encourage the patient to attempt active range of motion of the neck without assistance. If significant pain is encountered, the neck should be immobilized and the patient further evaluated.

D. Neurologic examination

1. **Sensory examination.** This examination should include tests of sharp versus dull discrimination, light-touch sense, deep pressure, vibration, and position sense in all extremities.

2. **Motor examination.** Muscular strength should be assessed and graded in all limbs. Reflexes should also be graded in all limbs.

3. **Rectal examination.** In cases of spinal cord injury, the rectal examination is the most important part of the examination and can help the clinician discriminate between complete and incomplete spinal cord lesions after the resolution of spinal shock. (Note: This procedure, although important, is not part of the on-site evaluation.)

VI. RADIOGRAPHS

A. **Standard cervical spinal radiographs** include anteroposterior, lateral, oblique, and odontoid views. If there is no evidence of fracture or dislocation, a flexion–extension view of the cervical spine is also obtained. Active neck flexion and extension are always performed by the patient without assistance and should not be pushed beyond the patient's reported comfort level. The spinal column is considered unstable when vertebral body subluxation in excess of 3.5 mm or an angular deformity of 11 degrees or more exists.

B. **Supplemental radiographs** consist of pillar views to evaluate the lateral masses. Computed tomography (CT) scan can be used to detect subtle fractures and evaluate the spine for rotatory subluxation. Magnetic resonance imaging (MRI) is also very useful in the evaluation of soft-tissue abnormalities (ligamentous disruption and disc protrusion).

VII. TREATMENT.

The most important aspect of the management of cervical spinal injury is **immobilization.** Neck immobilization should be maintained until a definitive diagnosis has been made. For example, football-related cervical spinal injuries are managed by transporting the patient (with helmet in place) on a backboard. The patient is log rolled onto a backboard with vigilant head stabilization. The face guard is left in place unless respiratory difficulty is encountered, in which case it is removed. The neck is never moved passively until a fracture or dislocation is ruled out. (Note: In cases of spinal cord injury, the administration of **methylprednisolone** intravenously should be strongly considered because this agent has been shown to improve neurologic recovery if given **within 8 hours** of injury.)

VIII. COMMON CERVICAL SPINAL PROBLEMS

A. **"Burners" or "stingers."** These injuries represent a stretch of the brachial plexus with a transient loss of motor power and transient pain radiating down the arm(s). This phenomenon usually occurs in football players. Most often, the symptoms are temporary and usually resolve within 1 to 2 minutes. The individual can generally return to play the day of injury. With more severe brachial plexus injuries (i.e., persistent pain or weakness), nerve damage may result. Consequently, neurologic loss and pain will persist. These athletes cannot return to play and should be carefully examined in a controlled, off-field setting.

B. **Ligamentous sprain.** These injuries occur when a force moves a joint through an abnormal range of motion. This condition presents with localized neck pain and muscle spasm. The neurologic and radiographic examination findings are usually normal. Treatment consists of immobilization (semirigid collar), local heat, muscle relaxants, anti-inflammatory medicines, and restriction of activity. Athletes can return to play when the symptoms resolve.

C. **Cervical spinal fractures—stable.** These types of fractures include C1 burst fractures (Jefferson's fracture), most odontoid fractures, traumatic C2 spondylolisthesis (hangman's fracture), compression fracture of a vertebral body without comminution, and spinous process fracture (clay shoveler's fracture). Most of these fractures are treated with rigid immobilization (halo vest) until healing is complete.

D. **Cervical spinal fractures and subluxation—unstable.** Cervical spinal subluxation/dislocation usually presents with neurologic loss. These injuries require immediate immobilization and should ultimately be reduced. MRI is useful for assessing soft-tissue damage in these cases. Cervical traction or surgical reduction and stabilization are frequently indicated.

E. **Cervical disc herniation.** This phenomenon is uncommon in young athletes but may be seen in axial compression injuries sustained during rugby or football. Again, MRI is the best diagnostic modality for assessing patients for potential disc problems.

THORACOLUMBAR SPINE

Repetitive stresses to the ligamentous and bony supports of the thoracic (dorsal) spine can result in an overuse syndrome with subsequent acute or chronic back pain. **Spondylolysis** is a unilateral or bilateral fracture of the pars interarticularis. This lesion is frequently nontraumatic and may represent a congenital lesion or stress fracture. However, spondylolysis can occur acutely, especially in gymnasts, weight lifters, and football linemen. **Spondylolisthesis** is a fracture of the pars interarticularis, which is associated with translation of one vertebral body over another. It is frequently observed in the lumbar spine, especially at the L5–S1 junction.

I.   **HISTORY.** Pain is usually localized to the lower back and, less commonly, to the buttocks and posterior thighs. Radicular symptoms are uncommon.

II. **PHYSICAL EXAMINATION.** Hamstring tightness is common. Point tenderness may be noted along the dorsal thorax.

III. **DIAGNOSTIC STUDIES.** Oblique views of the lumbosacral spine usually demonstrate the spondylolytic lesion (lucency at the neck of the "Scotty dog"). A stress fracture of the pars interarticularis that is not obvious on plain radiographs may be demonstrated by means of bone scintigraphy.

IV. **Treatment** consists of local measures, including heat, nonsteroidal anti-inflammatory drugs (NSAIDs), muscle relaxants, and rest during the acute period. Modification of activity or bracing is usually required. Surgical fusion is indicated only in cases of severe spondylolisthesis or unrelenting pain.

 SHOULDER

Sports that require repetitive overhead arm motion (baseball, racquet sports, and swimming) place unusual stresses on the supporting structures of the shoulder. Injuries to the shoulder capsule, rotator cuff musculature, biceps tendon, scapular stabilizers, and shoulder musculature are common. Most of these problems are discussed in Chapter 21. Additional shoulder problems, unique to overhead athletes, are discussed in this section.

I.   **Little Leaguer's shoulder** typically affects adolescents and teenagers and represents a separation of the proximal humeral epiphysis. The observed physical abnormality is likely to have been caused by repetitive forces associated with the acceleration phase of the pitching cycle (extreme humeral abduction and external rotation to forward flexion and internal rotation).

   A. **History.** These typically young patients complain of arm pain during and after throwing.

   B. **Radiographs** reveal widening of the proximal humeral growth plate and demineralization and fragmentation adjacent to the epiphyseal plate. Occasionally, loose bodies are noted in the glenohumeral joint.

   C. **Treatment** is conservative. Patients are prohibited from throwing until clinical and radiographic healing has occurred.

II. **Rotator cuff tendinitis** usually occurs as a result of overuse or in cases of subtle glenohumeral subluxation. It responds well to conservative measures (ice packs, NSAIDs, and rest). Rehabilitation is most effective in relieving symptoms.

III. **Posterior capsular tears, which occur in throwers,** can result in ossification of the posterior capsule near the glenoid labrum. These lesions occur secondary to traction on the capsule during the acceleration and follow-through phases of the pitching cycle. Treatment initially consists of rest, NSAIDs, strengthening exercises, and restriction of pitching.

IV. **Internal impingement syndrome** typically occurs in baseball pitchers. Lesions occur at the posterosuperior margin of the glenoid in the undersurface of the rotator cuff tendons (partial tears). These lesions are attributed to impingement of the rotator cuff on the bony margin of the glenoid during the cocking phase of the pitching motion (abduction and external rotation). Treatment is conservative (activity modification and NSAIDs). Recalcitrant cases may require debridement of the lesion.

V.   **INSTABILITY.** Global instability (anterior, posterior, and inferior) of the shoulder can occur in overhead athletes because of microtrauma to the shoulder capsule. The shoulder usually does not frankly dislocate but rather feels "loose" to the patient. Many cases can be treated with physical therapy; surgical stabilization may be necessary in severe cases.

ELBOW

The diagnosis and treatment of problems of the elbow require an understanding of the anatomy and function of the joint.

I.   **ANATOMY AND FUNCTION.** The elbow is a hinge joint. Elbow flexion and extension occur at the articulation of the humerus and ulna. Rotation takes place at the proximal radioulnar and radiocapitellar joints.

II. **JOINT STABILITY.** During valgus stress, primary stability is derived from the bony fit of the ulnohumeral and radiocapitellar joints. Secondary stability is derived from the restraint provided by the medial (ulnar) collateral ligament. The lateral (radial) collateral ligament and the anconeus muscle provide some resistance to varus loads; however, bony constraint is much more important in resisting these forces. Most throwing activities subject the elbow to valgus stress.

III. **COMMON ELBOW PROBLEMS.** Overhead athletes (throwers and tennis players) place tremendous, repetitive valgus forces on the medial side of the elbow. These forces result in the application of compressive forces on the lateral elbow during the acceleration phase of throwing. Forceful extension during follow-through (extension overload) leads to posterior compartment lesions (loose bodies and osteophytes). Medial elbow tension-overload injuries include acute valgus instability and chronic valgus instability, both of which can be complicated by ulnar neuropathy.

A. **Acute valgus instability**

   1. **Flexor mass tears.** These lesions occur at the elbow in association with sudden forced wrist flexion and pronation. Tenderness and pain at the point of the tear are noted with resisted wrist or finger flexion. Partial tears are initially treated with rest, ice packs, and NSAIDs. This is followed by resistive exercises at the wrist. Complete tears present with a palpable soft-tissue defect distal to the flexor muscle origin and may require surgical reattachment.

   2. **Medial (ulnar) collateral ligament tears (acute).** These lesions present with pain and tenderness during valgus stress of the elbow. Laxity with valgus testing at 30 degrees of flexion confirms the diagnosis. MRI is useful in distinguishing between complete and partial medial collateral ligament injuries. Partial tears are treated with ice packs, rest, early motion, and a gradual return to full activity. Complete tears require surgical repair/reconstruction in high-level athletes who wish to continue throwing.

   3. **Little Leaguer's elbow.** Repetitive valgus stresses in children can cause epiphyseal avulsion of the medial epicondyle rather than ligamentous rupture. Treatment is usually conservative (ice packs, rest, and early motion).

   4. **Athletes at risk** are pitchers, catchers, and javelin throwers.

B. **Chronic valgus instability** is common in athletes involved in throwing sports. Medial collateral ligament laxity develops slowly over time and occurs secondary to the microtrauma associated with repetitive throwing. Traction spurs at the distal insertion of the medial collateral ligament and calcification within the ligament can occur. Chronic ligamentous laxity may require surgical excision of calcified deposits and spurs, debridement, and reefing of the medial collateral ligament or reconstruction with use of the palmaris longus tendon. Loose bodies can also form within the elbow joint as a result of this condition, so that elbow arthroscopy is generally performed on patients undergoing reconstruction of the medial collateral ligament.

C. **Ulnar neuropathy** can develop secondary to ulnar nerve compression at or near the elbow (cubital tunnel). Affected patients present with pain along the ulnar groove, with radiation of pain and paresthesias into the fourth and fifth fingers. In most patients, Tinel's sign is positive at the elbow. Electromyographic and nerve conduction studies may be required to confirm the diagnosis. Studies have demonstrated that this condition often accompanies chronic laxity of the medial collateral ligament of the elbow. Initial treatment consists of rest and NSAIDs. Decompression of the cubital tunnel and nerve transposition may be required.

D. Lateral compartment injuries
  1. **Osteochondritis dissecans.** Valgus forces at the elbow result in compressive loading of the lateral side. Osteochondritis dissecans of the humeral capitellum frequently occurs in male adolescents aged between 12 and 14 years.
     a. **History.** The thrower presents with pain, motion loss, and catching or locking symptoms.
     b. **Radiographs** usually reveal flattening of the capitellum (most common site) or fracture.
     c. **Differential diagnosis** includes Panner's disease, which has a similar radiographic appearance but is found in younger patients (6 to 9 years) and is not related to trauma.
     d. **Treatment** of osteochondritis dissecans depends on the size of the lesion. Small osteochondral lesions are managed by activity modification and anti-inflammatory medications. Large lesions or loose bodies may require surgical debridement (elbow arthroscopy).
  2. **Lateral epicondylitis (tennis elbow)** causes pain at the lateral humeral epicondyle. Although commonly found in participants in racquet sports, this malady also occurs in individuals who do not play tennis.
     a. **Pathogenesis.** The site of pathology is generally found at the origin of the extensor muscle (extensor carpi radialis brevis) at the lateral epicondyle. The period of peak incidence is the fourth decade of life. This finding suggests a degenerative process in the tendon aggravated by repetitive stress, which leads to macroscopic and microscopic tears of this extensor muscle origin. Approximately 40% of these patients will have other sites of soft-tissue degenerative problems (shoulder bursitis and rotator cuff tendinitis).
     b. **History.** Patients typically present with lateral elbow pain that is exacerbated by wrist extension. They commonly complain of pain while they are using a screwdriver, shaking hands, making a fist, or lifting a weight. The pain radiates from the dorsum of the forearm to the fingers. Tennis players often complain of accentuated pain during backhand strokes. Numbness or paresthesias may occur. Such complaints should alert the physician to consider other causes of elbow pain (i.e., cervical radiculopathy). A history of fluoroquinolone antibiotic (i.e., ciprofloxacin) use may also be reported.
     c. **Physical examination.** Point tenderness at the lateral epicondyle is typical. Tenderness may also be present distally along the extensor muscle sheaths. Resisted wrist extension with the elbow straight and the hand and forearm pronated should reproduce symptoms.
     d. **Radiographs.** Calcification may be seen in the region of the lateral epicondyle, but the elbow joint itself is normal.
     e. **Differential diagnosis**
        i. **Medial epicondylitis (golfer's elbow)** is an inflammatory condition that leads to pathology within the origin of the flexor/pronator muscle groups and pain at the medial epicondyle.
        ii. **Intra-articular pathology.** A patient with elbow pathology [loose bodies, rheumatoid arthritis (RA), and osteoarthritis] may present with lateral elbow pain. Limitation of elbow motion and radiographic changes can clarify the diagnosis.
        iii. **Gout.** Differentiation is not difficult because the acute, inflammatory signs of gout (erythema and swelling) are not usually present in tennis elbow. Crystals found on joint aspiration will confirm the diagnosis of gout.
        iv. **Cervical spinal disease** may cause referred pain to the elbow. MRI of the cervical spine can be useful in clinching the diagnosis.
        v. **Posterior interosseous nerve (branch of radial nerve) entrapment** may mimic lateral epicondylitis. Tenderness is more volar than in lateral epicondylitis and lies over the entrance of the nerve into the supinator muscle.

f. **Treatment** is initially conservative. Activities that accentuate the pain are avoided for 8 to 12 weeks. Oral NSAIDs should be given for pain relief in the acute phase. Should symptoms persist, injection of 40 mg of methyl-prednisolone acetate (Depo-Medrol) with 1 mL of 1% lidocaine into the point of maximum tenderness usually provides some relief. When the acute pain has subsided, exercises directed at strengthening the extensor muscles are started. A flexibility program is also started, and an ice pack is used judiciously. A forearm band may reduce tension on the extensor muscle origin and provide relief in some patients. A volar wrist splint may also be helpful. Surgical excision of the degenerative tissue at the origin of the extensor carpi radialis brevis may be necessary in patients who fail conservative treatment.

g. **Prevention**

   i. **Awareness.** Warm-up, stretching, exercise, and weight lifting programs serve as prophylactic measures and should be encouraged.

   ii. **Warm-up.** Abrupt physical stresses may predispose certain muscle groups to injury. Appropriate warm-up activity should precede vigorous racquet sports. For example, the first 15 to 20 minutes of tennis should consist of low-intensity volleying. Speed and duration should be gradually increased. Stretching and ice application for 15 minutes should follow all activities.

   iii. **Technique.** Poor technique is one of the main causes of tennis elbow. Patients with lateral epicondylitis should pay specific attention to handgrip on the racquet and the technique of backhand strokes. Lighter racquets, large grip size, and less taut stringing (52 lbs) have all been reported to be helpful. Clay is a better surface, and opponents who hit at lower speeds may be safer to play against, should tennis elbow develop.

 HAND

The hand is exposed to many forces that may result in significant injury in the course of athletic activity.

I. **Bennett's fracture** is a fracture of the base of the first metacarpal.

   A. **History.** The mechanism of injury is a direct blow against a partially flexed metacarpal, or a fall on an outstretched hand, clutching a ski pole in that hand.

   B. **Physical examination.** Swelling and tenderness are present at the carpometacarpal joint and deformity of the thumb is present, particularly if the joint is dislocated.

   C. **Radiographs.** The fracture line characteristically separates the major part of the metacarpal from a small volar lip fragment, disrupting the carpometacarpal joint.

   D. **Treatment.** Closed or open reduction with pinning is required to re-establish articular congruity.

II. **ULNAR COLLATERAL LIGAMENT INSUFFICIENCY (GAMEKEEPER'S THUMB).** Rupture of the ulnar collateral ligament of the metacarpophalangeal joint of the thumb can be acute or chronic.

   A. **History.** A sudden valgus (abduction) stress applied to the metacarpophalangeal joint of the thumb results in partial or complete disruption of the ulnar collateral ligament. Falling with a ski pole in one's hand predisposes a skier to this injury.

   B. **Physical examination.** The patient presents with a painful, swollen metacarpophalangeal joint of the thumb. An abduction stress (45 degrees of flexion) should reveal laxity in comparison with the normal side. The stress test may also be performed under local anesthesia in more severe cases.

   C. **Imaging.** An avulsion fracture from the base of the proximal phalanx may be associated with the injury. A stress test with radiographs confirms the diagnosis. MRI can also aid in the diagnosis and confirm the presence of a Stener's lesion (interposition of the adductor aponeurosis) between the free ends of the torn ulnar collateral ligament.

   D. **Treatment.** Partial tears are treated nonoperatively with a molded thumb spica cast/splint. Complete tears are surgically repaired.

KNEE (LIGAMENTOUS INJURIES)

I. **ANATOMY.** Stability of the knee occurs in several planes: anteroposterior, medial, lateral, and rotational. Medial and lateral stability is imparted by the medial collateral ligament, lateral collateral ligament, and anterior cruciate ligament. Anteroposterior stability is imparted by the anterior cruciate and posterior cruciate ligaments. Other structures that contribute to knee stability include the knee joint capsule, menisci, and surrounding muscles.
   A. The **medial collateral ligament** prevents medial opening of the knee with valgus stress. The anterior cruciate ligament and posterior capsule are secondary stabilizers against medial opening with valgus stress.
   B. The **lateral collateral ligament** prevents lateral opening with varus stress. Secondary stabilizers against varus stress are the anterior cruciate ligament, posterior cruciate ligament, and popliteus muscle.
   C. The **anterior cruciate ligament** prevents anterior displacement of the tibia relative to the femur. Secondary stabilizers are the medial meniscus and medial collateral ligament.
   D. The **posterior cruciate ligament** prevents posterior displacement of the tibia relative to the femur. Secondary restraint to posterior displacement is imparted by the medial collateral ligament.

II. **CLASSIFICATION OF LIGAMENTOUS INJURIES OF THE KNEE**
   A. **Grade 1 (first-degree/mild) sprain.** Characterized by local pain and swelling, without instability. Joint opening of 0 to 5 mm is found on examination. This injury is represented microscopically by a mild tear in the collagen fibers of the ligament; however, full continuity of the ligament is maintained.
   B. **Grade 2 (second-degree/moderate) sprain.** Characterized by pain, swelling, and minimal to moderate instability. Joint opening of 6 to 10 mm is found on examination. A more substantial tear of collagen fibers is found, with some loss of continuity in the ligament.
   C. **Grade 3 (third-degree/severe) sprain.** Characterized by swelling and marked instability. Joint opening of more than 10 mm is noted at examination. There is complete disruption of ligament continuity.

III. **HISTORY**
   A. **History of prior injury.** An apparent acute tear of a ligament may actually represent the last of many recurrent episodes, each of which has damaged the involved ligament.
   B. **Mechanism of injury.** Determine the nature of the knee injury. Valgus stress versus varus stress? Hyperflexion injury versus hyperextension injury? If a ski injury, ask the patient in which direction the ski pointed at the time of injury. If a football injury, determine how the foot was planted at the time of impact and the site and direction of the force of injury.
   C. **Pain.** Collateral ligament injuries are most painful at the site of damage. Cruciate ligament injury usually results in capsular distension (hemarthrosis) and vague knee pain.
   D. **Ability to continue sports.** An athlete who, at the time of injury, could not resume activity as a result of pain or instability usually has more severe pathology than one who was able to continue.
   E. A **"pop" or "snap"** immediately followed by swelling is characteristic of anterior cruciate ligament injuries.
   F. **Swelling** that occurs immediately following injury usually indicates acute hemorrhage into the joint (hemarthrosis) and should raise suspicion of intra-articular fracture or cruciate ligament damage. Swelling that appears during the first 24 hours is more common in grade 1 or 2 collateral ligament injuries. Often, joint swelling will be less in a grade 3 collateral ligament injury because the complete disruption allows the joint fluid to escape into the periarticular soft tissues.
   G. **"Giving way"** is typical in patients with clinically significant knee instability (i.e., anterior knee instability secondary to anterior cruciate ligament insufficiency). "Locking" or "catching" is more representative of meniscal pathology.

IV. PHYSICAL EXAMINATION

A. Inspection

1. **Gait.** Patients with an acute ligamentous injury often walk with a limp, a flexed knee, or the two in combination.
2. **Swelling/effusion.** Is there suprapatellar fullness in the standing or prone position? Is the joint taut with fluid?
3. **Ecchymosis.** Collateral ligament injuries often show external signs of hemorrhage into soft tissue, which can present along the calf or ankle secondary to gravitational flow along muscle sheaths.

B. Range of motion is frequently limited, secondary to pain. Lack of extension secondary to effusion should not be confused with the locked knee of meniscal etiology. Intra-articular effusion is palpated for by compressing the suprapatellar pouch and ballottement of the patella.

C. Neurovascular status. A knee evaluation must include an assessment of popliteal and distal pulses, as well as a thorough neurologic examination. The peroneal nerve is particularly susceptible to damage, especially in varus stress injuries that stretch the lateral structures of the knee.

D. Ligament stress testing. The patient should be supine and must be relaxed, as spasm and apprehension can obscure the diagnosis. The collateral ligaments should be tested with the knee in 0 and 30 degrees of flexion. At 30 degrees, the test is more specific for the collateral ligaments. During full extension, secondary stabilizers tighten to stabilize the joint; if the knee should "open" in extension, the injury is severe. Occasionally, 1% lidocaine injected into the site of pain or even general anesthesia may be needed to evaluate the knee properly.

1. The **medial collateral ligament** stabilizes the joint against medial opening and therefore protects against a valgus stress. To test this ligament, the limb is grasped with one hand while the femur is stabilized with the other, and a valgus stress is applied. Instability, if present, is more often sensed than seen. If the ligament has torn completely, the usual firm, abrupt end point will be absent. If the ligament is injured but not completely torn (grade 2), the end point from the remaining intact fibers is present; however, the excursion of motion may be increased.
2. The **lateral collateral ligament** should be tested with a varus stress in the same manner. Additionally, the lateral collateral ligament can be palpated easily with the leg crossed in a figure-4 position.
3. The **anterior cruciate ligament** is tested by translating the tibia anteriorly versus the femur.
   a. The **Lachman's test** is easily performed with the knee at approximately 30 degrees of flexion by stabilizing the femur and distal thigh with one hand while an anterior force is applied to the back of the tibia. The examiner notes both the amount of excursion and the sense of end point. The absence of a normal crisp end point, even in the face of only minimal excursion, is usually indicative of an anterior cruciate ligament tear.
   b. The **anterior drawer test** is performed with the hip flexed 45 degrees and the knee flexed 90 degrees with the patient's foot flat on the table. The examiner sits by the foot and places the hands around the proximal tibia and ensuring hamstring relaxation, applies an anterior force to the tibia, noting both the amount of excursion and quality of end point. This test is difficult to perform in the acute setting with associated knee swelling and is less accurate than the Lachman's test.
   c. The **pivot shift test** notes anterior and rotational translation of the lateral tibial plateau with respect to the lateral femoral condyle. It is performed by having the patient relax fully and applying a valgus force to the knee with varying degrees of internal and external rotation of the tibia with respect to the femur. As the knee is brought from an extended to a flexed position, a sense of movement or jump takes place that in a chronic setting will reproduce the patient's sense of instability. Grading of the pivot shift is as follows: absent, 1+ (slide); 2+ (jump); 3+ (lock). It is very difficult to perform

a pivot shift maneuver in an acute setting without sufficient anesthesia. Similarly, if a patient is apprehensive, it is a difficult maneuver to reproduce even in chronic settings.

4. The **posterior cruciate ligament** is the primary restraint to posterior translation of the tibia with respect to the femur. The posterior drawer test is performed with the patient's hip flexed at 45 degrees and the knee flexed at 90 degrees. First visual inspection from the side may note less prominence of the tibial tubercle on the affected side with more prominence of the distal femoral condyles. On a posteriorly applied force to the tibia, the examiner will sense increased translation and absence of an end point. This is interpreted as a positive posterior drawer test. (Note: When examiners perform a Lachman's maneuver with the knee at 30 degrees of flexion and sense a large increase in amount of translation but a normal end point associated with a normal anterior cruciate ligament, they should suspect that they are really feeling a knee that has suffered a posterior cruciate ligament tear. What the examiner is actually doing is bringing the tibia back to its normal position under the femur.)

5. An evaluation of rotational stability includes an assessment of the **popliteal tendon and lateral collateral ligament complex.** These tests are performed at both 30 and 90 degrees of knee flexion. The patient lies prone and the degrees of external rotation of the affected and unaffected sides are compared. Increases in the amount of external rotation are noted.

V. **DIAGNOSTIC STUDIES**

A. **Radiographs.** Standard knee radiographic findings are usually negative but are useful to exclude a fracture. Avulsion fractures can sometimes be seen at ligamentous insertions (e.g., the tibial spine for anterior cruciate ligament injuries).

B. **Stress radiographs.** The joint opening is best viewed anteroposteriorly by applying mild stress.

C. **Arthrograms** are most useful for definite meniscal tears but may also demonstrate tears of the cruciate ligaments and more severe tears of the collateral ligaments. Leakage of dye from the joint usually indicates a complete collateral ligament disruption. This test is mostly of historical significance since the ascendency of the MRI as the imaging modality of choice.

D. **MRI** has become increasingly accurate in the diagnosis of knee injuries and is easier for the patient to undergo in the acute setting. This is the study of choice for delineating soft-tissue injuries.

VI. **DIFFERENTIAL DIAGNOSIS**

A. **Meniscal tear.** The history of a twisting injury followed by swelling, locking, medial or lateral pain, and a limp suggests a collateral ligament injury; however, the Lachman's test or anterior drawer test findings are negative. Tenderness is usually along the joint line; patients are usually unable to perform a deep knee bend. The combination of meniscal damage with collateral or cruciate ligament injuries is common and should always be suspected when an acute knee injury is evaluated.

B. **Patellofemoral subluxation or dislocation** will often present as acute knee pain. Inherent abnormalities of the patellofemoral mechanism usually result in most patellofemoral injuries. These patients will complain of patellar apprehension and usually respond to physical therapy. However, surgical realignment of the extensor mechanism may be necessary in recurrent cases.

VII. **TREATMENT**

A. **Collateral ligament injuries** without cruciate involvement are treated according to the degree of injury. However, most isolated injuries of the medial collateral ligament are treated in a conservative fashion.

1. **Grades 1 and 2.** Protected weight bearing based on the degree of the pain followed by early range of motion and rehabilitation of quadriceps musculature is indicated. Bracing is also used. MRI may be indicated to rule out concomitant meniscal pathology.

2. **Grade 3.** These injuries seldom occur as an isolated event but still can be treated in a conservative manner. Attention should be directed at range of motion, as flexion contractures will easily develop in the immediate postinjury period in

patients with significant medial collateral ligament pathology. Collateral hinge bracing is indicated. Early range of motion of the knee is instituted. If concomitant cruciate injury dictates surgical repair, surgery should be delayed until range of motion, specifically restoration of full extension, is obtained.

B. Cruciate ligament injury

1. **Injuries to the anterior cruciate ligament,** when complete, usually lead to anterior instability in the knee. Whether patients are affected by that instability or not is dictated by their activity level and age. For an individual whose lifestyle places high demands on the knee, surgical treatment is indicated. If a patient is willing to avoid activities that involve deceleration and cutting and jumping maneuvers, then anterior cruciate ligament injuries may be treated in a conservative fashion. MRI or arthroscopic investigation should be performed to rule out concomitant meniscal pathology.

2. **Injuries to the posterior cruciate ligament,** although they leave the knee with a characteristic instability, are often tolerated on a functional basis and are treated in a conservative fashion, with attention directed primarily at restoration of quadriceps muscle power.

3. Cruciate injuries that have an associated injury to the posterolateral structures of the knee **(popliteus, lateral collateral ligament, and joint capsule)** will lead to functional disability even in day-to-day activities in sedentary individuals. These injuries are also very difficult to treat when they become chronic. The best results are obtained with early surgical reconstruction of the cruciate ligaments and repair of the posterolateral corner.

VIII. RESUMPTION OF ATHLETICS. Patients should not be allowed to resume their usual athletic activities until the knee is stable, the pain minimal, and the range of motion adequate. They should be able to run in place, hop on the affected leg without difficulty, run figure-8 patterns in both directions, and start and stop quickly. Muscle strength should be 80% or more of that of the contralateral extremity, and muscle atrophy should be less than 1 cm (comparative circumference).

RUNNING INJURIES

Most running injuries to the musculoskeletal system are overuse-type problems that are typically preventable. A proper therapy program for any specific injury should include a conditioning regimen to prevent the recurrence of such injuries.

I.   ETIOLOGY OF INJURY

A. Biologic fatigue. Jogging or running requires repetitive motion that exposes the musculoskeletal system to severe stress. Even the most conditioned runner reaches a point of fatigue and biologic failure. Limitations and proper preparation are important in preventing running injuries.

B. Improper training. The "once-a-week" runner is the perfect candidate for a running injury. When muscle groups are inadequately conditioned, the repetitive forces associated with running can lead to injury. Excessive mileage, a sudden increase in mileage, and inadequate warm-up can lead to overuse injuries.

C. Anatomic variability. Patients with increased ligamentous laxity may be susceptible to sprains while running. The abnormal distribution of stresses on the feet of runners with flat feet or high arches makes them prone to specific problems related to the arch of feet. The likelihood of patellar problems is increased in an individual with congenital abnormalities of the patellofemoral joint. The "Q angle" of the female hip may also predispose women to certain overuse running injuries.

II.   HISTORY

Important questions

A. Weekly mileage?

B. Type of shoe worn—any change in shoe type recently?

C. Duration, location, and quality of pain?

III. PHYSICAL EXAMINATION

A. Medical examination. A complete respiratory and cardiovascular examination is mandatory for all patients, particularly those aged more than 40 years.

B. Musculoskeletal examination
1. **Observation** for joint swelling, muscular atrophy, and ecchymosis.
2. **Joint alignment**
   a. In runners, it is important to evaluate the foot and ankle. Flat feet (pes planus) and high-arched feet (pes cavus) will be subjected to different stress patterns that predispose to different forms of injuries. The knee examination should include an assessment of ligamentous stability and patellar tracking.
   b. **It is important to** always observe the patient while he/she walks or runs. Such activity will best demonstrate overall joint alignment in a functional, weight-bearing position.
3. **Palpation.** Areas of maximum tenderness should be noted.
4. **Range of motion** (active and passive) of the involved joint should be compared with that of the contralateral limb.
5. **Neurovascular status**

C. Type of shoe. If available, the runner's shoe should be examined.
1. **Fit.** The shoe should be both wide and long enough to allow space for the toes. This reduces blistering and the formation of subungual hematomas. The tongue of the shoe should be well padded to prevent extensor tendinitis and irritation of the dorsum of the foot.
2. **Cushioning** should be thick enough to reduce impact stresses.
3. The **heel** should be wide, thick, and soft. Many runners use a "heel–toe" type of gait. Impact tends to concentrate on the heel. Increasing the width of the heel increases the contact area and decreases the transmitted stresses.
4. **Rigidity** is needed for support and flexibility for foot motion. The shoe should be flexible at the metatarsophalangeal region, where "push-off" occurs but rigid at the arch (midfoot).
5. The **counter** must be high enough to avoid injury to the Achilles tendon and long enough medially to prevent hindfoot valgus and counteract forefoot pronation.

IV. IMAGING STUDIES
A. Radiographs. Many running injuries involve the soft tissues. However, stress and avulsion fractures, which occur quite frequently in runners, may be visualized on routine films. Joint alignment is best visualized with weight-bearing films.
B. Bone scans may afford the earliest diagnosis of a stress fracture, which may not be apparent on routine films for several weeks.
C. MRI and ultrasonography can aid the clinician in chronic cases of refractory Achilles tendinitis (tendinosis).

V. SPECIFIC INJURIES
A. Foot and ankle problems
1. **Corns, calluses, and blisters.** Painful, hypertrophic skin changes are caused by abnormal pressures and stresses. Pain is usually centered on the plantar surface of the metatarsal heads or the dorsum of the interphalangeal joints of toes. There are usually underlying structural foot deformities, such as flat feet (pes planus) or high-arched feet (pes cavus).
   a. **Treatment** is directed toward obtaining proper footwear, including padding to reduce stress on the area.
   b. **Prevention.** A gradual increase in the running distance is recommended.
2. **Subungual hematoma** is a traumatic hemorrhage under the nail bed with associated severe pain. Clotted blood under the nail causes it to lift off. Subungual hematoma is caused by poorly fitting footwear with a tight toe box. It is often noted in long-distance runners (marathon).
   a. **Treatment.** Therapy ranges from observation to decompression (placement of a hot wire through the nail to evacuate the hematoma). Removal of the nail may be needed secondarily.
   b. **Prevention.** Well-fitting footwear with sturdy, high, wide toe boxes will prevent the injury.
3. **Metatarsalgia** is a syndrome of pain under the metatarsal heads, with the first to third metatarsal head being the most commonly involved. Pain usually follows an episode of prolonged running. Tenderness is noted directly under

the involved metatarsal head, and an underlying structural deformity (pes cavus and hammertoes) may be present.

   a. Radiographs may reveal the underlying foot deformity.

   b. Treatment consists of a modification of footwear to include adequate cushioning and insertion of orthotics to redistribute weight from the metatarsal heads (metatarsal pad/bar).

   c. Prevention. The running gait should be changed to a heel–toe pattern.

4. **Stress fractures,** which are fatigue fractures of bones secondary to repetitive stresses, are common in runners. There is a sudden or gradual onset of pain with swelling and tenderness at the site. The condition is often confused with "shin splint." The tibial shaft and the first to third metatarsals are most commonly involved. A recent change in the running distance or the terrain run on is commonly reported by the patient.

   a. Radiographs may demonstrate periosteal callus 7 to 14 days after the appearance of symptoms, and the bone scan will demonstrate increased uptake within 3 to 5 days.

   b. Treatment consists of abstaining from running until symptoms cease. This is followed by a gradual increase in mileage. Stress fractures of the tarsal navicular, and the base of the fifth metatarsal, present unique problems and often require more aggressive forms of treatment.

   c. Prevention includes an adequate stretching program, avoidance of hard surfaces, no abrupt changes in running technique, and adequate footwear.

5. **Plantar fasciitis** is inflammation of the plantar fascia, usually at its medial calcaneal origin. It is the most common cause of heel pain in runners. The patient usually experiences pain with the first few steps taken in the morning. There is usually tenderness at the anteromedial calcaneal margin, and tightness of the Achilles tendon may be present.

   a. Radiographs may reveal a calcaneal spur, but this is not diagnostic.

   b. Treatment

      i. Achilles tendon stretch program.

      ii. Heel pads and/or heel cups.

     iii. NSAIDs.

      iv. Application of ice after running.

      v. Adhesive strapping.

      vi. Injection of 20 to 40 mg of methylprednisolone acetate at the site of maximum tenderness.

     vii. In rare cases, surgical release of the plantar fascia at the heel with removal of the spur may be needed.

   c. Prevention includes an adequate stretching program, avoidance of hard surfaces as running terrain, avoidance of abrupt changes in the running technique, and adequate footwear.

6. **Achilles tendinitis** is a painful inflammation of the Achilles tendon resulting from repetitive stresses. Pain is present near the insertion of the Achilles tendon. Tenderness may be noted along the length of the tendon. Increased warmth and swelling are often present, and in severe cases, crepitus, and a tendon nodule may develop.

   a. Predisposing factors include tightness of the Achilles tendon, cavus foot, functional talipes equinus, or a pronated foot secondary to forefoot or hindfoot varus or tibia vara. Running on hills and uneven terrain inflicts small cumulative tears in the tendon that produce the inflammatory response seen clinically.

   b. Treatment. Acute symptoms are treated by limitation of running, ice packs, and NSAIDs. A gradual return to running with a vigorous stretching program before and after running is essential. Local steroid injection may lead to tendon rupture. Rarely, surgical tenolysis or excision of a tender nodule is indicated.

c. Prevention
    i. The runner should avoid hills and banked roads.
    ii. The running shoe must have a flexible sole, a well-molded Achilles pad, a heel wedge at least 15 mm high, and a rigid heel counter.
    iii. An aggressive Achilles tendon stretching program should be undertaken.

B. Leg problems

  1. Shin splint, characterized by pain along the inner distal two-thirds of the tibial shaft, is an overuse syndrome of either the posterior or anterior tibial muscle-tendon units.

    a. History. The patient experiences aching pain after running, usually in the posteromedial aspect of the leg; pain may be severe enough to prevent running.

    b. Physical examination. Tenderness is present along the involved muscle unit, and no neurovascular deficits are found on examination.

    c. Predisposing factors include poor conditioning, running on hard surfaces, and abnormal foot alignment, including hyperpronation.

    d. Treatment. Ice pack and rest are the initial measures. Alternating hot and cold soaks are helpful.

    e. Prevention includes avoidance of hard surfaces, a warm-up and stretching program, and, if needed, orthotic devices to prevent hyperpronation.

  2. Stress fracture. Tibia and fibula stress fractures present as sudden or gradual onset of pain in the leg. These fractures usually are a result of excessive training. Other etiologic factors include running too far and too fast, often with improper shoes on hard surfaces. A history of a recent increase in mileage is common. Point tenderness is noted at the site of fracture. The proximal posteromedial tibia and the distal fibula are two common sites.

    a. Radiographs. A stress fracture may not appear on a radiograph for 3 to 4 weeks after the onset of symptoms. Results of a bone scan will be positive within 3 to 5 days.

    b. The **treatment** of all stress fractures is the avoidance of running. Running is resumed gradually after the patient has been asymptomatic for at least 6 weeks and radiographic healing has occurred.

    c. Prevention includes gradual changes in the running regimens, a vigorous stretching program, and orthotics for underlying structural foot problems.

  3. Exertional (chronic) compartment syndrome. This malady represents a common cause of leg pain in young individuals. It is caused by a transient increase in muscular compartment pressure in response to exercise. The anterior and lateral compartments of the leg are most commonly involved.

    a. History. Increasing and progressive pain in the anterior or lateral aspect of the leg is reported with varying levels of exercise. Rest relieves symptoms. Numbness and paresthesias in the foot are common.

    b. Physical examination. Before exercise, findings are normal. Exercise causes the onset of symptoms. Occasionally, neurologic symptoms and signs become evident during the examination.

    c. Compartmental pressure measurement represents the mode by which a definitive diagnosis is made. An absolute value above 30 mm Hg or a relative increase in pressure of at least 20 mm Hg, after exercise, is usually diagnostic.

    d. Treatment. Conservative measures are always indicated initially (activity modification, orthotics, and stretching). Surgical decompression (fasciotomy) of the compartment may be needed in refractory cases.

C. Thigh and hip problems

  1. Hamstring strain (pull) represents an injury to the musculotendinous unit. Symptoms may occur suddenly or develop slowly and are usually caused by inadequate stretching of these muscles before running activities. Patients with tight hamstrings are at an increased risk. Tenderness is present in the region of the hamstring in the back of the thigh or at the hamstring origin from the pelvis. Ecchymosis may be noted in more severe injuries.

   a. Radiographic findings are usually negative but may show an avulsion fracture or periosteal reaction at the origin of the hamstring.

   b. Treatment

   i. Acute. Ice pack, rest, and modification of activity.

   ii. Chronic. Stretching program, heat therapy, and ultrasound.

   c. Prevention includes a warm-up and stretching program.

2. **Stress fracture of the femoral neck** presents as acute or insidious onset of pain in the hip or pelvis. Running accentuates the pain. Tenderness is usually present over the pubis or ischium in patients with pelvic stress fractures. Pain on hip motion (particularly internal rotation) may indicate a stress fracture of the femoral neck. The fracture occurs in novice runners or in runners whose training regimen is changed abruptly.

   a. Radiographs. A stress fracture may not appear on radiographs for 3 to 4 weeks after the onset of symptoms. Results of a bone scan will be positive within 3 to 5 days.

   b. Treatment consists of a reduction in activity and no weight bearing for a hip stress fracture, with a gradual return to normal activity after 6 to 8 weeks. In refractory cases, surgical fixation may be required to protect the femoral neck (pinning).

   c. Prevention includes proper training, a stretching program, avoidance of abrupt changes in training habits and assessment of bone density, if indicated.

3. **Iliotibial band friction syndrome** is an overuse injury involving the iliotibial band and lateral femoral condyle. Pain is noted during knee flexion over the lateral condyle, where the friction occurs. Excessive iliotibial band tightness is prevalent in these patients; excessive foot pronation, genu varum, and tibial torsion may also be found. Climbing stairs and running (especially downhill) cause symptoms.

   a. Physical examination. Point tenderness is noted over the lateral condyle and sometimes the greater trochanter. Ober's test should be performed to assess iliotibial band tightness. Patients lie on their side with the unaffected limb flexed at the hip and down on the table, and the involved knee is flexed to 90 degrees and the hip extended. An excessively tight iliotibial band will prevent the affected limb/knee from dropping below the horizontal plane between the two limbs.

   b. Radiographs. There are no significant findings.

   c. Treatment consists of rest, ice packs, NSAIDs, and stretching of the iliotibial band. Equipment change (i.e., shoes and bicycle seat) or foot orthotics may be helpful. More resistant cases may require ultrasonography treatment or steroid injection. Surgical excision is performed only in the rarest of circumstances.

   d. Prevention consists of thorough iliotibial band stretching before activities.

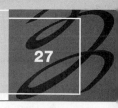

THE FEMALE ATHLETE

Lisa R. Callahan, Jo A. Hannafin, and Monique Sheridan

27

*R*egular exercise has been shown to decrease the risk for multiple diseases, including coronary heart disease, hypertension, osteoporosis, obesity, depression, and some cancers of the reproductive system. The U.S. Preventive Services Task Force and the Office of Disease Prevention and Health Promotion have emphasized that physical activity and fitness must be viewed as a health goal priority among the older population (with women comprising the majority).

Additionally, studies have demonstrated that girls who play high school sports are less likely to have an unwanted pregnancy or use drugs, are more likely to graduate from high school and have lower levels of depression. Clearly, encouraging an active lifestyle among women is critical to the long-term health of our country.

Although many aspects of physical activity are similar in both male and female populations, some issues require special consideration in the female athlete.

 PHYSIOLOGIC CONSIDERATIONS

I. **BODY STRUCTURE**
   A. Skeletal growth reaches its peak at an earlier age in girls (10.5 to 13 years of age) than in boys (12.5 to 15 years of age). Skeletal maturity occurs by the age of 17 to 19 years in girls, and by the age of 21 to 22 years in boys.
   B. The female pelvis is wider than the male pelvis, causing an increased quadriceps (Q) angle, which commonly contributes to anterior knee pain (also called "patellofemoral syndrome").
   C. Women develop thinner, lighter bones than do men, which may predispose them to osteoporosis and stress fractures.

II. **BODY COMPOSITION**
   A. In general, women have approximately 10% more body fat than men do, and 60% to 85% of the total muscle cross-sectional area of men. Because muscle is more metabolically active than fat, women have, on average, a resting metabolic rate that is 5% to 10% lower than that of men.
   B. In response to weight training, women experience similar relative increases in strength as in men. Because muscle hypertrophy depends on hormones, as well as on training program type and volume, levels vary for each athlete. However, male athletes have greater absolute strength and muscle hypertrophy (owing to their hormonal environment) than female athletes have. Even with training, women have 30% to 50% less upper body strength than men have.
   C. The percentage of body fat can be estimated by a variety of methods; ideal body fat composition varies with age and sex. Efforts have been made to establish a healthy minimum body fat percentage, but factors vary in women. However, athletes with a body fat percentage below 15% should be examined for any indications of the female athlete triad.

III. **CARDIORESPIRATORY SYSTEM**
   A. Women have a smaller thoracic cage and heart size, resulting in lower lung capacity and maximal cardiac output.
   B. Maximum oxygen composition (Vo_2 max) is lower in women, largely because of differences in body composition and oxygen-carrying capacity. Vo_2 max is similar in boys and girls before puberty.

IV. CIRCULATORY SYSTEM

   A. Women have a smaller blood volume, smaller iron stores, and lower concentrations of hemoglobin. These factors are associated with a lower oxygen-carrying capacity and they also increase the risk for anemia.

   B. Both male and female elite athletes tend to have lower levels of hemoglobin than their sedentary counterparts. This may be secondary to both a low dietary intake and exercise-related blood loss, such as that which occurs from the gastrointestinal tract.

V. ENDOCRINE SYSTEM

   A. There is no evidence that the phase of the menstrual cycle influences athletic performance.

   B. Female athletes may experience a wide array of alterations in the menstrual cycle, ranging from suppression of the luteal phase to amenorrhea. The latter is especially prevalent in athletes at risk for the "female athlete triad."

   C. Pregnancy results in many physiologic changes, including increases in cardiac output, in blood volume, and in oxygen demand. The American College of Obstetrics and Gynecology (ACOG) recently revised guidelines regarding exercise and pregnancy. The ACOG indicated that recreational and competitive female athletes with uncomplicated pregnancies can remain active, but those who exercise strenuously should seek close medical supervision. Athletes with a history of or risk for preterm labor or fetal growth restriction are advised to reduce physical activity in the second and third trimesters. Recent research also indicates that certain types of activities, such as diving (owing to changes in pressure underwater), exercise in the supine position (owing to restriction in large blood vessels), and any activity associated with risk for blunt abdominal trauma (contact sports and skiing) should be limited and/or avoided during pregnancy.

 THE FEMALE ATHLETE TRIAD

I. GENERAL CONSIDERATIONS

   A. The female athlete triad refers to the inter-relatedness of three conditions: disordered eating, amenorrhea, and osteoporosis.

   B. Traditionally, female athletes whose activity emphasized leanness for aesthetic reasons (ballet and gymnastics), who associated low body weight with improved performance (distance running), and those who were classified by weight (rowing and judo) were the ones thought to be at risk. However, women at risk have been found in many other sports, including swimming, soccer, volleyball, and cycling, and also in health clubs.

II. DISORDERED EATING

   A. It is important that the clinician differentiates disordered eating from the eating disorders of anorexia nervosa and bulimia nervosa, which are psychiatric diagnoses with specific diagnostic criteria. Disordered eating is a much more common phenomenon, and restricting awareness to the extremes of anorexia and bulimia will result in failure to recognize girls at risk for the triad.

   B. Disordered eating behaviors include the following:
      1. Food restriction.
      2. Fasting/skipping meals.
      3. Binging (which may or may not be followed by purging).
      4. Use of diet pills, diuretics, and laxatives.

   C. Girls with eating disorders are often
      1. preoccupied by thoughts of food.
      2. plagued by distorted body image.
      3. afraid that any weight gain is the equivalent of "getting fat."
      4. feeling guilty about eating before/after meals.
      5. compulsive exercisers.

III. AMENORRHEA

   A. Primary amenorrhea is defined as the absence of menarche by the age of 16 years.

   B. Secondary amenorrhea is the absence of three to six consecutive menstrual cycles in women who have experienced menarche.

    C. It is believed that exercise in the setting of inadequate calorie consumption may contribute to an "energy-deficient" state, which may lead to amenorrhea.

    D. In this setting, amenorrhea represents a hypoestrogenic state, which can predispose one to osteoporosis.

    E. Exercise-related amenorrhea is a diagnosis of exclusion. Other causes of amenorrhea (such as pregnancy) must be considered before it is assumed that cessation of menses in an athlete is exercise-driven.

IV. OSTEOPOROSIS

    A. Osteoporosis refers to bone loss in addition to inadequate bone formation, which results in lower bone mass, increased skeletal frailty, and increased risk of fracture.

    B. Premature osteoporosis occurring in the female athlete may be irreversible, even when treated with calcium supplementation, hormonal replacement, and correction of amenorrhea.

    C. Pharmacologic treatment of osteoporosis in the premenopausal female athlete is difficult. Bisphosphonates, which are indicated in postmenopausal women, have not been well-studied in the premenopausal population or in pregnancy. Although some physicians treat the amenorrhea and osteoporosis of the female athlete triad with oral contraceptive pills, such treatment has not been shown to actually improve bone density and mineralization.

    D. Stress fractures may occur with more frequency and severity in female athletes at risk for the triad; although there are no current guidelines regarding screening, one should consider evaluation of bone density to screen for premature osteoporosis in an athlete identified as being at risk for the female athlete triad.

 ORTHOPEDIC ISSUES

Current knowledge suggests that most injuries sustained by athletes are sport-specific rather than gender-specific (see Chapter 26). However, several orthopedic issues of special concern in the female athlete deserve specific mention.

I. ANTERIOR CRUCIATE LIGAMENT (ACL) INJURIES

    A. Epidemiologic data suggests that the incidence of severe knee injuries, especially ACL injuries, is higher in women than in men, particularly in the sports of soccer, basketball, and lacrosse (threefold to fivefold increase).

    B. The causes of increased ACL injuries are unclear. Factors thought to contribute to the higher rate of ACL injury are both intrinsic and extrinsic.

        1. Intrinsic factors

            a. Ligament size.

            b. Intercondylar notch dimensions.

            c. Muscular strength and coordination.

            d. Limb alignment.

            e. Hormonal influences.

        2. Extrinsic factors

            a. Shoe–floor interface.

            b. Level of skill and experience.

            c. Inadequate training and coaching.

    C. Data suggest that women are more likely to tear their ACL during the first half of the menstrual cycle than the second half. The explanation for this difference in incidence is unclear, but it may be related to neuromuscular and proprioceptive functions.

    D. Programs designed to decrease noncontact ACL injury risk, which have demonstrated a significant decrease in the incidence of injury in both high school and collegiate athletes, are available. The common factors in these training programs include balance, strength, proprioception, and plyometric training. The best characterized and studied programs are the Sportsmetrix and Prevent Injury, Enhance Performance (PEP) programs.

II. PATELLOFEMORAL PAIN

    A. Injuries to the patellofemoral joint are more common in women. Patellofemoral pain is often thought to be secondary to a variation in limb alignment ("miserable malalignment syndrome") consisting of a combination of increased anteversion of the femoral head, internal rotation of the femur, external rotation of the tibia, and foot pronation. Other anatomic features often considered to be causing patellofemoral pain include an increased quadriceps angle and hypermobility of the patella.

B. Patellofemoral pain should be differentiated according to whether the patella is hypermobile or "tight" (lateral patella compression syndrome). This distinction is important because treatment varies depending on whether the patella needs to be restrained (in the case of hypermobility) or "loosened" (in the case of tight lateral structures causing lateral compressive pain). In the case of the hypermobile patella, strengthening of the medial quadriceps (vastus medialis obliquus) aids in restraining the patella. In the patient with tight lateral structures causing lateral pull of the patella, stretching lateral structures, including the lateral retinaculum and iliotibial band, is recommended. A patellar tracking brace may be helpful in the patient with hypermobility of the patella but may actually exacerbate pain in the patient with lateral patella compression syndrome.

III. SHOULDER PAIN

A. Adhesive capsulitis is an idiopathic inflammatory synovitis in the glenohumeral joint. It occurs three to seven times more frequently in women than in men. The cause is not well-understood, but the clinical entity is frequently associated with other conditions, such as diabetes, hypothyroidism, trauma, and menopause. Four distinct stages have been recognized, which reflect the degree of synovitis. The cornerstones of treatment include intra-articular steroid injection and a rehabilitation program to maintain strength and range of motion. Manipulation under anesthesia and arthroscopy may be required.

B. Impingement syndrome, an overuse injury to the rotator cuff, occurs frequently in both male and female patients. However, in women, causative factors are often related to underlying glenohumeral laxity. Increased capsular laxity requires an increase in rotator cuff activity, leading to overuse and impingement. Another factor, especially in the novice female athlete, is deconditioning and weakness of the upper extremity, which leads to rapid fatigue of the rotator cuff, particularly in those involved in overhead activity.

IV. STRESS FRACTURES

A. Although stress fractures occur in both male and female athletes, they are clinically considered more common in female athletes, especially in certain sports such as running and gymnastics. The risk for stress fractures is clearly greater in women than in men, but there is great variability in reporting of incidents. Studies indicate a range of increased risk from 1.5 to 13 times greater in women than in men.

B. The tibia is the most common site of stress fracture for all athletes; stress fractures of the pelvis, femur, and metatarsals are reported more frequently in female athletes.

C. Spondylolysis (secondary to stress fracture) and spondylolisthesis should be considered in those athletes who perform repetitive flexion and extension activities and complain of low back pain.

D. Variables related to the increased rate of stress fractures in women include the following:

1. Menstrual irregularity/amenorrhea.
2. Low bone mineral density and bone size.
3. Training errors.
4. Inadequate shoes/equipment.
5. Biomechanical alignment of the lower extremity.
6. Decreased muscle strength in the lower extremity.
7. Diet/nutrition.

E. Evaluation of the female athlete with a stress fracture **must** include a careful menstrual history; loss of menses or any change in frequency or duration of the menstrual cycle requires further evaluation.

MEDICAL CONSIDERATIONS

Achieving fitness through moderate exercise has been linked to lower risks of heart disease, hypertension, cancer, depression, and osteoporosis—disorders that affect both women and men. General guidelines suggest that both women and men should be evaluated by a physician before embarking on an exercise program, especially after 40 years of age. Although most medical considerations in the athlete are not gender-specific, a few issues are of special concern to those caring for the female athlete.

I. OSTEOPOROSIS. Moderate exercise may help decrease the risk of osteoporosis, but exercise in the face of disordered eating and amenorrhea may contribute to premature osteoporosis. Low estrogen levels are associated with an increase in urinary loss of calcium and a decrease in calcium absorption from the gastrointestinal tract, which lead to less calcium deposition in bone. In the female athlete, a stress fracture may be a warning sign of osteoporosis and warrants thorough evaluation. Additionally, illnesses such as hyperthyroidism (whether overt, subclinical, or iatrogenically induced by excessive replacement of thyroid hormone) are more common in women and may contribute to osteoporosis.

II. RHEUMATOLOGIC DISEASE. Most rheumatologic diseases, such as lupus, rheumatoid arthritis (RA), and fibromyalgia, are reported to occur two to ten times more frequently in women than in men. Often, the first manifestation of such an illness is mistaken for an athletic injury. The physician should be alert to this fact and should include rheumatologic diseases in the differential diagnosis of musculoskeletal pain, especially in women. RA and systemic lupus erythematosus (SLE) are systemic inflammatory disorders, and the inflammatory and immunologic processes that are active lead to premature atherosclerosis and osteoporosis.

III. CARDIOVASCULAR ISSUES
  A. Factors affecting the risk for sudden death include the following:
    1. Age and, to a small degree, cholesterol level (both sexes).
    2. Hematocrit, vital capacity, and glucose level (women only).
  B. In women, the incidence of false-positive findings on electrocardiographic exercise testing is much higher than in men; therefore, the use of additional imaging modalities is especially important in the female athlete suspected of having cardiovascular disease.

IV. EXERCISE-RELATED ANEMIA. Anemia is more common in female athletes than in male athletes, and in fact is more common in female athletes than in the general population.
  A. Dilutional pseudoanemia is a physiologic dilution of hemoglobin that occurs because of the increase in plasma volume associated with regular exercise. In general, the dilution leads to a hemoglobin drop of 0.5 to 1 g/dL but may be larger in most elite athletes. It is often called "sports anemia" and is benign.
  B. Exertional hemolytic anemia (also called foot strike hemolysis) has been reported but the exact cause is not known. Although initially described in runners, it has since been reported even in nonimpact sports like swimming. Possible mechanisms include acidosis induced by exercise, turbulence caused by increased output demands, and foot strike.
  C. Iron deficiency anemia is most common and may be caused by gastrointestinal, sweat, urinary, or menstrual losses; impaired absorption; and inadequate intake of iron. This type of anemia has an adverse effect on performance and requires treatment. The Centers for Disease Control (CDC) recommend iron supplementation for 3 months.
  D. Female athletes do not appear to be at greater risk than the general female population for low iron stores. Low ferritin levels without actual anemia also may affect performance. Although no evidence-based recommendation exists, it is common practice to supplement ferritin levels less than 20 ng/mL with iron 325 mg/day; ferritin levels between 20 and 40 ng/mL are frequently treated with a multivitamin containing iron.

V. INFECTIONS. Physicians treating female athletes should be aware that certain types of infections, such as urinary tract and vaginal/genital infections, are related to gender and anatomy and therefore are more common in women.

 # NUTRITIONAL CONCERNS

Good nutrition is essential to athletic performance, and the basics of good nutrition are not gender-dependent. However, female athletes need to pay particular attention to a few special considerations.

I.   CALCIUM
   A. As mentioned previously, calcium is essential for bone health.
   B. The recommendations for daily intake (RDI) are 1,000 to 1,200 mg in premenopausal women, and 1,500 mg in postmenopausal women and adolescents.
   C. While calcium supplements are beneficial, many experts believe that intake of calcium-rich foods is a more effective method of meeting calcium RDI.
II.   IRON
   A. See section **IV** under Medical Considerations.
   B. Iron deficiency is often secondary to inadequate diet in addition to frequent losses, such as those through menstruation.
   C. A thorough evaluation is warranted before iron supplementation is prescribed. When taken with calcium supplements, iron absorption has been shown to decrease considerably. However, vitamin C enhances iron absorption.
   D. It is not known whether female athletes have a higher daily iron requirement than the current U.S. Food and Drug Association (FDA) recommendations.
III.   PROTEIN
   A. Protein is essential for the development and recovery/repair of muscles.
   B. Female athletes may tend to avoid protein-rich foods, because of their fat or caloric content, in order to avoid weight gain. Protein deficiencies can create fatigue, cause injury during athletics, and reduce immune system efficiencies.
IV.   OTHER DIETARY INSUFFICIENCIES. Female athletes may have inadequate intake of total calories, protein, fiber, and fat in efforts to avoid weight gain. Vegetarian diets often do not contain sufficient nutritional content as well. Such dietary inadequacies are known to contribute to poor bone health and may contribute to increased rates of certain injuries and possibly decreased rate of healing. Extreme restriction of intake may not only affect performance but also have negative effects on health, similar to those seen in the patient with anorexia nervosa.
V.   HYDRATION
   A. Like all athletes, female athletes must maintain appropriate hydration. Athletes can easily lose 2% to 5% of their body water in an intense exercise session. A loss of 2% affects performance.
   B. Electrolytes (primarily sodium and potassium) lost through exercise can be replaced by adequate diet.
   C. Female athletes, in an effort to avoid weight gain and/or suppress hunger pains, may drink excessive amounts of water and develop hyponatremia, also called "water intoxication." The condition is most prevalent in distance runners and triathletes. The resulting depletion of the athlete's blood sodium can be potentially fatal, and symptoms resemble those of other exercise-related disorders. Consumption of sports drinks is a recommended method of prevention.

EQUIPMENT AND SHOES

I.   EQUIPMENT. Only recently has the athletic equipment industry begun to design exercise equipment intended for use by female athletes. In developing and choosing equipment, the physiologic differences between women and men, mentioned briefly at the beginning of this chapter, should be kept in mind. These factors should influence the future design of equipment such as bicycles, skis, racquets, and weight machines.
II.   SHOES. A woman's foot is different from that of a man, in both shape and size. It is only recently that shoe manufacturers have begun to take such factors into consideration, which has resulted in greatly improved technology that is specific to the female athlete's anatomy and biomechanics, as well as specific to the sport.

BURSITIS AND TENDINITIS

Paul Pellicci and Richard R. McCormack

BURSITIS

I. ANATOMIC CONSIDERATIONS

A bursa is a closed sac that contains a small amount of synovial fluid and that is lined with a cellular membrane similar to synovium. Bursae are present in areas where tendons and muscles move over bony prominences; these structures facilitate such motion. Approximately 160 formed bursae are present in the body, and others may form in response to irritative stimuli. Descriptions of the clinically important bursae follow.

A. Shoulder
1. The **subacromial** bursa lies between the acromion and the rotator cuff.
2. The **subdeltoid** bursa lies between the deltoid muscle and the rotator cuff.
3. The **subcoracoid** bursa lies at the attachment of the biceps, coracobrachialis, and pectoralis minor tendons to the coracoid process.

B. Elbow
1. The **olecranon** bursa lies over the olecranon process.
2. The **radiohumeral** bursa lies between the common wrist extensor tendon and the lateral epicondyle.

C. Hip
1. The **iliopsoas** bursa may communicate with the hip joint and lies between the hip capsule and the psoas musculotendinous unit.
2. The **trochanteric** bursa surrounds the gluteal insertions into the greater trochanter.
3. The **ischiogluteal** bursa separates the gluteus maximus from the ischial tuberosity.

D. Knee
1. The **prepatellar** bursa lies between the skin and the patellar tendon.
2. The **infrapatellar** bursa lies deep to the insertion of the patellar ligament.
3. There are many **popliteal** bursae. The largest bursa lies between the semimembranous muscle and the medial head of the gastrocnemius muscle.
4. The **pes anserine bursa** lies between the medial collateral ligament and the sartorius, gracilis, and semitendinosus tendons.

E. Foot
1. The **Achilles** bursa separates the Achilles tendon insertion from the posterior aspect of the calcaneus.
2. The **subcalcaneal** bursa is located at the insertion of the plantar fascia into the medial tuberosity of the calcaneus.

II. ETIOPATHOGENESIS

A. Direct trauma to a bursal area may lead to an inflammatory response in the bursa, with its attendant hyperemia and the exudation of fluid and leukocytes into the bursal sac. Bursal fluid can be clear, hemorrhagic, or xanthochromic.

B. Chronic overuse or irritation of a bursal area.

C. A **systemic disorder,** such as rheumatoid arthritis (RA) or gout. In this case, the bursal fluid can be cloudy or purulent, depending upon the level of inflammation.

D. Septic bursitis may occur secondary to **puncture wounds,** from trauma, or to an overlying rash, such as psoriasis, a surrounding cellulitis, or after a **local therapeutic injection.** The organisms most frequently responsible are staphylococci (*Staphylococcus aureus* and *Staphylococcus epidermidis*) and streptococci.

DIAGNOSTIC INVESTIGATIONS

A. **Localized pain** is the presenting complaint, with radiation of the pain into the involved limb as an occasional feature.

B. **Swelling** is common in olecranon bursitis but is usually not seen in subdeltoid bursitis.

C. **Erythema** may be present and does not necessarily indicate sepsis.

D. **Tenderness** is always present.

E. **Pain** is usually elicited when the patient is asked to execute a maneuver that stresses the involved motor unit; for example, abduction of the hip against gravity will cause pain in trochanteric bursitis.

F. **Radiographs** may, on occasion, demonstrate deposits of calcium in the region of the bursae. Calcific bursitis and calcific tendinitis may be indistinguishable, both clinically and radiographically.

IV. **TREATMENT**

A. **Rest**

1. The region experiencing pain should be immobilized for 7 to 10 days.

2. For 1 to 2 weeks, the patient should be told to discontinue activities that aggravate the symptoms. An ergonomic assessment of the work areas in office or home can be helpful in defining those activities that lead to irritative inflammatory bursal reactions.

B. **Ice compresses** applied to the acutely inflamed area reduce swelling and provide relief from pain.

C. **Anti-inflammatory medications**

1. For mild to **moderate** symptoms, 600 mg of ibuprofen orally three times daily with food or other nonsteroidal anti-inflammatory drugs (NSAIDs) in appropriate doses is helpful.

2. For **severe** symptoms, 25 mg of indomethacin orally four times daily with food is recommended. This treatment should not be continued for more than 5 to 7 days.

D. Swollen subcutaneous bursae, such as the olecranon bursa, should be **aspirated.** Reaccumulation of fluid is common, and it is not unusual for two or three aspirations to be required to resolve the problem. The fluid should be cultured and a crystalline evaluation should be performed.

E. **Injecting** the offending bursa with 3 mL of 1% lidocaine mixed with 40 mg of methylprednisolone acetate (Depo-Medrol) is usually successful in relieving symptoms.

F. **Surgery** to excise a bursa is rarely necessary. However, if the procedures outlined in **A** through **E** have been repeatedly unsuccessful and the disability is significant, surgery may provide relief.

G. If **infection** is suspected (i.e., red, warm, bursa-yielding, cloudy, or purulent fluid associated with a cellulitis and/or fever), the bursa must be aspirated and the fluid must be smeared for direct Gram stain and sent for microbiologic culture. Pending results, patients with mild symptoms may be treated as outpatients with 500 mg of dicloxacillin or cephalexin orally four times daily. Patients who demonstrate no improvement or worsening with oral antibiotics and with bursal aspirations, who have more severe infections, or who are markedly symptomatic should be hospitalized and treated intravenously with nafcillin or cephalexin. In the presence of chronic bursitis refractory to antibiotics, bursectomy may be indicated.

 TENDINITIS

Tendinitis is a general term used to describe any inflammation associated with a tendon. The inflammation may occur within the substance of the tendon (intratendinous lesion) or may be associated with the tenosynovial sheath (tenosynovitis). Because bursae are often located near tendons, the terms tendinitis and bursitis are often used interchangeably to represent the same affliction (see preceding discussion on bursitis). Together, these entities are the most common causes of soft tissue pain.

I. ETIOPATHOGENESIS

    A. Intratendinous lesions occur primarily later in life as the vascularity of the tendon diminishes. They are usually associated with repetitive motion and are thought to represent microtrauma, or limited macrotrauma short of rupture, within the substance of the tendon. Local signs and symptoms of inflammation are caused by the reparative process of vascular infiltration with acute and chronic cellular responses. During the reparative process, calcium salts, which are visible on radiographs, may be deposited in degenerated portions of the tendon—hence the term calcific tendinitis. Tennis elbow, calcific tendinitis in the supraspinatus, and trochanteric tendinitis are examples of intratendinous lesions.

    B. Acute or chronic paratendinous inflammation or tenosynovitis may have several etiologies.

        1. Repetitive motion with injury is by far the most common etiology. Synovial tendon sheaths are located in areas where tendons pass over bony surfaces and where large tendon excursions are found, most commonly above the wrist and ankle. Repetitive motion causes inflammation with edema. The result is decreased excursion and painful motion of the affected tendon, often with signs of mechanical blocking, such as may be seen with de Quervain's disease and trigger finger.

        2. These paratendinous inflammations may also be triggered by **direct or microtraumatic intratendinous injuries** and result from the reparative process initiated in the tenosynovium.

        3. Systemic inflammatory disorders such as RA may be associated with prominent tenosynovitis of the hands and feet.

        4. Acute tenosynovitis may also be of **septic origin.** Most commonly, this disorder involves a direct wound contaminating the sheath. Alternatively, it may result from a generalized sepsis, especially in a compromised host, and may be multifocal. Neisserial organisms such as *Neisseria gonorrhoeae* typically can cause this type of inflammation. Because the vascular supply is poor, infection due to nongonococcal organisms is not well controlled with antibiotics alone, and surgical drainage is usually necessary.

II. PHYSICAL EXAMINATION

    A. The classic sign of inflammation within the tendon or tendon sheath is **pain on motion,** especially with passive stretch or contraction of the affected motor tendon unit against resistance.

    B. Local **swelling, warmth, and tenderness** are usually present. Tenderness may be elicited along the course of the tendon. On deep structures, such as the supraspinatus or gluteus medius tendons, deep-point tenderness in a specific and reproducible location may be elicited.

    C. Erythema may or may not be present, depending on the depth of the structure and the acuteness of the process. Because most tendons cross joints, tendinitis must be distinguished from acute **inflammatory or septic arthritis.** In the case of septic arthritis, the range of motion will be more severely restricted. Systemic signs may be present, and capsular tenderness should be distinguished from tenderness directly over the tendon. In doubtful cases, diagnostic arthrocentesis will resolve the matter.

III. TREATMENT

    A. The treatment of tendinitis is similar to that of bursitis.

    B. Immobilization is the most important therapy. Methods are as follows:

        1. A **splint** or cast for the affected region in the distal upper and lower extremities.

        2. A **sling** for lesions of the proximal upper extremity.

        3. Crutches for lesions of the proximal lower extremity.

    C. As the inflammation resolves, **gentle physical therapy** within the limits of pain should be started to avoid permanent stiffness.

    D. Local heat is helpful in relieving symptoms and in alleviating the painful muscle spasm associated with tendinitis. Hot packs, warm soaks, skin counterirritants (e.g., balms), ultrasound, or hot wax treatments are equally effective and should be utilized.

E. Anti-inflammatory drugs

 1. **NSAIDs** in appropriate doses are used for acute inflammation.

 2. **Corticosteroids,** given systemically or locally as injections with a local anesthetic, can also be beneficial in certain cases. The injected area should be cooled with ice for 24 hours after injection, and adequate analgesics should be prescribed to counteract the pain experienced when the local anesthetic wears off. The use of a long-acting local anesthetic such as **bupivacaine** can minimize the pain associated with corticosteroid injections. A suspension of 20 to 40 mg of methylprednisolone acetate is the most frequently used preparation. Not more than three injections should be administered over weeks or months. Steroid preparations are contraindicated in the presence of infection. At times, ultrasound-guided steroid injections can be quite helpful in cases previously unresponsive to "blind" injections.

F. Surgery is the treatment of choice when nonoperative therapy has failed. It involves repair of a degenerative tendon, as in tennis elbow; release of fibro-osseous tunnels, as in de Quervain's disease; and tenosynovectomy for chronic wrist tenosynovitis, a common manifestation of RA.

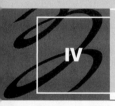

IV *Diagnosis and Therapy*

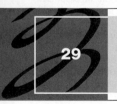

29 RHEUMATOID ARTHRITIS
Ioannis Tassiulas and Stephen A. Paget

■ KEY POINTS

■ Rheumatoid arthritis (RA) is a systemic inflammatory disease that affects predominantly the joints.

■ Proinflammatory cytokines tumor necrosis factor-α (TNF-α) and interleukin-1 (IL-1) are major mediators of the disease.

■ Highly specific anti-cyclic citrullinated peptide (anti-CCP) antibodies may be used for early diagnosis in atypical disease presentations and to predict the outcome.

■ Extra-articular manifestations should be recognized early and be treated aggressively.

■ Early initiation of treatment with an aim to achieve a stage of disease remission prevents future complications and improves prognosis.

INTRODUCTION

I. **Rheumatoid arthritis** (RA) is a chronic, systemic, immune-mediated inflammatory disease that affects at least twice as many women as men. Although RA affects predominantly the joints, epidemiologic studies have unearthed disturbing information about the true potential of this disease: RA leads to joint damage within the first 2 years; causes marked functional limitation; and shortens life by 5 to 7 years due to premature atherosclerosis.

II. **Rheumatoid factor (RF) and anti-cyclic citrullinated peptide (anti-CCP):** RF is an immunoglobulin M (IgM) antibody against the Fc portion of an IgG molecule, and is the main serologic marker of the disease found in 75% to 80% of patients. Another important disease-specific auto antibody, anti-CCP antibody has been recognized and serves as a sensitive and specific diagnostic and prognostic tool in the early stages of the disease, when patients may not yet have developed RF in their serum.

III. **Cytokines and immune cell networks** have been identified as important mediators in the pathogenesis and perpetuation of inflammation in RA. This information has been successfully translated into the development of new and significantly more effective targeted treatments in the form of tumor necrosis factor-α (TNF-α) and interleukin-1 (IL-1) antagonists.

ETIOPATHOGENESIS

I. **NO CLEAR ETIOLOGY HAS BEEN DEFINED.** There is substantial experimental evidence that the initiation of RA is a T-cell–mediated, antigen-specific process. The arthritogenic antigen has not yet been defined but it could be either an exogenous antigen, such as a viral protein, or an endogenous protein such as citrullinated peptides.

II. **The synovial membrane** in patients with RA is characterized by hyperplasia, increased vascularity, and an infiltrate of inflammatory cells, primarily CD4+ T cells, which are the main orchestrators of cell-mediated immune responses. The histologic appearance of the synovium in RA is not specific, as a similar picture is seen in other inflammatory arthritides, such as psoriatic arthritis. One characteristic feature of RA is the invasion of and damage to cartilage, bone, and tendons by an infiltrating inflammatory synovial tissue mass called the pannus.

III. **CELLULAR IMMUNITY**

A. CD4+ T cells constitute most T cells in the rheumatoid synovium. Often they form lymphoid aggregates in the subintimal area. B lymphocytes are also present in the synovium, where they are surrounded by T cells in follicle formation. B cells process autoantigen and contribute to the inflammatory process. B cells can differentiate into plasma cells and produce RF under the influence of T cells and cytokines, such as IL-6 and B-lymphocyte–stimulating factor (BLyS), which are found in rheumatoid synovium.

B. Activated macrophages and dendritic cells, both important in antigen presentation, are also found and are important sources of proinflammatory cytokines such as TNF-α and IL-1. Neutrophils are found predominantly in the synovial fluid, and are important mediators of tissue damage via the release of various enzymes.

IV. **CYTOKINES AND OTHER SOLUBLE MEDIATORS.** Cytokines are local protein mediators involved in cell growth and activation, inflammation, immunity, and differentiation. The important role of cytokines in the pathogenesis of RA has been demonstrated by the effectiveness of therapies that target TNF-α and IL-1, and emerging data have identified additional cytokines such as IL-6 and IL-15 as potential therapeutic targets in RA.

A. TNF-α and IL-1 are produced mainly by monocytes/macrophages and are potent stimulators of mesenchymal cells such as synovial fibroblasts, osteoclasts, and chondrocytes that release tissue-destroying matrix metalloproteinases (MMPs). TNF-α is considered to be the master regulator of the inflammatory cascade in rheumatoid synovium.

B. A number of anti-inflammatory cytokines such as IL-10, IL-4, and TGF-β are also detected in the rheumatoid synovium and synovial fluid, but are unable to downregulate the inflammatory response either because they are present in low concentrations or their action is blocked or altered in this inflammatory environment.

C. Enzymes, such as MMPs, which degrade matrix proteins, and complement proteins, which participate in acute inflammation, are effector molecules that mediate tissue destruction.

V. AUTOANTIBODIES

A. RFs are antibodies that bind to the Fc portion of IgG. The mechanisms initiating RF production and its exact role in disease pathogenesis have still not been established. RF is found in the serum of 75% to 80% of patients with RA (who are therefore called "seropositive"), is locally produced in the synovial membrane, and may be present in the serum of patients with other diseases characterized by B cell or immune hyperactivity, such as chronic hepatitis C infection, bacterial endocarditis, and systemic lupus erythematosus (SLE). The presence of high RF titers is associated with severe, erosive disease, a worse functional outcome, rheumatoid nodules, other extra-articular disease manifestations, and human leucocyte antigen (HLA)-DR4 positivity.

B. Anti-CCP antibodies are detected in up to two-thirds of patients with RA sera and in less than 5% of controls. Anti-CCP antibodies show the highest disease specificity (95%) for RA of any antibody known. They are already present in patients with early RA and predict the development of more severe disease. Their sensitivity is comparable to RF occurring in 50% to 75% of patients with established disease. Their role in the pathogenesis of RA is unknown.

VI. GENETIC FACTORS

A. Twin and family studies. Family studies have shown that siblings of individuals affected with RA have a twofold to fourfold risk of developing disease themselves, when compared with unrelated individuals. Studies of mono- and dizygotic twins have shown disease concordance rates of 12% to 15% and 4%, respectively. These twin concordance figures show that the risk of disease in relatives of affected individuals is conferred by shared genetic factors but also emphasizes that genetics is not the sole determinant.

B. The major histocompatibility complex (MHC). In genetic studies, RA is strongly linked to haplotypes containing the MHC class II antigens HLA-DR4 and HLA-DR1. On further molecular characterization, the association was confined to a short sequence in the HLA-DRβ1 gene that codes for the RA epitope in amino acid positions 67 through 74 (the "shared epitope"). Some of the HLA-DRβ1 alleles (HLA-DRβ1 *0401, *0404, and *0408, in general populations and some others in specific ethnic groups) are RA-associated alleles. The main function of MHC class II molecules is to present antigenic peptides to CD4+ T cells. These MHC genes are related not only to the initiation of the disease but also to its course and severity.

 PREVALENCE

Most studies of the prevalence of RA are based on cross-sectional population studies. Several estimates of between 0.5% and 1% have been obtained in studies across Europe, North America, Asia, and South Africa. There is a greater prevalence of the disease in certain native North American populations. In contrast, RA appears to be exceptionally rare in rural African black populations, and in certain Chinese groups. RA is two to three times more common in women than in men, but over the age of 50 years, the distribution of disease frequency becomes more equal between the two sexes. Although the disease is most common between the ages of 40 and 60 years, in one-third of patients, RA develops after the age of 60 years.

CLINICAL MANIFESTATIONS

I. **CLINICAL EVALUATION.** A careful clinical evaluation is the most important step in the diagnosis and successful management of RA.

   A. **History.** Diffuse, symmetric joint pain and swelling affecting the small peripheral joints are the most common presenting symptoms. These symptoms are often associated with prolonged (>1 hour) morning stiffness and generalized fatigue. Interestingly, RA is not associated with fever. If fever is a prominent clinical manifestation, alternative diagnoses such as viral arthritis, systemic infections, or SLE should be entertained. A history of RA in other members of the family should heighten suspicion that the patient's symptoms could be an expression of early RA. Evaluation of the patient's functional status using a number of self-report questionnaires, such as the Stanford Health Assessment Questionnaire (HAQ), is very important because it has been shown to correlate significantly with disease activity, mortality, pain, functional outcome, and psychosocial factors.

   B. **Musculoskeletal system.** The key signs of early joint inflammation in RA are those of tenderness and swelling. These may be associated with local heat, but erythema is not a common feature of rheumatoid inflammation. Although the disease may begin in an asymmetrical or monoarticular fashion, RA will eventually evolve within weeks or a few months into a symmetric inflammatory arthritis involving the wrists, the metacarpophalangeal (MCP) and proximal interphalangeal (PIP) joints of the hands, elbows, shoulders, hips, knees, ankles, and the small joints of the feet. The joint is considered "active" if it is tender on pressure or painful on passive movement. Joint swelling may be periarticular or intra-articular. Intra-articular swelling is associated with the detection of a joint effusion. Early changes include prominence of the ulnar styloid, and later deformities resulting from combinations of joint and tendon damage may evolve, including ulnar deviation, boutonniere, and swan neck deformities. Flexor tenosynovitis can lead to triggering of the fingers and eventually there may be rupture of tendons. Extensor tenosynovitis is seen as swelling over the dorsum of the wrist. Carpal tunnel syndrome may result from pressure on the median nerve by swollen flexor tendons, and may present as paresthesias, pain, or motor dysfunction in the radial aspect of the hand. Similarly, cubital tunnel syndrome or tarsal tunnel syndrome can occur as the result of compression of the ulnar nerve at the elbow or of the posterior tibial nerve at the ankle, respectively. Olecranon bursitis often presents as swelling at the tip of the elbow; synovial extensions, known as Baker's cysts, project from the knee to the medial calf region; occasionally, these cysts may rupture and the fluid may dissect inferiorly, resulting in a clinical picture that may mimic phlebitis. Spinal disease is usually limited to the cervical region, and in patients with severe and longstanding disease may lead to atlanto–axial subluxation and cord compromise.

II. **CRITERIA FOR THE CLASSIFICATION OF RA.** The 1987 revised American Rheumatology Association criteria for the classification of RA were developed for epidemiologic purposes (Table 29-1). However, because of the high sensitivity and specificity of these criteria in the classification of RA they are useful to consider at the time of clinical diagnosis. Of the seven criteria, the presence of four is sufficient for classifying a patient as having RA. The first four criteria must be present for at least 6 weeks. The natural history of individuals who do or do not meet the criteria for classification for RA may vary greatly from self-limiting disease, to mild, to severe form of the disease (Table 29-2). When faced with a patient with polyarthritis, the physician must keep in mind the many other conditions resembling RA. It is important to distinguish such disorders from RA as early as possible, because the correct and timely diagnosis of RA is fundamental to the application of optimal management.

III. **EXTRA-ARTICULAR MANIFESTATIONS.** In the past, extra-articular disease manifestations occurred in 40% of patients during the course of the disease. More recently, in the setting of more aggressive treatment early in the course of RA, these have become much less common.

   A. **Subcutaneous nodules** appear in 5% to 10% of seropositive patients. Nodules develop most commonly on pressure areas, including the elbows, finger joints, ischial

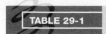

TABLE 29-1	Criteria for the Classification of Rheumatoid Arthritis

Criterion	Definition
Morning stiffness	Morning stiffness in and around the joints lasting at least 1 h before maximal improvement
Arthritis of three or more joint areas	At least three joint areas simultaneously have had soft tissue swelling or fluid observed by a physician. The 14 possible areas are right or left PIP, MCP, wrist, elbow, knee, ankle, and MTP joints
Arthritis of hand joints	At least one area swollen in a wrist, MCP, or PIP joint
Symmetric arthritis	Simultaneous involvement of the same joint areas on both sites of the body
Rheumatoid nodules	Subcutaneous nodules, over bony prominences, or extensor surfaces, or in juxta-articular regions, observed by a physician
Serum rheumatoid factor	Demonstration of abnormal amounts of serum rheumatoid factor by any method for which the result has been positive for <5% of normal control subjects
Radiographic changes	Radiographic changes typical of rheumatoid arthritis on posteroanterior hand and wrist radiographs

MCP, metacarpophalangeal; MTP, metatarsophalangeal; PIP, proximal interphalangeal.

and sacral prominences, occipital scalp, and Achilles tendon and are associated with active and more severe disease. Nodules may regress during treatment with disease-modifying drugs [disease-modifying antirheumatic drugs (DMARDs)], usually as RA improves. Paradoxically, methotrexate treatment may result in an increase in nodules, particularly over finger tendons, despite improvement in the overall disease activity. Capillary nailfold infarcts may be seen if rheumatoid vasculitis develops.

   B. Eye involvement. Keratoconjunctivitis sicca (dry eyes) is the most common eye abnormality, but scleritis and scleromalacia perforans may be associated with extensive disease activity.

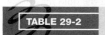

TABLE 29-2	Mild, Moderate, and Severe Rheumatoid Arthritis

Mild disease
- Fewer than 10 actively inflamed joints
- No impairment of daily activities
- No radiographic evidence of erosions or joint space narrowing
- No joint deformities
- No extra-articular manifestation

Moderate disease
- 10–15 actively inflamed joints
- Symptomatic fatigue or some limitations of daily activities
- Radiologic evidence of erosions or joint space narrowing
- Mild/moderate joint deformities
- Mild extra-articular manifestations (e.g., anemia of chronic disease and nodules)

Severe disease
- More than 15 actively inflamed joints
- Significant impairment of daily activities
- Significant joint destruction and/or need for surgery
- Serious extra-articular manifestation (e.g., vasculitis)

C. Pulmonary involvement. Pleurisy and pleural effusions may be bilateral in 25% of patients. Parenchymal pulmonary nodules, diffuse interstitial pulmonary fibrosis and bronchiolitis obliterans, and organizing pneumonia are associated with severe active disease. Upper airway obstruction in RA may be caused by inflammation of the cricoarytenoid joint and presents with sore throat, hoarseness, dysphagia, pain with speech, sensation of a foreign body in the throat, and difficulty with the inspiratory phase of respiration.

D. Cardiac manifestations include pericarditis, myocarditis, valvulitis, nodule formation with arrhythmia, amyloidosis, and vasculitis. More than 40% of patients with RA have premature atherosclerosis.

E. Peripheral neuropathy and central nervous system disease can be manifestations of rheumatoid vasculitis.

F. Felty's syndrome (granulocytopenia, splenomegaly, and recurrent infection) and **Sjögren's syndrome** may coexist with RA and often occur in patients with active, systemic disease.

G. A rare but potentially organ-threatening and life-threatening polyarteritis nodosa (PAN)-like systemic vasculitis called RA vasculitis or malignant RA is occasionally seen in patients with high serum titers of RF and nodules.

H. Adult-onset Still's disease. Adult-onset Still's disease is a systemic inflammatory disorder characterized by quotidian, spiking fevers typically accompanied by a salmon-colored evanescent rash, arthritis, and multiorgan involvement.

   1. Etiopathogenesis. Although the etiology of the disease is not known, various viruses [rubella, mumps, cytomegalovirus (CMV), Epstein-Barr virus (EBV), human herpesvirus 6 (HHV6)] and bacteria (*Mycoplasma pneumoniae, Chlamydia pneumoniae,* and *Yersinia enterocolitica*) have been suggested as triggers of the disease in genetically susceptible individuals. A number of cytokines have been suggested to be important mediators in this condition such as IL-18, IFN-γ, IL-1, TNF-α, and IL-6.

   2. Clinical manifestations. Transient quotidian fever accompanied by an evanescent, salmon-pink maculopapular eruption is the hallmark of the disease. Arthralgias and arthritis are found in 65% to 100% of patients. Arthritis is typically symmetrical and polyarticular and can lead to wrist fusion. Most frequently affected joints are the knees, wrists, and ankles. Hepatomegaly and abnormalities in liver function tests (LFTs), are seen in 50% to 75% of patients, and reflect inflammatory cell infiltration of the liver. Other disease manifestations include: lymphadenopathy, splenomegaly, pleuritis, pericarditis, interstitial nephritis, amyloidosis, cranial nerve palsies, aseptic meningitis, and seizures.

   3. Laboratory tests. There is no diagnostic test for adult-onset Still's disease. The presence of a significant leukocytosis and marked elevation of acute phase reactants [erythrocyte sedimentation rate (ESR) and C-reactive protein (CRP)] in the absence of antinuclear antibody (ANA) and RF are characteristic laboratory findings of the disease. Serum ferritin levels are also high.

   4. Treatment. Corticosteroids and nonsteroidal anti-inflammatory drugs (NSAIDs) are the mainstay therapy. DMARDs such as methotrexate, cyclosporine A, azathioprine, hydroxychloroquine, gold, and cyclophosphamide have been used with mixed results. Lately, the use of anti-TNF agents and an IL-1 receptor antagonist (IL-1ra) have been proved to be effective in cases refractory to standard therapy (NSAIDs, corticosteroids, and/or methotrexate).

DIAGNOSTIC INVESTIGATIONS

I. LABORATORY TESTS. Laboratory data can be used to support the diagnosis of RA and to monitor the course of the illness and its response to treatment.

A. Anemia and thrombocytosis are the most common abnormalities in complete blood counts of patients with RA. The white blood count is usually normal or mildly elevated.

B. The **ESR and CRP** are good indicators of the state of inflammation and can be used to monitor the response to treatment. However, they are very nonspecific markers of inflammation and increases in either ESR or CRP can occur in the setting of infections, malignancy, and tissue injury.

C. RF is detected in the serum of 75% to 80% of patients with RA. RF is not specific to RA and can be seen in other conditions such as hepatitis, endocarditis, as well as other rheumatic diseases. Further, approximately 20% of patients with RA test negative for RF (and are therefore called "seronegative"). In contrast to RF, anti-CCP antibodies show high specificity for RA (approximately 95%) and have been shown to predict worse outcomes in some studies. Anti-CCP antibodies are increasingly used for diagnostic and prognostic purposes.

II. IMAGING STUDIES. Baseline x-rays of the hands and feet are important in defining the severity of the RA and in determining the therapeutic approach. These should be repeated in 6-month to 1-year intervals to determine progression of the disease. Important radiographic findings in RA are: symmetric polyarticular disease of synovial joints of the appendicular skeleton, fusiform soft tissue swelling, regional or periarticular osteoporosis, marginal and central osseous erosions and cysts, and diffuse loss of joint space. Magnetic resonance imaging (MRI) and ultrasonography can reveal erosions 1 year earlier than plain x-rays but are not routinely performed as a screening test because of the imaging cost involved.

DIFFERENTIAL DIAGNOSIS

Other diseases must be excluded before the diagnosis of RA is made. A careful clinical examination is a powerful diagnostic tool. RA is a symmetrical polyarthritis involving the small joints of the hands and feet, wrists, elbows, shoulders, hips, knees, and ankles. A positive RF and radiographic presence of bone erosions make diagnoses other than RA unlikely. A number of other systemic connective tissue diseases and systemic infections can present in a similar clinical manner and should be excluded.

I. SLE can present with a symmetric polyarthritis indistinguishable from RA. The absence of characteristic skin rashes, mucosal ulcers, cytopenias, nephritis, and specific serologic tests effectively exclude SLE. Bone erosions are not usually seen in SLE, although a "Rhupus" overlap syndrome characterized by joint erosions and positive lupus serologies (i.e., anti-dsDNA antibodies) may occur.

II. Scleroderma, polymyositis/dermatomyositis, and systemic vasculitides, such as PAN and Wegener's granulomatosis, can present with a polyarthritis, but they commonly have or will develop their classic disease manifestations such as Raynaud's phenomenon, tight skin, and esophageal dysmotility with scleroderma; muscle weakness, Gottron's papules, and the heliotrope rash with polymyositis/dermatomyositis; fever, mononeuritis multiplex, and skin lesions with PAN; and a triad of sinus, lung, and kidney disease with Wegener's granulomatosis.

III. Polymyalgia rheumatica (PMR) may be difficult to differentiate from elderly-onset RA because the latter can have prominent proximal joint symptoms and a negative RF test. Some rheumatologists believe that late-onset RA and PMR are the same disorder and both respond to low-dose steroids. The presence of the signs and symptoms of giant cell arteritis supports the diagnosis of polymyalgia rheumatica.

IV. The **spondyloarthropathies** such as psoriatic arthritis, reactive arthritis, and the arthritis associated with inflammatory bowel disease usually present as asymmetrical mono- or oligoarthritis of the large joints, and involvement of the sacroiliac joint and low back. Psoriatic arthritis can frequently involve the small joints of the hands, but the involvement is usually asymmetric and it can be differentiated from RA by its prominent distal interphalangeal (DIP) joint involvement. Other characteristic manifestations of these disorders such as psoriatic skin lesions, urethritis, keratoderma blennorrhagicum, and enthesitis (prominent inflammation at the sites of tendon and ligament insertions) help in establishing the diagnosis. It is particularly important to differentiate seronegative RA from the spondyloarthropathies, which are also negative for RF.

V. Polyarticular gout or pseudogout can be misdiagnosed as RA. A history of acute episodes of monarticular inflammation, an elevated serum uric acid level and the finding of characteristic crystals in synovial fluid on polarizing microscopy go to make the definitive diagnosis.

VI. **Osteoarthritis** itself can easily be differentiated from RA by its late age of onset, involvement of the DIP and PIP joints, monoarticular involvement of a single hip or knee, the propensity to involve the neck and low back, and the absence of joint inflammation and constitutional symptoms.

VII. **INFECTIOUS ARTHRITIS**

A. Viral arthritides, such as rubella or rubella vaccine-induced arthritis, hepatitis B, hepatitis C as part of the RF-positive mixed cryoglobulinemia, and parvovirus B19, may often present as a self-limited symmetric polyarthritis usually lasting from days to a few months. Careful history of recent exposure and specific serologic tests establish the diagnosis.

B. Bacterial arthritis is usually monoarticular, although disseminated gonococcal disease may be characterized by a migratory polyarthritis. Whipple's disease may present as a symmetric, migratory, peripheral, seronegative polyarthritis, with gastrointestinal manifestations, and lymphadenopathy occurring simultaneously with the polyarthritis or preceding it by a wide interval.

C. Lyme disease rarely presents in an RA-like fashion. In its early phase, it can manifest by migratory polyarthralgias but not frank arthritis. A recurrent mono- or oligoarticular arthritis of large joints is characteristic of late, tertiary Lyme disease.

 TREATMENT

The goal in managing RA is to achieve remission, because RA is an aggressive disease that adversely alters and shortens the patient's life. During the last 10 years, improved understanding of the pathophysiology of RA has led to several key changes in the approach to therapy.

I. Early diagnosis and treatment are important. Joint damage occurs early in the course of the disease; 30% of patients have radiographic evidence of bony erosions at the time of diagnosis, and its proportion increases to 60% by 2 years. Initiation of treatment with DMARDs within 3 months of the diagnosis of RA is crucial.

II. The use of DMARDs in combinations is highly effective, particularly anti-TNF medications with methotrexate.

III. Agents that target cytokines such as TNF-α and IL-1 are highly effective in most patients.

IV. The assessment of treatment outcomes should include an analysis and control of coexisting illnesses, such as osteoporosis and cardiovascular disease.

 MEDICATIONS THAT ARE USED TO TREAT RHEUMATOID ARTHRITIS

Medications are divided into three main classes: NSAIDs, corticosteroids, and DMARDs (traditional, synthetic, and biologic).

I. **NSAIDs** are particularly helpful at any time during the course of the disease because they provide partial relief of pain and stiffness. NSAIDs suppress inflammation but do not slow the progression of the disease; therefore, in long-term care NSAIDs should be used together with DMARDs.

A. **Mechanism of action.** NSAIDs interfere with the metabolism of arachidonic acid released from cellular membrane phospholipids in response to inflammatory stimuli. They prevent the formation of proinflammatory prostaglandins and other lipid mediators that are important in the initial phase of the inflammatory reaction.

B. **The main toxicities of NSAIDs** relate to inhibition of prostaglandin production in the gastric mucosa and kidney, tissues where prostaglandins play important physiologic roles. Long-term administration of NSAIDs may result in gastrointestinal ulcer, perforation, hemorrhage, and arterial hypertension. The risk of these complications increases with old age, corticosteroid use, and a history of peptic ulcer disease.

C. Patients vary greatly with regard to favorable response or adverse effects to specific drugs. It is common to try several NSAIDs before settling on a preferred agent. When making treatment decisions, it must be noted that it usually takes 3 weeks for an NSAID to optimally work and 3 to 4 days for any effectiveness to wane on withdrawal of the NSAID.

D. The efficacy of the COX-2 inhibitor celecoxit is no better than that of the older and less expensive NSAIDs. Both traditional NSAIDs and COX-2 inhibitors have been associated with increased fluid retention, exacerbation of hypertension, and impairment of renal function in susceptible individuals. Thrombotic events such as myocardial infarctions and strokes have been reported in patients who are taking COX-2 inhibitors and traditional NSAIDs. This is particularly important in patients with RA who have an increased propensity for premature atherosclerosis due to the spillover effects of its systemic inflammation on blood vessels. Cost-benefit decisions must be carefully made with all medications but particularly with this group of drugs.

II. Corticosteroids are potent suppressors of the inflammatory response in RA but their dose-dependent side effects are major and familiar to all clinicians. There still is controversy about if, when, and how these compounds should be used to treat RA. Data from recent and older trials have clearly established that corticosteroids decrease the progression of RA as detected radiographically. What is agreed upon is the knowledge that the "double-edged sword" of these medications demands that if their use is absolutely indicated they must be used in the lowest dose and for the shortest period of time possible.

A. Mechanism of action. The anti-inflammatory effects of corticosteroids are mediated through their action on nearly all components of the immune and inflammatory systems, as well as many cellular targets of the immune system. Corticosteroids inhibit the production of proinflammatory cytokines, such as TNF-α, IL-1, IL-2 by monocytes/macrophages and lymphocytes. They interfere with the signal transduction pathway of interferons and induce apoptosis of lymphocytes. They inhibit lymphocyte proliferation and delayed-type hypersensitivity by interfering with antigen presentation. Corticosteroids inhibit phospholipase A_2 and block the production of proinflammatory prostaglandins, leukotrienes, and reactive oxygen intermediates.

B. Corticosteroids in low doses (e.g., <10 mg of prednisone/daily) are used to treat 30% to 60% of the patients, either in short courses or in the long term. In moderate to severe disease, intramuscular methylprednisolone (Depo-Medrol) 120 mg or short 4-day courses of daily prednisone beginning at 20 mg will reset the inflammatory process and allow other drugs to work faster and better. This is particularly useful in the window period that is normally required before a favorable therapeutic effect of DMARD therapy is achieved (i.e., weeks to months).

C. Minipulses of intravenous methylprednisolone (Solu-Medrol) (250 mg to 1,000 mg intravenously daily for 1 to 3 days) can be used for severe disease that is refractory to more conventional treatment or in patients with visceral involvement or RA vasculitis.

D. Intra-articular corticosteroid injections [e.g., methylprednisolone (Depo-Medrol) 10 to 80 mg, depending on the joint being treated] are often helpful in suppressing the inflammation in single joints that is resistant to systemic treatment. The possibility of infection should always be considered and excluded before the intra-articular corticosteroid injection.

E. Predictable side effects of corticosteroids include thinning of the skin, cataract formation, osteoporosis, hypertension, and hyperlipidemia. The last three conditions may be preventable with aggressive management of osteoporosis and cardiovascular risk factors. All patients taking corticosteroids should receive supplemental calcium (1 to 1.5 g/day) and vitamin D_3 (800 IU/day). Bisphosphonates are very effective in reducing vertebral fractures in patients taking corticosteroids and should be prescribed for patients who have low bone density. Other side effects include infection, diabetes, mood changes, myopathy, and osteonecrosis.

III. **Methotrexate** has been clearly identified in several clinical trials as the synthetic DMARD that is most likely to induce a long-term response. It has demonstrated efficacy and durability, a long-term track record of acceptable toxicity, and low cost. It has been shown that patients with RA who have been treated with methotrexate have a significantly lower mortality rate than those who have not been treated with methotrexate.

   A. Mechanism of action. Methotrexate is a dihydrofolate reductase inhibitor, a critical enzyme in the purine biosynthesis pathway, which is vital for the survival of proliferating cells. Methotrexate reduces polymorphonuclear cell chemotaxis, decreases the production of IL-1 and IL-2, and increases the release of adenosine that has anti-inflammatory actions.

   B. The **initial dose** of methotrexate is 7.5 mg to 10 mg/week; however, the dose at which most patients demonstrate a well-defined clinical response ranges between 20 and 30 mg/week, which is achieved over a 1- to 2-month period. Concomitant administration of folic acid (1 to 3 mg/day) or folinic acid (2.5 to 5 mg given 12 to 24 hours after methotrexate) significantly decreases many toxic effects without a measurable decrease in efficacy and has improved the tolerability of methotrexate.

   C. Bioavailability of methotrexate is less predictable after oral administration but is above 90% if given subcutaneously or intramuscularly. Therefore, if oral methotrexate produces a suboptimal response or gastrointestinal intolerance, a trial of subcutaneous or intramuscular methotrexate is indicated.

   D. Side effects of methotrexate include gastrointestinal intolerance, liver inflammation or scarring, oral ulcers, and rashes, many of which can be prevented by the concomitant administration of folic or folinic acid. More serious toxicities include myelosuppression and hepatotoxicity, and so complete blood counts and serum liver function tests (LFT) need to be monitored every 4 to 6 weeks. Patients with pre-existing liver abnormalities or a history of heavy alcohol intake or hepatitis virus infections should not be treated with methotrexate. Baseline or follow-up liver biopsies are not recommended, unless persistent or recurrent elevations of levels of transaminases or decreases in albumin occur on the LFT panel. Methotrexate treatment has rarely been associated with the development of non-Hodgkin's B-cell lymphomas, some of which resolve when methotrexate is stopped.

   E. Teratogenicity and induction of abortion. Methotrexate must be discontinued 3 months prior to a planned pregnancy. Methotrexate is an abortifacient, and women taking it should be made aware of this fact and counseled regarding the need to use appropriate birth control techniques while taking this medication. Men should conform to the same period of 3 months because of the potential effect of methotrexate upon sperm function and counts.

IV. **Leflunomide (Arava)** has been shown to have similar efficacy to sulfasalazine or moderate-dose methotrexate in the treatment of RA in controlled clinical trials. As compared with placebo, leflunomide slowed progression, as measured radiographically, over a period of 6 to 12 months. Leflunomide can be used as monotherapy or in combination therapy with methotrexate in the treatment of RA.

   A. Mechanism of action. Leflunomide is a competitive inhibitor of dihydroorotate dehydrogenase, the rate-limiting enzyme for the *de novo* synthesis of pyrimidines. It targets activated lymphocytes because they are dependent on the *de novo* synthesis of pyrimidines. *In vitro* it has been shown to interfere with inflammatory and cytokine signal transduction pathways.

   B. Leflunomide is a prodrug that, after oral administration, undergoes rapid chemical conversion to its primary active metabolite, A77 1726, which accounts for more than 95% of the levels of the drug in the circulation. This metabolite is highly protein-bound and has a long half-life of 15 to 18 days. Therefore, without a loading dose, it may take as long as 2 months to achieve steady-state concentrations. Because of its extensive enterohepatic recirculation, it may take up to 2 years for the amount of drug in the plasma to decrease to an undetectable level. Renal excretion appears to be limited, and the dose needs no adjustment in patients with decreased renal function.

   C. Because of its complex pharmacokinetics, a loading dose of 100 mg/day for 3 days is recommended at initiation of treatment. The maintenance dose is 20 mg/day. Leflunomide inhibits cytochrome P-450 2C9 (CYP2C9) *in vitro*, and therefore may increase the anticoagulant activity of warfarin. Rifampin raises the concentration of the active metabolite of leflunomide by 40% and the dose may have to be adjusted. Leflunomide reduces serum uric acid concentrations in treated patients by increasing renal urate excretion.

D. **The most important side effects** of leflunomide are hepatic. Patients with pre-existing liver abnormalities or a history of heavy alcohol intake or hepatitis virus infections should not be treated with leflunomide. The combination of leflunomide with methotrexate increases the risk of hepatotoxicity, demanding close monitoring of liver function. Other reported side effects include weight loss, diarrhea that can be severe and lead to hyponatremia, reversible alopecia, pancytopenia, hypertension, and peripheral neuropathy.

E. Preclinical studies indicated that leflunomide causes fetal death or is teratogenic; therefore, women of child-bearing potential must have a negative pregnancy test before beginning treatment with leflunomide and must use reliable contraception. Because of the long half-life of the drug, discontinuing treatment before conception is inadequate. An elimination protocol of oral cholestyramine, 8 g three times daily (daily is probably best or three times a day if that is appropriate) for 11 days, is recommended before conception.

V. **Sulfasalazine (Asulfadine)** was the first DMARD that was developed specifically to treat RA and has an efficacy similar to that of methotrexate. Sulfasalazine is the most commonly used initial DMARD in Europe and in the United States as part of a combination DMARD therapy.

A. The mechanism of action is unknown, but possibilities include inhibition of prostaglandin production, ability to modify proreactive oxygen species released from activated macrophages, reduction of activated circulatory lymphocytes, and effects on the metabolism of folic acid and adenosine.

B. The initial dose of sulfasalazine is 500 mg/day given with breakfast. The dose is then raised by 500 mg/week after a complete blood count and LFTs are checked and record normal results. The optimal dose range is between 2 and 3 g/day, usually taken as 1,000 to 1,500 mg with breakfast and dinner. Sulfasalazine is usually given as part of a combination treatment with methotrexate or with methotrexate and hydroxychloroquine.

C. The most common **side effects** are gastrointestinal, mainly nausea and vomiting. This problem is usually avoided with the use of enteric-coated tablets of sulfasalazine, and administration of the drug with meals. A serious side effect is leukopenia and granulocytopenia, both occurring as idiosyncratic reactions. Therefore, after the initial monitoring for dosing, complete blood counts and differential counts are repeated at the end of the first month and then every 6 to 8 weeks along with estimation of serum levels of aspartate aminotransferase (AST) and alanine aminotransferase (ALT).

VI. **Hydroxychloroquine (Plaquenil)** is the least effective slow-acting antimalarial drug that is most commonly used as part of combination DMARD therapy.

A. Its mechanism of action is probably related to accumulation of the drug in the acid vesicular lysosomal system of mononuclear cells, granulocytes, and fibroblasts. In macrophages, antimalarials may inhibit antigen presentation and IL-1 release.

B. Hydroxychloroquine is used mainly in combination with methotrexate in patients with RA. The initial dose is 200 mg/day and the recommended maintenance dose is 200 mg twice daily. Six weeks to 6 months of therapy may be required before a therapeutic effect is evident.

C. The most common side effects of hydroxychloroquine are allergic skin rashes and gastrointestinal disturbances. Eye toxicity because of accumulation of the drug in the retina is the most serious adverse effect. Ophthalmologic evaluation before the start of the treatment and every 6 months thereafter helps to prevent visual loss by detecting early disease while in a reversible stage. Although it is traditionally contraindicated in pregnancy, many years of experience in its use in patients of SLE suggest that it is safe during this period.

VII. **Minocycline** has been proven in controlled clinical trials to be moderately effective in the treatment of RA. The mechanism by which minocycline works is incompletely understood but probably involves immunomodulation, suppression of matrix metalloproteinases (MMPs), and suppression of nonspecific infections that would otherwise stimulate inflammatory cytokine production. It is used alone at a dose of 100 mg twice daily or as part of a combination DMARD therapy in RA. It should be avoided in pregnant women as it can cause dizziness and photosensitivity. Minocycline is not approved by the United States Food and Drug Administration (FDA) for the treatment of RA.

VIII. TNF-α ANTAGONISTS. Three biologic products that inhibit the actions of TNF-α (infliximab, etanercept, and adalimumab) are now available to treat RA. Only infliximab needs to be used in combination with methotrexate because without the combination, antibodies to the mouse component of the drug will decrease its effectiveness. While the other two anti-TNFs do not need to be used along with methotrexate, their effectiveness in improving function and rectifying joint damage is significantly better when they are used in combination with methotrexate.

   While uniquely effective in RA, all anti-TNF medications cost approximately $13,000/year. Higher costs will exist at higher doses, some of which may have to be absorbed by the patient and not the insurance company. Most insurance companies will pay for these drugs but only after a patient has failed to respond to or developed side effects while taking full doses (25 mg/week) of methotrexate or other DMARDs.

   These biologic agents seem to work in only 70% of patients. However, a switch to an alternative anti-TNF medication will likely yield a clinical response.

A. Infliximab (Remicade) is a chimeric IgG1 anti-TNF-α antibody containing the antigen-binding region of the mouse antibody (one-fourth of the molecule) and the constant region of the human antibody. It binds both soluble and membrane-bound TNF-α with high affinity, impairing the binding of TNF-α to its receptor. Infliximab also kills cells that express TNF-α through antibody-dependent and complement-dependent cytotoxicity. Infliximab is given as a 2-hour intravenous infusion of three loading doses of 3 mg/kg at week 1, 2 weeks later and at week 6, followed by maintenance dosing every 8 weeks in combination with methotrexate. Patients who do not have an adequate response or who have an initial response followed by a relapse may have a better response either if the interval between infusions is decreased gradually to every 4 weeks or if the dose is increased. Such dose adjustment may eventually bring the regimen to 10 mg/kg every 4 weeks.

B. Etanercept (Enbrel) is a soluble TNF-receptor fusion protein composed of two dimers, each with an extracellular, ligand-binding portion of the higher affinity type 2 TNF receptor (p75) linked to the Fc portion of human IgG1. This fusion protein binds both TNF-α and TNF-β, thereby preventing each from interacting with its respective receptors. Etanercept is given subcutaneously once (50 mg) or twice (25 mg) weekly, either as monotherapy or in combination treatment with methotrexate.

C. Adalimumab (Humira) is a recombinant human IgG1 monoclonal antibody that binds to human TNF-α with high affinity, both impairing cytokine binding to its receptors and lysing cells that express TNF-α on their surface. Adalimumab is given subcutaneously at a dose of 40 mg every other week and the dose can be increased to weekly. Adalimumab appears to have additive effects when used with methotrexate.

D. Adverse effects of anti-TNF medications

   1. Infections. Serious bacterial infections, tuberculosis, atypical mycobacterial infection, aspergillosis, histoplasmosis, and other opportunistic infections have been reported in patients treated with TNF antagonists. Tuberculosis has been reported in association with all TNF antagonists and most often arises from the reactivation of latent infection and usually occurs within the first 2 to 5 months of treatment. Extrapulmonary and disseminated disease is common, and atypical presentations may lead to delayed diagnosis and increased morbidity. All patients should be screened with a purified protein derivative (PPD) test, and if positive followed by chest x-ray for latent tuberculosis before anti-TNF therapy is begun. If the PPD is positive and the chest x-ray normal, the anti-TNF medication can be given, but isoniazid (INH) 300 mg and vitamin B_6 50 mg should be given in combination for a period of 9 months. All anti-TNF medication should be withheld during upper respiratory tract or other common infections and then started again after the problem has cleared and/or after antibiotics have been stopped. Because of the role of TNF in preventing or controlling skin infections, the infections and ulcers of the skin should be cleared before the institution of these anti-TNF medications. Episodes of septicemia probably reflect a major breakdown in the ability of the immune system to control infections while on anti-TNFs and reinstitution of this drug may be risky. Anti-TNFs are usually withheld 1 to 2 weeks before surgery and then started again 1 to 2 weeks after the wound is clean and healing.

2. **Lymphoma** of the non-Hodgkin's large B-cell type has been reported in association with all three TNF antagonists. Whether or not there is a causal relation is debated because there is a tenfold increase in these types of lymphoma in RA patients not treated with anti-TNFs. Apart from lymphoma, the incidence of cancer is not significantly altered.

3. **Autoantibodies.** Antinuclear antibodies and antibodies to double-stranded DNA have been reported to develop in patients treated with all three available TNF antagonists, especially when given along with leflunomide. However, drug-induced lupus is rare. Antibodies against the biologic agents have been reported to develop with all three TNF antagonists and decrease their efficacy over time. The concomitant use of methotrexate with infliximab and adalimumab decreases the formation of these antibodies significantly.

4. **Multiple sclerosis.** Exacerbation of previously quiescent multiple sclerosis and new-onset demyelinating neurologic disease have been reported. The range of symptoms included paresthesias, optic neuritis, and confusion. TNF antagonists should be avoided in patients with any demyelinating disorder and therapy should be discontinued if such an illness develops.

5. **Injection reactions.** Minor redness and itching at the injection site, lasting a few days, are common among patients who receive etanercept and adalimumab. Symptoms, most often headache and nausea, occur in 20% of patients during the infusion of infliximab and appear to be controllable with the use of antihistamines or by slowing the infusion rate. Symptoms suggestive of an immediate hypersensitivity response, such as urticaria or bronchospasm, occur in 2% of patients and may demand higher doses of steroids. Serious anaphylaxis is uncommon but has been described in patients with Crohn's disease who were treated with infliximab.

6. **Abnormal LFT and cytopenias** demand an every 6-weekly blood test for screening.

IX. **IL-1ra (Anakinra)** is a recombinant protein that targets the type I IL-1 receptor that is expressed in many tissues. IL-1ra is a natural IL-1 inhibitor that competes for binding to IL-1 receptors. Anakinra alone or in combination with methotrexate has been shown to be more effective than placebo in the treatment of RA and may be useful in patients who have no response to or are unable to tolerate methotrexate, leflunomide, or TNF antagonists. This medication has been much less effective than the anti-TNFs and should never be used along with anti-TNFs because of an increased risk of infection.

A. Daily injections are required because of the short half-life of anakinra. It is excreted predominantly through the kidneys; therefore, dose adjustment is required in patients with impaired kidney function. Hemodialysis and peritoneal dialysis do not appear to remove substantial amounts of anakinra.

B. The most common adverse event is dose-dependent skin irritation at the injection site. Most reactions appear to be mild, and resolve within a few weeks. The risk of infections, primarily bacterial, appears to be increased. No opportunistic infections were observed in clinical trials. Reversible neutropenia and thrombocytopenia have been reported and therefore monitoring the complete blood count is recommended.

NEW BIOLOGIC TREATMENTS FOR RHEUMATOID ARTHRITIS

Treatments for RA continue to advance rapidly, and many new drugs are under investigation. Some of them have shown promising results in phase I/II/III clinical trials. These include:

I. **RITUXIMAB (RITUXAN).** This chimeric monoclonal antibody against the CD 20 molecule on B lymphocytes has been very effective in the treatment of refractory, B cell, non-Hodgkin's lymphomas. In view of the newly appreciated, important role of B lymphocytes in the pathogenesis of RA, rituximab, along with methotrexate, has now been used with clinical efficacy in RA patients unresponsive to methotrexate alone. It causes B cell depletion for more than 6 months but has not been associated with significant side effects in phase II studies. The drug is administered intravenously. The optimal dose, treatment schedule, and need for concomitant use of methotrexate and steroids remain to be defined.

II. **CTLA4-Ig or abatacept (Orencia)** is a fully humanized biologic agent that blocks the activation of T lymphocytes and their downstream proinflammatory effects in RA. It has been shown, in phase III studies, to have significantly positive clinical and radiologic effects in RA patients unresponsive to methotrexate. Its dose will likely be 10 mg/kg given intravenously initially for three infusions administered every 2 weeks and followed by monthly treatments thereafter. When used alone or with methotrexate, it has a good safety profile but when given along with anti-TNF medications, it is associated with unacceptably high levels of infections.

III. **ANTI-IL6.** How these drugs will eventually fit into the armamentarium of RA will remain to be seen. However, the introduction of additional effective therapies for RA will improve the outlook for patients since even with the range of therapies currently available, some patients still have poorly or incompletely controlled disease.

 TREATMENT STRATEGY IN RHEUMATOID ARTHRITIS

Establishing a diagnosis as early as possible and then starting DMARD therapy is the foundation for successful treatment of patients with RA (Table 29-3).

I.   Most rheumatologists select methotrexate at a dose of 7.5 to 15 mg given orally once a week as the initial therapy for most patients. If patients continue to have active disease (i.e., lack of 80% in clinical improvement), the dose should be increased in 5 mg increments every 2 weeks or a month, to reach 20 to 30 mg/week. If patients continue to have active disease despite optimal methotrexate therapy, other DMARDs should be added. Clinical trials have shown that TNF blockade with etanercept in patients with early RA is equally effective to methotrexate in controlling the disease at 1 year, but etanercept was more effective in rapidly suppressing disease activity.

II. Patients with inadequate response after 2 to 3 months of methotrexate at a dose of 20 to 30 mg/week should be given another DMARD in addition to methotrexate. The most economic initial choice is the addition of sulfasalazine, hydroxychloroquine, or both. If active disease persists after 3 months of these DMARD combinations, leflunomide or a TNF antagonist should be added to methotrexate.

III. Clinical outcomes should be defined by the improvements in the number and severity of inflamed joints, the functional status of the patient, employing the HAQ (see Appendix C), and follow-up imaging as indicated (i.e., plain x-rays, ultrasonography, or MRI).

IV. Treatment of risk factors for atherosclerosis such as hypertension, lipid abnormalities, obesity, smoking, and hyperhomocysteinemia plays an important role. Patients with RA should be treated like diabetics regarding risk of premature atherosclerosis and enteric-coated baby aspirin is appropriate.

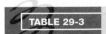 **TABLE 29-3**   **Optimizing Treatment in Rheumatoid Arthritis**

Make an early diagnosis
Start DMARD therapy within 3 mo after onset of symptoms
Aim for remission and the attainment of a "no evidence of disease" state in all patients, employing an aggressive therapeutic approach
Use corticosteroids as a "bridge" to effective DMARD therapy
Recognize and treat coexisting illnesses

DMARD, disease-modifying antirheumatic drugs.

SURGICAL THERAPY

In general, the main goals of surgery in RA are to alleviate pain, preserve function, and restore function (see Chapters 59 and 60). The frequency of joint replacement surgery in RA has profoundly decreased over the past 20 years, mostly because of the early, aggressive treatment approach to this disease. Spinal fusion for treatment of cervical instability is the one procedure accompanied by the greatest sense of urgency and is an example of surgery that can prevent loss of function and, possibly, death.

 NONPHARMACOLOGIC THERAPY AND REHABILITATION

A number of nonpharmacologic and physical/occupational therapy approaches can enhance the benefit of medical and surgical therapies. The primary goals of these therapies include pain control, preservation of function, joint protection, and psychologic well-being.

Many nonpharmacologic modalities are available for palliation, including heat and ultrasound massage for relief of stiffness and spasm, cold for reduction of inflammation, and electrical nerve stimulation for management of chronic pain. Physical therapy including range of motion exercises and muscle strengthening is essential for preserving overall joint function. Psychotherapy can often help patients to live and cope with a chronic and physically demanding disease in a healthy and adaptive manner.

 PROGNOSIS

I.   Life span is shortened in RA, mainly because of premature atherosclerosis related to the persistence of inflammation and other cardiac risk factors. Therefore, optimal disease control must aim at "no evidence of disease (NED) or inflammation" along with avoidance of cardiac risk factors.

II. The long-term prognosis for patients with RA depends not only on how well their joint disease is treated but also on how well their coexisting illnesses are addressed. There are three coexisting conditions that have the greatest effect on morbidity and mortality in RA: infection (particularly pulmonary infection), osteoporosis, and cardiovascular disease.

   A. The clinician who is caring for patients with RA should be aware of the risk of infection. All patients should have yearly influenza vaccinations and should receive the pneumococcal vaccine at appropriate intervals. Live vaccines should be avoided in patients who are receiving immunosuppressive medications. Both clinicians and their patients with RA should be vigilant with regard to avoiding infections and to treating them early and aggressively. Stopping or withholding drug treatment during infections is critical.

   B. The incidence of osteoporosis is doubled in patients with RA, and baseline bone density studies should be performed in all patients, particularly in those who will receive corticosteroids. If osteoporosis is present bisphosphonate therapy, which is reported to decrease the risk of fracture by 70%, despite the coadministration of corticosteroids, should be used.

   C. Cardiovascular disease accounts for most of the excess mortality associated with RA. Risk factors for atherosclerosis should be aggressively sought and addressed. In particular, cessation of smoking is essential, since smoking has also been associated with increased severity of arthritis.

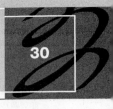

SYSTEMIC LUPUS ERYTHEMATOSUS

Jane E. Salmon and Robert P. Kimberly

30

$\mathcal{S}$ ystemic lupus erythematosus (SLE or lupus) is a multisystem disease with a spectrum of clinical manifestations and a variable course characterized by exacerbations and remissions. It is a uniquely complex illness both clinically and immunologically and no two individuals present in the same way. Lupus is marked by both humoral and cellular immunologic abnormalities, including multiple autoantibodies [e.g., anti-C1q, anti-N-methyl-D-aspartate (NMDA)] that may directly participate in tissue injury or may indirectly lead to tissue damage by activating Fc receptors and complement. Antinuclear antibodies (ANAs), especially those to native DNA, are common immunologic abnormalities found in the disease.

Identification and characterization of abnormal autoantibodies continue to be major areas of clinical and immunochemical interest. The development of sensitive laboratory tests for autoantibodies has enabled the recognition of milder forms of SLE, with a consequent change in both reported prevalence and prognosis. The broad clinical spectrum of SLE challenges the diagnostic and therapeutic acumen of the physician.

 ETIOPATHOGENESIS

I. **GENETICS.** The presence of a genetic component in SLE is supported by family studies.
   A. **Clinical disease.** Family members of patients with SLE are more likely to have lupus or some other connective tissue disease.
      1. The risk for development of SLE in a sibling of individuals affected by SLE, called the sibling risk ratio (λs), is approximately 20 times higher than that in the general population.
      2. Concordance of disease among monozygotic twin pairs may be as high as 50%. Fraternal twins, with a concordance rate of 2% to 5%, do not have a higher frequency of SLE than do other first-degree relatives.
      3. Asymptomatic (or healthy) family members are more likely to have a false-positive test result for syphilis, positive ANAs, antilymphocyte antibodies, and hypergammaglobulinemia.
   B. **Studies of major histocompatibility complex (MHC) genes**
      1. Lupus and lupuslike syndromes are associated with inherited abnormalities of the MHC class III genes for complement components (most commonly the C4-null allele, and also deficiencies of C2; deficiencies of other complement components are rare).
      2. Although the strength of the association varies by ethnicity, SLE is associated with the serologically determined MHC class II allo-antigens human leukocyte antigens (HLA)-DR2 and HLA-DR3. The association with HLA-DR2 reflects the DR2 allele DRB1*1501 in whites, DRB1*1502 in Asian populations, and the unique DRB1*1503 allele in African Americans. HLA-DR3 is primarily associated with patients with lupus having a northern European ancestry.
   C. **Non-MHC genes**
      1. Genetic variants of opsonins (mannose binding protein and C-reactive protein), opsonin receptors [complement receptors and immunoglobulin (Ig) receptors], lymphocyte cell surface and signaling molecules (PDCD1 and PTPN22), and cytokine genes [tumor necrosis factor-α (TNF-α) and interleukin-10] have been associated with SLE susceptibility.

2. Fcγ-receptors (FcγR) are important in immune complex clearance. Allelic variants of FcγR which differ in their capacities to bind IgG, alter the function of mononuclear phagocytes and thereby provide a mechanism of inherited differences in immune complex handling. The low IgG binding alleles of FcγR have been associated with increased risk for lupus nephritis.

3. Variants of PDCD1 and PTPN22 may be associated with lymphocyte hyperfunction.

II. IMMUNOLOGY

A. **Humoral immunity.** Hyperactivity of the humoral component of immunologic responsiveness is manifested by hypergammaglobulinemia, autoantibodies, and circulating immune complexes.

1. **Various autoantibodies** may contribute to tissue injury. Attempts to correlate specific clinical patterns of the disease with specific types of autoantibodies have been partially successful. The following provide examples:

   a. Anti-DNA antibodies have been found in renal glomerular lesions.

   b. Sicca syndrome with SLE has been associated with La (SS-B) antibodies.

   c. Ro (SS-A) and La antibodies have been associated with neonatal lupus, congenital complete heart block, and subacute cutaneous lupus.

   d. Positive result of lupus anticoagulant test and anticardiolipin antibodies are associated with thrombosis, thrombocytopenia, and fetal wastage.

   e. Although the titer of ANAs does not necessarily correlate with disease activity, the levels of anti-DNA antibodies may vary with clinical disease. Because results vary, this test cannot be used as the sole guide to therapy.

2. **Circulating immune complexes** are commonly found in active SLE and are often associated with **hypocomplementemia** measured as component proteins (C3 and C4) or hemolytic function (CH50). Immune complex deposits are found in many tissues. Isolated determinations of circulating complexes do not consistently correlate with disease activity. Sequential patterns of change may be of value in individual patients.

B. **Cellular immunity.** SLE is characterized by lymphopenia and often by monocytosis. The normal intricate immunoregulatory balance among cells is lost.

1. Anergy, evidenced by diminished delayed hypersensitivity skin testing reactions, is common.

2. Ig-producing B cells are hyperactive; perhaps reflecting enhanced stimulatory factors [e.g., BAFF/B-lymphocyte stimulator (BLyS)].

3. T-cell subsets are altered, and mononuclear phagocytes elaborate increased amounts of various cytokines. Circulating leukocytes show an mRNA expression profile suggesting interferon α stimulation, but the primary defect has not been identified.

C. **Provocative agents.** Although the etiologic agent(s) in SLE have not been identified, several factors may exacerbate the disease.

1. **Ultraviolet light.** Exposure to sunlight may precipitate either the onset or a flare of clinical disease, causing both dermatologic and systemic manifestations in about one-third of patients. Because complete avoidance of sunlight is impractical, patients should use sunscreens and should wear long-sleeved shirts, trousers rather than shorts, and wide-brimmed hats. Many effective sunscreens are available commercially; however, none of these can completely obviate the potential of significant exposure to sunlight to exacerbate SLE.

2. **Situational stresses.** Some patients may experience increased disease activity during periods of fatigue or emotional stress (e.g., when encountering school examinations or interpersonal conflict). The significance of such factors should not be overlooked, and such stress should be reduced as much as possible.

3. **Infection.** Viral infection has been suggested as an etiologic event in SLE. Although unproven as such, viral infection may provoke a flare of disease by an unknown mechanism, perhaps involving the triggering of tolllike receptors of the innate immune system and the eventual stimulation of the adaptive immune system by interferon α. Although vaccination provides exposure to foreign antigen, studies with influenza and pneumococcal vaccines suggest that such

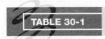

TABLE 30-1	Drugs Implicated in Drug-induced Lupuslike Syndrome

Anticonvulsants	■ Streptomycin	**Other drugs**
■ Carbamazepine[a]	■ Sulfonamides	■ Penicillamine[a]
■ Hydantoins[a]	■ Griseofulvin	■ Chlorpromazine[a]
■ Ethosuximide[a]	■ Nitrofurantoin	■ Phenylbutazone
■ Primidone	**Antiarrhythmics**	■ Thiazides
■ Trimethadione	■ Procainamide[a]	■ Oral contraceptive pills
Antihypertensives	■ Quinidine[a]	■ Levodopa
■ Hydralazine[a]	**β-Adrenergic blockers**	■ Lithium carbonate
■ Methyldopa[a]	■ Labetalol	■ HMG-CoA reductase
■ Captopril	■ Acebutolol	agents
Antibiotics	■ Pindolol	■ TNF-α inhibitors
■ Isoniazid[a]	**Antithyroidals**	
■ Sulfasalazine[a]	■ Propylthiouracil	
■ Penicillin	■ Methylthiouracil	
■ Tetracyclines		

[a]Association is well established.

vaccination provides protection without causing increased SLE disease activity. Specific antibody responses may be lower in patients with SLE, especially those on immunosuppressive agents, than in healthy subjects.

4. **Drugs.** Many drugs have been associated with the development of ANAs and, in some cases, a clinical lupuslike syndrome (Table 30-1); procainamide and hydralazine were the most commonly implicated, and now, minocycline and anti-TNF medications are increasing in significance. However, the potential to induce such serologic changes in patients without SLE does not preclude the use of these drugs in patients with SLE when clinically appropriate. Although most physicians prefer to avoid them if an alternative drug is available, the use of these drugs in SLE has not been associated with documented exacerbation of disease activity.

III. **PATHOLOGY.** Although no histologic feature is pathognomonic for SLE, several features are very suggestive: (a) fibrinoid necrosis and degeneration of blood vessels and connective tissue; (b) the hematoxylin body [the *in vivo* lupus erythematosus (LE) cell phenomenon]; (c) "onion skin" thickening of the arterioles of the spleen; and (d) Libman-Sacks verrucous endocarditis.

IV. **HISTOPATHOLOGY.** Routine histologic examination of tissue specimens reveals a broad range of findings.

A. **Skin biopsy** may demonstrate a leukocytoclastic angiitis, especially in palpable purpuric rash. The typical lupus rash usually shows epidermal thinning, liquefactive degeneration of the basal layer with dermal–epidermal junction disruption, and lymphocytic infiltration of the dermis. Rheumatoidlike nodules with palisading giant cells are uncommon, and panniculitis is rare.

B. **Synovium.** Synovial biopsies may show fibrinous villous synovitis. The presence of pannus formation or bone and cartilage erosions is rare.

C. **Muscle biopsies** usually show a nonspecific perivascular mononuclear infiltrate, but true muscle necrosis, as seen in polymyositis, can occur.

D. **Kidney.** The kidney has been the most intensively studied organ in SLE. The entire range of glomerulonephritis (membranous, mesangial, proliferative, etc.) is seen (Table 30-2). Crescentic and necrotizing vasculitic lesions may be found. Interstitial abnormalities are often present. No single renal lesion is diagnostic of SLE. Tubuloreticular structures are not restricted to SLE.

1. Renal biopsy provides one indicator of prognosis, characterizing patients with diffuse membranoproliferative lesions as having the poorest 5-year kidney survival (40% to 85% depending on the studies).

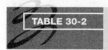

TABLE 30-2	The International Society of Nephrology (ISN)/Renal Pathology Society (RPS) Classification of Glomerulonephritis in Systemic Lupus Erythematosus (SLE) (Revised 2003)
Class I	Minimal mesangial LN
Class II	Mesangial proliferative LN
Class III	Focal LN[a]
Class IV	Diffuse segmental (IV-S) or global (IV-G) LN[b]
Class V	Membranous LN[c]
Class VI	Advancing sclerosing LN

Indicate the grade (mild, moderate, and severe) tubular atrophy, interstitial inflammation and fibrosis, severity of arteriosclerosis or other vascular lesions.
[a]Indicate the proportion of glomeruli with active and with sclerotic lesions.
[b]Indicate the proportion of glomeruli with fibrinoid necrosis and cellular crescents.
[c]Class V may occur in combination with class III or IV in which case both will be diagnosed.
LN, lupus nephritis.
Adapted from Weening JJ, D'Agati VD, Schwartz MM, et al. The classification of glomerulonephritis in systemic lupus erythematosus revisited. *J Am Soc Nephrol* 2004;15:241–50.

  2. Marked chronic changes (glomerular sclerosis, fibrous crescents, interstitial fibrosis, and tubular atrophy) indicate a poor prognosis.
  3. Recognition that the histologic class of the biopsy specimen may not be static and may either deteriorate or improve has emphasized the need for defining renal disease activity sequentially.
 E. **Central nervous system (CNS).** Multifocal cerebral cortical microinfarcts associated with microvascular injury are the most common abnormalities associated with neuropsychiatric SLE. CNS lesions usually reflect vascular occlusion as a consequence of noninflammatory vasculopathy, leukoagglutination, thrombosis, vasculitis (rarely), and antibody-mediated neuronal injury.
  1. Normal brain tissue is often present despite clinical abnormalities.
  2. Cytoid bodies, seen as white fluffy exudates on funduscopic examination, represent superficial retinal ischemia.
 F. **Other viscera**
  1. Other visceral pathologic findings include Libman-Sacks verrucous endocarditis with redundant mitral valvular leaflets and lengthened chordae tendineae, pulmonary fibrosis, and nonspecific pleural thickening.
  2. Necrotizing vasculitis may be present in the viscera and lead to secondary events, including bowel infarction, myocardial infarction, pancreatitis, and accelerated atherosclerosis.
  3. In the spleen, the concentric periarterial fibrosis of small arteries (onion skin lesions) may be an end-stage consequence of earlier vasculitis.
  4. Premature atherosclerosis can be found in coronary arteries and elsewhere.
V. **IMMUNOPATHOLOGY**
 A. **Skin.** Immunofluorescence shows deposits of Igs and complement at the dermal–epidermal junction (lupus band test) in 80% to 100% of lesional and 36% to 100% of nonlesional skin specimens.
  1. Attempts to correlate a positive lupus band test result with active SLE, or the presence of lupus nephritis have given inconsistent results. Positive lupus band test results are not specific for lupus
  2. Positive lupus band test is commonly associated with bullous pemphigoid and dermatitis herpetiformis (IgA). Dermal–epidermal immunofluorescence may also be seen in patients with rheumatoid arthritis, scleroderma, dermatomyositis, lepromatous leprosy, multiple sclerosis, cystic fibrosis, chronic active hepatitis, primary biliary cirrhosis, amyloidosis, and according to some reports, also in healthy individuals.

B. Kidney. Glomerular immunofluorescence to determine the distribution, pattern, and density of Ig, Ig class, and complement components does not appear to have prognostic or therapeutic significance. The presence of immunofluorescence for Ig or complement is not restricted to SLE; however, it is compatible with immune complex-mediated disease and its presence differentiates between SLE and ANCA-related disorders that do not demonstrate glomerular immunofluorescence and are therefore designated as "pauci-immune" nephritides.

PREVALENCE

I.   **SEX.** A female-to-male ratio of 9:1 is seen in most series of adult patients. The female predominance is less striking in SLE that occurs in childhood (disease onset preceding puberty) and in elderly patients with SLE.

II. **AGE.** First symptoms usually occur between the second and fourth decades of life, but may be seen in any age group. The presentation of SLE in the elderly (as much as 10% of the total population with lupus in some series) may differ from that in younger patients.

III. **ETHNIC DISTRIBUTION.** Although lupus occurs in all races, its prevalence is not equally distributed among all groups. SLE occurs more commonly in blacks than in whites, and Hispanic and black patients have been noted to have more severe disease. The average annual incidence in the United States is approximately 27.5 in 1 million for white women and 75.4 in 1 million for black women. The reported prevalence figures for women vary widely, from 1 in 100 to 1 in 10,000.

CLINICAL MANIFESTATIONS

I.   **SLE is a multisystem disease** in which the diagnosis rests on the recognition of a constellation of clinical and laboratory findings. No single finding makes the diagnosis, although some findings, such as antibodies to double-stranded DNA or a characteristic malar rash, are more suggestive than others.

II. **American College of Rheumatology (ACR) criteria for classification** of SLE have been devised to ensure at least minimum uniformity for disease classification in clinical studies (see Appendix A). The presence of four criteria (not necessarily occurring simultaneously) is required to classify a patient as presenting with SLE.

III. **Fever** is a common manifestation of active SLE. Although above 103°F at times, sustained fever of such magnitude is not common and should stimulate a search for infection. Acute severe disease ("lupus crisis") may be accompanied by fever of up to 106°F.

IV. **CUTANEOUS**
   A. Facial erythema is more common than the classic "butterfly" eruption as an acute cutaneous manifestation; photosensitivity dermatitis and bullous lesions may also occur. Subacute cutaneous LE includes both annular and papulosquamous lesions.
   B. Chronic discoid lesions with central atrophy, depigmentation, and scarring or non-scarring alopecia are common occurrences in 20% to 30% of patients.
   C. Mucous membrane lesions with ulcers of the hard palate and nasal septal perforations may be present.
   D. Raynaud's phenomenon may be associated with acrosclerosis and, rarely, with digital ulceration.
   E. Purpura and ecchymosis may occur as a result of either the disease (e.g., thrombocytopenia) or the corticosteroid treatment.

V.   **MUSCULOSKELETAL SYSTEM**
   A. **Arthritis** is common and affects both small and large joints in a symmetric pattern. The axial spine is not involved. Even in the face of longstanding arthritis, bony erosions are uncommon. Reducible joint deformity is caused by capsular laxity and by both tendinous and ligamentous involvement, which lead to partial subluxation. Tendon ruptures may occur.

B. Septic arthritis can occur due to the immunosuppressed state of the patient and the presence of joint damage due to osteonecrosis.

C. Osteonecrosis, an important cause of disability in late lupus, presents with acute pain, most commonly in the hip, but more than 50% of patients have involvement of multiple joints.

D. Inflammatory myositis may occur in 5% to 10% of patients. Muscle weakness may also reflect corticosteroid-induced myopathy, chloroquine-induced myopathy as a rare occurrence, or a myasthenia gravislike syndrome associated with SLE.

VI. CARDIOVASCULAR SYSTEM. The major cardiovascular morbidity associated with SLE appears to be accelerated coronary artherosclerosis and ischemic coronary disease.

A. Atherosclerotic cardiovascular disease occurs in excess of that predicted by conventional cardiovascular risk factors and is considered to be related to systemic inflammation associated with SLE.

B. Pericarditis is the most common cardiovascular manifestation. Pericardial effusions demonstrable by echocardiogram may be present in up to 60% of patients. Symptomatic pericarditis occurs in approximately 25% of patients. Tamponade is rare.

C. Myocarditis should be suspected in patients who present with arrhythmia, cardiomegaly without heart failure, or unexplained tachycardia.

D. Verrucous endocarditis (Libman-Sacks endocarditis) is a pathologic diagnosis, because it rarely causes clinically significant valvular lesions or embolic complications. It most commonly affects the posterior leaflet of the mitral valve and may predispose the patient to bacterial endocarditis.

E. Peripheral vascular manifestations include vasculitis that usually affects small arteries, arterioles, and capillaries, especially those of the skin. Phlebothrombosis and thrombophlebitis may occur and recur in some patients as a sign of disease activity, and in relation to antiphospholipid antibodies. Gangrene is rare. Raynaud's phenomenon may be a feature in up to 25% of patients.

VII. PULMONARY SYSTEM

A. Pleuritis is the most common pulmonary symptom. Pleural effusions may occur in up to 50% of patients and pleuritic pain in 60% to 70% of patients. Effusions may be secondary to processes other than active SLE, including infection and pulmonary emboli.

B. Pneumonitis as evidenced by rales on physical examination and patchy infiltrates or platelike atelectasis on chest radiography is a diagnostic problem. Because patients with SLE are often compromised hosts, infection by either common or uncommon agents must be considered.

1. "Lupus pneumonitis" does occur, but this diagnosis requires exclusion of other processes. Progressive lupus pneumonitis ending in acute pulmonary insufficiency is uncommon. Lung biopsy may be required to establish a diagnosis, especially in the setting of persistent or progressive findings despite therapy.

2. Abnormal findings on pulmonary function tests such as moderate restrictive and obstructive deficits are common, but patients may have mild or no associated symptoms.

C. Pulmonary hemorrhage presenting with cough and hemoptysis or as a pulmonary infiltrate is an uncommon and serious feature of SLE.

D. Pulmonary hypertension may occur without relation to overall disease activity. The clinical presentation is similar to that of idiopathic pulmonary hypertension, although with a higher incidence of Raynaud's phenomenon.

E. Shrinking lung syndrome is characterized by unexplained dyspnea, small lung volumes with restrictive pulmonary function tests, and normal lung fields with elevated diaphragms on chest radiographs.

VIII. GASTROINTESTINAL SYSTEMS. Abdominal pain is a common complaint and may reflect gastrointestinal disorders associated with medications or intrinsic SLE-related pathology.

A. Sterile peritonitis (serositis) and mesenteric vasculitis may be difficult to document. Intestinal perforation, especially in patients on corticosteroids that can mask symptoms, must be considered in addition to spontaneous bacterial peritonitis.

B. Pancreatitis may also occur.

C. Hepatomegaly may occur in one-fourth of patients, but abnormal liver function tests are often drug-related [i.e., nonsteroidal anti-inflammatory drugs (NSAIDs) and/or steroids] rather than being indicative of intrinsic lupus-associated liver damage. Chronic active hepatitis with positive tests for LE cells or ANAs (lupoid hepatitis) is not part of the spectrum of SLE.

D. Splenomegaly may be found in the setting of active disease and splenic infarcts can occur.

IX. **OTHER SYSTEMS**

  A. Lymphadenopathy is common but obviously not specific.

  B. A broad spectrum of eye disorders can occur including conjunctivitis, keratoconjunctivitis sicca, episcleritis, and retinal vasculitis with exudates (cytoid bodies).

  C. Parotid enlargement with or without a dry mouth (xerostomia) is reported in up to 8% of patients.

 DIAGNOSTIC INVESTIGATIONS

I. **LABORATORY TESTS**

  A. Autoantibodies to nuclear and cytoplasmic antigens occur in SLE. Their detection is diagnostically significant, although the sensitivity and specificity for SLE vary with each specific autoantibody (Table 30-3).

  1. Because these autoantibodies participate in immunologically mediated tissue damage, correlation between disease activity and antibody titer has been sought with the hope that antibody level (especially anti-DNA antibody level) might provide an index of disease activity and a guide to therapeutics. This is problematic in individual patients, because some may have persistently elevated anti-DNAs in the absence of active disease clinically and others may have flares of disease without elevated anti-DNA antibody titers.

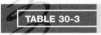 **TABLE 30-3** | Autoantibodies in Systemic Lupus Erythematosus

Antigen source	Antibody nomenclature	Incidence in SLE (%)	Specificity for SLE
Nuclear			
All determinants	ANA	100	—
dsDNA	Anti-DNA (double-stranded or native)	80–90	High
ss-DNA	Anti-DNA (single-stranded)	80–90	—
Acidic nucleoproteins	Anti-Sm	30	High
	Anti-RNP	30–40	—
	Anti-Ro (SS-A)	25	—
	Anti-La (SS-B)	15–20	—
Cytoplasmic ribonucleoproteins	Anti-rRNA, rRNP, Ro, La, and P	Uncertain	—
Cell surface determinants			
RBC	Direct Coombs'	30	—
WBC	Antilymphocyte antibodies	Common	—
	Antineutrophil antibodies	Uncommon	—
Platelets	Antiplatelet antibodies	Common	—
Others			
Phospholipid binding plasma protein complex	Anticardiolipin antibody	10–25	—

ANA, antinuclear antibody; dsDNA, double-stranded DNA; ss-DNA, single-stranded DNA; RBC, red blood cell; rRNP, ribosomal ribonucleoprotein; SLE, systemic lupus erythematosus; WBC, white blood cell.

2. The different technologies available for measuring any given autoantibody do not necessarily provide comparable results.

3. Although both IgM and IgG rheumatoid factors may occur in up to one-third of patients, their presence does not correlate with the presence of articular disease.

B. Serum complement is often abnormally low in conjunction with elevated autoantibody titers.

1. Hypocomplementemia *per se* is not specific to SLE and may reflect in any immunologically mediated disease accompanied by complement consumption, a hereditary complement component deficiency, impaired synthesis, or an improperly handled serum sample.

2. Hypocomplementemia is often, but not invariably, associated with nephritis. Like anti-DNA antibody levels, complement titers are valuable as a therapeutic guide in some, but not all, patients.

C. Routine laboratory examination may reveal abnormalities.

1. **Anemia** occurs in more than 50% of patients, especially when the disease is active. Most anemias in SLE are of the chronic disease type (normochromic, normocytic with low serum iron and total iron binding capacity). Patients may have more than one cause of anemia.

   a. Direct Coombs' test may be positive in approximately 25% of patients; true hemolytic anemia occurs in 10% of patients. The Coombs' test result may represent cell surface IgG, complement (C3, C4), or both.

   b. Anemia from blood loss or microangiopathic hemolytic anemia must always be considered.

2. **Leukopenia.** Patients with SLE are often leukopenic, especially during periods of disease activity. Lymphopenia caused by antilymphocyte antibodies is the most common type, but antibody-mediated neutropenia can also occur. Antistem cell antibodies are rare.

3. **Thrombocytopenia.** Antiplatelet antibodies have been demonstrated by a direct test similar to Coombs' test.

4. **Prolongation of the partial thromboplastin time (PTT).** Antibodies to both individual components of the clotting cascade (VIII, IX, XII) and to the prothrombin-converting complex have been described. Antiphospholipid antibodies may cause the prolongation of PTT, which does not cause bleeding, but does lead to an increased propensity to venous and arterial thrombosis. Rarely, antiprothrombin (factor II) antibodies can occur in the presence of a positive result of lupus anticoagulant test; a condition that is associated with the prolongation of both PTT and prothrombin time (PT) as well as bleeding (lupus anticoagulant hypoprothrombinemia syndrome).

5. **False-positive reaction to serologic test for syphilis.** A small percentage of biologic false-positive reactions show a "positive" fluorescent treponemal antibody, which can be distinguished from a true positive one by its beaded appearance. Antiphospholipid antibodies are associated with a false-positive reaction to the serologic test for syphilis.

6. **The erythrocyte sedimentation rate** is frequently elevated but is an inconsistent index of disease activity. It is not useful in differentiating active SLE from an intercurrent process, such as infection.

7. **Biochemistry.** Apart from hypergammaglobulinemia, routine biochemical screening (i.e., elevated creatinine and liver function test abnormalities) reflects the pattern and degree of organ involvement. Mild hyperkalemia in the absence of renal insufficiency may reflect an SLE-related renal tubular defect or the use of angiotensin converting enzyme inhibitors.

8. **Kidney studies.** Assessment of the urinalysis may define proteinuria, hematuria, or the presence of cellular casts and support the possibility of a nephritic or nephrotic disorder. A follow-up 24-hour urine sample for creatinine clearance and protein can be helpful in establishing the presence of nephrotic range proteinuria or renal insufficiency.

II. IMAGING STUDIES

Plain radiographs can define the presence of pulmonary infiltrates or effusions, cardiomegaly, osteonecrosis, or osteoporotic compression fractures. Computerized transaxial tomography can demonstrate pulmonary infiltrates or pleural disease, brain infarcts or bleeding, intestinal inflammation, or the presence of peritoneal fluid. Magnetic resonance imaging is effective in showing brain or spinal cord infarcts, osteonecrosis, or bone infections. All these findings can support the clinical possibility of a superimposed infection or a lupus-related disorder.

 DIFFERENTIAL DIAGNOSIS

I. The **diagnostic strategy** for SLE involves recognition of a multisystem disease, the exclusion of infection and malignancy as causes, the presence of certain serologic findings, and the absence of any other recognized disease processes that can, cumulatively, explain the findings.
   A. Not all clinical and laboratory findings are of equal specificity. Acute pericarditis, psychosis, proteinuria, and leukopenia can have many causes other than SLE. Conversely, a discoid lupus rash and high titers of antinative DNA antibodies or anti-Smith antigen antibodies strongly support the diagnosis.
   B. The art of diagnosis rests in recognizing a constellation of findings and giving each the appropriate clinical weightage. Because the presentations of SLE are many and varied, the full differential diagnosis includes most aspects of internal medicine.

II. The **most common presentation** is that of a young woman with polyarthritis; however, SLE is not the most likely cause of her symptoms.
   A. Rheumatoid arthritis or an infectious arthritis, such as gonococcal arthritis, must be considered first, since specific or curative therapy is available.
   B. The single most useful laboratory test to evaluate the possibility of SLE is the ANA determination. Although not completely specific, it is highly sensitive (Table 30-4). A positive test result is a signal to consider the diagnosis further, and a negative test result in a patient in the setting of active clinical manifestations of inflammatory disease makes the diagnosis highly unlikely.

III. **Organ systems that may be affected** by SLE include skin and mucous membranes (rash, mouth, or nasal ulcerations, and alopecia), joints (nondeforming, often symmetric RA-like polyarthritis), kidneys (glomerulonephritis), serosal membranes (pleuritis, pericarditis, and abdominal serositis), blood (hemolytic anemia, leukopenia, and thrombocytopenia), lungs (infiltrates and serositis), and the nervous system (seizures, strokes, psychosis, and peripheral neuropathies).

IV. **OTHER RHEUMATIC DISEASES.** Patients with multisystem disease and ANAs may have a condition other than SLE. Up to 40% of patients with rheumatoid arthritis may have ANAs. Systemic sclerosis (scleroderma), mixed connective tissue disease, and chronic active hepatitis must also be considered.

V. **THE MOST COMMON DIAGNOSTIC CHALLENGES**
   A. **Symmetric polyarthritis.** Conditions that look similar include rheumatoid arthritis (no fever, visceral disease, or anti-DNA); systemic sclerosis (tight skin, Raynaud's phenomenon, and different serologies); Wegener's granulomatosis (prominent triad of sinus, lung, kidney, and ANCA serologies); and infectious arthritis due to viruses like parvovirus B19 (self-limited and may be associated with rashes and fever).
   B. **Fever of unknown origin.** The differential diagnosis is wide, including infections of all types, malignancies, other connective tissue disorders, vasculitides, allergic reactions, inflammatory bowel disease, and granulomatous disorders such as sarcoidosis. It is usually the other disease manifestations, rather than fever, that define the illness.
   C. **The combination of kidney and lung disease.** Wegener's granulomatosis, Churg-Strauss vasculitis, Goodpasture's syndrome, and microscopic polyangiitis syndrome.
   D. **The combination of CNS and renal disease.** Thrombotic thrombocytopenic purpura.
   E. **Pancytopenia.** Malignancy, infectious disorders, drug reactions, and aplastic anemia.

VI. **DRUG-INDUCED SLE-LIKE SYNDROME** (Tables 30-1 and 30-4). Certain drugs trigger systemic lupus, and the inflammatory process usually resolves when steroids are given and the offending agent is stopped. Such patients rarely develop CNS or renal disease and commonly have antihistone antibodies in their serum. These same drugs can be given to patients with spontaneous lupus without fear of exacerbating the illness.

TABLE 30-4 Differential Diagnosis of Common Serologic Tests

	Antinuclear antibodies	Anti-DNA antibodies	Low CH50	Rheumatoid factor
SLE incidence	~100%	80%	80%	20% to 40%
Diseases with high incidence	Discoid lupus	Drug-induced LE (single-stranded)	Hereditary complement deficiency	Rheumatoid arthritis
	Drug-induced LE		Hereditary angioedema	Sicca syndrome
	Sicca syndrome		Membranoproliferative glomerulonephritis	
	Systemic sclerosis		Cryoglobulinemia	
Diseases with occasional incidence	Rheumatoid arthritis	Chronic active hepatitis	Rheumatoid arthritis	Dermatomyositis
	Dermatomyositis	Sicca syndrome	Serum sickness	Juvenile idiopathic arthritis
	Idiopathic pulmonary fibrosis	Rheumatoid arthritis	Serious infection:	Systemic sclerosis
	Chronic active hepatitis	Systemic sclerosis	Gram-negative sepsis, pneumococcal sepsis	Subacute bacterial endocarditis
	Aging	Dermatomyositis		Idiopathic pulmonary fibrosis
				Aging
Diseases with rare incidence	Necrotizing vasculitis	Necrotizing vasculitis	Necrotizing vasculitis	Insulin-dependent diabetes
				Healthy subjects

CH50, hemolytic complement; LE, lupus erythematosus; SLE, systemic lupus erythematosus.

TREATMENT

I. **Treatment must be individualized** and the therapeutic strategy must consider both the pattern and the severity of the inflammatory process and the extent of organ system involvement. The poor prognosis reported in the earliest series of patients with lupus has been altered because of an overall improvement in general medical care, judicious and balanced use of medications, and the capability of diagnosing milder forms of the disease. General measures include adequate rest, avoidance of sunlight, and avoidance of stress.

II. The **armamentarium** for treating lupus includes single or combination drug therapy that is crafted to the problem and might include:
   A. Nonsteroidal anti-inflammatory drugs;
   B. Antimalarial drugs that are employed in disease control, specifically of joint inflammation, skin rash and fatigue;
   C. Corticosteroids in the form of:
      1. Oral prednisone in varying doses
      2. Intravenous Solumedrol:
         a. To replace oral doses in patients who cannot tolerate oral medications or absorb them from the gastrointestinal tract;
         b. Three times daily in high doses for disease flares;
         c. "Pulse" of 250 to 1,000 mg for 1 to 3 days for the most severe disease flares.
   D. Immunosuppressive agents used for control of severe disease and visceral dysfunction:
      1. Azathioprine (Imuran)
      2. Methotrexate
      3. Mycophenolate mofetil
      4. Cyclophosphamide
      5. Rituximab
   E. Miscellaneous medications used for disease control:
      1. Intravenous gamma globulin
      2. Thalidomide
      3. Dapsone

III. **Corticosteroids.** The diagnosis of SLE does not demand the use of steroids. However, when they are needed, they are employed in various doses and dose regimens, as guided by the severity of the clinical presentation, prior response or lack of response to other medications including steroids, co-morbidities, and prior steroid-related side effects. A careful balance and dose titration are always demanded between that needed to control the lupus problem at hand and the avoidance of cumulative steroid-related side effects. Steroids are the classical "double-edged sword" because, while they are profoundly strong in controlling inflammation, they can lead to major side effects such as:
   A. **Physical appearance** is altered by weight gain that produces truncal fat deposition (moon facies and buffalo hump), hirsutism, acne, easy bruising, and purple striae. Although individual patients differ in their susceptibility to these changes, reduction of the steroid dosage will eventually reduce the severity of these manifestations.
   B. **Infection** occurs with greater frequency in patients treated with corticosteroids. Corticosteroids may mask both local and systemic signs of infection. Minor infections have a greater potential to become systemic. Latent infections, especially mycobacterial varieties, may become activated, and opportunistic agents such as fungi, *Nocardia*, *Cryptococcus*, and *Pneumocystis carinii* may cause serious clinical problems. Skin testing for delayed hypersensitivity to *Mycobacterium tuberculosis* should be performed before the initiation of corticosteroid therapy. However, a negative reaction may reflect the altered immunity of active SLE rather than lack of previous exposure to *M. tuberculosis*.
   C. **Mental function** may be altered. Minor reactions include irritability, insomnia, euphoria, and inability to concentrate. Major reactions may include severe depression, mania, and paranoid psychoses.
   D. **Glucose intolerance** may be induced or exacerbated by corticosteroids. Insulin may be required to control hyperglycemia and should be adjusted as the corticosteroid dosage is changed.

E. Hypokalemia may be caused by preparations that have mineralocorticoid activity. Serum potassium should be checked frequently, especially if congestive heart failure, nephrosis, or peripheral edema producing secondary hyperaldosteronism is present. Hyperkalemia can occur in the setting of pulse steroid therapy.

F. Sodium retention, edema, and hypertension may be induced by all corticosteroid drugs. When these effects become clinically significant, agents with fewer salt-retaining properties can be used. Alternative steroid preparations are listed in Appendix E. Because steroids should be given only for major SLE manifestations, it is usually not feasible to control hypertension by a reduction in dosage; therefore, blood pressure must be controlled by appropriate antihypertensive therapy.

G. Myopathy may occur in patients receiving long-term, high-dose steroids. The muscles are not tender, and unlike inflammatory myositis, steroid-induced myopathy is usually not characterized by elevated serum muscle enzymes. Proximal weakness is the most common symptom and it can affect the diaphragm and intercostal muscles. Weakness of the pelvic girdle is more common than the shoulder girdle. Drug-induced myopathy will gradually improve with a reduction of corticosteroid dosage.

H. Skeletal abnormalities

   1. Decreased bone density and osteoporosis

      a. Corticosteroids may reduce gastrointestinal calcium absorption, induce secondary hyperparathyroidism, and also reduce collagen matrix synthesis by osteoblasts.

      b. Compression fractures in the vertebral spine represent a major secondary complication, especially in older patients. They occur in approximately 15% of patients treated with steroids.

      c. Prophylactic vitamin D_3 (400 U twice daily) and calcium (1,500 mg/day from dietary and supplemental sources) are recommended.

      d. Patients receiving long-term corticosteroid therapy (for more than 1 month) should undergo baseline and yearly bone density evaluations and treatment with suitable bisphosphonates or other agents if necessary (see Chapter 53).

   2. Osteonecrosis occurs most frequently in weight-bearing joints, especially the femoral heads. The mechanism is unknown (therapy is discussed in Chapter 52). Reduction in corticosteroid dosage is desirable whenever possible, although it is unlikely to affect established osteonecrosis.

I. Hypoadrenalism may occur during periods of physiologic stress in patients with suppression of the hypothalamic–pituitary–adrenal axis resulting from exogenous steroid administration.

   1. During episodes of surgery or major intercurrent illness, it is advisable to provide supplemental steroid therapy to patients who are receiving corticosteroid therapy or who have discontinued such therapy within the previous year. Hydrocortisone (300 mg/day or equivalent dosage in three divided doses) may be given intravenously or intramuscularly during the period of maximum stress and subsequently tapered over a period of 5 days.

   2. The stress of major nonsurgical illness may be managed with an increase in daily steroid dose to at least the equivalent of 30 mg of prednisone.

J. Other side effects of corticosteroids include increased intraocular pressure, which may precipitate glaucoma, and the occurrence of posterior subcapsular cataracts. Although dyspepsia may accompany the use of steroids, it usually responds to antacids or H2 blockers, proton pump inhibitors, and administration of medication along with meals. Gastrointestinal ulcers may occur and diverticulitis or cholecystitis can be exacerbated. Menstrual irregularities, night sweats, and pancreatitis have been associated with corticosteroid therapy. Pseudotumor cerebri associated with rapid steroid dosage reduction is a rare complication.

TREATMENT RECOMMENDATIONS BY ORGAN SYSTEM OR PROBLEM

I. FEVER. Persistent or high fever without other manifestations of lupus (e.g., arthritis and rash) is uncommon and should always stimulate a search for infection, particularly in patients on steroids or immunosuppressive agents. NSAIDs (e.g., 500 mg of naproxen twice daily, 400 to 800 mg of ibuprofen four times daily, 25 to 50 mg of indomethacin three times daily) and acetaminophen are effective antipyretics. Corticosteroids, the most potent fever-controlling medications, are rarely used for fever alone, but are commonly used and are effective in clinical situations in which fevers accompany other active lupus manifestations.

II. **SKIN RASH.** Avoidance of exposure to ultraviolet light to prevent exacerbation of both cutaneous and systemic disease is paramount. Sunscreens, wide-brimmed hats, long sleeves, and long pants should be used by all patients. Highly protective sunscreen lotions should be applied liberally before exposure to sunlight and reapplied after any swimming or sustained sweating.

   A. **Topical therapy.** Active skin disease should be treated with topical corticosteroid preparations (e.g., hydrocortisone, triamcinolone, or fluocinonide two to three times daily) rather than with systemic corticosteroids. Occlusive dressings with cellophane wrap may be used at night, particularly on the upper extremities. Tacrolimus topical cream may also be effective.

   B. **Systemic therapy.** The antimalarial hydroxychloroquine (200 mg orally twice daily) is used to supplement topical treatment of extensive lesions. Quinacrine (100 mg orally daily) is also effective and at times both are used. Regular ophthalmologic examinations at 6-month intervals should include a slit-lamp examination and measures of light and color perception thresholds. The drug should be tapered as soon as disease control permits. Systemic corticosteroids and immunosuppressive therapies are rarely needed for the treatment of severe and refractory lupus skin lesions. Dapsone is sometimes used for bullous lesions and thalidomide for severe vasculitic skin lesions.

III. **ARTHRITIS**

   A. **NSAIDs.** NSAIDs can be quite effective for the treatment of the RA-like polyarthritis. However, gastrointestinal intolerance and the presence of renal disease may limit therapy with NSAIDs in some patients. Occasionally, large elevations of liver enzymes may occur and require either reduction or termination of therapy. Transient changes in renal function may occur with any NSAID and, in general, patients with nephritis should avoid these medications. Fever and aseptic meningitis may be caused by nonaspirin NSAIDs.

   B. **Antimalarial drugs,** including both hydroxychloroquine and quinacrine, may be effective in the treatment of joint pain and inflammation, fatigue, and skin rash. These drugs can also be used as steroid-sparing agents.

   C. **Systemic corticosteroids.** Oral prednisone (10 to 20 mg/day) is reserved for patients with accompanying constitutional symptoms unresponsive to NSAIDs.

   D. **Methotrexate or azathioprine** is effective for the treatment of persistent arthritis, rash, or serositis, which are unresponsive to NSAIDs, antimalarial agents, or low-dose glucoco. Methotrexate dose reductions are necessary for patients with renal insufficiency.

IV. **Serositis** can be treated with an NSAID as outlined for arthritis. At times, severe pericarditis may require a short course of steroids. Rarely, a large pericardial effusion necessitates therapy with high-dose prednisone (20 mg three times daily), or may demand pericardiocentesis or pericardial stripping.

V. **PNEUMONITIS.** Infection with routine or opportunistic organisms and pulmonary emboli must be considered when a patient with lupus presents with a pulmonary infiltrate.

   A. Infiltrates secondary to SLE may require steroid therapy, especially if they are associated with other signs of disease activity or are associated with dyspnea or desaturation.

   B. Fulminant pneumonitis with hemorrhage, which is rare, requires aggressive therapy with high-dose intravenous corticosteroids (1 mg of methylprednisolone/kg/day) and often cytotoxic agents (1 to 3 mg of azathioprine/kg/day, or 0.5 g/m^2 of cyclophosphamide/kg/day).

VI. **HEMATOLOGIC ABNORMALITIES**

   A. **Anemia.** This can be due to immunologic damage to erythrocytes, blood loss through the gastrointestinal or genitourinary tracts, decreased production due to the anemia of chronic disease or renal dysfunction, or combinations of these.

      1. **Hemolytic anemia** is uncommon but may be severe and require corticosteroid therapy. Depending on the level of hemoglobin or other symptoms, 40 to 60 mg

of prednisone is given daily in two to three divided doses when required, and tapered as quickly as possible, with the hemoglobin and reticulocyte count used as guides.

2. **Microangiopathic hemolytic anemia** (elevated lactate dehydrogenase and schistocytes) may be associated with SLE vasculitis and is often treated with high-dose steroids.

B. **Immune thrombocytopenia** secondary to SLE usually responds to corticosteroid therapy. Platelet counts of 80,000 to 100,000, however, are considered adequate and do not demand treatment.

1. Life-threatening thrombocytopenia (i.e., platelet counts <30,000) unresponsive to dosage of several weeks of 60 mg of prednisone given daily may improve with intravenous gamma globulin (IVIG) therapy (0.4 g/m^2/day for 5 days consecutively), which usually leads to an immediate (2 to 3 days) rise in the platelet count.

2. Rituximab is now commonly used for steroid-unresponsive thrombocytopenia. Other medications that include danazol, azathioprine, vincristine, vinca alkaloid-loaded platelets, and intravenous "pulse" cyclophosphamide have been used on occasions for steroid-resistant thrombocytopenia. Splenectomy is often the final recourse; it works in approximately 50% of cases and demands immunization for pneumococcal and *Hemophilus influenza* before the procedure, and often administration of IVIG in order to optimize the platelet count for the surgery.

C. **Leukopenia** in SLE usually represents lymphopenia rather than neutropenia and is not associated with the serious risk for infection that accompanies the leukopenia of cancer chemotherapy. Leukopenia usually does not warrant specific treatment *per se*, but it does improve when steroids are used to treat other disease manifestations.

VII. **VASCULITIS.** Small-vessel cutaneous vasculitis, usually found on the digits and palm of the hand, may be managed with low-dose prednisone (20 mg/day). Medium-vessel and large-vessel vasculitis, although uncommon, require 60 mg/day in divided doses, often with concomitant immunosuppressive therapy. Thalidomide in doses of 50 to 200 mg/day can be very helpful for the treatment of refractory vasculitic skin rashes.

VIII. **NEUROLOGIC DISEASE**

A. **Seizures.** Remember that seizures in a patient with lupus can be due to either the lupus itself, or related to hypertensive encephalopathy, CNS infection or bleeding, or metabolic abnormalities. They require the use of anticonvulsant drugs, usually in consultation with a neurologist. Refractory cases in patients with active systemic disease may need to be treated with high-dose steroids.

B. **Psychosis** may be secondary to either steroid therapy or SLE.

1. **Steroid-induced psychosis, a problem that usually occurs in a patient receiving 40 to 60 mg of prednisone and not 5 to 10 mg,** will improve with prudent tapering of systemic corticosteroids. Psychotic manifestations should be treated in consultation with a psychopharmacologist. If the patient needs high-dose steroids in the future, reconsultation with the psychiatrist is mandatory and prophylactic psychotropic medication is often needed, as is optimal medication to enable the patient to sleep. Pulse steroids are often free of such psychological problems.

2. **SLE-related psychosis.** The occurrence of SLE-related psychosis does not necessarily require an increase in steroid therapy. If adequate behavioral control is achieved with major tranquilizers and no organic signs are present on either physical examination or cerebrospinal fluid analysis, corticosteroids are not initiated or increased. However, at times, high-dose steroids are needed if the psychosis occurs in the setting of active systemic disease and does not respond to psychotropics.

C. **Parenchymal CNS disease**

1. CNS manifestations such as headache, new neurologic abnormalities, altered mental status, visual changes, problems with cognition and seizures, alone or in combination, can be due to lupus itself or due to factors listed:

a. CNS infection such as meningitis, encephalitis, or septicemia.

b. Hypertensive crisis related to renal disease.

    c. Medications such as indomethacin, other NSAIDs, and steroids.

    d. Metabolic abnormalities such as diabetic ketoacidosis, hyponatremia, and hepatic encephalopathy.

  2. If the above possibilities have been excluded and the problem is thought to be lupus itself, in the presence of new focal neurologic findings, 20 mg of prednisone is given three times daily until either improvement or toxicity is observed. Some neurologic lesions are not responsive to steroids. If no improvement is evident after approximately 3 to 4 weeks of high-dose therapy, prednisone is tapered to avoid complications. Dosages of prednisone higher than 60 to 80 mg/day rarely produce additional therapeutic benefit but markedly increase the risk of serious side effects. Any trial of very high-dose prednisone in severe disease should be continued only for a predetermined, limited period of time.

  3. Pulse methylprednisolone therapy may be helpful for patients who do not respond to standard therapy.

  4. Cytotoxic agents such as intravenous cyclophosphamide have been used in patients with SLE and with severe CNS disease who are unresponsive to steroids.

D. Peripheral nerve disease. Peripheral neuropathy is common. Mononeuritis multiplex usually represents small-vessel vasculitis. If the patient is unresponsive to 60 mg of prednisone daily in three divided doses, then 1 to 3 mg of azathioprine/kg or 1 to 2 mg of cyclophosphamide/kg may be initiated.

IX. RENAL DISEASE

A. Assessment of disease

  1. For the initial management of active renal disease, as defined by active urinary sediment including red blood cells and red cell casts, proteinuria, and a decrease in creatinine clearance, the intensity of therapy is often defined by the severity of presentation and extrarenal manifestations of disease.

  2. Response to a chosen treatment is assessed by serial urinalyses, 24-hour urine testing (or spot protein/creatinine ratios), and determination of levels of serum complement and anti-DNA antibodies.

  3. Although renal biopsy is helpful in characterizing the type of renal lesion and the extent of acute and chronic change, it is not mandatory. It is, however, usually performed prior to instituting cyclophosphamide therapy. Some rheumatologists recommend kidney biopsies initially, and also when there is lack of response to a treatment regimen. Patients with diffuse proliferative or membranoproliferative glomerulonephritis have the worst prognosis, but the natural history of clinically silent, diffuse proliferative disease with normal renal function has not been determined. Chronic changes of fibrosis and atrophy suggest little reversible disease and a poor prognosis.

  4. Any therapeutic regimen must consider both short-term and long-term effects encountered during the management of chronic nephritis.

  5. Infection, prerenal and postrenal and drug-related causes of renal abnormalities must be sought and corrected. Vigorous control of blood pressure and avoidance of nephrotoxins is mandatory.

B. Corticosteroid therapy is the mainstay of treatment of active nephritis. The dosage, route of administration, and duration of therapy vary depending on the initial presentation, the type of nephritis (see Table 30-2), presence of comorbidities, and prior treatment modalities. Milder forms of nephritis such as class I, II, and V often respond to the steroid regimen employed for the treatment of other SLE manifestations. Two approaches have been employed for the management of severe forms of class III and class IV lupus nephritis.

  1. Prednisone (60 mg/day in divided doses) for 1 to 2 months. Resolution of signs of active disease commonly permits tapering of prednisone. A recurrence of active urinary sediment, increased proteinuria, and decreased kidney function may prompt an increase in steroid dosage, a switch to "pulse" steroids, or a decision to perform a kidney biopsy in preparation for consideration of immunosuppressive therapy with cyclophosphamide.

  2. High-dose, "pulse" methylprednisolone. This regimen is defined by dosages of 1,000 mg/day for 3 days monthly for 6 months, with 0.5 mg of oral prednisone/kg between pulses, to control both renal and extrarenal manifestations. It is used as (a) initial therapy for active nephritis, (b) sole therapy to avoid cumulative side effects of long-term daily steroids, or (c) therapy for exacerbations of severe disease that do not respond to daily oral steroids. Although prednisone clearly helps to relieve acute exacerbations of disease, long-term corticosteroid therapy is associated with serious side effects.

C. **Cytotoxic drugs** are used in either severe corticosteroid-resistant disease or in the context of unacceptable steroid side effects.

    1. In patients with diffuse proliferative glomerulonephritis, **cyclophosphamide** has been shown to retard progression of scarring in the kidney and reduce the risk of end-stage renal failure. Induction therapy with monthly infusions of intravenous "pulse" cyclophosphamide (0.5 to 1.0 g/m^2 of body surface area) preserves renal function more effectively than do corticosteroids alone, but the rate of relapse following a 6-month induction course alone is high. Most patients require extended immunosuppressive maintenance therapy with intravenous cyclophosphamide at the same dose every 3 months for a total of 1.5 years. To optimally balance the positive and negative effects of cyclophosphamide, rheumatologists are now employing an initial induction phase with cyclophosphamide for approximately 6 months, which is followed by the use of daily azathioprine or mycophenolate mofetil thereafter.

    2. Potential toxicities with cyclophosphamide are substantial: nausea and vomiting (often requiring treatment with antiemetic drugs); alopecia (reversible); ovarian failure (nearly universal in patients older than 30 years) or azoospermia; and hemorrhagic cystitis, bladder fibrosis, and bladder transitional cell or squamous cell carcinoma. Intermittent intravenous cyclophosphamide may decrease the incidence of bladder complications associated with daily oral therapy.

    3. **Azathioprine** (Imuran; 1 to 3 mg/kg/day) is a far less toxic drug that avoids the potential complications of alopecia, sterility, and hemorrhagic cystitis associated with cyclophosphamide.

    4. **Mycophenolate mofetil** (CellCept; up to 3 g/day) is being used more and more either as the initial treatment of diffuse proliferative nephritis or as the maintenance drug after nephritis control has been established with cyclophosphamide. Each agent requires careful monitoring of complete blood cell counts. The long-term toxicity of these agents may include both hematopoietic malignancy and solid tumors (lymphomas with azathioprine, bladder carcinoma with cyclophosphamide).

D. **Other regimens.** Controlled trials of plasmapheresis have not shown benefit in most cases. Currently, clinical experience is being gathered with methotrexate, but no controlled studies are available. Clinical experience with cyclosporin A (3 to 6 mg/kg/day) suggests that it might be useful in membranous glomerulonephritis. Side effects, particularly hypertension and renal toxicity, appear to be infrequent.

SPECIAL MANAGEMENT CONSIDERATIONS

I. **DRUG-INDUCED LUPUS.** Medications associated with drug-induced lupus (see Table 30-1) have been used extensively and effectively in patients with idiopathic SLE. Although the risk for exacerbating the underlying disease is often discussed, such risk has not been established and does not contraindicate the use of an otherwise indicated medication.

II. **PREGNANCY.** The effects of pregnancy on SLE are variable and are discussed in detail in Chapter 38.

III. **CONTRACEPTION**

    A. Because SLE is a disease of women of childbearing age, contraception is an important issue. Barrier protection condoms and a diaphragm are preferable because they have no adverse effects. However, the patient's willingness to use these methods effectively must be considered.

    B. Because hormonal manipulation might theoretically exacerbate SLE, oral contraceptives with progesterone only or with a combination containing the lowest estrogen dose are preferable. However, a recent prospective double-blind study of patients with SLE who did not have risk factors for increased thrombosis (i.e., no antiphospholipid antibodies) revealed no increase in mild, moderate, or severe flares in patients randomized to triphasic combined oral contraceptives compared to those randomized to placebo.

IV. HEMODIALYSIS. Patients with SLE appear to tolerate long-term hemodialysis equally well as any population with chronic renal failure. Clinical impressions suggest that patients with SLE may have more quiescent disease when on dialysis, but they may still occasionally experience SLE disease activity.

V. TRANSPLANTATION. Patients with SLE may undergo renal transplantation without any apparent increase in morbidity in comparison with other populations undergoing renal transplantation, and often with good control of the lupus itself. Recurrences of lupus in transplanted allografts are uncommon.

 PROGNOSIS

I. The prognosis of SLE has improved, not only because milder forms of disease are recognized and treated early but also because of the availability of potent antibiotics, the judicious use of corticosteroids and immunosuppressive agents, and improvements in general medical care.

II. Prognosis depends on the pattern of organ involvement; patients with renal and CNS disease have the worst 5-year survival rates. Infection and cardiovascular disease continue to be major causes of death. Nonetheless, 5-year survival rates now approach approximately 90%.

III. Premature atherosclerosis due to the systemic inflammation associated with lupus itself, in addition to traditional risk factors, have a profoundly important impact upon survival. Therefore, vigorous control of the disease, lipids, blood pressure, weight, smoking, and diabetes is mandatory.

 SPECIAL VARIANTS OF LUPUS

I. DRUG-INDUCED LUPUS. Many drugs (see Table 30-1) have been implicated in the induction of a lupuslike syndrome, with manifestations ranging from an isolated positive ANA test result to a clinical lupus syndrome. In the past, procainamide and hydralazine were the drugs most frequently reported to produce a lupuslike syndrome; more recently, it is likely to be anti-TNF medications and minocycline.

    A. Clinical features. Skin rash, arthritis, pleural and pericardial effusions, lymphadenopathy, splenomegaly, anemia, leukopenia, elevated erythrocyte sedimentation rate, and transient false-positive serologic tests for syphilis may all be included. Pleuropulmonary disease is prominent, and renal and CNS diseases are characteristically absent. Most manifestations resolve after discontinuation of the drug.

    B. Laboratory studies. The laboratory profile of a patient with drug-induced lupus may help distinguish the syndrome from spontaneous SLE. Serum complement is rarely reduced in the drug-induced syndrome, and antibodies to native (or double-stranded) DNA are usually absent. However, antibodies to single-stranded DNA are often present, in addition to antibodies to histones and ribonucleoproteins.

    C. Treatment of drug-induced lupus involves discontinuation of the offending agent and symptomatic management of the clinical manifestations, often requiring steroids. Because most manifestations are reversible, therapy is usually of short duration. A positive ANA test result alone should prompt review of the indications for use of the inciting agent, but does not *per se* require the addition of therapeutic agents.

II. DISCOID LUPUS ERYTHEMATOSUS

    A. Clinical presentation. Disease may be limited to the skin and assume the chronic discoid form, with scaling red plaques and follicular plugging. Healing of these lesions is associated with central scarring and atrophy. Although chronic discoid LE remains primarily cutaneous in most patients, SLE will develop in a small percentage (approximately 5%). Conversely, patients with SLE may have discoid lesions among the cutaneous manifestations of their disease. Certain types of skin lesions, such as those of subacute cutaneous LE, may reflect a specific immunogenetic predisposition.

B. Therapy follows the same principles as those outlined for skin disease in SLE. Avoidance of sunlight and ultraviolet exposure and use of topical steroids and hydroxychloroquine (see Chapter 16 for more information regarding discoid LE).

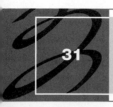

ANTIPHOSPHOLIPID SYNDROME
Doruk Erkan and Lisa R. Sammaritano

■ KEY POINTS

- ■ The origin of antiphospholipid (aPL) antibodies is unknown but is hypothesized to be an incidental exposure to environmental agents inducing aPL in susceptible individuals.

- ■ Concomitant prothrombotic risk factors may promote clotting in an additive manner in aPL-positive patients.

- ■ The clinical manifestations of aPL represent a spectrum [from asymptomatic to catastrophic antiphospholipid syndrome (APS)]; therefore, patients should not be evaluated and managed as having a single disease manifestation.

- ■ Stroke and transient ischemic attack are the most common presentation of arterial thrombosis; deep vein thrombosis (DVT), often accompanied by pulmonary embolism (PE), is the most common venous manifestation of APS.

- ■ The effectiveness of high-intensity anticoagulation in patients with APS and with vascular events is not supported by prospective controlled studies.

- ■ Some patients are surviving on a very tenuous balance between a nonclotting and a clotting state. These have to be watched carefully in the setting of surgery.

$\mathcal{T}$**he antiphospholipid syndrome** (APS) is defined as vascular thromboses and/or pregnancy morbidity occurring in persons with antiphospholipid antibodies (aPL) [most commonly anticardiolipin antibodies (aCL), positive results for lupus anticoagulant (LA) test, and anti-β_2-glycoprotein-I (β_2GPI) antibodies].

I.   The clinical manifestations of aPL represent a spectrum (Tables 31-1 and 31-2); therefore, patients should not be evaluated and managed as having a single disease manifestation.

   A. The presence of aPL in the absence of typical clinical complications does not indicate a diagnosis of APS, and aPL-positive patients may remain asymptomatic for a long period.

   B. aPL-related vascular events range from a superficial thrombosis to life-threatening multiple-organ system thromboses developing over a short period (i.e., catastrophic APS).

II.   APS may be seen in patients with autoimmune diseases such as systemic lupus erythematosus (SLE) or in otherwise healthy persons (i.e., primary APS).

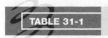

TABLE 31-1	Clinical Manifestations of the Antiphospholipid Syndrome

Arterial thrombosis: Extremity gangrene, stroke, myocardial infarction, aortic occlusion, and other visceral infarctions
Venous thrombosis: Peripheral venous thrombosis, pulmonary emboli, and visceral venous occlusion (e.g., Budd-Chiari syndrome, portal vein)
Renal: Arterial or venous occlusion and thrombotic microangiopathic glomerular disease
Cardiac: Valvular disorders, early myocardial infarction, and intracardiac thrombus
Cutaneous: Livedo reticularis[a], pyodermalike leg ulcerations, distal digital cyanosis, and distal gangrene
Hematologic abnormalities[a]: Thrombocytopenia, Coombs'-positive hemolytic anemia, and thrombotic microangiopathic hemolytic anemia
Nonthrombotic neurologic[a]: Transverse myelitis, migraine, chorea, multiple sclerosislike syndrome, and seizure
Obstetric: Fetal loss, recurrent (pre)embryonic losses, intrauterine growth retardation, and (pre)eclampsia
Catastrophic antiphospholipid syndrome: Sudden multisystem thromboses

[a]Not included in the Sapporo criteria.

 ETIOPATHOGENESIS

I. **The aPL are a family of autoantibodies** directed at phospholipid-binding plasma proteins, most commonly the natural anticoagulant β_2GPI.
   A. Physiologic phospholipids include cardiolipin, phosphatidylserine, phosphatidylinositol, and phosphatidylethanolamine.
   B. Phospholipid-binding plasma proteins are not limited to β_2GPI and include prothrombin, thrombomodulin, high- and low-molecular-weight kininogen, antithrombin III, protein C and S, and annexins I and V.

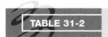

TABLE 31-2	Sapporo Classification Criteria for Antiphospholipid Syndrome

Clinical criteria
   Vascular thrombosis:
   ■ Arterial, venous, or small vessel thrombosis, in any organ or tissue
   Pregnancy morbidity:
   ■ One or more unexplained deaths of morphologically normal fetus at or beyond the tenth week of gestation or
   ■ One or more premature births of a morphologically normal neonate at or before the thirty-fourth week of gestation because of severe pre-eclampsia or eclampsia, or severe placental insufficiency or
   ■ Three or more unexplained consecutive spontaneous abortions before the tenth week of gestation
Laboratory criteria
   Anticardiolipin antibody of IgG and/or IgM isotype in blood, present in medium or high titer, on two or more occasions, at least 6 weeks apart and/or
   Positive lupus anticoagulant test on two or more occasions at least 6 weeks apart

Definite APS: one clinical and one laboratory criteria.
Ig, immunoglobulin.

II.   **The origin of aPL is unknown** but it is hypothesized that an incidental exposure to environmental (primarily infectious) agents induces aPL in susceptible individuals (i.e., a molecular mimicry mechanism).

   A.   Most infection-induced aPL are not truly pathogenic (β_2GPI-independent). Furthermore, infection-induced aPL that can occur during infections, such as syphilis, Lyme disease, and viral infections, especially HIV and hepatitis C, are usually transient and in low titers.

   B.   The aPL can also be induced by certain drugs (such as chlorpromazine, procainamide, quinidine, and phenytoin) and malignancies (such as lymphoproliferative disorders). In these cases, aPL are usually in low titer, of the IgM isotype, and are reversible once the inducing drug is discontinued. They are rarely associated with thrombosis.

III.   **The pathogenesis of aPL-related thrombosis is unknown;** any or all of the major components of the clotting system may be involved, and laboratory and clinical research suggest that more than one mechanism may be at work.

   A.   Possible aPL mechanisms of pathogenic actions include inhibition of coagulation cascade reactions catalyzed by phospholipids (such as inhibition of activation of the protein C and S); activation of the endothelial cells or platelets; aPL-induced increase of tissue factor (a physiologic initiator of coagulation) expression on monocytes; and interaction between aPL and an annexin V anticoagulant shield in the placenta.

   B.   Complement activation is necessary for the induction of fetal loss by aPL; in animal models, blocking certain complement components prevents fetal loss.

IV.   **The strength of association between aPL and thrombosis varies considerably among studies** (from none to strong), depending largely on the aPL and the clinical populations studied. There is substantial support that the presence of other thrombotic risk factors in aPL-positive individuals influences the risk of thrombosis.

   In the currently accepted "second-hit hypothesis," a second trigger event (such as cigarette smoking, oral contraceptive usage, surgical procedures, prolonged immobilization such as a long duration plane travel, or a genetic prothrombotic state), which by itself may not be sufficient to initiate thrombosis, may be necessary for an aPL-positive patient to develop a vascular event.

V.   **Familial occurrence of aPL has been reported.** Suggested associations include HLA-DR4, DR7, DRw53, and C4 null allele; however, none of these data are as yet compelling for a strong genetic predisposition and these tests need not be performed routinely.

 PREVALENCE

The prevalence of aPL among the general population is 2% to 5%, and its incidence increases with age (generally low-titer aCL). aPL are present in 12% to 34% of patients with SLE.

I.   Although it is difficult to accurately estimate the risk of thrombosis annually, on the basis of the limited number of uncontrolled studies available, asymptomatic aPL-positive patients have a 0% to 3.8% risk.

II.   Approximately 50% of patients who are younger than 50 years and affected with stroke and up to 20% of patients with idiopathic deep vein thrombosis (DVT) possess aPL. However, the true significance of the association is unknown.

 CLINICAL MANIFESTATIONS

I.   **ARTERIAL EVENTS.** Stroke and transient ischemic attack are the most common presentations of arterial thrombosis and make up almost one-fourth of initial presenting events in APS. Recurrent stroke may lead to multi-infarct dementia. Thrombosis in peripheral arteries, such as mesenteric or extremities, may lead to bowel ischemia or digital or extremity gangrene. Myocardial infarctions (MIs) and aortic occlusion can also occur in aPL-positive patients.

II. VENOUS EVENTS. DVT, often accompanied by pulmonary embolism (PE), is the most common manifestation of APS. Pulmonary hypertension may develop because of recurrent PEs or small vessel thrombosis. Unusual venous distributions may be affected, leading to ocular vascular disease, renal or splenic vein thrombosis, Budd-Chiari syndrome, portal vein, saggital sinus, and mesenteric thrombosis, as well as adrenal insufficiency due to thrombosis and resulting "paradoxical" hemorrhage.

III. RENAL MANIFESTATIONS. Thrombosis may develop at any location within the renal vasculature, including the renal artery, intrarenal arteries or arterioles, glomerular capillaries, and renal veins. aPL-associated glomerular disease histopathology is similar to the thrombotic microangiopathy seen in thrombotic thrombocytopenic purpura and usually presents with proteinuria, hypertension, and a decrease in creatinine clearance. Urine sediment is usually inactive, although progression to renal failure may occur.

IV. CARDIAC MANIFESTATIONS. Valvular heart disease (vegetations and/or valve thickening) is the most common aPL-related cardiac involvement. Libman-Sacks endocarditis can be seen in patients with both aPL-positive SLE and primary APS. Prevalence of valvular heart disease is estimated at 32% to 82% of patients with aPL.

    A. Intracardiac thrombosis (case reports) may mimic myxoma in their embolic characteristics.

    B. Aortic and mitral insufficiencies are common and lead to valve replacement in severe cases.

    C. Coronary artery disease is reported, and prospective studies support aPL as a risk factor for MI, especially in young individuals. An association of aPL with increased risk of atherosclerosis has been suggested but is controversial.

V. CUTANEOUS MANIFESTATIONS. Livedo reticularis, a latticelike pattern of superficial skin veins, is the most common cutaneous manifestation. Cutaneous necrosis and pyodermalike ulcerations have been reported.

VI. HEMATOLOGIC MANIFESTATIONS. Thrombocytopenia (usually platelet count $>100 \times 10^9$/L is common; Coombs'-positive hemolytic anemia and Evan's syndrome (thrombocytopenia and hemolytic anemia occurring together) may occur. Microangiopathic hemolytic anemia is also reported.

VII. NONTHROMBOTIC NEUROLOGIC MANIFESTATIONS. Although controversial and relatively uncommon, these may include chorea, transverse myelitis, multiple sclerosis-like syndrome, and seizures. Migraines, a nonspecific symptom, are common. Furthermore, cognitive dysfunction independent of cerebrovascular disease can occur secondary to aPL.

VIII. OBSTETRIC COMPLICATIONS. See Chapter 38 for the discussion of aPL-related obstetric complications.

IX. CATASTROPHIC ANTIPHOSPHOLIPID SYNDROME (CAPS). CAPS is a rare, life-threatening complication of aPL, which occurs in multiple organs over a short period of days. Multiple thromboses of small and medium-size vessels may occur despite adequate anticoagulation. Mortality is estimated at 50% with therapy.

    Definite catastrophic APS is diagnosed when all four criteria in Table 31-3 are met. **Probable catastrophic APS** is considered when any three of the criteria in Table 31-3 are met.

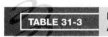

TABLE 31-3	International Classification Criteria for Catastrophic Antiphospholipid Syndrome

Evidence of involvement of three or more organs, systems and/or tissues
Development of manifestations simultaneously or in less than a week
Confirmation by histopathology of small vessel occlusion in at least one organ or tissue
Laboratory confirmation of the presence of aPL (LA and/or aCL and/or anti-β_2GPI antibodies)

Definite catastrophic antiphospholipid syndrome: all four criteria.
aCL, anticardiolipin antibodies; aPL, antiphospholipid antibodies; β_2GPI, β_2-glycoprotein-I; LA, lupus anticoagulant.

Figure 31-1. Livedo reticularis.

PHYSICAL EXAMINATION

I.   **No physical examination findings** are specific for aPL or APS.
II. The manifestation of **livedo reticularis** (Fig. 31-1), especially in young patients with a history of vascular events or pregnancy, should alert the physicians for the possibility of the presence of aPL. However, livedo reticularis is not specific for APS and may be a normal variant.

DIAGNOSTIC INVESTIGATIONS

An international consensus statement on the preliminary classification criteria for definite APS was published in 1999 after a workshop in Sapporo, Japan (see Table 31-2). The purpose of the criteria is to facilitate studies of treatment and causation; however, the Sapporo criteria are currently the best available tool for the diagnosis of APS.

I.   Definite APS is diagnosed when at least one clinical and one laboratory criteria are met.
II. Manifestation of livedo reticularis, cardiac valve disease, thrombocytopenia, cognitive dysfunction, chorea, transverse myelitis, and multiple sclerosislike disease, in the absence of a recognized vascular event or pregnancy, do not classify a patient as having APS according to the Sapporo criteria, but clinicians recognize these findings while managing aPL-positive patients.

LABORATORY TESTS

I.   **Sapporo criteria require a positive LA test and/or medium-to-high titer IgG aCL** to confirm the diagnosis of APS; a false-positive test result for syphilis (although sometimes seen) does not fulfill the laboratory criteria.
   A. Laboratory tests should be repeated, at least 6 weeks apart, to rule out the presence of transient infection-induced antibodies.
   B. Low-titer aCL are not included in the Sapporo criteria because of high differences among interlaboratory test results at low titers and the lack of concordance between low-titer aCL and clinical manifestations. Although there is no consensus among APS experts about what constitutes medium-to-high titer aCL, several studies have

concluded that aCL titer higher than 40 U is more predictive of thrombotic events than aCL titer lower than 40 U.

II. **LUPUS ANTICOAGULANT.** aPL prolong phospholipid-dependent coagulation steps *in vitro* by competing with coagulation factors for binding to phospholipid. The LA test is a functional coagulation assay that measures the ability of aPL to inhibit the conversion of prothrombin to thrombin.

   A. The most sensitive and commonly performed initial assays for the LA test are the kaolin clotting time (KCT) and the dilute Russell's viper venom time (dRVVT).

   B. Final diagnosis requires demonstration of a failure to correct the prolonged coagulation time by mixing studies, correction of the prolonged coagulation by addition of excess phospholipids, and the exclusion of other coagulopathies.

   C. A positive LA test result is even more strongly associated with thrombosis than IgG aCL.

III. **aCL** are detected by aCL enzyme-linked immunosorbent assay (ELISA). Presence of β_2GPI is a requirement for binding of autoimmune aCL to cardiolipin-coated plates in the standard ELISA.

   A. IgG aCL is more strongly associated with clinical events than IgM aCL, and the risk of thrombosis increases with higher levels of both IgG aCL and IgM aCL.

   B. IgA aCL, as well as low titers of IgG aCL and IgM aCL, are rarely associated with clinical events.

IV. **Anti-β_2GPI antibody** is also detected by ELISA, is found in the sera of many aCL-positive patients, and has been suggested to be more specific than aCL in predicting complications. However, the anti-β_2GPI test requires further standardization before it replaces the aCL test.

V. **aPL assays other than LA test and aCL ELISA** are currently neither well standardized nor widely accepted.

 RADIOLOGIC STUDIES

Radiologic findings are not specific for aPL or APS; however, radiology studies are commonly used to demonstrate the presence of thrombosis associated with aPL.

 DIFFERENTIAL DIAGNOSIS

I. **CONCOMITANT PROTHROMBOTIC RISK FACTORS MAY PROMOTE CLOTTING IN AN ADDITIVE MANNER.** The presence of other acquired risk factors (e.g., hypertension, smoking, pregnancy, surgical procedures, malignancy, nephrotic syndrome, oral contraceptive use, or hormone replacement therapy) and genetic risk factors (e.g., factor V_{Leiden}, prothrombin 20210, and MTHFR mutations; homocystinemia; and protein C, protein S, or antithrombin III deficiencies) should also be investigated in aPL-positive patients when possible, and the investigation results may aid in directing treatment and in recommendations.

II. **EXCLUSION OF CONFOUNDING CONDITIONS ARE IMPORTANT IN aPL-POSITIVE PATIENTS WITH PREGNANCY MORBIDITIES.** Gynecologic conditions such as uterine abnormalities, hormonal imbalance (e.g., luteal phase defect), maternal and paternal karyotype abnormalities, fetal genetic abnormalities, or presence of a heritable procoagulant state may mimic APS. Diagnosis also requires exclusion of chronic infections, systemic diseases, and alcohol and drug abuse.

III. **Histologic examination** of the vessels, skin, kidney, or other tissue biopsies shows thrombus formation without surrounding inflammation. Inflammatory vasculitis should suggest concomitant SLE or other connective tissue disorders.

IV. **Other** conditions such as sepsis, vasculitis, disseminated intravascular coagulation, heparin-induced thrombocytopenia, and thrombotic microangiopathies (such as thrombotic thrombocytopenic purpura and hemolytic uremic syndrome) can be challenging in the differential diagnosis of CAPS.

TREATMENT

See Table 31-4 for a summary of treatments for aPL-related manifestations.

I. THROMBOTIC EVENTS

   A. Retrospective studies suggest that high-intensity (INR 3 to 4) warfarin be used to prevent recurrent thromboembolic events, with a high risk for recurrent thrombosis in the 6 months following discontinuation of warfarin. However, the necessity for high-intensity anticoagulation has become controversial and is not supported by recent prospective studies.

   B. A prospective randomized controlled trial of two intensities of warfarin concluded that both low-intensity (INR 2 to 3) and high-intensity (INR 3 to 4) anticoagulation are similarly effective for patients at a low risk for APS. This study suggests that less intense anticoagulation is acceptable for patients with APS and with venous events; however, the debate on arterial events continues because patients with arterial events comprised only one-fifth of studied patients.

   C. The Anti-Phospholipid Antibody and Stroke Study (APASS) found no difference in recurrence rate of stroke in aPL-positive patients randomized to aspirin versus warfarin; however, patients with low-titer aPL were included, and target INR was moderate rather than high-intensity.

   D. APS patients with venous and arterial vascular events usually receive life-long warfarin. However, it is unclear whether patients who develop a vascular event in the presence of other hypercoagulable risk factors (e.g., surgery or oral contraceptive pills) should be kept on warfarin indefinitely.

II. PREGNANCY MORBIDITIES. See Chapter 38 for the discussion of the management of aPL-related obstetric complications.

III. TREATMENT OF aPL MANIFESTATIONS THAT ARE NOT INCLUDED IN THE SAPPORO CRITERIA

   A. Platelet counts greater than 50×10^9/L due to APS require no specific therapy. Corticosteroids and/or intravenous immunoglobulin are the first-line treatments for platelet counts less than 50×10^9/L. In addition to intravenous immunoglobulin, danazol or even splenectomy may be considered in corticosteroid-resistant cases.

   B. Very few studies address the treatment of the nonthrombotic manifestations of APS. Most of these manifestations, such as cardiac valve involvement and cognitive dysfunction, are generally managed with low-dose aspirin initially, although no published data strongly support this approach.

   C. Recent prospective studies suggest that aspirin and/or heparin treatment in patients with positive aPL and failed *in vitro* fertilization (IVF) cycles does not improve IVF outcome.

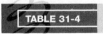

TABLE 31-4	Management of the Antiphospholipid Antibodies-related Manifestations

Clinical manifestation	Treatment
Venous thrombosis	Warfarin (INR 2.0–3.0)
Arterial thrombosis	Warfarin (INR 3.0)[a]
Recurrent thrombosis	Warfarin (INR 3–4) + low-dose aspirin
Thrombocytopenia >50,000 × 10⁹/L	No treatment
Thrombocytopenia ≤50,000 × 10⁹/L	Corticosteroids
	Intravenous immunoglobulin
Catastrophic antiphospholipid syndrome	Anticoagulation + corticosteroids + intravenous immunoglobulin or plasmapheresis
Asymptomatic aPL-positive patients	No treatment[b]

[a]The intensity of anticoagulation is controversial.
[b]Low-dose aspirin or hydroxychloroquine may be given.
aPL, antiphospholipid antibodies; INR, international normalized ratio.

IV. CATASTROPHIC APS

    A. The highest survival rate is achieved with the combination of anticoagulation, corticosteroids, and plasma exchange or intravenous immunoglobulins.

    B. Plasma exchange with fresh frozen plasma should be especially indicated if symptoms of microangiopathic hemolytic anemia (i.e., schistocytes) appear.

V. ASYMPTOMATIC aPL-POSITIVE PATIENTS

    A. Primary thrombosis prevention lacks an evidence-based approach; controlled, prospective, and randomized studies are in progress.

    B. Modification of other reversible thrombotic risk factors (such as smoking or oral contraceptive usage) and prophylaxis during high-risk periods (such as surgical interventions or prolonged immobilization) are crucial.

    C. Low-dose aspirin is generally used in clinical practice. However, until further studies are available, physicians should be aware of the fact that the necessity and/or the effectiveness of low-dose aspirin is not yet fully supported by the current literature.

 PROGNOSIS

I. **During long-term follow-up**, serious morbidity and disability occur in an unpredictable proportion of patients with APS, who experience a major vascular event and in those for whom diagnosis and treatment is delayed.

II. **Factors associated with worse prognosis** include pulmonary hypertension, neurologic involvement, myocardial ischemia, nephropathy, gangrene of extremities, and catastrophic APS.

III. **Patients with APS who have only pregnancy morbidities** are at high risk for future vascular events based on retrospective data.

IV. **Catastrophic APS** recurrence is unusual and generally patients who survive have a stable course with continued anticoagulation.

V. **Serious perioperative complications may occur despite prophylaxis** and patients with APS are at additional risk for thrombosis when they undergo surgery.

    Perioperative strategies should be clearly identified before any surgical procedure, pharmacologic and physical antithrombosis interventions should be vigorously employed, periods without anticoagulation should be kept to an absolute minimum, and any deviation from a normal course should be considered a potential disease-related event.

DERMATOMYOSITIS, POLYMYOSITIS, AND INCLUSION BODY MYOSITIS 32

Petros Efthimiou and Lawrence J. Kagen

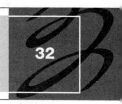

■ KEY POINTS

- Chronic, idiopathic skeletal muscle inflammation can be considered under three general types: dermatomyositis (DM), polymyositis (PM), and inclusion body myositis (IBM).

- All three entities present with progressive muscle weakness and loss of function, caused by persistent muscle inflammation that eventually leads to skeletal muscle loss and atrophy.

- DM is distinguished clinically from PM by the presence of a characteristic rash.

- IBM presents insidiously, mainly in elderly male patients, thereby delaying diagnosis and treatment.

- An often occult, underlying malignancy can be present, especially in DM.

- Cardiopulmonary complications, dysphagia, and calcinosis are serious complications.

■ Serum muscle enzyme level elevations; presence of autoantibodies; and magnetic resonance imaging (MRI), ultrasonographic, and electromyography (EMG) studies can provide valuable clues to diagnosis.

■ Treatment options include systemic and topical corticosteroids, often in conjunction with immunomodulators, and intravenous immunoglobulin (IVIG).

Polymyositis (PM), dermatomyositis (DM), and inclusion body myositis (IBM)** represent nosologic forms of the rare "idiopathic inflammatory myopathy" (IIM) disease group, which is characterized by chronic, acquired skeletal muscle inflammation. These disorders are all marked by progressive weakness, loss of function, and pathogenic processes, which likely involve immunocompetent cells and cytokine production. **A number of infectious agents, drugs, and toxins must be excluded** before the diagnosis of any of these idiopathic disorders can be established. **Recognition of this group of disorders by the clinician is important** because these disorders represent the largest group of acquired, and potentially treatable, myopathies in both children and adults.

 ETIOPATHOGENESIS

I. **The causes and pathogenesis of human inflammatory myopathies** remain unclear. There is evidence of an autoimmune process, in which both cellular and humoral components are involved in capillary and muscle fiber injury. Altered expression of matrix metalloproteinases and cytokines/chemokines also play an important role in the pathogenesis.

II. **Genetic factors predispose** to autoimmunity, and relatives of patients with myositis have increased susceptibility to myositis and other autoimmune diseases. Associations of PM with major histocompatibility complex (MHC) genes human leucocyte antigen (HLA)-DR3, DRB1*0301, and DQA1*0501 have been reported.

III. **Environmental factors** have long been suspected to act as disease triggers in a genetically predisposed host. A variety of infections, drugs, and toxins can induce a syndrome resembling PM.

IV. **Lymphocytic muscle infiltrates** have a prominent role in the pathogenesis of human inflammatory myopathies. Characterization of the infiltration pattern and of cell surface markers in muscle biopsies can provide valuable clues about which form of inflammatory myopathy is present. In DM, B cells and CD4+ cells predominate in the perivascular regions, whereas in PM and IBM, cytotoxic CD8+ T lymphocytes invade the endomysium and appear to have the primary pathogenic role.

   PM is considered an antigen-driven T-cell–mediated disease, in which CD8+ cells invade skeletal muscles, proliferate in a clonal fashion, and release toxic enzymes such as perforin and granzyme-B. Target myofibrils may be capable of engaging CD8+ cells by demonstrating MHC class I molecules on their surface. Macrophages are present in areas of necrosis and can also contribute to cytokine and enzyme release.

V. **Humoral immune** mechanisms are implicated in the pathogenesis of DM, in which the primary antigenic target seems to be the vascular endothelium. Vasculopathy mediated by complement through the membrane attack complex (MAC and C5-9) deposition leads to ischemic injury and perifascicular atrophy. Vasculopathy occurs not only in muscles but also in other areas of the body including the skin and the gastrointestinal tract.

VI. **Cytokines and chemokines** have attracted increased attention as contributors in the complex inflammatory cascade that leads to capillary and muscle fiber damage.

   A. **Proinflammatory cytokines** such as tumor necrosis factor-α (TNF-α), TNF-β, IL-1α, IL-1β, IL-2, and interferon-γ (IFN-γ) have been shown to be present in elevated levels in myositis biopsy tissue. TNF-α and TNF-β may contribute to the pathophysiology by being directly toxic to the existing muscle fibers and by preventing myofiber regeneration.

   B. **Chemokines,** monocyte chemotactic protein 1 (MCP-1), macrophage inflammatory protein-1α (MIP-1α), MIP-1β, and regulated on activation of normal T cell expressed and secreted (RANTES) present in infiltrating inflammatory cells and extracellular matrix can perpetuate the autoimmune attack against muscle antigens by amplifying lymphocyte activation and migration.

VII. **Amyloid-containing inclusions are present in IBM muscle biopsies.** They are derived from β amyloid precursor protein and phosphorylated tau protein. Various hypotheses exist about the pathogenic process. Proteosomal abnormalities marked by the increased deposition of mutated ubiquitin, defects in oxidative processes, and mitochondrial abnormalities have all been implicated. The role of the aging process is also of undoubted importance.

 ## PREVALENCE

I. **DM and PM are rare disorders (incidence of 5 to 7.6 in 1 million)** and affect all age groups, with a peak frequency in childhood before the age of 18 years and again another adult peak between ages 55 and 69 years. Prevalence for DM and PM varies from 5 in 10,000 to 11 in 10,000. The relative frequency of DM may increase in latitudes near the equator. More women are affected than men (female-to-male ratio is 2:1) and African American women are more frequently affected than white women (African American women-to-white women ratio is 2.8:1).

II. **IBM has an incidence of 2.2 in 1 million** and a prevalence of 4.9 in 1 million. When adjusted for age, the prevalence rises to 16 in 1 million inhabitants older than 50 years. Men are affected twice as commonly as women.

 ## CLINICAL MANIFESTATIONS

I. **DM**
   A. **DM usually begins with a characteristic rash.** Often sun-sensitive and pruritic, the rash tends to be erythematous and macular over flat body surfaces and heaped up or papular at bony prominences.
      1. **There is swelling and a purplish discoloration around the eyes,** with telangiectasia of the upper lids—the "heliotrope sign" or "lilac" suffusion.
      2. **Over the dorsal surface of the hand and finger joints,** the rash is papular (Gottron's papules). Similar manifestations can also be seen at the elbows, knees, and ankles (Fig. 32-1).
      3. **Large macular areas of rash** are also seen on the upper outer anus and thighs, as well as on the anterior neck and chest (V-sign), and over the shoulders and upper thorax (shawl sign).
   B. **The rash usually precedes the recognition of myopathy.** In some cases, this interval may be quite long, rarely lasting months or even years. Patients with rash alone are designated as having **amyopathic** DM, although careful observation will often disclose subtle clinical or laboratory signs of myopathy in most patients.
   C. **The myopathy of DM manifests as pain and weakness** of the proximal musculature. Muscles innervated by cranial nerves are not affected, and distal musculature is generally less affected.

II. **PM. This type of inflammatory myopathy does not have rash** and begins with proximal muscle weakness (see Table 32-1 for clinical characteristics of DM, PM, and IBM).

III. **IBM. This illness, most common among elderly patients, begins insidiously** with weakness in both proximal and distal musculature. The involvement of the musculature may be asymmetrical. Because of its subtle onset in elderly people, it may be present for a long while before the patients realize that this weakness is not a natural accompaniment of the normal aging process. This results in a delay in the diagnosis and a poor response to therapy.

IV. **ASSOCIATED DISORDERS**
   A. **Malignancy may develop in approximately one-fourth of patients with DM.** In some instances, malignancy precedes the appearance of rash and myopathy; in others it occurs simultaneously; and in still others, malignancy may develop later,

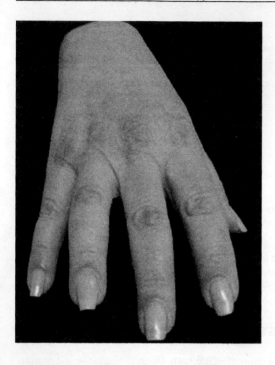

Figure 32-1. Gottron's papules.

TABLE 32-1	Idiopathic Inflammatory Myopathy

Disease	Demographics	Biopsy	Clinical picture
DM	Rare (incidence 5/10^6) female:male = 2:1 Two peaks: age <18 and 50–69	CD4+ T cells in perivascular area Complement (C5-9) vascular wall deposition Vasculopathy Muscle atrophy	Rash: V-sign, shawl sign, Gottron's papules Photosensitivity Fatigue Often occult malignancy Muscle weakness, atrophy Dysphagia Polyarthritis Calcinosis Interstitial lung disease
PM	Same as DM	CD8+ T cells invade endomysium causing myofiber necrosis	Muscle weakness, atrophy Dysphagia Polyarthritis Calcinosis Fatigue Interstitial lung disease
IBM	Age usually >50	CD8+ T cells invade endomysium attacking myofibers Eosinophilic inclusions	Muscle weakness, proximal and distal Asymmetrical involvement Insidious onset

DM, dermatomyositis; IBM, inclusion body myositis; PM, polymyositis.

during the course of inflammatory myopathy. The risk for occult malignancies in patients with PM and IBM, although increased when compared to the normal population, is significantly lower than in DM.

The type of malignancies is varied, including carcinomas, sarcomas, and both liquid and solid tumors of the blood-forming and lymphoid system. Ovarian carcinoma has been preponderant in reported series. Because neoplasms may often be occult, careful examinations bearing this fact in mind are warranted, especially in patients with DM.

B. **Interstitial pulmonary disease or fibrosing alveolitis** can occur in association with myositis. Although infection, hypoventilation, retention of secretions, and medication toxicity (e.g., secondary to methotrexate or cyclophosphamide) may be etiologic factors, in patients with PM/DM, interstitial pulmonary disease may actually precede the overt appearance of myopathy, making it an associated disorder rather than a secondary disorder. Lung infiltrates interfere with oxygen diffusion and transport and may lead to hypoxemia.

C. **The antisynthetase syndrome** encompasses a subset of patients, generally with PM, who possess antibodies to the enzymes that bind transfer RNA (tRNA) to amino acids for transporting the amino acids to the ribosome for protein synthesis. A number of these anti–tRNA synthetases have been observed, the most common being anti-Jo1, the antihistidyl-tRNA synthetase. [See Table 32-2 for a list of myositis-specific antibodies (MSA) and associated clinical syndromes.]

Patients with the antisynthetase syndrome frequently have interstitial pulmonary disease, Raynaud's phenomenon, small joint arthritis, and skin thickening (mechanic's hands) in addition to inflammatory myopathy.

D. **Dysphagia,** although uncommon, represents a potentially serious complication of inflammatory myopathy. It may lead to aspiration pneumonia, thereby negatively affecting prognosis. Causes of dysphagia include weakness of the muscles of deglutition and esophageal peristalsis, peristaltic incoordination (cricopharyngeal achalasia), and/or obstruction due to a neoplastic process.

Treatment of dysphagia is generally aimed at the underlying disorder. In the case of cricopharyngeal achalasia, however, myotomy, and, in some centers, injection of botulinum toxin, have reversed this severe complication.

TABLE 32-2	Myositis-specific Antibodies		
Antibody	**Antigen**	**%**	**Clinical subgroup**
Antisynthetases			**Antisynthetase syndrome[a]**
Anti-Jo1	Histidyl-tRNA synthetase	15–40	
Anti-PL-7	Threonyl-tRNA synthetase	<3	
Anti-PL-12	Alanyl-tRNA synthetase	<3	
Anti-OJ	Isoleucyl-tRNA synthetase	<2	
Anti-EJ	Glycyl-tRNA synthetase	<2	
Anti-KS	Asparaginyl-tRNA synthetase	<1	
Other			**Acute, severe PM ILD and Raynaud's DM**
Anti-SRP	Signal recognition particle	<5	
Anti-KJ	Unidentified translation factor	<1	
Anti-MI-2	Nuclear helicase		

[a]Fever, arthritis, Raynaud's, "mechanic's hands," and ILD.
DM, dermatomyositis; ILD, interstitial lung disease; PM, polymyositis.

E. **Calcinosis** may complicate the course of inflammatory muscle disease, occurring most commonly in DM and in the PM-scleroderma overlap variant. It may take several forms:

  1. **Excrescences of calcium,** as hard, pebbly masses or as soft pastelike accumulations, may appear generally in the digits and elsewhere. When these calcifications are found in the breast tissue, diagnostic dilemmas may arise, which require clearing through biopsy.

  2. **Masses** of calcium may accumulate in the connective tissue that surrounds muscle and its subcomponents, resulting in severe limitations of function.

  3. **"Tumoral calcinosis"** is the phenomenon in which large calcium masses occur in the torso and extremities, thereby causing deformities and loss of function.

  4. **Occasionally, surface eruptions** of calcium may become the site of infections.

 DIAGNOSTIC INVESTIGATIONS

I. **LABORATORY TESTS**

  A. **Several sarcoplasmic enzymes are released from the muscle cell** as a consequence of injury or inflammation, with corresponding increases in their activities in the circulation.

  B. **Creatine kinase (CK) is the most sensitive and specific** of these enzymes, and variations in its serum level can be used to monitor the course of myositis. CK is a dimer consisting of M and B subunits. Skeletal muscle contains more than 95% of the CK-MM dimers; however, during the disease course of myopathy the MB form is also expressed and can be found in elevated concentrations in the serum. Both CK-MM and CK-MB are found in cardiac muscle.

   1. **CK-BB** is found in smooth muscle and in the central nervous system.

   2. **Mitochondrial CK** is a large polymer, almost never found in the serum, except in certain rare catastrophic circumstances.

  C. **Aspartate aminotransferase (AST), alanine aminotransferase (ALT), and aldolase A can also be found in skeletal muscle,** and their serum activities increase during the course of myositis.

  D. **Occasionally, patients with myositis present with normal serum enzyme values.** The reason is unclear, although in some instances circulating inhibitors may interfere with the detection of enzyme activity.

  E. **The serum concentrations of myoglobin** can also be used to assess severity of the disorder and to monitor disease activity. This oxygen-binding heme-protein is found only in skeletal and cardiac muscles and, therefore, has greater specificity for myopathy than the enzymes do. In addition, persistent, marked elevations of myoglobin levels in the circulation may in rare instances be associated with myoglobinuria and may pose a risk of secondary renal failure.

  F. **Creatine,** which is synthesized in extramuscular locations, is taken up by muscle and is used as a vehicle for energy transport. Its rate of uptake and retention by diseased muscle is below normal. Loss of myofibrils also contributes to a lower uptake of creatine from the circulation. As a result, creatinuria occurs in myositis and other myopathies as well. However, there are currently insufficient data linking this finding with other disease activity and severity indices.

II. **RADIOLOGIC STUDIES**

  A. **Magnetic resonance imaging (MRI)** has proven to be of use in detecting abnormalities in muscle of patients with myositis. This is largely based on the detection of edema, or increased water content, in affected inflamed muscle, especially when T2-weighted images are used. Atrophy can also be assessed. The thigh muscles are the most often studied. MR signal intensity can vary with disease activity, making it a useful index to monitor therapeutic response.

  B. **Ultrasonography** also has been utilized in these disorders. Ultrasonographic examination can assess atrophy in affected musculature and, when combined with the use of power Doppler techniques, can detect hyperemia, a surrogate indicator of inflammation.

    C. Both MRI and US can be employed not only for diagnostic assessment but also for selecting a site for biopsy, corresponding to an area of increased muscle inflammation and responsiveness to treatment.

III. ELECTROMYOGRAPHY (EMG)
    Muscle affected by inflammation produces short, low-amplitude polyphasic potentials on contraction. Additionally, acute inflammation may be associated with irritative phenomena. EMG is of value in differentiating myopathies from neurogenic causes of muscle weakness and, as with the imaging techniques, can be used as a guide in the selection of the site for muscle biopsy. Because needle artifacts may be produced by EMG, the contralateral symmetrical muscle, which has not been instrumented by EMG, is usually chosen for tissue sampling by biopsy.

 DIFFERENTIAL DIAGNOSIS

I.   **The first step** in differential diagnosis is to ascertain whether the symptoms and signs are those of myopathy. Chapter 15 presents a categorization of etiologic groups to be considered. Among the most common factors in this connection are medications (e.g., the statins and D-penicillamine), excessive alcohol or illicit drug use, endocrinopathies (e.g., thyroid disorders), and genetic and metabolic abnormalities.

II.   **Muscle biopsy** is extremely helpful in demonstrating findings of inflammation in the myositic disorders. In addition, the presence of vacuoles and inclusions, as in IBM; hypertrophic fibers, as in the dystrophies; fiber type grouping, as in neuropathic disorders; vasculopathy, as in DM; and mitochondrial abnormalities will allow the pathologist to identify findings of diagnostic importance.

 TREATMENT

I.   **The goal of treatment is to suppress inflammation** and to thereby prevent myofiber damage and loss.

II.   **To the present, corticosteroids represent the mainstay of therapy.** Oral therapy is generally begun at approximately 30 to 50 mg/day of prednisone or its equivalent and is then tapered down when physical and laboratory response is noted. Parenteral corticosteroids, including pulse Solumedrol 1,000 mg/day for 3 consecutive days, given periodically, have also been successfully employed in select patients. It must be appreciated that steroids, in the doses used in these disorders, can lead to myopathy, and this can lead to diagnostic difficulties and therapeutic conundrums.

III.   **Immunomodulatory agents** such as azathioprine, methotrexate, cyclophosphamide, cyclosporine, and mycophenolate mofetil (MMF) have all been used in conjunction with steroids to control inflammation, thereby allowing for a decrease in the steroid dose needed. Methotrexate, which can have pulmonary toxicity, should be used with caution if pulmonary disease is present or suspected. The primary use of cyclophosphamide is in patients with pulmonary involvement.

IV.   **Intravenous immunoglobulin (IVIG),** in a total dose of 2 g/kg, given over 2 to 5 days, has demonstrated efficacy in DM and probable benefit in IBM, in double-blind, crossover, placebo-controlled studies. Although there have been no similar studies for PM, case reports and small series describe success in this disorder as well.

V.   **Hydroxychloroquine** has been useful in the treatment of both skin and muscular components of the myositic syndromes.

VI.   **Topical medications** used in conjunction with systemic therapies for the treatment of DM rash include steroid applications and/or tacrolimus or pimecrolimus ointments.

VII.   **Physical therapy** is also important in maintaining the functioning of joints and in preventing joint contractions, which may occur after extended periods of disuse of joints.

VIII. **The treatment of calcinosis** is problematic. Many therapies including warfarin, colchicine, bisphosphonates, intralesional steroid injections, phosphate-binding antacids, probenecid, and calcium channel blockers have all been reported to be helpful. The natural history of calcinosis syndromes complicating myositis is thus far not known. Large calcific masses, or calcifications complicated by infection, may require surgical intervention.

IX. **Experimental therapies** currently under study include biologic therapies targeting T-cell regulatory pathways, costimulatory molecules, cytokines, B cells, and monoclonal antibodies targeting adhesion molecules. TNF-α antagonists have been helpful in some refractory cases.

PROGNOSIS

I. **All studies of prognosis agree that the earlier the treatment is instituted,** the better the chances of improvement are. This may explain, in part, why IBM, which often begins insidiously in the elderly people, has a poor response to therapy. Many affected individuals delay medical evaluation, believing aging to be the cause of weakness.

II. **In addition to delay in therapy, a number of factors negatively affect prognosis.**
   A. Disease severity.
   B. Cardiopulmonary complications.
   C. Underlying malignancy.
   D. Ulcerating skin lesions on the torso of patients with DM.
   E. Disease chronicity.
   F. Dysphagia, especially with aspiration.
   G. Antisynthetase syndrome.

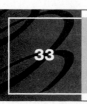

SJÖGREN'S SYNDROME
Stuart S. Kassan

33

■ KEY POINTS

■ Sjögren's syndrome (SS) is a common autoimmune disease that may occur alone or in combination with any of the other autoimmune diseases such as rheumatoid arthritis (RA), systemic lupus erythematosus (SLE), and progressive systemic sclerosis (PSS).

■ Ninety percent of patients with SS are women.

■ The differential diagnosis includes conditions and medications that can produce dry eyes and mouth, including diabetes mellitus, amyloidosis, sarcoidosis, viral infections, trauma, irradiation, psychogenic conditions, certain vitamin deficiencies, and the use of certain antihypertensives, antihistamines, and psychotherapeutic agents.

■ Non-Hodgkin's lymphoma has been found to occur more often in patients with SS, in whom the relative risk is 44 times greater than expected.

■ Patients of SS with parotid enlargement, splenomegaly, lymphadenopathy, palpable purpura, leg ulcers, low C4 levels and mixed cryoglobulin, and cross-reactive idiotypes of monoclonal rheumatoid factors may indicate the future development of lymphoma.

*S*jögren's syndrome (SS) is a common, slowly progressive, systemic autoimmune disease associated with exocrine gland dysfunction due to lymphocytic infiltration (epithelitis).

I. **The most commonly accepted definition of SS** has been the presence of two of the following findings: (a) keratoconjunctivitis sicca (dry eyes), (b) xerostomia (dry mouth), and (c) one of the connective tissue disease syndromes.

II. **Primary SS** includes patients with keratoconjunctivitis and xerostomia in the absence of any other definable connective tissue disease. They have certain clinical, serologic, and genetic differences from the secondary SS that are associated with connective tissue disorders. These differences suggest varying etiologies for similar clinical manifestations of disease.

III. **Secondary SS** is defined as keratoconjunctivitis and xerostomia in the setting of another connective tissue disease. Rheumatoid arthritis (RA) is the most common connective tissue disease seen in association with secondary SS, but other diseases have been well-documented and include systemic lupus erythematosus (SLE), scleroderma, polymyositis, mixed connective tissue disease, and juvenile idiopathic arthritis (JIA).

IV. **Pathologic evidence** that differentiates between primary and secondary SS has also been developed and has been employed along with the clinical designations noted in the subsequent text.

 ETIOPATHOGENESIS

I. **ABNORMALITIES OF HUMORAL IMMUNITY**
   A. **Anti-salivary duct antibody** is present more frequently in secondary SS (70% positive) than in primary SS (10% positive). No differences in other organ-specific antibodies (e.g., antithyroid and antigastric parietal cell antibodies) have been found.
   B. **Non–organ-specific autoantibodies**
      1. **Immunoglobulin M (IgM) rheumatoid factor (RF)** is the most common type of RF in all cases of SS and is present in nearly 100% of patients with SS.
      2. **Levels of IgG and IgA rheumatoid factors** seem to be elevated in primary SS more often than in secondary SS.
      3. **Antinuclear antibody (ANA)** positivity was found in 64% to 68% of all SS cases. ANA patterns tend to be speckled because of the anti–SS-B antibodies found in SS.
   C. **Antibodies to soluble acidic nuclear antigens** (e.g., Ro and La) extracted from lymphoid cell lines.
      1. **Anti–SS-A** (or anti-Ro) antibodies are present in the following percentages:
         a. Primary SS—70%.
         b. SS with RA—1%.
         c. SS with SLE—33%.
      2. **Anti–SS-B** (or anti-Ha, anti-La) antibodies are present in the following percentages:
         a. Primary SS—50% to 70%.
         b. SS with RA—3% to 5%.
         c. SS with SLE—73%.

II. **GENETICS.** Histocompatibility testing of patients with SS has demonstrated a genetic dichotomy between patients with primary SS (SS alone) and those with secondary SS (SS associated with another connective tissue disease, generally RA).
   A. **Primary sicca syndrome** has a significantly increased association with human leucocyte antigen-B8 (HLA-B8) and HLA-DR3.
   B. HLA associations discussed in the preceding text are usually not found in patients with **secondary sicca syndrome.** In the case of patients with SS and RA, there is an increased incidence of the HLA-DR4 antigen (that antigen found most often in seropositive RA alone).
   C. **Family studies** show that relatives of patients with SS may have an increased incidence of serum autoantibodies, positive results on Schirmer's test, elevated γ globulin levels, and RA.

III. **ABNORMALITIES OF CELLULAR IMMUNITY AND IMMUNE REGULATION IN SS**
   A. Evidence suggests the presence of a serum-blocking factor that may decrease the percentage of T cells. Natural cell-mediated cytotoxicity is depressed in both primary and secondary SS. Overall, it seems that B-cell activation is the most consistent immunoregulatory aberration in patients with SS. It may begin as a polyclonal activation, evolving to oligoclonal and monoclonal activation, and may end in a transformation to a malignant monoclonal proliferation. Elevated levels of immune

complexes and abnormal clearance of these complexes by the reticuloendothelial system have been demonstrated in active SS. Their role in the pathogenesis of disease is unclear, but they may be important in vasculitic states and glomerulonephritis.

B. Graft versus host disease (GVHD)-related SS resembles spontaneous SS, suggesting a possible pathophysiologic mechanism for the development of SS and other connective tissue diseases.

C. Viral studies. Tubuloreticular structures have been identified in labial salivary gland tissue and renal endothelium from patients with SS. No successful viral isolation from salivary gland tissues has been accomplished. Patients with **human immunodeficiency virus (HIV)** infection may manifest a clinical picture indistinguishable from that of SS. These patients usually do not demonstrate antibodies to Ro (SS-A) or La (SS-B) cellular antigens, and the intralesional T cells are CD8+, as opposed to CD4+ in autoimmune SS.

PREVALENCE

I. **SEX.** At least 90% of the patients with SS (primary or secondary) are women.

II. **AGE.** Most patients with the disease are older than 40 years, but the disease may be encountered in persons in their second and third decades of life.

III. When various populations of patients with SS have been evaluated for the presence of other connective tissue diseases, the results are as follows:
   A. RA—30% to 55%.
   B. Scleroderma—5% to 8%.
   C. SLE—5% to 10%.
   D. Polymyositis—2% to 4%.
   E. Hashimoto's thyroiditis, mixed connective tissue disease, chronic active hepatitis, Raynaud's disease—the incidences of these disorders in patients with SS is unknown.

IV. Alternatively, when evidence of SS is specifically sought in patients with other connective tissue diseases, the results are quite different.
   A. SLE—more than 50%.
   B. RA—20% to more than 50%.
   C. Scleroderma—40% to 50%.

CLINICAL MANIFESTATIONS

I. **GLANDULAR INVOLVEMENT IN SS.** Eighty percent of patients with SS have major salivary gland enlargement. Focal lymphocytic infiltration with linear destruction may be seen in minor salivary glands in the labial, nasal, and hard palate mucosa. Involvement of the exocrine glands of the upper and lower respiratory tracts, gastrointestinal tract, vagina, pancreas, and skin has been found in SS, and each area of involvement can be associated with dryness-related symptoms and complications.

II. **Ocular symptoms** may not be present in one-third to one-half of patients at any one given time during the course of their disease despite definite pathologic ocular changes. However, approximately 95% of patients with SS will manifest ocular symptoms at some time.

III. **Xerostomia** is an infrequent presenting sign of SS, but approximately 90% of patients will have sialographic abnormalities of the parotids. Salivary gland enlargement, primarily of the parotid gland, is present in one-third of patients with SS and is usually bilateral. Lacrimal gland enlargement is unusual (4%).

IV. **EXTRAGLANDULAR INVOLVEMENT.** In the case of primary SS, these extraglandular manifestations may be directly associated with SS and be a function of the epithelitis in the specific organs or tissues. In the case of secondary SS, some of these extraglandular manifestations may be a reflection of the other connective tissue disease with which SS is associated.
   A. Gastrointestinal disorders in SS have included the following:
      1. Esophageal stenosis.
      2. Atrophic gastritis.
      3. Pancreatitis.

B. Hepatic disorders in patients with SS have included the following:
1. Abnormal liver function test results (especially elevated levels of alkaline phosphatase and γ glutamyl transpeptidase) in 45% of patients.
2. Primary biliary cirrhosis.
3. Chronic active hepatitis.
4. Cryptogenic cirrhosis (15% of patients with SS in one study).

C. Renal disorders have been found in as many as one-third of patients with SS and include the following:
1. Renal tubular acidosis type 1.
2. Nephrogenic diabetes insipidus.
3. Chronic interstitial nephritis.
4. Immune complex glomerulonephritis.

D. Pulmonary disorders may be found in 4% to 15% of patients with SS and include the following:
1. Chronic obstructive pulmonary disease.
2. Pulmonary infiltrates (e.g., pseudolymphoma).
3. Fibrosing alveolitis.

E. Myositis, often of an indolent nature, may be encountered in SS. Up to 50% of patients have been found to exhibit, on random muscle biopsy specimens, abnormalities consisting of interstitial and perivascular fibrosis, inflammatory infiltrates, or both.

F. Vasculitis is present in less than 10% of patients with SS. It may be seen in association with the following:
1. Myositis.
2. Mononeuritis multiplex.
3. Axonal neuropathy.
4. Central nervous system involvement (in which immune vasculopathy and anti-SS antibodies may play a pathogenetic role).
5. Purpura.

V. MALIGNANCY IN SS

A. Non-Hodgkin's lymphoma has been found to occur more often in patients with SS (primary or secondary), with a relative risk of 44 times the expected incidence. An increased risk of lymphoma occurs in patients with a history of parotid enlargement, splenomegaly, lymphadenopathy, palpable purpura, leg ulcers, serologic changes of low levels of C4 complement, mixed cryoglobulin, and cross-reactive idiotypes of monoclonal rheumatoid factors.

B. Waldenström's macroglobulinemia appears to be more frequent in SS, but its true incidence is unknown.

C. Pseudolymphoma in SS is characterized by the extraglandular extension of lymphoproliferation that is clinically and histologically benign. The incidence of pseudolymphoma in SS is not known.

D. Other malignancies reported to coexist with SS include Kaposi's sarcoma, immunoblastic lymphadenopathy, and immunoblastic sarcoma.

 DIAGNOSTIC INVESTIGATIONS

I. SPECIFIC TESTS

A. Tests of functional glandular abnormalities
1. **Schirmer's test.** Five millimeters of unstimulated wetting of filter paper in 5 minutes is considered normal (17% false-positive and 15% false-negative results).
2. **Parotid salivary flow rate**
3. Results of **radionuclide scan** of the parotid glands (pertechnetate ^{99m}Tc) may be falsely abnormal as a result of other abnormalities of the parotid gland.
4. **Parotid gland sialography** is performed by introducing radiopaque dye into the parotid duct system. The abnormalities seen in SS include acinar and duct atrophy with puddling of dye, main duct enlargement, and retention of contrast material. All the above abnormalities may be seen in chronic parotitis with causes other than SS.

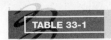 TABLE 33-1	American–European Consensus Group Modification of the European Community Criteria for Sjögren's Syndrome

- Symptoms of dry eye
- Signs of dry eye (abnormal results of Schirmer's or Rose bengal test)
- Symptoms of dry mouth
- Tests of salivary glandular function (abnormal flow rate, scintigram, or sialogram)
- Minor salivary gland biopsy (focus score of >1)
- Autoantibodies (SS-A or SS-B)

Definite Sjögren's syndrome requires the fulfillment of four criteria, one of which must be either a positive biopsy finding or autoantibody screen.
Adapted with permission from Kassan and Moutsopoulos.

   B. Tests of anatomic abnormalities
      1. Rose bengal staining of the cornea may be helpful in confirming the diagnosis but is not specific (4% false-positive and 5% false-negative results).
      2. Parotid gland sialography
   C. Biopsy
      1. Lip biopsy of minor salivary glands. Abnormalities include the presence of lymphocytic infiltrate and the characteristic epimyoepithelial islands.
      2. Lacrimal glands and parotid glands. Abnormalities are similar to those found in the minor salivary glands of the lip. Because of the relative lack of morbidity associated with lip biopsies, this procedure is preferred over lacrimal or parotid gland biopsies as a diagnostic tool.
II. **NONSPECIFIC LABORATORY ABNORMALITIES.** These changes are also often seen in other states of inflammation and in many autoimmune diseases.
   A. Elevated erythrocyte sedimentation rate—80%.
   B. Anemia—40%.
   C. Leukopenia—less than 30%.
   D. Hypergammaglobulinemia—80%.
   E. Positive RF—more than 90%.
   F. Positive ANA—70%.
   G. Circulating cryoglobulins may be 30%.
III. **CLASSIFICATION CRITERIA.** An international consensus statement was published in 2002 after numerous meetings of the American–European consensus group. Classification criteria for SS were proposed by this group as a revision of the previous criteria sets (Table 33-1).

 DIFFERENTIAL DIAGNOSIS

The salivary gland involvement in SS, including glandular swelling, pain, tenderness, and sicca symptoms, may be confused with numerous other conditions.
I. **INFECTION OF SALIVARY GLANDS**
   A. Viral. Coxsackie virus infection, mumps, cytomegalovirus inclusion disease, and HIV infection.
   B. Bacterial. Acute sialadenitis is often seen in dehydrated, debilitated patients. Chronic bacterial sialadenitis is frequently associated with obstruction of the salivary ducts by inspissated saliva.
   C. Fungal. Actinomycosis or histoplasmosis.
   D. Tuberculosis. Rare.
II. **GRANULOMATOUS DISEASE.** Sarcoidosis.
III. **OTHER INFILTRATIVE DISORDERS**
   A. Primary neoplasms of the parotid gland.
   B. Leukemia.

    C. Amyloidosis.

    D. Lymphoma of intraparotid lymph nodes.

    E. Burkitt's lymphoma.

    F. Pseudolymphoma.

IV. SYSTEMIC DISEASES

    A. Cirrhosis.

    B. Diabetes mellitus.

    C. Hyperlipoproteinemias (types 3, 4, and 5).

    D. Obesity.

    E. Pregnancy and lactation.

    F. Gouty parotitis (rare).

    G. Cushing's disease.

    H. Cystic fibrosis.

V. NUTRITIONAL DEFICIENCY

    A. Starvation.

    B. Vitamin B_6 deficiency.

    C. Vitamin C deficiency.

    D. Vitamin A deficiency.

VI. Drugs associated with the development of dry mouth

    A. Sedatives.

    B. Hypnotics.

    C. Narcotics.

    D. Phenothiazine.

    E. Atropine.

    F. Propantheline.

    G. Antiparkinsonian drugs.

    H. Antihistamines.

    I. Ephedrine.

    J. Epinephrine.

    K. Amphetamines.

 TREATMENT

The general approach to treatment in SS centers around the manifestations of xerostomia and xerophthalmia and the extraglandular manifestations of SS and/or the other autoimmune disease in the case of secondary SS. In the exocrinopathy of SS, the therapies are specific to the local problem (see in subsequent text). In regard to the extraglandular manifestations of the disease, the treatment is often focused on the specific organ involvement, which may be due to SS (primary) or due to one of the other autoimmune diseases associated with SS (secondary). No controlled trials have been undertaken in the therapy for the systemic manifestations of SS. In general, the approach to treatment has been empiric. Vasculitis, renal disease (immune complex-mediated or otherwise), myositis, alveolitis, cryoglobulinemia, and other manifestations have mostly been treated in the past with corticosteroids, immunosuppressive agents, or both, depending on the severity of disease. Because the cytotoxic drugs are immunosuppressive and because patients undergoing renal transplantation and others treated with these agents have an increased incidence of lymphoma (as do untreated patients with SS), it is advisable to avoid their use in SS.

I.   **OCULAR ABNORMALITIES.** Artificial tears are the mainstay of treatment. Solutions consisting of methylcellulose and polyvinyl alcohol are useful. The dosage varies from two drops four times daily to every 15 minutes, depending on the clinical state. Inserts placed into the conjunctival sac that release small amounts of methylcellulose over many hours are presently available and may be beneficial in some patients. Lacrimal duct occlusion, temporary or permanent, may enhance local moisture. Bromhexine, a secretagogue, is presently being studied in clinical trials for use in the United States.

II.   **XEROSTOMIA.** Pilocarpine hydrochloride (Salagen tablets) and cevimeline (Evoxac tablets) are indicated for the treatment of symptoms of xerostomia secondary to salivary gland hypofunction. As a cholinergic parasympathetic agent, pilocarpine can increase secretion of the salivary glands. The usual initial dose is 5 mg three times a day. It is contraindicated in patients with asthma, iritis, and narrow-angle glaucoma. Side effects include abdominal cramps and sweating. Cevimeline is a cholinergic agent that binds to muscarinic receptors and increases secretions of exocrine glands such as salivary and sweat glands. The dosage is 30 mg three times daily. Side effects include sweating, nausea, exacerbation of asthma, and cardiac abnormalities. Lubrication of the mouth and mild secretagogues, such as lemon-flavored juice or lubricating agents (water and methylcellulose), are useful. More potent secretagogues may exacerbate the signs and symptoms of parotitis. Prevention of states of dehydration in SS is very important because dehydration may enhance the formation of parotid ductal calculi. Avoidance of drugs that may aggravate oral dryness (e.g., narcotics, antihistamines, and anticholinergics) is also important.

III. **PAROTID ENLARGEMENT.** In the past, numerous modes of therapy have been employed to treat parotid enlargement.

    A. Surgical removal is often technically difficult, and resultant nonhealing fistulae and facial nerve damage preclude this mode of therapy.

    B. Drug therapy for symptomatic inflammatory parotid enlargement

        1. Nonsteroidal anti-inflammatory drugs. Useful regimens include 25 to 50 mg of indomethacin four times daily or 600 mg of ibuprofen four times daily.

        2. Corticosteroid therapy should be limited to those with severe, recalcitrant disease because of the risk for corticosteroid toxicity. The regimen is 20 to 40 mg/day, with dosage tapering as soon as a clinical response is obtained.

        3. Oral pilocarpine and cevimeline therapy have been recently approved by the U.S. Food and Drug Administration for use in SS. They may be helpful in patients with sicca symptomatology in dosages of 5 mg three or four times daily for pilocarpine and 30 mg three times daily for cevimeline.

        4. Hydroxychloroquine use has also been studied in SS, and its effects have been very modest in treating the sicca symptoms and the fatigue symptoms.

    C. Cytotoxic therapy (specifically azathioprine, cyclophosphamide, chlorambucil, and methotrexate) does not seem to offer any significant benefit unless a true malignancy (lymphoma) or an invasive form of pseudolymphoma in SS is being treated.

    D. Antitumor necrosis factor therapy has been recently studied and found to be ineffective in patients with SS, especially for the treatment of the sicca symptoms.

 PROGNOSIS

I. In long-term follow-up, local mucous membrane damage may occur involving eyes, mouth, vagina, trachea, and so on, if moisturization is not maintained effectively.

II. Systemic involvement of lungs, kidneys, nervous system, and skin may develop as part of the epithelitis or with vasculitic involvement.

III. The predictors for the development of lymphoma are noted in the preceding text.

IV. The exocrinopathy of SS may be relatively stable or may exhibit a slow progression of secretory alteration physiologically over the course of 5 to 10 years.

V. Patients treated aggressively to maintain secretory function may have a beneficial effect on exocrine gland function, which emphasizes the need for vigorous therapy stretching over prolonged periods in patients with SS.

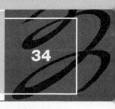

SYSTEMIC SCLEROSIS AND RELATED SYNDROMES

34

Robert F. Spiera

▪ KEY POINTS

- Scleroderma is a systemic fibrosing disease in which underlying vasculopathy plays a major role.
- Raynaud's phenomenon is nearly ubiquitous in scleroderma, and its absence should make the clinician question the diagnosis.
- The pattern of skin involvement, in particular, limited versus diffuse disease, is important in predicting the organ systems that may become involved and has prognostic implications.
- There is no proven treatment of the disease itself, but organ-based therapies have vastly improved the quality of life and survival in patients with scleroderma.
- In patients with diffuse disease, aggressive blood pressure monitoring is essential, particularly in the early years, because early detection of hypertension and appropriate prompt aggressive treatment with angiotensin-converting enzyme (ACE) inhibitors can usually successfully prevent progression to renal failure.
- Visceral disease, in particular cardiac involvement, is a predictor of poor survival in patients with scleroderma.

I. **Systemic sclerosis** is a systemic disorder characterized by microvascular injury and fibrosis in the affected organs.
   A. Skin involvement is a defining feature.
   B. Raynaud's phenomenon is almost universally found in patients with systemic sclerosis.
   C. Nomenclature. Other terms include morphea for isolated skin disease, CREST syndrome for limited disease, and progressive systemic sclerosis for diffuse progressive disease.
II. **Various patterns of scleroderma** are recognized, often with distinct serologic associations and prognostic implications; patients can be roughly categorized on the basis of the pattern of skin involvement.
   A. Localized cutaneous disease (morphea)
   B. Limited disease. The acronym **CREST** syndrome is often used for patients with limited disease in whom **C**alcinosis, **R**aynaud's phenomenon, **E**sophageal dysmotility, **S**clerodactyly, and **T**elangiectasias are prominent features and in whom cutaneous involvement is mostly of the distal extremities.
   C. Diffuse disease
III. **Visceral involvement** can occur particularly in patients with diffuse disease and can be organ- and/or life-threatening.

 ETIOPATHOGENESIS

I. **The etiology of scleroderma** is unknown; it is idiopathic in most instances.
   A. Some environmentally associated sclerodermalike syndromes have been described as occurring after particular exposures, including to bleomycin, vinyl chloride, and silica dust.
   B. No strong genetic associations have been recorded, but familial clusters have been recognized in some populations.

II. **PATHOGENESIS.** The interplay between microvascular injury, inflammatory response, and fibrosis contribute to the pathogenesis of scleroderma.

   A. Microvascular injury with fibrosis and excess deposition of extracellular matrix, particularly collagen, is recognized. Endothelial injury has been hypothesized as the primary process, with resultant tissue ischemia and secondary fibrotic changes eventually resulting in the clinical phenotype of scleroderma. Vascular luminal narrowing secondary to intimal proliferation has been demonstrated.

   B. Vasoactive mediators are abnormally expressed in patients with scleroderma. Elevated circulating levels of endothelin-1 and diminished levels of nitric oxide have been reported. These may ultimately be targets of therapeutic interventions.

   C. Inflammation plays an important role, particularly early in the disease process. Inflammatory perivascular infiltrates with a T cell predominance, particularly at the border dividing the reticular dermis and subcutaneous fat, can be demonstrated.

   D. Evidence of cellular immunity is supported by the predominance of T cells in the early tissue infiltrates, as well as by the correlations between interleukin-2 (IL-2) and soluble IL-2 receptor levels and disease activity.

   E. There are similarities between scleroderma and graft versus host disease. Investigators have demonstrated cellular mosaicism in women with scleroderma, with retention of fetal cells in skin lesions and in the peripheral blood of women with systemic sclerosis. This suggests the possibility that a graft versus hostlike reaction induced by fetal cells contributes to the pathogenesis in these patients.

   F. Autoantibodies are found in up to 95% of patients, although no direct pathogenic role has been demonstrated. These may be the epiphenomena of immune system activation and tissue injury.

   G. Cytokines, including those of transforming growth factor-β (TGF-β), IL-1, IL-2, and platelet-derived growth factor, have been implicated in fibroblast dysregulation and in excess collagen production.

 PREVALENCE

I. **Scleroderma** is a relatively uncommon disorder. The incidence is estimated to be between 10 and 20 cases in 1 million annually. Prevalence rates of 4 to 253 in 1 million individuals have been reported.

II. **Scleroderma affects women** more commonly than men.

III. **Disease onset** is often recognized in the third or fourth decade of life but can occur in childhood as well.

 CLINICAL MANIFESTATIONS

I. **Vascular disease is nearly universal in scleroderma.** The distribution of vascular disease largely determines the organ system that will be affected.

   A. Raynaud's phenomenon occurs in 95% of patients, and its absence should caution the clinician to question the diagnosis. The typical changes are pallor and cyanosis followed by erythema in response to cold stimuli. Episodes can also be precipitated by stress and smoking or may occur spontaneously.

   B. Intimal hyperplasia and adventitial fibrosis can result in attenuation of vessel lumen. Vasoconstriction in already compromised vessels can result in ischemia with digital ulcers, infarcts, and even autoamputation.

   C. Visceral Raynaud's phenomenon may occur in the heart and kidney.

II. **Skin disease is the hallmark of systemic sclerosis.** It is the most identifiable, nearly universal feature.

   A. An early edematous phase is characterized by puffy swelling of the hands and fingers.

   B. With disease progression, the skin thickens and binds down, with loss of normal structures such as hair follicles. Spontaneous loosening of the skin can occur later in the course of the disease. Pruritus is a common complaint.

C. Skin discoloration is common, with areas of erythema early in the disease course and subsequent areas of hypopigmentation or hyperpigmentation.

D. Skin breakdown, particularly over the extensor surfaces of the joints of the hands, can result in ulcerations, which heal poorly and may become secondarily infected.

E. Skin changes often begin distally in the hands and progress more proximally to the trunk.

F. The pattern of skin involvement has allowed stratification into two distinct subgroups with differing serologic association, clinical course, and pattern of organ involvement (Table 34-1).

III. Pulmonary disease is a major cause of mortality in scleroderma. Interstitial lung disease often begins at the bases of the lungs and can be progressive. It can occur early in the course of diffuse scleroderma; in patients with limited disease, it can be a late and indolently progressive feature.

A. Symptoms include dyspnea and a nonproductive dry cough.

B. Pulmonary involvement can be complicated by secondary pulmonary hypertension in patients with advanced interstitial lung disease.

C. Pulmonary hypertension can occur early in patients with limited scleroderma in the absence of interstitial lung disease and can similarly present with dyspnea, particularly on exertion.

IV. Renal disease can occur relatively early in the disease course in patients with diffuse disease. Hypertensive renal crisis is characterized by a hyper-reninemic state, with associated hypertension, rapidly progressive renal insufficiency, microangiopathic hemolysis, and consumptive thrombocytopenia.

A. Hypertensive retinopathy, encephalopathy, and renal failure can occur if the syndrome is unrecognized and untreated.

B. The occurrence of the syndrome may be associated with corticosteroid use.

C. The syndrome can occur, uncommonly, in the absence of measurable arterial hypertension. Also, it may exist in patients with minimal or no sclerodermal skin changes (i.e., scleroderma sine scleroderma).

D. Early recognition is crucial because this complication of scleroderma is treatable.

TABLE 34-1	Limited and Diffuse Scleroderma: Clinical Associations	
	Limited	**Diffuse**
Serologies	Anticentromere antibody (70%)	Antitopoisomerase-I (30%)
Skin	Distal extremities—can extend to forearms	Progressive, involving arms, face, legs, and trunk
	Calcinosis	May regress later in disease course
Vascular	Raynaud's, severe	Raynaud's
	Telangiectasias	Telangiectasis later in course
Pulmonary	Uninvolved early; fibrosis later in some	Early involvement
Cardiac	Pulmonary hypertension in absence of interstitial lung disease	Cardiomyopathy, myocarditis, and pericarditis
		Pulmonary hypertension late, secondary to interstitial disease
Gastrointestinal	Mostly upper tract; pyrosis and dysphagia	Diffuse involvement including upper and lower tract
Renal	Generally spared	Involvement usually early
Musculoskeletal	Flexion contractures hands, usually late	Arthralgias, tendon friction rubs
		Bland myopathy and overt myositis

V.   **Gastrointestinal (GI) involvement** can cause clinical symptoms in more than 50% of patients with scleroderma. Early changes can include vasculopathy and smooth muscle atrophy and fibrosis, which eventually result in dysmotility. Neuropathic changes contributing to disordered myoelectric function can predate the atrophic or fibrotic changes.

   A. Esophageal disease is the most common complaint, often related to lower esophageal sphincter incompetence and impaired esophageal motility. Dysphagia, odynophagia, pyrosis, erosive esophagitis, and strictures can occur.

   B. Stomach involvement characterized by gastroparesis can cause bloating and early satiety. Gastric telangiectasias can be an important source of GI bleeding.

   C. Small intestinal involvement can cause bloating, cramping abdominal pain, bacterial overgrowth, malabsorption, and diarrhea.

   D. Colonic manifestations include constipation and pseudo-obstruction and can cause wide-mouthed diverticulae, which are of common occurrence but often not of clinical importance.

VI.   **Cardiac involvement** can be an important cause of mortality in patients with systemic sclerosis.

   A. Pulmonary hypertension can occur in the setting of fibrotic lung disease, particularly in patients with diffuse disease; it can occur as a primary vascular problem, particularly in patients with limited scleroderma.

   B. Myocardial fibrosis is a poor prognostic feature. The appearance of the lesion is similar to the contraction band necrosis, likely related to microvascular disease and to intermittent ischemia resulting from vessel spasm. Fibrotic replacement of myocardium can cause arrhythmias, which are an important cause of mortality.

   C. Effusive pericarditis can occur. Pericardial effusions have been associated with an increased risk for developing subsequent hypertensive renal crisis.

VII.   **Musculoskeletal problems** are important contributors to functional limitation in patients with scleroderma.

   A. Arthralgias are common, related to involvement of periartricular structures more commonly than to arthritis *per se.*

   B. Fibrosis of tendon sheaths or cutaneous involvement of overlying skin can result in contractures, particularly of the hands, and also of large joints, including the shoulders and elbows.

   C. Myopathy can occur, often related to fibrotic disease and atrophy, resulting in muscle weakness. Less commonly, an overt inflammatory myositis can occur.

 PHYSICAL EXAMINATION

I.   **Skin involvement** is the defining feature of scleroderma.

   A. The early edematous phase is characterized by puffiness and swelling, particularly of the hands and fingers.

   B. Subsequent development of thickened, bound-down skin, with loss of normal appendicular structures is more specific to scleroderma. Hyperpigmentation or hypopigmentation is common, especially later in the course of the disease. Cutaneous involvement often begins distally, extending proximally.

   C. Facial symptoms include pursing of the mouth and thinning of the lips, as well as the presence of telangiectasias.

   D. Subcutaneous calcific deposits (calcinosis) are seen most commonly in the hands or over bony prominences.

   E. Ulcerations on the extensor surfaces of contracted joints, particularly over the proximal interphalangeal (PIP) joints of the hands, are common.

II.   **Vascular disease is nearly ubiquitous,** characterized by acrocyanosis, especially precipitated by cold exposure.

   A. Distal tuft ulcerations and infarcts can be seen, and less commonly, autoamputation of distal phalanges can occur.

   B. Nailfold capillary changes including tortuosity of capillary loops and areas of loop dropout can be readily observed using an ophthalmoscope at $40\times$ power with oil immersion.

    C. Telangiectasias can involve the oral mucosa, face, lips, and hands and can represent the microvascular change.

III. **Pulmonary findings** relate to the underlying fibrosing disease. Typical dry "Velcro" rales can be auscultated. Early involvement can be undetectable on routine examination.

IV. **Cardiac examination findings** can include the detection of irregular heart rate in patients with arrhythmia, which is a poor prognostic sign. Prominence of the P_2 sound can suggest pulmonary hypertension.

V. **Musculoskeletal examination** can be striking in patients with scleroderma.
    A. Contractures of hands, shoulders, elbows, and loss of flexion in the knees can be seen particularly in patients with diffuse disease.
    B. Tendon friction rubs can be present, particularly in patients with diffuse disease.
    C. Weakness in proximal muscle groups, especially the hip flexors and shoulder abductors, is common and can relate to a low-grade fibrotic myopathy or less commonly to overt inflammatory muscle disease.
    D. Sclerodactyly with tapering of the digits is a typical finding.

DIAGNOSTIC INVESTIGATIONS

I. **LABORATORY TESTS**
    A. Autoantibodies are found in up to 95% of patients with systemic sclerosis. Antinuclear antibody (ANA) can be found in 90% of patients.
        1. Antitopoisomerase-I (SCL-70) antibodies are found in 30% of patients with diffuse disease.
        2. Anticentromere antibodies can be found in greater than 50% of patients with limited scleroderma (CREST syndrome).
    B. General laboratory evaluations are helpful in defining organ system involvement.
        1. Elevation in the levels of creatine kinase (CK) or aldolase can be seen in patients with inflammatory muscle involvement.
        2. Urinalysis abnormalities or serum creatinine level elevations can be seen in patients with renal disease.
        3. Anemia can be present and can be due to chronic disease, blood loss from the GI tract, and renal disease; microangiopathic hemolytic anemia can occur in patients with scleroderma hypertensive crisis (also called malignant scleroderma).

II. **IMAGING STUDIES**
    A. Musculoskeletal imaging can reveal features that are characteristic of scleroderma.
        1. Subcutaneous calcinosis often occurs over the extensor surfaces in patients with limited scleroderma (CREST) and are radiopaque on plain x-rays.
        2. Acro-osteolysis with resorption of the distal tufts of the phalanges is characteristic and relates to recurrent ischemic injury to the distal extremity.
        3. Erosive arthritis is not a common feature of scleroderma.
    B. Pulmonary disease is common, particularly in diffuse scleroderma; however, it also occurs late in the course of the disease in some patients with limited disease. A baseline chest x-ray is advisable in staging patients with diffuse disease, and a high-resolution chest computed tomography (CT) scan is often indicated, particularly if clinical symptoms or findings are present or if abnormalities are identified in the pulmonary function test results.
        1. Chest x-ray findings are typically those associated with interstitial lung disease with increased markings and fibrosis, often beginning at the bases.
        2. High-resolution chest CT scan is more sensitive in detecting and staging the lung involvement in scleroderma. Alveolitis is often suggested by a "ground glass" appearance on CT scan. Honeycombing is a sign of advanced fibrotic change.
    C. GI abnormalities are common in patients with scleroderma, causing clinical symptoms in up to 50% of patients. Imaging studies are helpful in defining involvement.
        1. Cine esophagography can reveal abnormalities of peristalsis that are typical of scleroderma and can be seen in both limited and diffuse disease; barium swallow often reveals reflux secondary to incompetence of the lower esophageal

sphincter. Upper pharyngeal function abnormalities can reflect inflammatory muscle disease and is less common.

2. Delayed gastric emptying and hypomotility reflecting gastroparesis and intestinal hypomotility can be seen in upper GI series with small bowel follow-through.

3. Colonic enlargement and even megacolon can be seen on x-ray or on barium swallow studies and are related to impaired colonic motility. Wide-mouthed colonic diverticulae are often seen but are not usually of clinical significance.

D. **Pulmonary function testing** is important in assessing patients with scleroderma and is often included in the baseline evaluation, particularly if any clinical symptoms or signs are suggestive of pulmonary disease. Even in the absence of clinical symptoms, many clinicians favor pulmonary function test evaluation at baseline and possibly in follow-up if any baseline abnormalities are detected.

Diminished diffusion capacity can be secondary to the presence of interstitial lung disease. In patients with limited disease, diminished single-breath diffusing capacity of the lung for carbon monoxide (DLCO) can be related to the presence of pulmonary hypertension even in the absence of parenchymal lung disease.

A. **Echocardiography** can reveal wall motion abnormalities related to myocardial involvement. Echocardiography with Doppler studies can also estimate the pulmonary arterial pressure and offers a noninvasive method of investigating the presence of pulmonary hypertension. Pericarditis can be seen in patients with diffuse disease, and its presence may be associated with an increased risk of the subsequent development of a hypertensive renal crisis.

 DIFFERENTIAL DIAGNOSIS

Scleroderma tends to be readily identifiable in the presence of the characteristic skin findings and Raynaud's phenomenon. A number of related syndromes, however, can mimic some of the findings of systemic sclerosis.

I. **Localized scleroderma,** or morphea, is characterized by plaques of asymmetric fibrotic dermal lesions that can be histologically indistinguishable from the lesions of scleroderma.

A. Localized scleroderma is not associated with visceral disease, and survival in this group does not differ from that of the general population.

B. Raynaud's phenomenon is not typically seen.

C. Different patterns of morphea have been recognized, including localized disease that can regress over time. Generalized disease is less common. Linear scleroderma occurring in children can be characterized by a linear indurated patch of dermal fibrosis often involving the lower extremity. Facial hemiatrophy with an *en coup de sabre* deformity is rare.

II. **Eosinophilic fasciitis** is characterized by thickening and inflammation of fascia with puckering and tightness of the overlying skin. This can result in pain, weakness, and contractures.

A. Diagnostic biopsy must be deep, including the fascial layer where eosinophilic and lymphocytic infiltrates can be identified.

B. Laboratory evaluation often reveals eosinophilia and the presence of acute phase reactants.

C. Skin changes can resemble scleroderma, but often Raynaud's phenomenon and sclerodactyly do not occur. Visceral disease and the presence of ANA are less common.

D. Distinguishing the syndrome from scleroderma is crucial because corticosteroids often afford remarkable response in patients with eosinophilic fasciitis, and the disease is often self-limiting.

III. **Chemically induced sclerodermalike illnesses** have been described.

A. Sclerodermalike fibrosing illness has been associated with exposure to bleomycin, vinyl chloride, and silica dust.

B. A sclerodermalike illness was described in Spain and was associated with prior ingestion of toxic rapeseed oil.

- **C.** In 1989, the eosinophilia-myalgia syndrome was described, which was characterized by myalgias, arthralgias, and neuropathy and often sclerodermalike skin changes and was related to ingestion of contaminated tryptophan.
- **D.** A possible association between augmentation mammoplasty and development of subsequent scleroderma had been suggested, but larger epidemiologic studies have not supported a causal relation.

IV. **Mixed connective tissue disease** is an overlap connective tissue disease demonstrating features of systemic lupus, systemic sclerosis, and polymyositis.
- **A.** Puffy hands and arthralgias similar to what is seen in the early phase of scleroderma are common.
- **B.** Raynaud's phenomenon, esophageal dysfunction, interstitial lung disease, and inflammatory myopathy can be seen in a pattern consistent with that seen in scleroderma and polymyositis.
- **C.** The presence of detectable and often very high titers of antibodies to anti-ribonucleoproteins (anti-RNPs) is a requisite criterion to fulfill.
- **D.** "Overlap" syndromes, even in the absence of anti-RNP antibodies, are recognized, with various features of rheumatoid arthritis, scleroderma, lupus, and polymyositis. The focus of treatment is usually on the most prominent and troublesome clinical manifestations.
- **E.** Skin features are ultimately the most helpful in defining the presence or absence of scleroderma.

V. **Metabolic and neurogenic diseases can mimic scleroderma** and should be considered in patients with sclerodermalike features, particularly if Raynaud's phenomenon is not present.
- **A.** Diabetic sclerodactyly and cheiroarthropathy can be associated with contractures of hands and shoulders, as well as with distal skin thickening. The absence of Raynaud's phenomenon or nailfold capillary changes, the lack of autoantibodies such as ANA, and the context of prior history of diabetes readily distinguishes this syndrome.
- **B.** Myxedema in the context of hypothyroidism can cause thickening and coarseness of skin, which can be confused with scleroderma. Again, the absence of Raynaud's phenomenon or abnormal serologies and the presence of other features of hypothyroidism help distinguish this syndrome.
- **C.** Reflex sympathetic dystrophy, also called the shoulder–hand syndrome, can lead to a sclerodermalike tightening of the hands. There is usually a history of some type of trauma, surgery, or illness that predates the causalgic arm pain and skin changes.

 TREATMENT

I. **No drug has been proven to have a disease-modifying role in the treatment of scleroderma** in altering the progression of the underlying disease process. Numerous agents have been tried, some with anecdotal benefit, but to date none has stood the scrutiny of prospective placebo-controlled clinical trials.
- **A.** D-Penicillamine interferes with cross-linking of collagen, and has been widely used in diffuse scleroderma. Retrospective studies suggested improvement in skin thickening and progression of lung disease, as well as survival in treated patients, compared with historical controls. A trial comparing low-dose (62.5 mg/day) with high-dose (750 to 1,000 mg/day) D-penicillamine did not show a benefit to treatment with the higher doses.
- **B.** Colchicine has antifibrotic properties *in vitro* but has not been adequately assessed in controlled clinical trials.
- **C.** Minocycline has been reported to be of benefit in one small case series, but its role in the treatment of scleroderma is as yet uncertain.
- **D.** Recombinant human relaxin was preliminarily felt to be of benefit in arresting the progression of skin disease, but this finding was ultimately not confirmed in large controlled clinical trials.

E. Some studies have suggested benefit with immunosuppressive agents including methotrexate and cyclosporine A, but the magnitude of the benefit was minimal, and toxicity can be substantial, particularly with the use of cyclosporine in cases in which renovascular concerns are of particular importance.

F. There may be benefit to treatment with cyclophosphamide, but its use has mostly been restricted to patients with progressive interstitial lung disease or inflammatory myocardial disease.

G. Photophoresis is being used in some centers but has not gained U.S. Food and Drug Administration (FDA) approval for use in scleroderma.

H. Ongoing trials of type 1 oral collagen, cyclophosphamide, and even high-dose immunosuppressive therapy and stem cell transplantation salvage are being explored in the treatment of scleroderma.

II. **Organ-specific complications** have been very amenable to therapeutic intervention in scleroderma and have afforded improved quality of life and survival to patients with systemic sclerosis.

III. **Vascular disease** is ubiquitous in scleroderma and can be ameliorated by topical or pharmacologic intervention. The vasospastic component is particularly amenable to treatment. New agents that address the processes of intimal hyperplasia and proliferation and the resultant narrowing of the lumen are being investigated.

A. Avoidance of smoking and exposure to cold are paramount.

B. Systemic vasodilators, particularly calcium channel blockers (e.g., extended-release nifedipine starting at 30 mg oral daily or long-acting diltiazem starting at 120 mg oral daily) and α-blockers (e.g., prazosin started at 1 mg twice daily), are helpful in reducing the severity and frequency of vasospastic episodes.

C. Topical nitrates have been used in some patients with benefit.

D. Iloprost, an intravenously administered prostacyclin analog, has been shown to be of value in patients with ischemic ulcerations related to Raynaud's phenomenon. It is not presently available in the United States.

E. Bosentan, an endothelin-1 antagonist, starting at 62.5 mg twice daily and increased up to 125 mg twice daily, may be of value in reducing the development of new ischemic ulcerations in patients with systemic sclerosis and Raynaud's phenomenon. Hastened healing of pre-existing lesions has not yet been demonstrated in clinical trials.

F. Phosphodiesterase inhibitors such as sildenafil have been anecdotally described as being of value in treating severe Raynaud's phenomenon in patients with scleroderma.

G. Sympathetic blockage can be effective in controlling severe or persistent vasospasm. Surgical digital sympathectomy may be useful in salvaging digits at risk. Surgical amputation is generally avoided. Autoamputation can occur but is often more digit sparing than surgical amputation.

H. Antiplatelet agents such as aspirin (81 to 325 mg/day), clopidogrel 75 mg/day, or even full anticoagulation may improve perfusion in patients with a low flow state in the context of a digit at risk.

IV. **Skin disease** has not been convincingly shown to be ameliorated by any specific systemic intervention in prospective controlled trials. Spontaneous skin softening tends to occur with time in most patients.

A. D-Penicillamine has been used in patients with rapidly progressive skin disease by many clinicians. Its use has been supported in retrospective case–control series. A prospective trial of high- versus low-dose D-Penicillamine did not demonstrate benefit to the use of the high-dose regimen.

B. Colchicine, potassium P-Aminobenzoate, dimethyl sulfoxide, and photophoresis have been anecdotally described as ameliorating skin disease but have not been proven to be of benefit in controlled trials.

C. Ultraviolet A (UVA) treatment of localized skin lesions (morphea) may be of benefit.

D. There are no pharmacologic remedies known to be of benefit in calcinosis. Colchicine 0.6 mg twice daily may be helpful in the setting of inflammatory ulcerating lesions. Diltiazem was suggested to be of benefit in one trial. Surgical debulking of calcinosis is generally not pursued because recurrence is common but can be of value in instances of recurrent infection or severe pain.

V. Pulmonary disease is a major cause of mortality in systemic sclerosis but may be amenable to treatment if detected and is treated in its early phase.

   A. Data from case-controlled studies suggests a beneficial impact of cyclophosphamide in patients with scleroderma and alveolitis, and an ongoing prospective controlled trial is addressing this issue. Bronchoalveolar lavage may be useful in determining whether inflammatory alveolitis warranting such aggressive therapy is present.

   B. Pulmonary vascular disease had traditionally been refractory to treatment. Standard agents included high-dose calcium channel blockers and anticoagulation, which afforded symptomatic benefit. More recently, administration of intravenous epoprostenol by infusion pump has been shown to improve function and survival in patients with primary pulmonary hypertension. Bosentan, an endothelin-1 antagonist, has been shown to be of value in improving function and hemodynamics in patients with pulmonary hypertension in trials including a subgroup of patients with scleroderma.

   C. Lung transplantation seems to be a viable option for select patients with scleroderma and advanced lung disease.

VI. Renal disease had previously been a major cause of morbidity in scleroderma. The use of angiotensin-converting enzyme (ACE) inhibitors has remarkably changed renal outcomes in this disease.

   A. Aggressive monitoring of blood pressure, particularly in patients with diffuse disease, early in the disease course is essential. The prompt and aggressive institution of treatment with ACE inhibitors can abrogate the hypertensive renal crisis complicating scleroderma.

   B. Patients may be temporarily dialysis-dependent but can, in some instances, recover adequate renal function to allow withdrawal of dialysis as much as 1 year after the institution of dialysis. It is imperative, therefore, that ACE inhibitors be continued, pushing the dose to the largest that can adequately be tolerated by blood pressure.

   C. Renal transplantation has been successfully performed in patients with scleroderma.

VII. GI involvement is common in scleroderma and is often palliated by pharmacologic intervention.

   A. The introduction of proton pump inhibitors has been a tremendous advance in the management of reflux in patients with scleroderma and may help prevent development of esophageal strictures.

   B. Prokinetic agents such as cisapride (10 mg four times a day) can help with early satiety and reflux, as well as with hypomotility. Erythromycin has been similarly used, particularly now that the availability of cisapride is limited in the United States because of concerns about cardiac toxicity.

   C. Erythromycin and octreotide may be of value in improving gastric and intestinal motility.

   D. Bacterial overgrowth causes bloating and diarrhea and can be treated with periodic, rotating, empiric courses of antibacterial agents; quinolones (such as ciprofloxacin 500 mg twice daily for 2 weeks) or tetracycline (250 mg twice daily for 2 weeks) have been useful.

VIII. Cardiac complications of scleroderma including arrhythmias and congestive heart failure are treated in standard medical manner.

   A. Pericarditis can be treated with nonsteroidal anti-inflammatory drugs, but caution must be used because of their potential renal and GI side effects. Corticosteroids, such as prednisone 30 mg/day, can be helpful but must be used with caution as the use of corticosteroids in these substantial doses have been associated with an increased risk of developing scleroderma renal crisis.

   B. Impaired contractility is often related to myocardial fibrosis, but if recognized in the context of markers of myocardial injury such as CK-MB or troponin elevations, some have advocated that treatment with glucocorticoids and cyclophosphamide can lead to clinical and functional improvement.

IX. Musculoskeletal disease is common in scleroderma and can be an important cause of disability.

   A. Arthralgias and tendon friction rubs can be treated with nonsteroidal anti-inflammatory drugs but with caution given the GI and renal concerns in this patient population. Low-dose corticosteroids (7.5 mg of oral prednisone or less daily) can similarly be helpful.

B. Physical therapy and occupational therapy are essential to treatment, with particular attention to maintaining range of motion, muscle strengthening, and splinting and the use of paraffin treatments when appropriate.

C. Surgical reconstruction can be helpful in select patients with severe contractures causing functional limitation or with refractory extensor surface ulcerations.

D. Inflammatory myositis is treated with substantial dosages of corticosteroids (often beginning with 40 to 60 mg of daily prednisone) and other immunosuppressive agents such as methotrexate and azathioprine as would be used in idiopathic myositis.

 PROGNOSIS

Systemic sclerosis has been associated with an increased risk of premature death, although the disease is heterogenous; it is recognized that particular clinical features can be identified that predict poor prognosis.

I. Diffuse cutaneous disease predicts worse survival than limited cutaneous involvement, but this may be related to increased risk of specific areas of organ involvement in patients with diffuse disease rather than being a truly independent risk factor.

II. Cardiac involvement has been the strongest predictor of decreased survival.

III. Pulmonary and renal involvement are associated with an increased mortality risk.

IV. The presence of antitopoisomerase-I has been associated with decreased survival.

V. There are subgroups of patients, particularly those with limited scleroderma without pulmonary hypertension, in whom survival is probably not different from the age-matched nondisease controls.

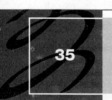

POLYMYALGIA RHEUMATICA AND GIANT CELL ARTERITIS
35

Richard Stern

■ KEY POINTS

Polymyalgia Rheumatica (PMR)

■ PMR is a common illness in individuals older than 60 years and is manifested by proximal arthralgia/myalgia, morning stiffness, gelling, and an elevated sedimentation rate.

■ Critical to the diagnosis of PMR is a dramatic response to low-dose corticosteroids.

■ The symptoms of PMR are nonspecific, and other myalgic illnesses should be excluded.

Giant Cell Arteritis (GCA)

■ GCA is a type of vasculitis, which affects the branches of the external and internal carotid artery, and it can cause permanent blindness when the retinal vessels are involved.

■ Although visual loss is the most well-known symptom of GCA, visual loss, in most cases, is preceded for some time by headache. Partial visual loss (amaurosis fugax and unilateral blindness) may precede total visual loss.

■ If GCA is suspected, the patient should immediately be started on high-dose steroids (60 to 80 mg prednisone daily). Moreover, treatment should not be delayed until a temporal artery biopsy is done.

- PMR frequently occurs in patients with GCA.
- GCA can also involve large elastic vessels causing claudication, aneurysms, or even coronary disease.

 POLYMYALGIA RHEUMATICA

Polymyalgia rheumatica (PMR) is a syndrome in elderly patients with an elevated erythrocyte sedimentation rate that is manifested by proximal aching, soreness, and stiffness that cannot be attributed to a defined rheumatic, infectious, metabolic, or neoplastic disorder.

I. **ETIOPATHOGENESIS.** There is an association between PMR and human leucocyte antigen-DR4 (HLA-DR4).

II. **PREVALENCE. PMR affects approximately 1 in 1,000 persons in the US population** who are older than 50 years.

III. **CLINICAL MANIFESTATIONS**
   A. **Sixty percent of the patients are women.** Most patients present after their fiftieth year, and the peak incidence is between ages 60 and 80 years. Rarely, cases have been observed in younger patients.
   B. **Proximal soreness and stiffness.** PMR is characterized by chronic, symmetric aching and stiffness of the proximal joints and muscles. These symptoms are most prominent in the shoulder and pelvic girdles and neck, but distal muscle groups may also be involved, although to a lesser extent. It is not unusual for symptoms to be restricted to the upper extremities. Aching and stiffness are worse in the morning, usually lasting more than 30 minutes and occurring after a period of inactivity (gelling). Aching may be severe and incapacitating. Strength is often difficult to evaluate because pain is present; however, this parameter should be normal.
   C. **Constitutional symptoms.** Patients with PMR frequently complain of malaise and fatigue. Fever is usually low-grade, but temperature may occasionally reach 102°F. Night sweats may occur. PMR may rarely present with a fever of unknown origin. Anorexia and weight loss may be prominent features and suggest malignancy; however, no direct association of PMR with neoplastic disease has been proven. Yet, an age-appropriate malignancy assessment is appropriate. Depression, usually mild, is not infrequent.
   D. **Joints.** Most patients have poorly localized tenderness over their joints, especially prominent over the shoulders and hips. Moderate bland effusions can be seen in the knees and occasionally in the wrists, but they do not dominate the clinical picture as they do in rheumatoid arthritis (RA). Carpal tunnel syndrome has also been noted. Ultrasonography and magnetic resonance imaging (MRI) have shown that proximal joint symptoms reflect soft tissue inflammation such as tendinitis and bursitis.
   E. **Giant cell arteritis (GCA), also called temporal (cranial) arteritis (TA).** PMR and GCA are companion disorders that are part of a continuum of an inflammatory disorder. It has been estimated that approximately 10% of patients with PMR may have GCA and 50% of patients with GCA may have characteristic PMR symptoms.

IV. **DIAGNOSTIC INVESTIGATIONS**
   A. **PMR should be considered in patients older than 50 years who complain of proximal arthralgia and myalgia associated with morning stiffness lasting over 30 minutes.**
   B. **Laboratory tests**
      1. **An elevated Westergren erythrocyte sedimentation rate** is the laboratory hallmark of PMR; it is usually in excess of 50 mm/hour and may exceed 100 mm/hour. There is evidence that PMR can occur with normal sedimentation rates (20 to 30 mm/hour) but sedimentation rates below 10 mm/hour would be very unusual.
      2. **Normocytic normochromic anemia** is seen in approximately 50% of patients.
      3. **Immunologic studies.** The frequency of rheumatoid factors, antinuclear antibodies, and other autoreactive antibodies is not higher than that of age-matched controls.
      4. **Muscle enzyme levels** (e.g., creatine kinase, serum glutamic-oxaloacetic transaminase, lactic dehydrogenase, and aldolase) are normal.

    C. Plain radiographic findings are normal but MRI and ultrasonography of proximal joints demonstrate soft tissue inflammation such as tendinitis and bursitis. These tests, however, are not routinely performed.

    D. Electromyographic findings have been normal, but this test is not a part of the diagnostic workup of this disorder.

    E. Muscle biopsy histology. Myositis is not seen.

    F. Synovial fluid and tissue studies

        1. Leukocyte counts in joint fluid range between 1,000 and 8,000 mm^3, with a preponderance of lymphocytes. It is rare to find synovial fluid in joints in PMR.

        2. Synovial biopsy specimens, rarely needed or available, reveal mild synovial proliferation with slight lymphocyte infiltration.

V. DIFFERENTIAL DIAGNOSIS. The diagnosis requires exclusion of other syndromes associated with significant proximal soreness and stiffness, erythrocyte sedimentation rate (ESR) elevation, and constitutional symptoms, such as the following:

    A. Neoplasia.

    B. Infectious syndromes such as endocarditis and viral illnesses.

    C. Rheumatologic conditions

        1. RA. Some experts believe that PMR and RA presenting in the elderly patients are the same disorder, both responsive to low-dose prednisone. The usual differential point is the prominence of inflammation in the small joints of the hands and feet in older patients with RA, some of whom have prominent proximal joint symptoms.

        2. Systemic lupus erythematosus. The usual joint presentation is RA-like, not proximal, and the accompanying serositis, rash, and renal disease are not seen in PMR.

        3. Vasculitides other than GCA. Polyarteritis nodosa (PAN) can present in a GCA manner, with clinical findings that mimic GCA. Temporal artery biopsy can also show inflammation but not the presence of giant cells. A rash and mononeuritis multiplex are characteristic of PAN.

        4. Muscle disease, such as polymyositis or thyroid myopathy.

        5. Plasma cell dyscrasias, bone pain, elevated ESR, and anemia.

        6. Fibromyalgia is a syndrome of generalized ache **not associated** with an elevated ESR (see Chapter 56).

VI. TREATMENT

    A. Prednisone. Initial therapy for PMR is usually 10 to 15 mg of prednisone daily, although on occasion an even lower dose may be effective. A prompt and dramatic clinical response is considered by some to be an absolute criterion for the diagnosis and a "retroactive" support of the pretreatment diagnosis.

        1. Response to treatment. Most symptoms resolve in 48 to 72 hours, and the ESR should normalize after 7 to 10 days. Unusually, a patient who fails to respond to prednisone may respond to another corticosteroid, such as methylprednisolone or dexamethasone. If a dramatic response does not occur after several days, an alternative diagnosis should be considered.

        2. Steroid taper. Following control of symptoms, the dose of corticosteroids should be reduced to the lowest level required to suppress symptoms because the morbidity associated with therapy often exceeds that associated with the underlying disease. Flares of PMR can often be treated with a brief boost in steroids stretched over several days; this is especially true of flares that occur after acute viral illnesses. The dose of prednisone should be increased only for recurrence of symptoms and not for elevation of the ESR alone. Some flares, especially after years of disease, manifest as severe fatigue only. Unfortunately, a proportion of patients with PMR will continue to have mild but smoldering PMR for 2 years or more.

        3. The physician should be cautious about the development of GCA symptoms in patients with "pure" PMR. It is important to let patients with PMR know that if they develop headache or visual symptoms at any time, they should call their physician immediately. The transition from pure PMR to GCA is not common but not unheard of. An increase in the dosage of steroids and a temporal artery biopsy should be considered if there are no other reasons for the development of new symptoms.

4. **Persistent ESR elevations** in a patient without PMR symptoms may indicate another diagnosis such as infection.
5. **Osteoporosis prevention.** Consideration should be given to ensure adequate calcium and vitamin D intake in these elderly patients who take corticosteroids and who are at risk for corticosteroid-induced osteoporosis (see Chapter 53). This is especially true for postmenopausal women who also should obtain a baseline bone densitometry test and be started on a bisphosphonate.

B. **Nonsteroidal anti-inflammatory drugs** may suppress rheumatic symptoms, but they do not reduce the risk for blindness if GCA is present.
C. **Steroid-sparing medications.** At times, an immunosuppressive agent such as methotrexate or azathioprine is needed to control PMR that is not fully responsive to steroids or in patients with significant cumulative steroid-related side effects. These drugs are not routinely used in PMR.

 GIANT CELL ARTERITIS

Also known as temporal or cranial arteritis, GCA is a systemic vasculitis that primarily affects cranial arteries, and its clinical manifestations are a reflection of the sequelae of vascular occlusion caused by a granulomatous vascular inflammation.

I. **ETIOPATHOGENESIS.** Like PMR, GCA is associated with HLA-DR4.
II. **PREVALENCE.** The incidence of GCA is half that of PMR, and it occurs more often in women than men. The age distribution of GCA is similar to that of PMR, with a peak incidence from 60 to 80 years of age; it rarely occurs in patients younger than 50 years and in African Americans.
III. **CLINICAL MANIFESTATIONS. GCA and PMR are companion inflammatory disorders that present along a clinical continuum from mild to severe.** GCA shares clinical features with PMR, including fatigue, malaise, fever, and weight loss. It is now recognized that arterial lesions may be widespread, and the varied clinical expressions of the syndrome can be analyzed according to the anatomic patterns of affected arteries.
   A. **Symptoms related to involvement of branches of the external carotid artery**
      1. **Headache** is probably the most frequent symptom of GCA, occurring in 50% to 75% of patients; it is often the first manifestation of the disease. Headache is described as being persistent and severe, with night awakening and dull, boring, and burning pain, and as being unresponsive to simple pain medications. Classically, patients complain of temporal headaches, and the inflamed temporal arteries on physical examination may be prominent, beaded, tender, and pulseless. Patients with occipital artery involvement may have difficulty combing their hair or may experience discomfort from the pressure of a pillow on their head.
      2. **Jaw claudication** occurs infrequently in GCA, but its presence is highly suggestive of the syndrome. Patients with involvement of the maxillary or lingual arteries may have jaw or tongue pain on chewing or talking. There are rare case reports of tongue gangrene.
      3. **Pain in the ear canal, pinna, or parotid gland** may be secondary to the involvement of the posterior auricular artery.
      4. Pain in the **temporomandibular joint** may be secondary to the involvement of the superficial temporal artery.
   B. **Symptoms related to the involvement of the internal carotid artery**
      1. **Ophthalmologic damage** secondary to arteritis is the most common serious consequence of GCA. Although it occurs in 20% to 50% of patients and is the presenting symptom **at diagnosis** in 60% of patients with GCA in whom visual loss develops, eye damage is rarely the earliest symptom. In most patients with visual loss, a careful history will reveal that headache, usually specific enough to suggest the diagnosis, preceded blindness in approximately 40% of

cases. Symptoms characteristic of PMR are early manifestations in approximately 30% of patients. Because loss of vision in GCA is often irreversible unless treatment is initiated within several hours following the onset of ocular symptoms, special attention must be directed toward early recognition of the syndrome.

2. **Ophthalmologic manifestations** vary according to the pattern of arterial branch involvement and can be the integrated effect of multiple vascular insults of the eye, chiasma, and brain. The central retina is supplied by the central retinal artery, which is the terminal branch of the ophthalmic artery. Also derived from the ophthalmic artery are the posterior ciliary arteries, which supply the optic nerve, and the muscular branches, which supply the extraocular muscles. Because the posterior ciliary arteries are the most frequently involved arteries in GCA, ischemic optic neuritis is by far the most common lesion and ischemic optic neuropathy is the telltale eye finding of GCA by the ophthalmologist. Results of the funduscopic evaluation will often be normal, or the examination will show only mild edema of the nerve head several days after the onset of symptoms. Because these patients often also have atherosclerosis, cholesterol embolic plaques, and not GCA, can be the cause of visual changes.
   a. **Amaurosis fugax** occurs in approximately 10% of patients with GCA, and permanent visual loss will develop in 80% of these patients if they are not treated.
   b. **Unilateral or incomplete blindness** occurs in approximately 30% to 40% of patients and, if untreated, may progress to complete blindness over a period of several days.
   c. **Bilateral blindness** occurs in 25% of patients with GCA and is often preceded by amaurosis fugax or partial blindness.
   d. **Diplopia or ptosis secondary to ischemic paresis** of the extraocular muscles occurs in approximately 5% of patients with GCA.
3. **Central nervous system (CNS) disease** is uncommon but can occur in GCA secondary to the involvement of any of the intracerebral arteries and can produce seizures, cerebral vascular accidents, or abnormal mental status. Peripheral nerve involvement is rare. As a result of the relative inaccessibility of intracranial vessels and the high prevalence of arteriosclerotic vascular disease in older patients, the frequency with which GCA leads to significant ischemic CNS disease is not known.

C. **Symptoms related to involvement of large arteries**
1. **Aortic arch and thoracic aorta.** Careful physical examination in patients with GCA often reveals bruits over the carotid, axillary, or brachial arteries. Limited pathologic studies have shown GCA in such vessels; however, because bruits secondary to arteriosclerotic vascular disease are common in elderly subjects, the frequency of aortic arch and aortic root involvement in GCA is not known. Nevertheless, GCA has been documented as a basis for aneurysms, dissections, and stenotic lesions of the aorta and its major branches and can occur more than 10 years after the illness has resolved clinically.
2. **Abdominal aorta.** Involvement of the abdominal aorta, like that of the thoracic aorta, can produce symptoms secondary to aortic aneurysms and intestinal infarction. For unknown reasons, renal involvement is rare.
3. **Large arteries of the arms and legs** can be occluded along long stretches, leading to claudication and to the absence of a palpable pulse or obtainable blood pressure readings. These often improve or return to the premorbid state with steroid treatment over a 6- to 12-month period.

D. **Symptoms related to PMR.** Patients with PMR without signs or symptoms of GCA should not be empirically treated with steroid regimens that are appropriate for GCA and do not need to undergo temporal artery biopsy.

IV. **DIAGNOSTIC INVESTIGATIONS**
A. **Laboratory tests—ESR.** As in PMR, the laboratory hallmark of GCA is the elevated ESR, and they also commonly have elevated C-reactive protein levels. The ESR (Westergren) is usually between 50 and 100 mm/hour, rarely below 40 mm/hour and

is commonly above 100 mm/hour. A normal ESR does not exclude GCA. A normocytic, normochromic anemia may be present. As in PMR, muscle enzyme levels are normal. The results of tests for rheumatoid factor, antinuclear antibodies, and anti-DNA antibodies are negative. Complement levels are normal, and cryoglobulins and monoclonal immunoglobulins are absent.

B. Radiographs. Temporal artery arteriography has no value.

C. Ultrasonography is a relatively accurate test for the identification of GCA. The "halo sign" representing edema of the superficial temporal artery wall has an overall sensitivity of 69% and specificity of 82% when compared to temporal artery biopsy. Arterial stenosis or occlusion is an almost equally sensitive marker compared to biopsy. However, not all studies have demonstrated these statistics, and the results differ depending on the technologic variations.

D. Superficial temporal artery biopsy. This continues to be the gold standard for the diagnosis of GCA. The biopsy specimen should always be taken from the temporal artery on the symptomatic side of the head. If a specific part of the artery is tender, beaded, or inflamed, the biopsy specimen should include that area. There is no information about whether the artery trunk or a distal branch specimen is best. At least 1 in. of the artery should be taken as the biopsy specimen. Because the process may be segmental, multiple sections should be taken. If the biopsy is negative on the first side, some do a contralateral biopsy to improve the yield. Histologically, the following are seen:

1. **An inflammatory infiltrate,** predominantly of mononuclear cells, involves the entire vessel wall. Fibrinoid necrosis is not a feature of the lesion.

2. **Fragmentation** of the internal elastic lamina.

3. **Giant cells** are almost always present and often seem to engulf parts of the internal elastic lamina. They are difficult to find in some cases, and their absence does not rule out the diagnosis.

4. **Intimal proliferation** is often marked, is a nonspecific feature in this age-group, and cannot, if found alone, be considered evidence of past or present arteritis. These findings are in contrast to those of the lesions of PAN, which are characterized by fibrinoid necrosis of the vessel and neutrophil infiltration. When GCA involves larger vessels, the lesions are indistinguishable from those seen in Takayasu's arteritis.

V. DIFFERENTIAL DIAGNOSIS. The diagnosis of GCA is made in a patient with a compatible history and physical findings. Polymyalgia need not be present, but the ESR is often above 50 mm/hour. A definite diagnosis of GCA requires a biopsy specimen showing the histologic changes described above. Finally, all symptoms should improve remarkably after steroid therapy; the exception is loss of vision, which is usually irreversible.

A. Arteriosclerotic vascular disease may be responsible for some clinical signs that can also be attributable to GCA, including a decrease in the temporal artery pulse, temporal artery thickening, and acute visual loss. Patients who have had only arteriosclerotic changes on temporal artery biopsy and have not responded to steroid therapy have been described with loss of vision, elevated ESR, and absent temporal pulses. Similarly, patients with previously documented and treated GCA may develop symptoms suggesting relapse that are actually secondary to arteriosclerotic vascular disease.

B. Takayasu's arteritis is a large-vessel disease and does not directly involve the temporal artery or other arteries of medium and small size. Although Takayasu's arteritis is pathologically indistinguishable from GCA involving large vessels, its clinical picture is different. Female patients predominate, and patients are usually from 20 to 50 years old. Although symptoms of arteritis may be preceded by a "prepulseless" stage (arthralgias and fatigue), the characteristic PMR symptoms are not common. Finally, the ESR has no consistent pattern, and the response to steroids is common but not predictable.

C. Systemic necrotizing vasculitis. The temporal arteries may occasionally be histologically involved in patients with polyarteritis (see Chapter 37); however, these arteries are rarely abnormal on physical examination, and clinical signs of GCA are rarely seen, even in patients with involvement of the temporal arteries. Finally, the kidney and the peripheral nervous system involvement is rare in GCA, even when large vessels are involved.

VI. TREATMENT

A. **The management of uncomplicated GCA (i.e., GCA without visual or CNS manifestations) is by prednisone 40 to 60 mg given orally daily in divided doses.** Treatment should **not** be withheld waiting for a biopsy since the pathologic findings are stable despite several weeks of corticosteroids.

B. **When acute visual changes thought to be secondary to GCA are present,** patients should be initially treated with 80 to 100 mg of intravenous methylprednisolone daily and in divided doses and then tapered to the conventional 60-mg oral dose of prednisone after 7 to 10 days. Pulse steroids (250 to 1,000 mg solumedrol daily for 1 to 3 days) are sometimes employed in the setting of visual or CNS problems. Alternate-day therapy is not effective in preventing visual loss.

C. **Symptoms (e.g., PMR, headache, and lethargy) should disappear in 36 to 72 hours on the prescribed drug regimen.** Elevated ESR and ischemic manifestations, such as temporal headache, jaw claudication, and localized temporal artery inflammation, should diminish over several days. The temporal artery pulse may not return, and visual loss may be permanent.

D. **High-dose steroids should be maintained only as long as necessary** until symptoms resolve and then should be tapered over a period of several weeks to a maintenance dose of 5 to 10 mg of prednisone daily. Most patients require at least 3 weeks of high-dose steroids. Both clinical signs and ESR may be used to follow the response. In patients with visual involvement, tapering should be slower.

E. **The average patient will require continued maintenance therapy with 5 to 10 mg of prednisone daily for 1 to 2 years,** but some patients may need treatment for as long as 5 years. Because the incidence of new visual damage appears to decrease with duration of disease, patients who relapse after 18 to 24 months should probably undergo a repeated temporal artery biopsy before being restarted on high-dose corticosteroids.

F. **There are conflicting opinions in the literature about whether low-dose weekly methotrexate will prevent relapses** and allow a quicker reduction in corticosteroid dose. In individual patients with refractory disease or excessive steroid co-morbidities, however, addition of RA-type dose of methotrexate or azathioprine are employed. Low-dose aspirin (81 mg/day) should be given to all patients with GCA because of its protective effect against visual loss or stroke.

G. **GCA continues to be a clinical diagnosis, supported by laboratory tests and biopsy.** Thus, at times, patients are treated for GCA with steroids despite a negative biopsy and in the setting of a very strong clinical suspicion of GCA. The same clinical parameters of improvement are seen in this group of patients.

H. **Tumor necrosis factor α antagonists.** Trials have failed to demonstrate benefits of infliximab.

CHILDHOOD RHEUMATIC DISEASES

Thomas J. A. Lehman

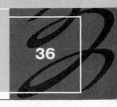

36

I.   **The rheumatic diseases of childhood represent a diverse group, both clinically and immunologically.** Their etiologies are varied and their pathogeneses are unclear. Lyme disease and acute rheumatic fever are the only two rheumatic diseases of childhood with a known infectious etiology, that is, *Borrelia burgdorferi* and group-A β hemolytic streptococci, respectively.

II. **Most childhood rheumatic diseases result from a combination of genetic predisposition, autoimmunity, and unknown environmental factors.** Most of these diseases are treated with a broad range of anti-inflammatory or immunosuppressive medications.

PREVALENCE

I.   **Reactive arthritis** (acute episodes of arthritis and arthralgia following an infectious illness) **is common in childhood, but chronic rheumatic diseases are infrequent.** Nonetheless, there are more than 250,000 children with arthritis in the United States. Prevalence estimates are confused between the number of children with juvenile rheumatoid arthritis (JRA) (100,000) and the number of children with any form of arthritis (250,000). This dichotomy is responsible for an ongoing process of redefinition and reclassification.

II. **The term JRA is being replaced by the term juvenile idiopathic arthritis (JIA).** However, it is important to remember that JIA does not describe a specific disease; rather, it is an umbrella term covering various forms of childhood arthritis that may have different etiologies, natural histories, best therapies, and underlying genetic predispositions. At present, eight distinct subtypes of JIA have been described, and it is expected that more subtypes will be delineated before the redefinition is complete.

III. **With this new definition, the spondyloarthropathies and many other types of arthritis that currently fall outside the spectrum of JRA will be included in JIA.** This is unfortunate because the etiology, natural history, and best therapy for spondyloarthropathies are distinct. Officially, however, spondyloarthropathies will be termed enthesitis-associated arthritis, which will be a subtype of JIA.

IV. **JIA** (including what was previously termed JRA and spondyloarthropathies), **Henoch-Schönlein purpura, Kawasaki's disease, systemic lupus erythematosus (SLE), dermatomyositis, and scleroderma** are the most common forms of chronic arthritis in childhood.

CLINICAL MANIFESTATIONS, DIAGNOSIS, AND DIFFERENTIAL DIAGNOSIS

A careful history and physical examination are crucial to the proper diagnosis of childhood arthritis. The examining physician must have a clear knowledge of the differential diagnosis because children are often poor historians. A useful algorithm is illustrated in Table 36-1. The examining physician must determine whether inflammation is present (i.e., objective pain, swelling, warmth, or limitation of motion), whether the inflammation is articular or periarticular, and whether the inflammation is acute or chronic.

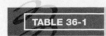

TABLE 36-1	Common Forms of Chronic Synovitis in Childhood

Juvenile Idiopathic arthritis (JIA) (previously juvenile rheumatoid arthritis)

A. **Oligoarticular-onset JIA** (typically 2 to 5 y old girls with fewer than four joints involved at onset). Note: Children with a family history of psoriasis, a positive RF, or enthesitis are automatically excluded from this category.
   1. ANA-positive children with high risk for iridocyclitis
   2. ANA-negative children
   3. Extended oligoarticular-onset—fewer than four joints at onset with progression later
B. **Polyarticular-onset JIA**
   RF-negative with at least five joints involved during the first 6 mo
   RF-positive on at least two occasions 3 mo apart; adolescent girls with typical adult-type RA
C. **Systemic-onset JIA**
   1. Definite-quotidian fever for at least 2 wk, evanescent rash and arthritis
   2. Probable-quotidian fever for at least 2 wk, evanescent rash and any two of generalized lymphadenopathy, hepatomegaly or splenomegaly, or serositis

Spondyloarthropathies-enthesitis–associated arthritis

Arthritis and enthesitis or arthritis plus two of the following: SI joint tenderness; HLA-B27; uveitis; inflammatory spinal pain; family history of either uveitis, spondyloarthropathy, or inflammatory bowel disease

A. Ankylosing spondylitis
B. Juvenile spondyloarthropathy
C. Reactive arthritis—full combination of arthritis, urethritis, and conjunctivitis occurs infrequently in childhood
D. Psoriatic arthritis subset with psoriasis-associated JIA-dactylitis, asymmetric joint inflammation and typical skin lesions or a family history of psoriasis (first- or second-degree relative)
E. Inflammatory bowel disease

Arthritis associated with primarily vasculitic conditions

A. Systemic lupus erythematosus
B. Dermatomyositis
C. Kawasaki's disease involving small joints
D. Sarcoidosis
E. Henoch-Schönlein purpura

Miscellaneous

A. Plant thorn synovitis (typically 1–5 y old)
B. Benign hypermobile joint syndrome
C. Immunization-associated arthritis
D. Arthritis associated with immunoglobulin deficiency
E. Linear scleroderma

Arthritis associated with metabolic and inherited conditions in childhood

A. Marfan's syndrome
B. Ehlers-Danlos syndrome
C. Cystic fibrosis

ANA, antinuclear antibody; HLA, human leucocyte antigen; JIA, juvenile idiopathic arthritis; RA, rheumatoid arthritis; RF, rheumatoid factor; SI, sacroiliac.

I. **WHEN NO OBVIOUS INFLAMMATION IS PRESENT**
   A. **Growing pains.** This is the most common and most misused diagnosis for musculoskeletal pain in childhood. The true syndrome of "growing pains" occurs in young children, peaking at the age of 4 to 5 years. Pain occurring in the popliteal fossa is a

classic example. It is relieved by gentle massage or by reassurance and occurs **only** at night. Pain during the day does not represent growing pains. Growing pains are benign and self-limiting. Often, there is a family history of similar complaints, which may aid in the diagnosis. Growing pains are typically relieved by acetaminophen and do not require specific therapy.

B. **Psychogenic rheumatism.** Joint pains and fatigue occur frequently as **somatization** disorders. It is worrisome when a child is unable to attend school or participate in normal activities despite an unremarkable physical and laboratory evaluation. Some children respond to gentle reassurance, but for others the complaints of pain mask a major psychological disorder. Children with persistent complaints of pain despite normal findings should be evaluated carefully by an experienced pediatric rheumatologist to exclude undiagnosed illness. If the physician is not able to find an objective source of the complaints of diffuse aches and pains with fatigue in a child, he or she should also consider the possibility that the child may be reacting to problems within the family. Often the families of such children reject an immediate recommendation of psychological counseling. However, physicians who establish a trusting relationship with the family may be able to bring about gradual resolution of the complaints or an acceptance of the need for psychological intervention.

C. **Reflex neurovascular dystrophy** represents an extension of psychogenic rheumatism in which the somatization has progressed to include hyperesthesias, often with mottled skin coloring and vascular instability. Reflex neurovascular dystrophy often begins with a well-documented injury that fails to improve. The syndrome typically occurs in "perfect" children under excessive parental pressure. Any psychological stress may initiate this syndrome. Excessive pressure to excel in sports or other activities is the most common cause, but sexual abuse is another well-recognized cause. Although the specific complaints may be resolved with intensive physical and occupational therapy, failure to resolve the underlying psychological issues often results in recurrence of similar problems within a short period.

II. **PERIARTICULAR INFLAMMATION.** Children with periarticular (i.e., soft tissue, tendon, ligamentous, or bursal) inflammation must be carefully evaluated for associated osseous disorders.

A. **Orthopedic disorders.** Acute periarticular pain may result from a stress fracture or osteomyelitis. Young children with fractures may not report trauma. Battering must be considered when a child presents with unsuspected fractures. Bone scan is often helpful in the evaluation of these entities.

B. **Neoplastic disorders** associated with infiltration of the bone marrow include leukemia, lymphoma, and neuroblastoma. All these conditions may present with difficulty in walking or with "joint pains." Disproportionate anemia, thrombocytopenia, hyperuricemia, lymphadenopathy, or hepatosplenomegaly should prompt further investigation and bone marrow aspiration.

C. **Rheumatic disorders.** The juvenile spondyloarthropathies often present with both periarticular and articular inflammation. The periarticular manifestations may predominate, but articular inflammation is usually present. Lumbar stiffness, enthesitis, and heel pain should be specifically sought. Often, these children are thought to have recurrent sprains or strains. The possibility of arthritis is often incorrectly dismissed by inexperienced physicians because the erythrocyte sedimentation rate (ESR) is normal.

III. **ARTICULAR INFLAMMATION.** Children with true articular inflammation must be subdivided depending on whether the inflammation is acute or chronic (of more than 6-week duration).

A. **Acute articular inflammation**

1. **Infection.** An acutely inflamed joint must be considered septic until proven otherwise. Staphylococci, streptococci, and *Hemophilus influenzae* are frequent causes of septic arthritis in childhood. Lyme disease is a systemic disease, usually presenting as arthritis in children and is frequent in areas where *Ixodes* ticks are endemic. Not infrequently, Lyme disease may involve several joints simultaneously. Septic arthritis typically presents with a single inflamed joint accompanied by fever and an elevated ESR. It is less common but not impossible for

other infectious agents to involve multiple joints. Children with reactive arthritis may also have an associated infectious process and multiple joints may be involved (see in the subsequent text).

2. **Reactive arthritis** may occur as a result of bacterial, viral, or fungal infections. Toxic synovitis is the most common type of reactive arthritis in children. The typical child with toxic synovitis is aged 3 to 5 years. He or she is well except, perhaps, for symptoms of an upper respiratory infection the prior evening. The following morning, the child awakens unable to walk, with a decreased range of mobility in one hip. There is only low-grade or no fever, without significant elevation of the white blood cell count or ESR. Unless an experienced physician is comfortable with the clinical picture, the joint must be aspirated to rule out bacterial infection. In experienced centers, ultrasonography may be adequate to discriminate a septic joint on the basis of the characteristics of the joint fluid and the degree of reaction in the surrounding tissues. The joint symptoms of a child with toxic synovitis typically begin to improve within a few hours; in contrast, those of a child with a truly septic hip often rapidly worsen. Reactive arthritis often follows the acute infectious episode and antibiotic therapy is unnecessary, but the infectious agent may still be present and the patient may require treatment even if the agent is not found in the inflamed joint (e.g., reactive arthritis in association with a gonococcal infection).

3. **Poststreptococcal reactive arthritis** deserves special consideration. This disorder is not classified as acute rheumatic fever because it does not fulfill the Jones's criteria. Nonetheless, children with arthritis and elevated ESRs should receive antibiotic prophylaxis following a documented streptococcal infection (see Chapter 49). Cardiac damage has been found with subsequent streptococcal infections in some children who did not receive such long-term prophylaxis.

4. **Acute expression of a collagen vascular disease.** Serum sickness, acute rheumatic fever, Henoch-Schönlein purpura, and the "chronic" collagen vascular diseases (e.g., SLE) may present with acute arthritis. Most of these conditions are discussed elsewhere in this manual; only those that are unique to childhood or have unique manifestations in children are discussed in this chapter.

B. **Chronic articular inflammation**

1. **Infection.** Chronicity does not exclude infection but makes it less likely. Tuberculosis is a frequent cause of smoldering septic arthritis, but other bacterial infections, including staphylococcal arthritis, may present with such a clinical picture. Additionally, physicians must remain aware that children with known collagen vascular disease, especially those on immunosuppressive drugs, may develop a complicating septic arthritis or osteomyelitis.

2. **Collagen vascular diseases.** All the chronic collagen vascular diseases may occur in children. Most are discussed elsewhere.

DISEASES WITH UNIQUE MANIFESTATIONS IN CHILDHOOD

I. **JUVENILE IDIOPATHIC ARTHRITIS (JIA) (PREVIOUSLY CALLED JUVENILE RHEUMATOID ARTHRITIS)**

A. **As noted in the preceding text, JIA has replaced the term JRA.** Although many will be confused by this new term, it has come into use because many children with arthritis have not fulfilled the classic criteria for JRA.

B. **JIA is an umbrella term used to describe any noninfectious or nontraumatic arthritis in childhood.** There are currently eight recognized subtypes, and it is expected that there will be more. It should be appreciated that JIA does not refer to a "specific" disease. Each subtype of JIA is distinct, most likely with its distinct etiology, pathogenesis, prognosis, and optimal therapy. Because the subtypes represent different diseases, it is important that the subtypes be properly differentiated from one another when studying pathogenesis, natural history, or therapeutic effectiveness of drugs.

C. Oligoarticular onset (four or fewer joints involved) and **polyarticular onset** are defined on the basis of the number of joints involved during the first 6 months after disease onset—not on the basis of the number of joints involved at the time the child is first seen by the physician.

1. **Oligoarticular-onset JIA** involves four or fewer joints. It most commonly occurs in young girls but may affect individuals of either sex. This group is divided into the subset that is antinuclear antibody (ANA)-positive, which is at greater risk for complicating eye disease (iridocyclitis), and the subset that is ANA-negative. Typical oligoarticular JIA is limited to the lower extremities. The condition of a child who has fewer than four joints involved during the first 6 months of disease, but who progresses to have more than four joints involved later, is termed as extended oligoarticular disease in the new nomenclature. Young girls with early involvement of small joints (i.e., finger and toe joints) are at high risk for progression to polyarticular involvement and have a poor prognosis. This is most likely a distinct entity.

   a. Some children have "sausage digits" and probably "psoriasis-associated arthritis" (psoriatic arthritis **sine** psoriasis), as described in the subsequent text. Children with a close family history of psoriasis or "nail pitting" may be differentiated as having psoriasis-associated arthritis. However, other children, who have neither a family history of psoriasis nor nail lesions, may also have arthritis with an identical appearance.

   b. Adolescents with involvement of four or fewer large joints are more likely to have a spondyloarthropathy (now called enthesitis-associated arthritis).

2. **Polyarticular-onset JIA** has at least two distinct subtypes: RF-positive and RF-negative. Rheumatoid factor (RF)-positive adolescent girls have typical, adult-type RA, whereas young children with polyarticular JIA are typically RF-negative. Both these entities carry a guarded prognosis.

3. **Systemic-onset JIA** presents with high spiking fever, leukocytosis, rash, and variable joint involvement. It occurs in a more equal sex ratio than the other forms of JIA, which have a female predominance. Children with systemic-onset JIA appear strikingly ill during episodes of fever and appear relatively normal between episodes. The fleeting salmon-pink rash and a temperature elevation, which falls to normal or below normal at least once each day, are characteristic. Although many children with systemic-onset JIA do well, in the others, the internal organs are involved to a great extent, or they progress to chronic destructive arthritis. Leukopenia or thrombocytopenia in a child with presumed systemic-onset JIA suggests either an incorrect diagnosis or a severe complication such as the macrophage activation syndrome.

II. SPONDYLOARTHROPATHIES. The spondyloarthropathies, occurring in both male and female patients, are now defined as enthesitis-associated arthritis. Their hallmark is asymmetric, large-joint arthritis associated with limited lumbar flexion and tenosynovitis. The children affected by this condition are typically ANA- and RF-negative. They are at risk for acute, painful iritis, but this generally does not progress to the chronic iridocyclitis that is seen in children with the oligo-onset disease. Human leucocyte antigen-B27 (HLA-B27) is present in approximately half of these children.

A. Ankylosing spondylitis (AS) is the "classic" spondyloarthropathy. It occurs predominantly in male patients who are positive for HLA-B27 and who have limited lumbar flexion. Because definite AS cannot be diagnosed in the absence of radiographic sacroiliitis, many children who are "suspects" fail to fulfill the diagnostic criteria. These children should be diagnosed as having juvenile spondyloarthropathy, as noted in the subsequent text. Some will ultimately fulfill the criteria for the diagnosis of AS, but many will not.

B. Juvenile spondyloarthropathy (seronegative enthesopathy/arthropathy syndrome). This condition occurs in children with asymmetric large-joint arthritis and with enthesopathic findings who do not meet the criteria for AS. They are easily differentiated from patients with other forms of JIA by their later age at onset (usually 10 years or older), the early presence of back or hip involvement, and the frequent occurrence of asymmetric metatarsal joint pain or Achilles tendinitis. Although many of these patients are boys who are positive for HLA-B27, girls and HLA-B27–negative individuals of either sex may also be affected. It was initially thought that classic AS would develop in most of the boys when they reached adulthood. It is presently thought that the disease will develop in many of the HLA-B27–positive boys to a significant extent but in only a small percentage of the others.

C. Reactive arthritis. The full triad of arthritis, urethritis, and conjunctivitis occurs infrequently in childhood. When it does, its manifestations are the same as in adults. It is not important to differentiate children with "incomplete" reactive arthritis from others with juvenile spondyloarthropathy because the therapy and prognosis are similar (see Chapter 42).

D. Psoriatic arthritis/"psoriasiform" arthritis, subset with psoriasis-associated JIA. True psoriatic arthritis with typical skin lesions and bony changes is infrequent in childhood. However, a subgroup of children without psoriatic skin changes present with asymmetric dactylitis (sausage digits), a family history of psoriasis in a first- or second-degree relative, and variable degrees of asymmetric joint inflammation. In contrast to the other spondyloarthropathies, this constellation of findings affects not only adolescents but also young girls who would otherwise be labeled as having oligoarticular JIA. Currently, the proper nomenclature for this group is psoriasis-associated JIA. As with other forms of psoriatic arthritis, the prognosis is guarded (see Chapter 41).

E. Inflammatory bowel disease. The arthritis accompanying inflammatory bowel disease is expressed as a typical spondyloarthropathy. Because arthritis may be the initial manifestation of inflammatory bowel disease, any child with a spondyloarthropathy in whom chronic or recurrent abdominal pain or persistent unexplained anemia develops should be carefully evaluated for the presence of Crohn's disease or ulcerative colitis (see Chapter 40).

III. MISCELLANEOUS CONDITIONS

Several forms of arthritis that occur predominantly in children are not easily characterized. Recognition of these conditions is important to prevent their being confused with more serious entities and to ensure proper therapy and counseling.

A. Plant thorn synovitis results from retention of a fragment of plant material within the joint following a puncture injury. This condition is diagnosed when such injuries are recalled and the condition is suspected. Confusion arises when a small child falls and the parents are unaware that the foreign matter might have entered the joint. The onset of joint swelling and limitation in range of motion is usually delayed by 4 to 6 weeks. The arthritis is often quite painful and unresponsive to the usual treatment. The proper diagnosis is often made following surgical biopsy of patients with intractable synovitis. The pathologic specimen reveals plant fibers under polarized light microscopy. Synovectomy is the treatment of choice.

B. Benign hypermobile joint syndrome typically occurs in girls during or just before early adolescence. They are most often gymnasts who practice extensively and have great flexibility that can be attributed to marked ligamentous laxity. As a result of their athletic activities and ligamentous laxity, their joints are subjected to repeated episodes of "microtrauma." Acute episodes may be treated with nonsteroidal anti-inflammatory drugs (NSAIDs), but more prolonged difficulty should prompt the review of the athletic program. Osteochondritis dissecans (particularly of the knee) may present in this group of patients. In rare cases, children who have continued their activities despite chronic pain have experienced permanent disability.

C. Immunization-associated arthritis. The development of a benign polyarthritis primarily affecting the small joints of the hands, 10 to 14 days following rubella immunization, is well-documented. The arthritis is typically mild and resolves within 7 to 10 days with only symptomatic therapy. Similar episodes have been reported less frequently with other viral immunizations.

D. Arthritis associated with immunoglobulin (Ig) deficiency. Children with IgA deficiency are most often asymptomatic, but this immunodeficiency occurs with a greater-than-expected frequency in children with arthritis. The arthritis commonly consists of benign recurrent joint effusions; however, some children present with typical erosive JIA. A benign arthritis may also occur in children with mild transient hypogammaglobulinemia. This arthritis may recur with viral infections, but ultimately it resolves as the child's immune system matures and as the Ig levels normalize. IgA deficiency will be detected only if quantitative immunoglobulins are routinely measured. Pan-hypogammaglobulinemia may be suspected if the total protein level is decreased with a normal serum albumin level.

E. Linear scleroderma occurring in childhood is a gradually progressive, bandlike tightening of the skin that may occur over the face, trunk, or an extremity. It typically does not cross the midline. There may be progressive loss of underlying muscle and bony tissue, with markedly disturbed growth when a limb is involved in a young child. Findings on laboratory evaluation are usually entirely normal. Physical therapy may be beneficial, but surgical intervention is required in extreme cases. Medical therapy with methotrexate has been beneficial for more severe cases in which the skin involvement crosses a joint line.

F. Linear scleroderma *en coup de sabre*. This entity is a variant of linear scleroderma characterized by primary involvement of one side of the scalp. It is incompletely differentiated from the Parry-Romberg syndrome of progressive facial hemiatrophy. Recognition of Parry-Romberg syndrome is important because affected children may be afflicted with neurologic disorders, including learning disability and seizures, findings that are not normally associated with linear scleroderma. Proper therapy for these conditions is uncertain.

IV. ARTHRITIS ASSOCIATED WITH PRIMARILY VASCULITIC CONDITIONS
Arthritis is a well-recognized complication of many forms of vasculitis that occur in childhood, including SLE, Wegener's granulomatosis, Takayasu's arteritis, and Henoch-Schönlein purpura. These diseases are not unique to childhood and are discussed elsewhere (see Chapter 37). Kawasaki's disease and juvenile-onset dermatomyositis are vasculitic diseases with unique manifestations in childhood.

A. Kawasaki's disease typically affects children in the first 5 years of life. It presents with fever accompanied by a pleomorphic rash, conjunctivitis, and cervical adenopathy. As the disease progresses, changes in the oral mucosa become evident, with dryness and cracking of the lips. Indurative edema of the hands and feet followed by peeling of the skin from the tips of the fingers or toes (but sometimes beginning in the perineal region) is characteristic. An acute arthritis may accompany the disease, but most often there is diffuse swelling of the hands or feet. Marked elevations of the ESR, white blood cell count, and platelet count evolve during the first 10 days of illness. Prompt recognition and echocardiographic evaluation are desirable. Untreated Kawasaki's disease is associated with a 1% to 3% mortality rate caused by aneurysmal dilatation of the coronary arteries, with subsequent thrombosis and myocardial infarction. The illness should be suspected whenever the characteristic findings are present. Early intervention with large doses of intravenous gamma globulin has been shown to decrease the frequency of aneurysms and to improve outcome. For children who fail to respond after two courses of intravenous gamma globulin, the diagnosis should be re-evaluated and consideration should be given to corticosteroid therapy. In addition to gamma globulin, NSAIDs are used to treat most children during the acute phase of their illness. While many investigators use aspirin, other NSAIDs have been shown to be effective.

B. Childhood-onset dermatomyositis most often presents with the gradual onset of weakness and fatigue but may have an explosive onset with fever, weakness, and vascular collapse. A heliotropic rash, although not always present, is characteristic of the disease. Childhood-onset dermatomyositis is divided into three subtypes.

1. Unicyclic disease usually presents with gradual onset of proximal muscle weakness, responds well to prednisone, and disappears completely within 1 year. Gottren's papules and nail fold capillary abnormalities are typically absent.

2. Polycyclic disease is similar to unicyclic disease but recurs whenever the corticosteroids are tapered. It may be associated with a poor prognosis secondary to chronic skin manifestations, subcutaneous calcification, or vasculitic involvement of internal organs. The presence of Gottren's papules and/or nail fold capillary abnormalities suggests polycyclic disease.

3. A third form of childhood dermatomyositis consists of prominent skin manifestations and muscle enzyme level elevation in children who are not extremely weak. These children often have persistent vasculitis.

Children with any form of dermatomyositis and evidence of dysphonia or cough while eating are at high risk for aspiration and should immediately be started on aggressive therapy.

V. **Arthritis associated with metabolic and inherited conditions in childhood.** Many inherited disorders, such as hemophilia, sickle cell disease, mucopolysaccharidoses, sphingolipidoses, and epiphyseal dysplasias, may present with arthritis or periarticular pain in childhood. Characteristic nonarticular manifestations usually predominate.

A. **Marfan's syndrome.** Children with Marfan's syndrome are characteristically tall with arachnodactyly. They typically exhibit ligamentous laxity and present with complaints similar to those with hypermobile joint syndrome. Characteristic findings are an arm span greater than the height and a leg length greater than trunk length. Recognition is important because these children are vulnerable to dissecting aortic aneurysms. Aortic root dilatation may be evaluated by routine echocardiography.

B. **Ehlers-Danlos syndrome.** Children with Ehlers-Danlos syndrome have an extreme form of joint hypermobility associated with abnormal connective tissue. Recurrent joint injury secondary to chronic subluxation is common. In typical cases, marked cutaneous laxity is present with characteristic "cigarette paper" scarring. However, milder cases that lack the cutaneous manifestations occur. These children, too, are subject to dissecting aortic aneurysms, which may be catastrophic. They are also vulnerable to early onset of osteoarthritis due to recurrent episodes of trauma.

C. **Cystic fibrosis** in childhood will be recognized by the pulmonary and gastrointestinal manifestations. Occasionally, however, benign effusions of the large joints or immune complex–related synovitis develops in these patients, which will prompt rheumatologic referral. Hypertrophic osteoarthropathy may also occur in children with cystic fibrosis.

 TREATMENT

I. **NSAIDs** are the first-line agents of choice for children with chronic synovitis. Although these drugs are often criticized because they are not "disease-modifying agents," this criticism is unjustified. NSAIDs directly modify disease outcome by reducing pain and inflammation. As a result of decreased pain and inflammation, the patient is able to preserve strength, range of motion, and endurance to a better extent, which in turn preserve function. Preservation of function has a definite positive impact on outcome. Therefore, NSAIDs definitely are disease-modifying agents, but they are not remission-inducing agents.

A. **Aspirin** remains the nominal drug of first choice because of its cost advantages, but it has been supplanted by naproxen and tolmetin in many centers because of less frequent dosing and reduced risk of both hepatotoxicity and Reye's syndrome. The dosage schedules and pharmacologic characteristics of the NSAIDs are discussed in Chapter 64.

B. **Indomethacin** deserves special mention in diseases in childhood because for many years it was regarded as being unsafe for use in children younger than 12 years. This restriction has been removed from recent issues of the *Physicians' Desk Reference*. Indomethacin is a potent NSAID that is effective for rheumatic diseases in childhood. It is frequently effective in children with severe, systemic-onset JIA or spondyloarthropathies that have not responded to other NSAIDs. Care must be taken while using indomethacin because of potential hepatotoxicity and gastric irritation. Headaches are a frequent side effect during the initial stages of therapy but usually respond to symptomatic therapy. The accepted dosage in childhood is 1 to 3 mg/kg/day.

II. **Slow-acting antirheumatic drugs** provide useful adjunctive therapy in children with chronic rheumatic disease.

   A. **Gold salts.** These are no longer in routine use; however, there is extensive literature about the long- and short-term efficacy of gold salts. Although the patient must be monitored carefully for evidence of toxicity, injectable gold salts (aurothioglucose and gold sodium thiomalate) are highly effective for children with specific subtypes of JIA. The accepted dosage of injectable gold salts in childhood is 1 mg/kg/week after initial evaluation of the response to a series of gradually increasing "test doses."

   B. **Methotrexate (Rheumatrex, Trexol)** is frequently used in the therapy for rheumatic disease in childhood. The short-term effectiveness of methotrexate is quite good, but it is difficult to wean patients from this agent. Long-term studies of efficacy and toxicity in childhood have not been completed. The accepted dosage regimen for methotrexate in childhood is 10 mg/m^2/week up to a maximum of 20 mg/m^2/week. Hematologic and hepatic toxicity require close monitoring. The long-term risks for hepatic cirrhosis or pulmonary fibrosis in childhood appear to be low. The major concern with methotrexate therapy is that in up to 50% of children, the disease flares when the methotrexate is withdrawn. Furthermore, a significant subset of these children does not improve when the methotrexate is reinstituted.

   C. **Hydroxychloroquine (Plaquenil)** has been used with success in children with chronic arthritis. However, the onset of action is extremely slow. The accepted dosage regimen is 7 mg/kg/day up to 200 mg/day. Children receiving hydroxychloroquine require ophthalmologic examinations every 6 months to monitor for evidence of retinal toxicity.

   D. **Etanercept (Enbrel),** a recombinant tumor necrosis factor-α blocker, is frequently used for children with severe arthritis. Administered at a dosage of 0.4 mg/kg as a subcutaneous injection twice weekly or 0.8 mg/kg/week, etanercept has not been associated with significant toxicity. At present, long-term efficacy and toxicity are unknown, and the drug is being used primarily in those who have not responded adequately to methotrexate. The full potential and proper utilization of etanercept in childhood diseases should become apparent within the next few years. Where the socioeconomic conditions and travel history warrant, routine purified protein derivative (PPD) testing is recommended before initiating therapy.

   E. **Adalimumab (Humira),** is a monoclonal antibody that binds with tumor necrosis factor-α both in the serum and on the cell surface. It has proven to be an effective agent for the treatment of JIA in children. It may be more effective than etanercept for children with severe uveitis.

   F. **Infliximab (Remicade)** is a third tumor necrosis factor blocking agent. It has the advantage of being given as an intravenous infusion monthly or less often. In addition, the dosage is easily customized to the individual patient. However, it is a partially humanized monoclonal antibody, and allergic reactions are more common than with other similar agents.

III. **SURGERY.** Replacement of severely damaged and painful hip, knee, and elbow joints is now routinely performed in adolescents at larger orthopedic centers. For younger and smaller patients, the procedures require a center with extensive surgical expertise, the ability to manufacture custom prostheses, and extensive rehabilitation facilities. Although there is a risk that further replacements may be required in future, the physical and psychological benefits of maintaining independent function throughout adolescence far outweigh the risks associated with the potential need for subsequent surgery. Soft tissue releases and synovectomies have been performed on many children with JIA. The loss of function associated with postoperative pain and loss of strength that accompanies these procedures must be weighed against the transient gains in alignment and range of motion. Arthroscopic synovectomy is associated with much less morbidity than open synovectomy and has led to renewed interest in this technique.

IV. **Physical and occupational therapy** are vital components of the care of children with rheumatic disease. Appropriate exercises to maintain strength and range of motion, coupled with splinting to maintain proper alignment, are important to the ultimate outcome.

V. **Family support** remains a major component of the overall program of care for children with chronic disease. The primary burden of family support may be carried by social workers, nurse clinicians, or psychologists in different institutions. Each group has different strengths to bring to these families, and optimally all will be available for the families. The presence of a child with chronic disease in the family creates profound stress in even the "best-adjusted" families. A program of care that does not provide for the emotional needs of the affected child's parents and siblings may result in profound psychological scarring.

VI. **OPHTHALMOLOGIC EVALUATION.** The ophthalmologist is a major participant in the care of children with rheumatic disease. All children with JIA are at risk for the development of iridocyclitis. Those with ANA-positive pauciarticular-onset JIA require slit-lamp evaluation every 4 months, and those who are ANA-negative should be checked every 6 months.

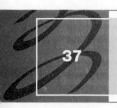

THE VASCULITIDES
Yusuf Yazici and Michael D. Lockshin

■ KEY POINTS

■ The major ischemic manifestations of vasculitides are defined by the type and size of the blood vessels involved and the tissue and organ damage caused by ischemia related to vascular occlusion.

■ Most diagnoses are defined by clinical rather than laboratory findings.

■ Treatment of most vasculitides involves corticosteroids usually along with immunosuppressive agents, especially when there is major organ involvement.

■ When there is a high suspicion of vasculitis, treatment should be started right away before waiting for definite laboratory or tissue evidence because major organ complications can develop quickly.

*T*he vasculitides are a heterogeneous group of systemic inflammatory disorders that have as their common manifestation the inflammation of blood vessels with demonstrable structural injury to the vessel walls.

The major ischemic manifestations are defined by the type and size of the blood vessels involved and the tissue and organ damage caused by vascular occlusion.

ETIOPATHOGENESIS

Although the specific cause of many of these disorders is not known, the inciting agents and disease mechanisms have been characterized in many. Infectious organisms, drugs, tumors, and allergic reactions are some of the defined triggers.

Pathogenetic factors include immune complex disease, antineutrophil cytoplasmic antibodies, antiendothelial cell antibodies, and cell-mediated immunity.

CLINICAL MANIFESTATIONS

I. **Although each of the vasculitic disorders has its own clinical signature** (see the specific disease discussions in subsequent text), they share clinical manifestations to one degree or another.

II. When the physician deals with a patient who has a multisystem disorder, and once infection and neoplasm have been ruled out appropriately, a vasculitic disorder should be strongly considered if combinations of the following manifestations are prominent:
   A. Constitutional symptoms, including fatigue, weight loss, fever, weakness, and failure to thrive.
   B. Skin rash.
   C. Joint inflammation.
   D. Muscle inflammation.
   E. Neuropathy or central nervous system disjunction.
   F. Pulmonary infiltrates or nodules.
   G. Sinus or nasal inflammation.
   H. Kidney inflammation or insufficiency.
   I. Gastrointestinal or liver inflammation.
   J. Laboratory abnormalities, including anemia, leukocytosis, thrombocytopenia, and elevated erythrocyte sedimentation rate (ESR), or C-reactive protein (CRP).

CLASSIFICATION

Although many clinical overlap syndromes may exist, the following clinical parameters can be employed to diagnose the disorder, define its severity, and then construct the correct therapeutic plan.

I. **VESSEL SIZE.** The occlusion of blood vessels as a consequence of inflammation leads to different clinical manifestations defined by the type and size of blood vessel involved and the tissue bed that is perfused by the vessel. Therefore, the physician can employ the findings the patient presents with as a diagnostic tool. For example, large-vessel involvement might cause blindness, stroke, or a myocardial infarction; medium-vessel disease can lead to renal or bowel dysfunction; and small-vessel disease can cause skin lesions and ischemia (Table 37-1).

II. **PATHOLOGY AND TYPE OF INFLAMMATION.** The types of inflammation involving blood vessels fall into two broad categories: necrotizing and granulomatous; however, overlaps can exist. In the necrotizing type, seen classically in polyarteritis nodosa (PAN), inflammatory lesions are focal and segmental and consist of macrophages, CD4+ T lymphocytes, and polymorphonuclear leukocytes. Fibrinoid necrosis may or may not exist, but disruption of the internal elastic lamina is expected. The granulomatous lesion of Wegener's granulomatosis (WG) in the lung reveals focal necrotizing lesions with or without granulomatous inflammation or multinucleated giant cells. It is important to note that vasculitides are commonly segmental, with areas skipped between active vessel inflammation and normal vessel. This demands multiple tissue sections. In PAN,

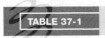

TABLE 37-1 Clinical Manifestations of Vasculitis According to Vessel Size

Vessel size	Disorder
Large vessels (aorta and its branches)	Giant cell arteritis
	Takayasu's arteritis
	Primary angiitis of the central nervous system
Medium-sized vessels (main visceral arteries)	Polyarteritis nodosa
	Kawasaki's disease
Small vessels (venules, capillaries, arterioles, and small arteries)	Churg-Strauss syndrome
	Wegener's granulomatosis
	Henoch-Schönlein purpura
	Microscopic polyangiitis
	Mixed cryoglobulinemia

inflammation can also occur in one section of the vessel and it is this asymmetry of vessel wall damage that can lead to aneurysms.

III. **CHARACTERISTIC CLINICAL PATTERNS.** WG—lung, sinus, and kidney; PAN—aneurysms and neuropathy; Henoch-Schönlein purpura (HSP)—rash, abdominal pain, and joint problems.

IV. **CLUES TO PATHOGENIC MECHANISMS.** Virus/immune complexes (hepatitis B and C)—PAN; cytoplasmic antineutrophil cytoplasmic antibodies (c-ANCA) and antiproteinase 3—WG; perinuclear antineutrophil cytoplasmic antibodies (p-ANCA) and antimyeloperoxidase—microscopic angiitis.

V. **LABORATORY ABNORMALITIES**

VI. **INCITING AGENTS.** Hepatitis B virus—PAN; hepatitis C virus—mixed (IgG–IgM) cryoglobulinemia; human immunodeficiency virus—PAN, leukocytoclastic vasculitis (LV).

DIAGNOSTIC INVESTIGATIONS

Most patients with vasculitis have nonspecific systemic symptoms, involvement of multiple organ systems, or both. They commonly present as diagnostic challenges. The diagnosis is based on a combination of clinical, serologic, histologic, and, for medium and large vessel disease, angiographic findings. **A complete history and physical examination are mandatory,** because most diagnoses are optimally defined by clinical rather than by laboratory findings.

Although the diagnosis of the vasculitides is usually based on the clinical presentation, certain supporting data are employed in solidifying the diagnosis, defining the extent of the disease and the degree of tissue damage, and guiding therapeutic choices. However, it must be appreciated that if the clinical picture dictates immediate therapeutic action, awaiting the results of more sophisticated tests or biopsies may not be appropriate.

LABORATORY TESTS

I. **The level of inflammation** can be defined by the presence of anemia, leukocytosis, thrombocytosis, and elevation of the ESR or CRP levels. All values may be abnormal on disease presentation and improve or normalize after therapy is instituted.

II. **ORGAN-SPECIFIC LABORATORY TESTING.** Testing for the presence and extent of organ involvement is often guided by the clinical manifestations and also includes routine blood testing and imaging.

A. **Renal involvement** can be clarified best with measurement of serum creatinine, urinalysis, and possibly a 24-hour urine collection for determination of creatinine clearance and protein. An elevated creatinine level and active urinary sediment with red blood cells, casts, and proteinuria commonly reflect active kidney inflammation, characteristic of small vessel vasculitis.

B. **Muscle inflammation.** An elevated creatine kinase level could represent muscle damage resulting from inflammation or myocardial infarction resulting from coronary vasculitis.

C. **Lung involvement.** A posteroanterior and lateral chest radiograph or computed tomography (CT) scan can be quite helpful in defining a pulmonary infiltrate cavity, nodule, pleural involvement.

D. **Liver involvement.** Abnormal results of liver function tests may reflect liver inflammation or associated infectious hepatitis.

E. **Sinus involvement.** A routine sinus series radiograph or CT scan may help define the presence and extent of mucosal inflammation.

III. **TESTING FOR TYPE OF VASCULITIS OR ITS ETIOLOGY.** These tests are used in specific clinical circumstances, as guided by the disease presentation and the results of the above routine tests.

A. **Consider an infectious trigger.** Hepatitis B or C and human immunodeficiency virus.

B. **Consider an immune complex disorder.** Complement consumption with low C3 and C4 levels and presence of cryoglobulins (e.g., hepatitis C).

    C. Consider an autoimmune disorder such as systemic lupus erythematosus (SLE). Antinuclear antibody (ANA) and anti-dsDNA testing.

IV. DISEASE-SPECIFIC LABORATORY TESTING

    A. Antineutrophil cytoplasmic antibody (ANCA). These antibodies are found in the serum of patients with specific types of vasculitis and are helpful as adjunctive diagnostic tools in the setting of a clinical picture consistent with WG, microscopic polyangiitis (MPA), and Churg-Strauss syndrome (CSS). Two different indirect immunofluorescence staining patterns characterize these antibodies: cytoplasmic (c-ANCA, reflecting antibodies to serine proteinase 3) and perinuclear (p-ANCA, reacting with myeloperoxidase). A few points about ANCA that are important are listed below.

        1. Most, but by no means all, patients with WG have c-ANCA positivity and most with MPA or CSS have p-ANCA positivity.

        2. The definite diagnosis of WG continues to be based on biopsy results, not on ANCA positivity.

        3. Decisions regarding disease activity should be based on clinical signs, not on the ANCA titer or the biopsy.

        4. Ten percent of patients may be negative for ANCA in the setting of active vasculitis.

    B. Tissue biopsy. Like any test, a tissue biopsy should be considered if it is needed to define a diagnosis, guide a therapy, or clarify the prognosis. In general, the simplest and safest procedure with the highest yield should be chosen, as defined by the specific clinical setting. At times, the severity of the disease and the comorbidities are such that one employs the clinical picture alone in guiding the treatment.

        Certain procedures are associated with both a high yield and low risk: skin biopsy in patients with dermatitis, temporal artery biopsy in giant cell arteritis (GCA), and muscle biopsy in PAN. Others entail a higher risk with a high diagnostic yield: lung biopsy in WG, kidney biopsy in MPA, muscle and nerve biopsy in PAN, and brain biopsy in primary angiitis of the brain.

IMAGING STUDIES

I. MAGNETIC RESONANCE IMAGING (MRI) AND COMPUTED TRANSAXIAL TOMOGRAPHY (CTT). These procedures may be needed to define the presence of specific organ involvement or extent of disease. Examples include MRI of the brain to assess for infarcts or CTT of the chest to characterize lung disease.

II. ANGIOGRAPHY. In special circumstances, this procedure can add greatly to diagnostic accuracy and to the definition of the type and the extent of vascular involvement. This is particularly true when diagnostic questions remain after the initial clinical evaluation of PAN and Takayasu's arteritis (TA). Magnetic resonance angiography (MRA) can be employed as a noninvasive method of evaluating vessel involvement. Angiograms are not helpful in small vessel vasculitis.

III. Positron-emission tomography (PET) scanning can be used in select cases for showing aortic and other vascular inflammation as part of a fever of unknown origin or vasculitis workup.

GIANT CELL ARTERITIS

GCA is a disease of aging adults, usually starting after the age of 50 years. It affects primarily whites, and women are twice as likely to be affected. GCA can accompany polymyalgia rheumatica (PMR), a syndrome characterized by proximal muscle aches and stiffness that is usually symmetric.

I. CLINICAL MANIFESTATIONS

    A. Common presenting symptoms are fatigue, headache, and tenderness of the scalp, particularly around the temporal and occipital areas. Jaw claudication (pain when chewing) is seen in two-thirds of patients. Headache is the presenting symptom in two-thirds of the patients, and half of them have the proximal soreness and stiffness, often severe, of PMR.

  B. Physical examination. Temporal arteries can be palpable, tender, and nodular, with reduced pulsation. In some series, visual disturbances have been reported in 20% of patients, but the frequency has declined over the years, probably because of earlier diagnosis and treatment. Transient ophthalmologic symptoms can lead to permanent blindness if not treated promptly.

II. **Diagnosis** of GCA should be considered in any patient older than 50 years with recent onset of headache, loss of vision, myalgia, fever of unknown origin, a high ESR, or anemia. It should be remembered that PAN can, but rarely, also affect the temporal arteries.

  A. Laboratory tests. The ESR is usually elevated, often over 100 mm/hour. A normal ESR is unusual but does not rule out GCA. Anemia and thrombocytosis are common. Similarly, the ESR is usually elevated in PMR, but a normal ESR does not rule out PMR.

  B. Temporal artery biopsy. Most rheumatologists recommend biopsy to define the presence of vessel inflammation. Some do bilateral biopsies initially and some recommend contralateral biopsy when the first side is negative. Things to keep in mind are as follows: Do not delay treatment awaiting the results of the biopsy; and remember that in one-third of patients biopsy results are negative because the lesions can involve the artery in a skipped fashion. Color duplex ultrasonography may have a place in the diagnosis of GCA; the most specific finding is a dark halo around the artery, which may represent edema. However, skill and experience of the ultrasonographer is important.

  C. Pathology shows granulomatous arteritis with giant cells and destruction of the internal elastic lamina.

III. **TREATMENT.** Most rheumatologists use an initial dosage of 10 to 20 mg of prednisone daily for **PMR** and 40 to 60 mg of prednisone daily for **GCA** because of the higher risk of arteritic complications in GCA. There is usually a dramatic response to steroids in patients with PMR, seen within days.

  A. Corticosteroid tapering begins after a month; most patients are on 5 to 10 mg of prednisone at 6 months. Although controversy exists over the length of treatment, patients will usually need to be on steroids for about a year, and some for as long as 2 years.

  B. Relapses are defined on clinical grounds, not solely by an elevation of the ESR, and are managed by increasing the dose of steroid. Side effects of corticosteroids should be kept in mind and may necessitate the use of steroid-sparing agents such as methotrexate or azathioprine.

  C. Low-dose aspirin (100 mg) has been shown to help prevent cranial ischemic complications of GCA.

 TAKAYASU'S ARTERITIS

TA is a chronic inflammatory disorder of unknown etiology affecting the aorta and its major branches. It predominantly affects women from ages 15 to 25 years, with a female-to-male ratio of 9:1.

I. **CLINICAL MANIFESTATIONS**

  A. TA is characterized by malaise, fever, night sweats, weight loss, myalgia, and symptoms of claudication, headaches, syncope, and visual disturbances.

  B. Physical examination can reveal arterial bruits over the involved vessels, and an absence of pulse is seen later in the disease. Hypertension is common but is often spuriously low in the arms, so that measurement of blood pressure in the legs is required.

II. **Diagnosis** of TA should be considered when symptoms of vascular insufficiency (claudication, transient visual disturbances, syncope) occur in the setting of bruits, weak pulses, and discrepancies of limb blood pressure in young women with constitutional symptoms.

A. Laboratory studies reflect the inflammatory state and include elevation of the ESR and CRP, anemia, and thrombocytosis.

B. Chest radiography might show a widened aortic shadow, irregularity of the descending aorta, and cardiac enlargement with hilar fullness. Arteriography is most helpful.

C. MRI may show a very thickened and altered aorta. Visualization of the whole aorta is needed because multiple parts may be involved. Suggestive findings include a segmental, smooth, tapered pattern of stenosis and complete occlusion of a large vessel, such as a subclavian. MRA is often diagnostic.

D. Differential diagnosis includes SLE, syphilitic aortitis, tuberculosis, mycotic aneurysm, aortitis secondary to rheumatic fever, Behçet's syndrome, and ankylosing spondylitis, all of which can involve the large vessels. In addition, GCA, congenital coarctation, thrombotic or embolic disease (as in endocarditis), antiphospholipid syndrome (APS), fibromuscular dysplasia, relapsing polychondritis (RP), and myxoma can sometimes mimic TA.

III. TREATMENT is primarily with oral corticosteroids. Untreated disease has a significant mortality rate.

A. Most patients respond to a dosage of 1 mg/kg/day, but there is also evidence that a starting dosage of 30 mg/day with a maintenance dosage of 5 to 10 mg/day is effective therapy. Cytotoxic therapy has been used in patients failing steroid treatment.

B. Vascular surgery and percutaneous transluminal angioplasty have also been used in cases of advanced disease with variable success.

C. Anticoagulation may be needed in the form of aspirin or warfarin.

D. Tuberculosis is sometimes associated with TA, so a PPD (purified protein derivative) skin test should be performed and prophylactic tuberculosis therapy given to patients with positive test results.

 ISOLATED ANGIITIS OF THE CENTRAL NERVOUS SYSTEM

Isolated angiitis of the central nervous system is a recently recognized vasculitic disorder localized to the central nervous system.

I. CLINICAL MANIFESTATIONS. Typical patients are in their 40s or 50s. Onset is highly variable, usually with a prodrome of 6 months.

A. The most common symptoms are headaches, often severe, which can spontaneously remit for long periods. Nonfocal neurologic deficits are characteristic, including a decrease in cognitive function.

B. Any anatomic area can be involved with signs and symptoms, which range from transient ischemic attacks, strokes, paraparesis, and cranial neuropathies to seizures.

II. DIAGNOSIS

A. Cerebrospinal fluid analysis findings are abnormal in more than 90% of patients and include modest pleocytosis, normal glucose levels, and increased protein. The cerebrospinal fluid should be cultured and infection should be ruled out.

B. MRI and CT scan have made diagnosis easier; suggestive findings include multiple, bilateral supratentorial infarcts. Angiography has proven to be less useful but is often performed by neurologists as part of the workup of "the worst headache of my life"; histologic confirmation of a granulomatous vasculitis through **leptomeningeal biopsy** is the gold standard.

III. Therapy is with corticosteroids and cyclophosphamide (CTX) and is usually continued for 6 to 12 months after remission. Mortality rate of this disease is high.

 POLYARTERITIS NODOSA

PAN is an acute necrotizing vasculitis of medium-sized and small arteries. Before the 1994 International Chapel Hill Consensus Conference, PAN also included MPA. After this conference, MPA was separated from PAN, with involvement of vessels smaller than arterioles indicating MPA and not PAN.

I. ETIOLOGIC FACTORS AND PATHOGENESIS

A. In most cases, the etiology of PAN is not known; in some cases, however, it is a consequence of hepatitis B viral infection. In France, hepatitis B–related PAN formerly accounted for about one-third of all cases of PAN, but there has been a decrease in the number of cases since the development of vaccines against hepatitis B and a safer blood bank. Other viruses (human immunodeficiency virus, cytomegalovirus, parvovirus B19, human T lymphotrophic virus type 1, and hepatitis C virus) are also implicated as etiologic agents.

B. The pathologic lesion that best defines PAN is a focal, segmental, sectoral necrotizing vasculitis of medium-sized and small vessels. The existence of uninvolved segments just next to the diseased areas is typical of PAN. The lesion may occur in any artery of the body, but involvement of the aorta and pulmonary arteries is rare. Arterial aneurysms and thromboses can occur at the site of the vascular lesion.

II. CLINICAL MANIFESTATIONS

A. Most patients present with constitutional symptoms (malaise, fever, weight loss), peripheral neuropathy, and gastrointestinal or cutaneous involvement.

B. Peripheral neuropathy is most often seen in the form of painful mononeuritis multiplex or multiple mononeuropathies, commonly with a dropped foot or hand.

C. Cutaneous lesions are present in 27% to 60% of patients. Vascular purpura is typically papulopetechial. Inflammatory lesions are infrequent, but when present they are the ideal site for biopsy. Livedo reticularis is common. When possible, the biopsy specimen should include the subdermis to detect medium-sized vessel involvement.

D. Myalgia and arthralgia are also common.

E. Kidney involvement is diverse and, in PAN as opposed to MPA, it is vascular, not glomerular.

F. Gastrointestinal involvement can be severe and present with abdominal pain, bleeding, and bowel perforation. Orchitis and epididymitis are also seen in PAN.

G. Although the spectrum of the clinical presentation may vary, most patients will have severe manifestations and appear acutely ill.

III. DIAGNOSIS

A. Laboratory tests. Patients are commonly anemic with leukocytosis and thrombocytosis. The ESR and CRP are usually high. Positivity for ANCA is rare in PAN. Hepatitis B surface antigen (HBsAg) should be sought in all cases.

B. Radiologic studies. Angiography often shows microaneurysms and stenoses in medium-sized vessels.

C. Biopsy. Although the diagnosis of PAN is clinical, it is useful to demonstrate vasculitis in biopsy specimens. Skin, skeletal muscle, nerve, and kidney are the usual sites. Biopsy specimens of apparently unaffected muscles may reveal vasculitis in a small fraction of patients.

IV. TREATMENT

A. Initial management of PAN without hepatitis B is with high-dosage corticosteroids (40 to 60 mg/day). CTX is added for severe cases. Traditionally, oral CTX has been used, but intravenous administration as an induction therapy can be as effective as the oral administration with fewer side effects. Induction therapy can be followed with azathioprine after 3 to 6 months.

B. In hepatitis-B–related PAN, corticosteroids and CTX may allow the virus to persist, which can lead to chronic hepatitis and liver cirrhosis. Good results have been reported treating these patients with antiviral agents, accompanied by plasma exchange, and short courses of corticosteroids.

C. Relapses are rare in patients who achieve remission.

 KAWASAKI'S DISEASE

Kawasaki's disease (KD) is an acute febrile disease occurring most commonly in infants and children under the age of 5 years (see Chapter 36). The first case was described in Japan in 1961.

I. The **etiopathogenesis** of KD is not known. Although many hypotheses involving an infectious cause have been proposed, none has been confirmed.

II. **CLINICAL MANIFESTATIONS**
    A. Vasculitis, especially of the coronary arteries, is the most serious and life-threatening complication.
    B. The onset is typically abrupt, with remitting or continuous high fever that generally lasts 1 to 2 weeks. Within 2 to 4 days of onset, bilateral conjunctival congestion occurs. Dryness, redness, and fissuring of the lips are observed within 2 to 5 days, and a "strawberry" tongue (as in scarlet fever) can be seen.
    C. The angiitis of KD usually lasts for approximately 7 weeks and is most commonly seen in the medium-sized and large arteries, including the coronary and iliac arteries.
    D. Painful cervical lymphadenopathy appears shortly before or simultaneously with the fever. Exanthema of the trunk and reddening of the palms and soles with consequent desquamation are usual.
    E. Cardiovascular involvement can include carditis with heart murmurs and electrocardiographic changes. Coronary artery lesions with dilatation or aneurysms may be seen on echocardiography.
    F. Other symptoms include abdominal pain, vomiting, diarrhea, and arthritis.

III. **DIAGNOSIS.** KD should be included in the differential diagnosis of all febrile illnesses (measles, scarlet fever, drug reactions, Stevens-Johnson syndrome, and viral exanthems) associated with rash in children.

IV. **TREATMENT.** Management is supportive in uncomplicated cases.
    A. Coronary artery involvement should be assessed with two-dimensional echocardiography weekly for the first month. If changes are detected, high-dose intravenous gamma globulin as a single infusion of 2 g/kg is given.
    B. Low-dosage aspirin (3 to 5 mg/kg/day) is used until the coronary artery changes regress.
    C. Long-term management should include coronary angiography or echocardiography and follow-up for coronary atherosclerosis.

 WEGENER'S GRANULOMATOSIS

WG is a relatively rare disease (3 in 100,000 cases in the United States) with the classic triad of necrotizing granulomatous vasculitis of the upper and lower airways, systemic vasculitis, and focal necrotizing glomerulonephritis. A milder and less aggressive form of WG exists (limited WG), with involvement predominantly in the lungs and an absence of glomerulonephritis; limited WG carries a better prognosis. WG affects male and female subjects at about the same rate, and approximately 80% to 90% of the patients are white.

I. **CLINICAL MANIFESTATIONS.** The diagnosis is usually made within 6 months of initial symptoms, but unusual presentations of the mild form may elude diagnosis for years. It is important to distinguish WG from other pulmonary-renal syndromes, such as Goodpasture's syndrome, SLE, MPA, and CSS.
    A. Most patients seek care for upper and lower respiratory tract symptoms. Sinus pain, purulent sinus drainage, nasal mucosal ulceration, and otitis media are common; tracheal inflammation can lead to subglottic stenosis.
    B. At presentation, 80% of patients have no renal involvement and 50% have no overt lung disease; however, pulmonary or renal problems or both eventually develop in more than 80% of patients. The glomerulonephritis is characterized by focal necrosis, crescent formation, and an absence or paucity of immunoglobulin (Ig) deposits. Identical "pauci-immune" necrotizing glomerulonephritis occurs in CSS and MPA, the other two ANCA-associated small-vessel vasculitides.
    C. Other WG manifestations include ocular inflammation, cutaneous purpura, peripheral neuropathy, arthritis, and diverse abdominal visceral involvement. Necrotizing granulomatous pulmonary inflammation produces radiographic densities and nodules, and the lesions may cavitate. Alveolar capillaritis can cause pulmonary hemorrhage with irregular infiltrates and the patient often presents with hypoxemia, decreased hemoglobin due to lung bleeding, and an elevated lactate

dehydrogenase (LDH). Massive pulmonary hemorrhage is a life-threatening manifestation and requires aggressive immunosuppressive treatment as well as intensive pulmonary therapy.

II. **DIAGNOSIS**
   A. Patients usually have normochromic, normocytic anemia, leukocytosis, thrombocytosis, and an elevated ESR and CRP.
   B. WG, in contrast to the immune complex vasculitides, is associated with ANCA, especially c-ANCA, which has a 98% specificity but much lower sensitivity. Elevated titers are usually associated with disease activity; consequently, only 30% to 40% of patients with limited WG or generalized WG in remission have c-ANCA positivity. There is not, however, a good correlation between c-ANCA titer and disease activity, which is best defined on clinical grounds. A minority (5%) can be positive for p-ANCA also. The limited form of the disease can be difficult to diagnose on clinical grounds, and the presence of c-ANCA may strongly influence the diagnosis.
   C. The strongest diagnostic evidence, nonetheless, comes from biopsy specimens of the involved tissues, which show granulomas. Lymphomatoid granulomatosis and necrotizing sarcoidosis may be confused with WG. The causative agent(s) leading to granuloma formation are unknown.

III. **TREATMENT.** Patients are initially given oral CTX (2 mg/kg/day) and oral prednisone (1 mg/kg/day).
   A. Prednisone is changed to an alternate-day regimen in approximately 4 to 6 weeks, and then the dosage is gradually tapered. CTX is continued for at least 1 year after complete clinical remission. Leukocyte count is a guide to CTX dose adjustment, and one should aim to keep the neutrophil count above 3,000/mm^3.
   B. An increased risk for infection, especially with *Pneumocystis carinii*, and bladder cancer should be kept in mind at all times. When compared with oral CTX and corticosteroids, pulse intravenous CTX and corticosteroids are equally effective in achieving initial remission; however, in the long term, treatment with pulse CTX does not maintain remission or prevent relapses to the degree that oral CTX treatment does.
   C. Methotrexate and azathioprine are alternatives to CTX in less severe forms of WG, and both have been used for maintenance after achievement of remission in generalized WG.
   D. Relapses are associated with respiratory tract infections and with chronic nasal carriage of *Staphylococcus aureus*. Some studies suggest that trimethoprim/sulfamethoxazole may be useful in the initial phases of WG or in preventing relapses.

 MICROSCOPIC POLYANGIITIS

MPA is a pauci-immune necrotizing vasculitis of the small vessels without evidence of granulomatous inflammation. p-ANCA positivity is common.

I. **CLINICAL MANIFESTATIONS.** Pulmonary and renal involvement are commonly seen, with approximately 90% of patients having glomerulonephritis. MPA is the most common cause of pulmonary-renal syndrome. Alveolar hemorrhage can complicate the picture. The onset is usually insidious and the prognosis is more guarded than in classic PAN.

II. **DIAGNOSIS**
   A. More than 80% of patients have ANCA, most often p-ANCA. This helps in distinguishing MPA from ANCA-negative small-vessel vasculitis but does not help in distinguishing it from other ANCA-related vasculitides. Pathologically, MPA can cause a necrotizing vasculitis identical to PAN.
   B. At the Chapel Hill Consensus Conference, MPA and PAN were distinguished by the absence of vasculitis in vessels other than arteries in PAN and the presence of vasculitis in vessels smaller than arteries (arterioles, venules, and capillaries) in MPA. By this definition, the presence of glomerulonephritis or pulmonary alveolar capillaritis would exclude a diagnosis of PAN.

III.   Treatment of MPA includes corticosteroids and cytotoxic agents; doses and duration of treatment are similar to those used for WG. High-dose intravenous steroids, followed by oral steroids and oral or intravenous CTX in cases with major organ involvement is a useful treatment strategy. About one-third of patients relapse and are treated with a repeated regimen similar to the induction therapy.

 CHURG-STRAUSS SYNDROME

CSS is a rare disorder characterized by hypereosinophilia, systemic vasculitis, and necrotizing granulomatous inflammation that occurs in individuals with asthma and allergic rhinitis.

I.   CLINICAL MANIFESTATIONS. Pulmonary infiltrates occur in up to 90% of patients, and a cutaneous eruption is seen in 70%. Cardiac manifestations (pericarditis, cardiomyopathy, and myocardial infarction) account for about half of the deaths. Peripheral neuropathy is found in 70% of patients; its occurrence in susceptible patients is highly suggestive of CSS. Renal disease, seldom seen, is generally mild.

II.   DIAGNOSIS

    A. Laboratory findings. Approximately 70% of patients have ANCA, more commonly p-ANCA; virtually all have eosinophilia. Anemia and an elevated ESR are also found with active disease. The diagnosis of vasculitis should be substantiated by biopsy of one of the involved tissues.

    B. The **differential diagnosis** of CSS includes WG, MPA, PAN, chronic eosinophilic pneumonia, and the idiopathic hypereosinophilic syndrome. Neither asthma nor a history of allergies is a prominent feature of WG; eosinophilia is rarely found in this condition. Renal involvement is less severe in CSS, and the histopathologic features of the granulomatous lesions of CSS and WG are very different. The absence of vasculitis or granuloma formation in chronic eosinophilic pneumonia and in the idiopathic hypereosinophilic syndrome helps differentiate these entities from CSS. At times, it is difficult to easily differentiate between CSS, MPA, and WG when they present with capillaritis and kidney disease.

III.   TREATMENT. Most cases of CSS respond well to corticosteroids. Initial management requires high dosage of prednisone (1 mg/kg/day) or the equivalent; methylprednisolone pulses have also been used. Life-threatening complications call for CTX or azathioprine in addition to steroids. Both oral and pulse intravenous CTX have been used, with differing rates of success. Relapses are rare after complete remissions.

 HENOCH-SCHÖNLEIN PURPURA

HSP is the most common vasculitis occuring in childhood. Half of the time, it is preceded by an upper respiratory tract infection, but the etiology remains unknown. Boys and girls are affected equally. The median age of onset is 4 years. It follows a self-limited course in most patients.

I.   CLINICAL MANIFESTATIONS

    A. The classic triad is palpable purpura with a normal platelet count, colicky abdominal pain, and arthritis. Palpable purpura occurs in 100% of patients but is the presenting symptom in only half. Dependent areas are usually involved, and involvement of the buttocks is common.

    B. Arthritis is transient and usually involves the knees and ankles; there are no permanent sequelae.

    C. Up to one-third of patients experience hematemesis and half have occult gastrointestinal bleeding, but serious hemorrhage is rare. Ten percent to 50% have renal involvement, ranging from transient isolated microscopic hematuria to rapidly progressive glomerulonephritis.

    D. HSP and IgA nephropathy are similar; the latter is confined to the kidney, whereas the former is a systemic disease.

II. **Diagnosis** is made on clinical grounds. Laboratory tests may indicate the organs involved and are mostly used to rule out other causes. Skin or kidney biopsies demonstrate IgA deposits.

III. **Treatment** is largely supportive and includes hydration and monitoring. Nonsteroidal anti-inflammatory drugs (NSAIDs) can be used for joint pain and will not aggravate the purpura. However, they should be avoided if renal insufficiency is present. Corticosteroids have been used in the management of abdominal pain, edema, and nephritis. Kidney disease can be quite refractory to all treatments.

 LEUKOCYTOCLASTIC VASCULITIS

LV is also known as hypersensitivity or allergic vasculitis, meaning blood vessel inflammation from a sensitizing source (see Chapter 16). Drugs, infections, and malignancies can be the cause. About half the cases are idiopathic, with drug-associated and infection-associated disease making up the rest. Allopurinol, β-blockers, sulfonamides, and thiazides are a few of the drugs from a long list of offenders. Lyme disease, gonococcemia, and viral exanthema should be kept in mind as possible infectious causes. HSP, mixed cryoglobulinemia, cholesterol emboli, PAN, and CSS are also in the differential diagnosis. It can be seen in the setting of SLE, RA, Sjögren's syndrome, and other vasculitides.

I. **CLINICAL MANIFESTATIONS.** The classic finding is the nonblanching palpable purpura caused by erythrocyte extravasation from damaged vessels.

   A. Skin lesions usually begin as petechiae and expand to palpable purpura. They usually resolve in 1 to 2 weeks.

   B. Lesions are more commonly seen in dependent areas, likely related to increased pressure and slowing of blood flow.

   C. Systemic signs may include fever, pericarditis, arthritis, headaches, nephritis, and retinal vasculitis in advanced cases.

   D. Typical **histopathologic** finding is migration of polymorphonuclear leukocytes to postcapillary venules, along with production of nuclear debris.

II. **DIAGNOSIS.** Laboratory evaluation should include tests to help in eliminating different causes. Biopsy of lesions usually are not diagnostic and show nonspecific vascular inflammation, including a predominantly neutrophilic infiltrate, sometimes with cell destruction and the liberation of "nuclear dust."

III. **TREATMENT.** Potentially precipitating agents should be discontinued and avoided in the future. Treatment depends on the extent of involvement. Pressure stocking is helpful for avoiding further lower extremity involvement. For mild skin disease, colchicine 0.6 mg 2 to 3 times a day or dapsone may be used. In severe disease steroids and immunosuppressive agents may have to be used and tapered slowly when the disease is in remission.

   For disease confined to the skin, the prognosis is very good. Disease confined to the skin initially rarely progresses to systemic manifestations.

 CRYOGLOBULINEMIC VASCULITIS

I. **INTRODUCTION.** Cryoglobulins are circulating immunoglobulins (Igs) that precipitate at low temperatures. They are grouped into three categories:

   A. Type 1, composed of a single monoclonal Igs, IgM, or IgG.

   B. Type 2, composed of a monoclonal component with activity toward polyclonal Igs.

   C. Type 3, composed of two or more polyclonal Igs.

   Both type 2 and 3 are composed of more than one Ig type, one of which is the rheumatoid factor, and are referred to as mixed cryoglobulins. Mixed cryoglobulins lead to immune complex disease by depositing in the vessels, activating complement, and causing inflammation.

II. **CLINICAL MANIFESTATIONS**

   A. The most frequent manifestations are palpable purpura, arthralgia, and nephritis. Histologic section reveals LV. Skin ulcers, Raynaud's phenomenon, hepatic abnormalities, and splenomegaly can also be seen. The main cause of morbidity is renal involvement.

B. Hepatitis C virus has been detected in more than 90% of patients with mixed cryoglobulins in various population studies.

C. Mixed cryoglobulins and rheumatoid factor are typically detectable in the serum. For reliable detection, blood must be maintained at 37°C during transport and clotting. Serum must then be stored at 4°C for at least 7 days for cryoglobulins to be observed.

III. DIAGNOSIS

A. Cryocrit, a method for detecting and quantifying cryoglobulins, measures the percentage of packed cryoglobulins in graduated test tubes after cold incubation and centrifugation of the serum. The cryocrit is usually between 1% and 3% in type 3 and between 2% and 7% in type 2, and it may be up to 50% in type 1 cryoglobulinemia. There is, however, no correlation between the cryocrit and disease severity.

B. Very low levels of C4 and normal or slightly low levels of C3 are common and aid in the diagnosis.

IV. TREATMENT

A. Mild disease with purpura and arthralgia is usually treated with NSAIDs.

B. Serious visceral involvement, such as glomerulonephritis, calls for treatment with corticosteroids and cytotoxic drugs such as CTX and azathioprine.

C. Plasmapheresis has also been used with some success. Recently, interferon-α has been successfully used in patients with cryoglobulinemic vasculitis associated with hepatitis C infection.

 PSEUDOVASCULITIS

These are conditions that obstruct blood flow in vessels without an accompanying inflammation of the vessel wall. They need to be kept in the differential diagnosis of any suspected vasculitis. A useful mnemonic to recall the more frequently seen pseudovasculitic conditions is **AMACEC** (APS, myxoma, amyloidosis, cholesterol emboli, endocarditis, and calciphylaxis).

I. **APS** causes both large- and small-vessel occlusions (arterial and venous), leading to gangrene, livedo, and skin ulcers. Signs of inflammation, including a raised ESR, are usually absent. It should be kept in mind that APS may also be seen in the setting of true vasculitis, as in patients with SLE.

II. **Myxomas** are benign cardiac tumors, most commonly found in the left atrium. They can cause extracardiac symptoms of petechial skin rashes, Raynaud's phenomenon, glomerulonephritis, arthritis, myositis, pleurisy, and pericarditis, often accompanied by fever, increased ESR, leukocytosis, hypocomplementemia, positivity for ANA, and thrombocytopenia. Diagnosis is usually made with echocardiography.

III. **Amyloidosis** can sometimes mimic vasculitis and be accompanied by PMR and GCA-type symptoms of scalp tenderness and claudication of the jaw. Histology shows amyloid deposits in the vessel walls.

IV. **Cholesterol embolism** is caused by the shedding of cholesterol crystals from atheromatous plaques. It is most commonly seen in elderly men. It is usually seen in the setting of recent onset of anticoagulation and diffuse atherosclerosis, commonly after abdominal surgery or diagnostic angiography, during which emboli become dislodged. When emboli occlude small arteries, the symptoms are indistinguishable from those of true vasculitis. Livedo reticularis in the lower extremities is common. More serious complications are occlusion of intestinal or coronary arteries. Renal failure may develop. Myalgia with muscle tenderness is common. The key element in diagnosis is clinical suspicion. Histologic demonstration of cholesterol emboli in skin, muscle, or bone marrow may be diagnostic. Steroids are not helpful, and anticoagulation should be avoided. Surgical removal of the part of the aorta involved, bypassing the area or grafting, can be used in severe cases with recurrent episodes.

V. **Infective endocarditis** is associated with a true vasculitis and embolic phenomena. True vasculitic lesions can be caused by an immune complex vasculitis. Emboli occluding the vessel lumen are more common. Skin, brain, spleen, and kidney are the organs frequently involved. Patients can also have arthralgia, arthritis, and an increased acute-phase response and be positive for rheumatoid factor, which makes diagnosis difficult; SLE may also be suggested, given that these patients commonly have valvular disease.

VI. Calciphylaxis is a rare and potentially lethal syndrome, almost always associated with chronic renal failure. Although calcifications develop in many patients with chronic renal failure, in some, a severe condition develops that is characterized by skin necrosis and gangrene of the extremities. Internal organ involvement can also occur. Calciphylaxis is thought to be an idiosyncratic reaction of unknown cause, involving parathyroid hormone, vitamin D, and hypercalcemia. Treatment is aimed at local management of skin ulcers and their common infections with gram-negative organisms and at keeping the calcium/phosphate product low.

RELAPSING POLYCHONDRITIS

RP is a rare disease characterized by inflammation of cartilage, mainly of the ears, nose, larynx, and joints.

I. CLINICAL MANIFESTATIONS. The most common clinical manifestation is a destructive auricular chondritis with sparing of the ear lobule. Articular symptoms are second in frequency and are usually self-limited, with a nonerosive oligoarticular or polyarticular peripheral arthritis.

    A. Inflammatory eye disease may also occur. LV causing skin lesions and aneurysms of the thoracic and abdominal aorta and cerebral artery can occur.

    B. In 30% of cases, there is an association with rheumatoid arthritis, Sjögren's syndrome, WG, MPA, and malignancies (including carcinoma of the lung, breast, and colon and myeloproliferative disorders).

II. DIAGNOSIS. There are no specific laboratory tests for RP. Ear biopsy is rarely done but may show basophilic staining of the cartilage matrix accompanied by perichondral inflammation at the interface of cartilage and soft tissue and fibrocyte and capillary endothelial cell proliferation.

III. TREATMENT. Although NSAIDs can control mild episodes of inflammation, corticosteroids are the mainstay of treatment, initially in dosages of 0.75 to 1 mg/kg/day. Immunosuppressive drugs are used as steroid-sparing agents in patients requiring long-term steroid therapy.

BEHÇET'S DISEASE

First described by Hulusi Behçet of Istanbul, this syndrome is a systemic vasculitis involving both arteries and veins.

I. Clinical manifestations are characterized by recurrent oral and genital aphthous ulceration, chronic relapsing uveitis, and a variety of skin manifestations, including the **pathergy reaction** (nonspecific hyperreactivity of the skin), erythema nodosum, and superficial thrombophlebitis. Uveitis can lead to blindness in up to 20% of patients with eye disease.

    A. Men and young patients have a more severe course than do women and older patients.

    B. Behçet's disease has been associated with HLA-B51 and is mainly observed in countries around the Mediterranean and in the Far East.

    C. The natural history of Behçet's disease is one of exacerbations and remissions.

    D. Disease manifestations, as a rule, usually become less severe with time.

II. Diagnosis is made on clinical grounds.

III. TREATMENT

    A. Mild oral and genital ulcers can be treated with local corticosteroids. Thalidomide has also been used successfully in treating mucocutaneous lesions.

B. Colchicine, which has traditionally been used for every aspect of Behçet's disease, seems to be effective mainly for the treatment of mucocutaneous lesions in female patients.

C. Immunosuppression is the mainstay of treatment of eye disease; azathioprine has been shown to maintain visual acuity and prevent new eye disease, and cyclosporine A is used for disease flares. Steroids are usually used in the short term for quick control of symptoms and for bridging therapy with immunosuppressive medications.

D. The role of heparin or anticoagulants for thrombophlebitis is still being debated. Antiplatelet drugs may be preferred for milder cases. Immunosuppressive therapy remains the standard of care.

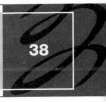

PREGNANCY AND CONNECTIVE TISSUE DISORDERS   38

Doruk Erkan and Lisa R. Sammaritano

KEY POINTS

■ Pregnancy-induced physiologic changes and the complications in pregnancy may make assessment of connective tissue disorder (CTD) activity during pregnancy difficult.

■ Most patients with CTD may safely complete pregnancy with good outcome. Both maternal and fetal outcome are better for patients with inactive disease at the time of conception.

■ Prepregnancy evaluation for patients with CTD should include the following:
  ■ Assessment of disease activity and disease-related organ damage.
  ■ Serologic assessment for the relevant autoantibodies.
  ■ Review of medications, with required adjustments before pregnancy is attempted.

■ Evaluation and monitoring of the patient with CTD, during pregnancy, requires participation of both a rheumatologist and an obstetrician capable of handling high-risk pregnancies.

■ Care and follow-up must continue through the postpartum period, as patients are at continued risk for complications, including disease flare or thrombosis.

■ Treatment with aspirin and heparin can have a profoundly positive effect in patients with prior pregnancy losses due to antiphospholipid (aPL) antibodies.

 ## INTRODUCTION

I. **Pregnancy is an altered physiologic state** characterized by particular signs, symptoms, and hormonal changes. Awareness of these changes is critical for appropriate assessment of patients with connective tissue disease (CTD) during pregnancy.

A. **Hemodynamic changes.** Intravascular volume increases approximately 30% during pregnancy, which may further stress previously compromised renal or cardiac function.

B. **Skin and musculoskeletal systems.** Palmar and facial erythema from increased cutaneous blood flow, generalized edema, and arthralgia are common in late pregnancy, and may mimic inflammatory rash or joint symptoms.

C. **Coagulation.** Pregnancy is a prothrombotic state. Fibrinogen, factor II, platelet activation inhibitor-1, prothrombin fragment 1 and 2, D-dimer, and tissue plasminogen activator levels increase, whereas free and total protein S decrease, during normal pregnancy. As a result of these changes, and in conjunction with the increased venous stasis, the risk of venous thromboembolism increases during pregnancy by a factor of five.

D. Hematologic changes. Moderate anemia due to hemodilution is frequent during pregnancy. Despite increased platelet production, increased utilization may lead to mild thrombocytopenia in up to 8% of uncomplicated pregnancies.

E. Erythrocyte sedimentation rate (ESR) increases during normal pregnancy, which makes this test less useful as a gauge of systemic inflammation.

II. **Pregnancy-induced complications are often difficult to distinguish from active CTD due to the similarity in signs and symptoms.**

A. **The pre-eclampsia (PEC) syndrome** includes hypertension in late pregnancy, (i.e., blood pressure higher than 140/90 mm Hg recorded after 20 weeks' gestation on at least two occasions), proteinuria (more than 300 mg/day), edema, and hyperuricemia. If seizures occur in this setting, the syndrome is defined as **eclampsia.**

B. **The HELLP syndrome** (**h**emolysis, **e**levated **l**iver enzymes, **l**ow **p**latelets) may be a severe variant of PEC. Patients with this life-threatening syndrome present with prominent hepatic enzyme abnormalities, fever, thrombocytopenia, and encephalopathy.

C. **Pregnancy loss** represents the most extreme pregnancy-related complication and can occur as: **pre-embryonic loss** (conception through week 4 of gestation); **embryonic loss** (week 5 through 9); **fetal loss** (tenth week of gestation until delivery); and **neonatal loss**. It is critical to differentiate pregnancy loss due to CTD [e.g., antiphospholipid antibody (aPL)-related loss] from other obstetric etiologies.

III. **Data on outcomes of pregnancy in many CTDs are limited** due to lack of prospective controlled studies. Maternal and fetal outcomes in selected CTDs will be discussed in the subsequent text.

 RHEUMATOID ARTHRITIS

I. **RISK OF DISEASE FLARE.** Pregnancy usually has a positive effect on rheumatoid arthritis (RA) symptoms. Up to three-fourths of patients experience some degree of clinical remission during pregnancy, even in the absence of medication.

A. Almost all patients relapse following delivery by the end of 8 months postpartum; most within the first 6 weeks.

B. The development of remission during pregnancy has been attributed to maternal-fetal disparity in certain human leukocyte antigen (HLA)-DQ loci.

II. **RISK OF DISEASE ONSET.** A large case-control study found a decreased risk of development of RA in women who had at any time been through a pregnancy. However, an increased risk of RA onset during the postpartum period has been noted in multiple studies.

III. **FETAL AND NEONATAL OUTCOMES.** Fertility and parity are not decreased in patients with RA and no conclusive increase in fetal morbidity or mortality has been demonstrated. Intrauterine growth retardation (IUGR) has been described in RA patients with severe disease activity and vasculitis.

IV. **MANAGEMENT.** Many patients do not require medications during pregnancy. Corticosteroid (CS) may be used for active disease. Most other medications [other than Hydroxychloroquine (HCQ)] are stopped due to safety concerns.

A. Cervical spine arthritis with atlanto-axial instability dictates careful management of patients under general anesthesia, because manipulation of the unstable spine may produce spinal cord compression.

B. Severe cricoarytenoid involvement may also be a relative contraindication to intubation with general anesthesia.

C. Assessment for adequate hip range of motion (native or prosthetic joints) should be done prior to vaginal delivery, especially if epidural anesthesia is planned.

SYSTEMIC LUPUS ERYTHEMATOSUS

I. **RISK OF DISEASE FLARE.** The definition of lupus flare during pregnancy is not uniform. Although recent case-control studies support little or no increased risk for flare during pregnancy, patients with systemic lupus erythematosus (SLE) may flare anytime during pregnancy, most commonly in the latter half and during the postpartum period.
   A. Inactive disease for the 6 months preceding pregnancy is associated with lower risk of disease flare.
   B. Hypertension and active kidney disease preceding pregnancy increase the risk of lupus kidney flare and PEC. Risk of significant decrease in renal function is greatest for patients with a creatinine clearance of less than 60 mL/minute. Assessing the degree of renal dysfunction is of more prognostic value than studying the precise renal histology.
   C. Differentiating lupus flare from PEC can be challenging (Table 38-1). Changes felt to represent SLE activity include an increase in anti–double-stranded DNA antibody level, lymphadenopathy, lupus rash, inflammatory arthritis, fever, and microscopic hematuria with erythrocyte casts. It is not uncommon for patients to have both a lupus flare and PEC—they are not mutually exclusive.

II. **RISK OF DISEASE ONSET.** The initial presentation of SLE with or without nephritis during pregnancy is rare.

III. **FETAL OUTCOMES.** Fertility is generally unimpaired unless the patient has been treated with cyclophosphamide. Fetal outcome is related more to the presence of renal involvement and the presence of aPL than the occurrence of lupus flare.
   A. If disease is quiescent for at least 6 months before conception, the pregnancy outcome improves. Pregnancy is inadvisable in the presence of uncontrolled hypertension, progressive renal failure, severe neurologic and cardiopulmonary involvement, severe thrombocytopenia, and during the use of teratogenic medications.
   B. Proteinuria higher than 0.5 g/24 hours is an independent predictor of poor fetal outcome.
   C. aPL, present in approximately 30% of patients with SLE, markedly increases the risk of fetal loss [see antiphospholipid syndrome (APS) section below]. Risk of fetal loss related to aPL appears to be similar for patients with SLE and primary APS.

IV. **Neonatal outcomes** depend on several factors: presence of aPL, presence of anti-Ro/SS-A and anti-La/SS-B autoantibodies, and maternal medications. Presence of aPL is associated with increased risk of prematurity and its attendant complications. Offsprings of the 30% of mothers with SLE who are positive for anti-Ro and anti-La are at risk for **neonatal lupus erythematosus (NLE)**, consisting of rash, thrombocytopenia, abnormal liver function tests, and congenital heart block (CHB). The risk for any manifestation of NLE in the offspring of a mother who is positive for anti-Ro is

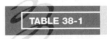 **TABLE 38-1**	Helpful and Unhelpful Measures for Defining Systemic Lupus Erythematosus (SLE) Activation during Pregnancy	

Helpful measures	Unhelpful measures
Inflammatory arthritis	Arthralgia, bland joint effusion
Lupus rash	Palmar or facial erythema
High anti-dsDNA antibody titers	Hypocomplementemia
Microhematuria, RBC casts	Proteinuria
Fever	Elevated ESR
Mucosal ulcers	Thrombocytopenia
Lymphadenopathy	

dsDNA, double-stranded DNA; ESR, erythrocyte sedimentation rate; RBC, red blood cell.

approximately 25%; however, the risk for cardiac involvement with irreversible CHB and myocarditis is less than 3%. The risk for development of SLE in a child of a mother with SLE is small; the risk for positive autoantibodies in the child is approximately 10%, and the risk for development of SLE is approximately 1%.

V. **MANAGEMENT.** Both the rheumatologist and an experienced obstetrician capable of handling high-risk cases should partner throughout the management of patients with SLE during their pregnancy.

   A. **Initial evaluation** should include an assessment of disease activity and disease-related organ damage, review of current medications, and discussion of specific risks with the patient and her partner.

   B. **Laboratory evaluation** should include complete blood count, biochemical profile, urinalysis, 24-hour urine for creatinine clearance and total protein, aPL, and anti-Ro and anti-La antibodies. Regular (monthly) follow-up of each of these tests is helpful, with the exception of the aPL and the anti-Ro and anti-La antibodies.

   C. **Fetal monitoring**
      1. Antepartum monitoring of the fetal heart rate (nonstress test) is often initiated at approximately 26 weeks; a nonreactive test (absence of appropriate heart rate response) is abnormal and may precede a decrease in fetal movement by several weeks. If fetal distress is noted and the fetus is considered viable, early delivery may prevent fetal death.
      2. Fetal echocardiography, generally at weeks 20 through 24, should be performed for evaluation of fetal heart rhythm, pericardial effusion, or myocarditis in mothers who are positive for anti-Ro and anti-La antibodies. More intensive monitoring is indicated for high-risk patients with a previous history of a child with NLE.

   D. **Treatment of flare in pregnant patients with lupus** does not generally differ from that of the patients who are not pregnant; CS is the first-line choice, with dose adjusted according to severity. HCQ and certain immunosuppressive medications may be continued if necessary (detailed in the subsequent text). Mild thrombocytopenia may respond to aspirin, but there is no evidence that treatment of mild thrombocytopenia improves maternal or fetal outcomes. CS and/or intravenous immunoglobulin (IVIG) can be used for severe thrombocytopenia.

   E. **Neonatal lupus.** Because of the low risk for CHB in the offsprings of mothers positive for anti-Ro and anti-La antibodies, prophylactic treatment is not indicated. Treatment of an abnormality with dexamethasone (which easily crosses the placenta) or, rarely, even plasmapheresis, may be helpful, although no large experience supports this.

ANTIPHOSPHOLIPID SYNDROME

I. **RISK OF DISEASE FLARE AND ONSET.** Cross-sectional studies and murine models demonstrate that the presence of aPL [positive lupus-anticoagulant test (LA) and/or anticardiolipin antibodies (aCL)] is a risk factor for pregnancy morbidities (see Chapter 31 for the discussion of APS and the definition of aPL-related pregnancy morbidities). Although the risk of pregnancy morbidity is unknown in asymptomatic (i.e., no history of vascular and/or other events during pregnancy) aPL-positive patients and in APS patients and with only a history of vascular events, it can be as high as 90% in untreated APS patients with a history of pregnancy morbidities.

II. **FETAL AND NEONATAL OUTCOMES**
   A. Fetal loss (≥10 weeks of gestation) is more strongly associated with aPL than are early pregnancy losses.
   B. Pre-embryonic and embryonic loss (<10 weeks of gestation) can occur in aPL-positive patients; however, since early pregnancy losses are common in the general population, the diagnosis of APS should be made only with three or more consecutive losses, in the absence of other identifiable etiologies. Overall, approximately half of the aPL-associated pregnancy losses occur in the first trimester.

    C. In addition to pregnancy losses, IUGR, premature delivery, PEC, eclampsia, and HELLP syndrome can be associated with aPL.

    D. The most frequent neonatal complication is prematurity. Neonatal thrombosis is extremely rare.

III. MANAGEMENT. Although numerous controversies exist in the management of aPL-positive patients, several points are generally agreed upon.

    A. Other causes of loss of pregnancy such as uterine abnormalities or hormonal imbalance should always be excluded in aPL-positive patients, especially in the presence of low titer aCL test results.

    B. Pregnancy is a prothrombotic state; thus management strategies should focus on prevention of both pregnancy morbidity and maternal thrombotic complications.

    C. High-dose prednisone alone worsens fetal outcome; although more efficacious when given in combination with low-dose aspirin (LDA) (81 mg), maternal morbidity is still significantly increased.

    D. Management strategies, including medications, are still controversial due to a limited number of well-designed controlled studies. Although it is difficult to have evidence-based recommendations, the current standard of care is given (Table 38-2).

        1. LDA and prophylactic dose heparin for patients fulfilling the Sapporo APS criteria based on a history of pregnancy loss or morbidity only (see Chapter 31 for APS criteria).

        2. LDA and therapeutic dose heparin for patients fulfilling the Sapporo APS criteria based on a thrombotic vascular event, regardless of a pregnancy history.

        3. Dose adjustments guided by midinterval (6 hours after injection) activated partial thromboplastin time (aPTT) for unfractionated heparin, or plasma antifactor Xa activity for low-molecular-weight heparin in high-risk patients (usually in consultation with a hematologist).

        4. LDA for asymptomatic (i.e., no history of vascular or pregnancy events) LA and/or medium-to-high-titer aCL-positive patients during pregnancy; however, no clinical data support this strategy. Given that pregnancy and the presence of aPL may be additive risk factors for vascular thrombosis, and that LDA has very few maternal or fetal side effects, LDA use seems justified and is usually given to these patients.

    E. If patients fail in their therapeutic response to the aspirin and heparin combination, a common next step is the addition of IVIG, shown to be efficacious in case reports only.

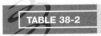 **TABLE 38-2**   **Management of aPL-Positive Patients during Pregnancy**

Asymptomatic aPL-positive patients	No treatment or LDA[a]
Single pregnancy loss <10 wk	No treatment or LDA[a]
Recurrent (pre) embryonic losses or fetal loss >10 wk **and** no history of vascular thrombosis	LDA+prophylactic dose heparin during the pregnancy, continue heparin for postpartum 6–12 wk and then switch to LDA[b]
Recurrent (pre) embryonic losses or fetal loss >10 wk **and** history of vascular thrombosis	LDA+therapeutic dose heparin during the pregnancy, switch to warfarin postpartum[b]
No history of pregnancy morbidity **and** history of vascular thrombosis	LDA+therapeutic dose heparin during the pregnancy, switch to warfarin postpartum[b]

[a]Although no data support the use of low-dose aspirin (LDA) in this situation, it is commonly given due to low risk of adverse events.
[b]**Prophylactic dose** such as enoxaparin 30 to 40 mg subcutaneously once daily; **therapeutic dose** such as enoxaparin 1 mg/kg subcutaneously twice daily or 1.5 mg/kg subcutaneously once daily.

POLYMYOSITIS AND DERMATOMYOSITIS

I. RISK OF DISEASE FLARE AND ONSET. Patients who are in remission prior to conception have roughly a 25% risk of exacerbation during pregnancy. Acute and severe onset of disease may occur during pregnancy or in the postpartum period; however, this is rare as the age of onset of polymyositis (PM)/dermatomyositis (DM) is most often during childhood or only after the age of 45 years.

II. FETAL AND NEONATAL OUTCOMES. Fetal outcomes are significantly worse in patients diagnosed during pregnancy compared to patients with established disease (50% vs. 20% rate of fetal loss). As with SLE, the timing of pregnancy in relation to disease onset or activity has a significant effect on pregnancy outcome. Only two newborns with high serum creatine kinase (CK) levels have been reported following pregnancies of patients with PM/DM.

III. MANAGEMENT. Prepregnancy evaluation of patients to assess disease activity is prudent. No evidence supports prophylactic CS treatment of patients in remission. In case of PM/DM flare, prompt diagnosis and therapy with CS may improve prognosis. In steroid-resistant cases, cyclosporine A, azathioprine, plasma exchange, or IVIG can be used.

SJÖGREN'S SYNDROME

I. RISK OF DISEASE FLARE AND ONSET. Sjögren's syndrome is often secondary to RA and other autoimmune diseases; little is known about the interaction of pregnancy with the primary syndrome.

II. Fetal and neonatal outcomes have been evaluated in patients with primary Sjögren's syndrome, and the results of the studies differ. One study suggested that pregnancies in patients with the primary syndrome have an increased risk of fetal loss, unrelated to aPL or anti-Ro/La antibodies. IUGR is uncommon. Risk of NLE is related to the presence of anti-Ro/La antibodies, independent of the underlying diagnosis; approximately 60% of patients with primary Sjögren's syndrome are positive for these antibodies (see SLE section).

III. MANAGEMENT

    A. The most common management issue is evaluation and monitoring for anti-Ro and anti-La antibodies to assess risk of NLE.

    B. Severe neurologic involvement in the pregnant mother, which is rare, may be treated with CS. Immunosuppressives (other than azathioprine or cyclosporine A) should not be used.

    C. Symptoms of mucous membrane dryness may worsen during pregnancy, and may be treated symptomatically.

SYSTEMIC SCLEROSIS

I. RISK OF DISEASE FLARE AND ONSET. Systemic sclerosis often affects women in their later reproductive years, and pregnancy during the stage of established disease is uncommon.

    A. In a combined analysis of early studies, about one-third of patients reported pregnancy-related aggravation of their disease; 10% died of pregnancy-related complications, mainly hypertension, renal failure, and cardiovascular complications.

    B. In a recent prospective study of 91 pregnancies in 59 patients with systemic sclerosis, maternal outcomes were generally good. There were three cases of renal crisis, all in women with early diffuse disease.

    C. Overall, 10% to 20% of patients may experience worsening of their disease during pregnancy, mostly Raynaud's phenomenon, arthritis, and skin thickening. Patients with severe cardiac and pulmonary involvement are at risk for significant morbidity and mortality.

II. **FETAL AND NEONATAL OUTCOMES.** Patients with scleroderma have been reported to have both decreased fertility and parity when compared with control populations.
   A. Early case–control studies showed twice the rate of spontaneous abortion and three times the rate of infertility compared to controls, as well as a significant incidence of IUGR and preterm births, which occurred with equal frequency before and after the diagnosis of systemic sclerosis.
   B. Recent prospective data on patients with a broad spectrum of disease severity show no increase in frequency of miscarriage except in those with longstanding diffuse scleroderma. Preterm births occurred in 29% of pregnancies, but neonatal survival was good.
   C. Patients with severe renal disease and hypertension are at risk for PEC.
III. **MANAGEMENT.** Treatment of pregnant patients affected with systemic sclerosis involves careful monitoring of renal function and treatment of hypertension.
   A. In general, angiotensin-converting enzyme (ACE) inhibitors should be stopped because of the risk of fetal renal toxicity. However, for true scleroderma renal crisis, which is a life-threatening complication, ACE inhibitors may be the only effective therapy.
   B. Because of delayed wound healing in patients with advanced systemic sclerosis, interventional or operative procedures should be minimized.

 THE VASCULITIDES

I. **WEGENER'S GRANULOMATOSIS (WG)**
   A. **Risk of disease flare and onset.** Pregnant patients with WG and whose disease is inactive have a 25% risk of disease flare during pregnancy. Onset of WG during pregnancy is rare; however, in case of its onset during pregnancy, it may have a more aggressive course
   B. **Fetal and neonatal outcomes.** Patients with active disease at conception have higher risk of fetal death. Premature delivery is a common feature in pregnant patients with active disease.
   C. **Management.** For patients with active disease presenting during pregnancy, CS alone or in combination with azathioprine should be considered. Other treatment options include plasmapheresis or IVIG. A small number of patients with life-threatening active disease in the late second or third trimesters of pregnancy have been successfully treated with cyclophosphamide with good neonatal outcomes.

II. **TAKAYASU'S ARTERITIS (TA)**
   A. **Risk of disease flare and onset.** Pregnancy-related exacerbation of hypertension, as well as PEC, is commonly observed in pregnant patients with TA, which probably increase the risk of neurologic events including stroke or seizure. The presence of severe aortic valvular disease or aortic aneurysms is a contraindication for pregnancy.
   B. **Fetal and neonatal outcomes.** Despite the significant vascular abnormalities, pregnancy outcomes in patients with TA are generally uncomplicated if appropriate antihypertensive therapy is administered. Infants may show evidence of IUGR related to the severity of the hypertension, extent of abdominal aorta and renal artery involvement, and the onset of PEC.
   C. **Management.** Usual management during pregnancy includes CS if indicated, careful monitoring and treatment of hypertension, and most importantly, aggressive hemodynamic and pharmacologic management in the peripartum period. Chronic disease may require vascular surgical intervention even during the course of pregnancy.
        Anesthesia management at the time of labor and delivery is critical. Both hypertension and hypotension should be avoided in TA due to vessel changes with marked variation in regional blood flow and, potentially, in organ perfusion. Epidural anesthesia may affect blood pressure.

III. POLYARTERITIS NODOSA (PAN)

    A. Risk of disease flare and onset. Pregnancy in association with PAN is relatively uncommon due to the older mean age at onset and the disease predominantly affecting the male population.

        1. Presentation of PAN during the initial stage of pregnancy results in significant maternal mortality, with better fetal than maternal outcome. This is likely to be due to difficulty with diagnosis; most reported cases of new-onset PAN during pregnancy have been diagnosed postmortem.

        2. Patients in remission prior to pregnancy have a low rate of exacerbation.

    B. Fetal and neonatal outcomes. Outcomes are significantly better for patients with established disease who are in clinical remission at the time of pregnancy. Both premature and low-birth-weight babies have been reported.

    C. Management. Serious manifestations are treated with CS. When PAN is diagnosed in early phases of the pregnancy, therapeutic abortion can be considered.

IV. CHURG-STRAUSS VASCULITIS (CSV)

    A. Risk of disease flare and onset. Pregnant patients with CSV and in whom the disease is inactive have 50% risk of disease flare (mostly asthma, mononeuritis multiplex, and rash) during pregnancy. Patients with CSV onset during pregnancy have a poor prognosis, including fetal and maternal death.

    B. Fetal and neonatal outcomes. Premature and low-birth-weight infants are commonly observed to be born to patients with CSV.

    C. Management. Patients with CSV flare are generally treated with CS and, for severe manifestations, immunosuppressive medications such as azathioprine are used.

V. BEHÇET'S DISEASE (BD)

    A. Risk of disease flare and onset. Review of the literature on BD and pregnancy reveals contradictory reports of the effect of pregnancy on disease activity, with documentation of both exacerbation (mostly oral and genital ulcers, arthritis, and eye inflammation) and remission.

    B. Fetal and neonatal outcomes. Fetal outcome is generally good, although infants with pustulonecrotic skin lesions and other manifestations have rarely been reported.

    C. Management. Patients with BD are generally treated with CS and, for severe manifestations, immunosuppressive medications such as azathioprine are used.

 OTHER RHEUMATOLOGIC DISORDERS

I. SPONDYLOARTHROPATHIES (SpA). Fetal outcome is not compromised in patients with SpA. On the basis of studies involving patients with ankylosing spondylitis (AS), axial disease remains unchanged, whereas peripheral arthritis and uveitis may be suppressed during pregnancy. Axial disease may worsen in some patients due to the mechanical stress caused by the pregnant state.

II. UNDIFFERENTIATED CONNECTIVE TISSUE DISORDER. Patients usually have uncomplicated pregnancy outcomes; however, close monitoring is required due to the possibility of a disease flare or the development of new CTD manifestations.

 MEDICATION SAFETY

I. MEDICATION SAFETY DURING PREGNANCY

    A. Acetaminophen is safe for simple analgesia, but can be insufficient to control pain and arthritis.

    B. Aspirin. Because of greater experience in its use in pregnancy, aspirin is preferred to the relatively newer nonsteroidal anti-inflammatory drugs (NSAIDs). Premature closure of the ductus arteriosus in the neonate is a theoretical concern, but this complication has not been reported with LDA. In addition, bleeding may occur in the neonate and in the mother with high daily doses.

    C. NSAIDs, especially newer agents, are avoided because of limited experience in their use during pregnancy. If NSAIDs are used, ibuprofen is preferred and is used in the lowest effective dose until the last 6 to 8 weeks of pregnancy. Use of NSAIDs after this period can result in prolonged labor, increased peripartum blood loss, premature closure of the ductus arteriosus, fetal pulmonary hypertension and impaired renal function, and reduced amniotic fluid volume.

D. Heparin. Heparin is generally used as an anticoagulant for the full 8 to 9 months of gestation, usually for patients with APS. Maternal complications may include excessive bleeding and the risk of osteoporosis. Both the fractionated and unfractionated heparin are too large to pass through the placental barrier and so do not reach the fetal circulation. **Low-molecular-weight heparin** (LMWH) has been increasingly used in patients with APS due to low risk of heparin-induced thrombocytopenia and heparin-induced osteoporosis, as well as convenience of use.

E. Warfarin use during pregnancy is associated with a high incidence of fetal loss and congenital malformations, and may also cause fatal hemorrhage in the fetus. The teratogenic effects (fetal warfarin syndrome) include nasal hypoplasia, stippled epiphyses, limb hypoplasia, low birth weight, hearing deficit, and ophthalmic anomalies. However, warfarin has been used for pregnant patients with mechanical heart valves and is thought to be safe when instituted **after** the embryonic period is completed (after week 10 of gestation). Two studies addressed the use of warfarin in pregnant patients with APS (between weeks 14 to 36 and 15 to 34 weeks of pregnancies, respectively) without any teratogenicity or significant maternal hemorrhage. The use of warfarin during pregnancy is more common in Europe than in the United States.

F. CS. In conventional doses, prednisone and methylprednisolone are safe for the fetus and are the CS of choice. The fetal effect (plasma level) in a woman taking a maternal dose of prednisolone of 20 mg/day or less is insignificant. Fluorinated CS (dexamethasone and betamethasone) easily cross the placenta and should not be used unless there is an intent to treat the fetus.

   1. CS may increase the risk for developing gestational diabetes, hypertension, and premature rupture of membranes.

   2. High-dose intravenous ("pulse") methylprednisolone does reach the fetus, with unknown effects.

   3. All patients with rheumatic disease and on chronic CS therapy should receive stress-dose steroid at the time of delivery, especially if by cesarean section.

   4. Patients with single joint arthritis or bursitis can be safely treated with intraarticular or intrabursal CS injections.

G. HCQ. Until recently, the relative safety of antimalarials was not established in pregnant patients and HCQ was usually stopped prior to pregnancy. However, it has now been well demonstrated that discontinuation of antimalarial drugs can precipitate a lupus flare and that HCQ is safe during pregnancy, with no reported fetal effects.

H. Sulfasalazine. In general, sulfasalazine may be continued during pregnancy. There have been rare case reports of congenital cardiovascular defects and oral clefts in the fetus with the first trimester exposure to the drug. Folate supplementation decreases the risk; the sulfasalazine dose should not exceed 2 g/day.

I. Azathioprine is widely used in pregnant patients with renal transplant, and is considered generally safe in pregnancy, although fetal cytopenias and malformations have been reported.

J. Methotrexate is contraindicated in pregnancy. It is an abortifacient and causes a characteristic fetal syndrome of craniosynostosis and other central nervous system malformations. Patients receiving methotrexate should not get pregnant until 3 months after stopping the medication.

K. Cyclosporine may cause maternal nephrotoxicity, but appears to be safe for the fetus.

L. Cyclophosphamide should not be administered during pregnancy, because it is teratogenic. Pregnancy should not be attempted until 3 months after stopping the medication.

M. Leflunomide is teratogenic in animals, but no human studies exist. Pregnancy should not be attempted until after elimination of the drug by treatment with cholestyramine.

N. Mycophenolate mofetil is not recommended during pregnancy, as there are limited animal data on it. However, at least five mothers are reported to have taken mycophenolate mofetil during pregnancy without fetal complications.

O. IVIG is safe and may be used during lupus-associated pregnancy for thrombocytopenia, and for aPL-associated pregnancy losses that are refractory to LDA and heparin.

P. Tumor necrosis factor-α (TNF-α)-inhibitors. All three TNF-α inhibitors (etanercept, infliximab, and adalimumab) are rated U.S. Food and Drug Administration (FDA) pregnancy category "B," meaning that animal studies reveal no fetal harm, but no adequate human studies are available. No adequate or controlled studies in pregnant women have been done for any of the TNF-α inhibitors, although a limited number of case reports in humans have not identified developmental problems.

II. POSTPARTUM PERIOD AND MEDICATIONS

A. Heparin, warfarin, CS, aspirin, and NSAIDs may be administered; however, the use of other drugs is discouraged.

B. A patient on prednisone or methylprednisolone should breast-feed just prior to ingestion of medication, which minimizes the infant's exposure to CS.

C. Antimalarial drugs are secreted in breast milk; however, they are generally thought to be safe during breast-feeding.

D. It is not known whether breast milk-transmitted autoantibodies are pathogenic; however, many investigators advise women with anti-Ro, anti-La antibodies against breast-feeding due to associated risk of NLE.

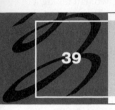

39 ANKYLOSING SPONDYLITIS
Eric S. Schned

▓ KEY POINTS

■ The diagnosis of ankylosing spondylitis (AS) should be strongly considered if four or more of the following clinical features are present: age of onset of back pain less than 40 years; insidious onset; low back pain lasting longer than 3 months; association with morning stiffness; improvement with exercise.

■ Radiologic imaging is the key to the accurate diagnosis of AS. Investigation should start with x-rays; if these are not diagnostic, computed tomography (CT) scans or magnetic resonance imaging (MRI) may be more sensitive and specific.

■ Spinal fracture is a serious complication of AS. Risk of fracture is increased by the presence of ankylosis of the spine, osteoporosis, and trauma. Acute back pain in a patient with AS after minor trauma should raise concern regarding a possible fracture.

■ Common disorders that need to be distinguished from AS are lumbosacral disc disease, degenerative arthritis of the spine, diffuse idiopathic skeletal hyperostosis (DISH), and osteitis condensans ilii.

■ Tumor necrosis factor-α (TNF-α) inhibitors are important to provide relief of symptoms in patients with AS who are unresponsive or inadequately responsive to nonsteroidal anti-inflammatory drugs (NSAIDs). Early evidence suggests that they may modify the outcome of AS.

*A*nkylosing spondylitis (AS) is a chronic inflammatory disorder of unknown etiology that primarily affects the spine, axial skeleton, and large proximal joints of the body. Distinctive features of the disease are the striking tendency toward ossification and ankylosis of the spine and involvement of entheses. There is a spectrum of clinical severity, ranging

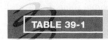

| TABLE 39-1 | Proposed Classification Criteria for Ankylosing Spondylitis |

Clinical criteria
- Low back pain and stiffness for more than 3 mo duration, improved by exercise, unrelieved by rest
- Limitation of motion of the lumbar spine in both sagittal and frontal planes
- Limitation of chest expansion relative to norms corrected for age and sex

Radiologic criteria
- Sacroiliitis with more than minimum abnormality bilaterally or
- Sacroiliitis of unequivocal abnormality unilaterally

Diagnosis
Definite AS is present if one of the radiologic criteria is associated with at least one clinical criterion
Probable AS is present if 3 clinical criteria are present or if one of the radiologic criteria is present without any signs or symptoms satisfying the clinical criteria

From van der Linden S, Valkenburg HA, Cats A, et al. Evaluation of diagnostic criteria for ankylosing spondylitis. A proposal for modification of the New York criteria. *Arthritis Rheum* 1984;27:366, with permission.

from asymptomatic sacroiliitis to immobilizing spinal encasement. The most common manifestations of the disease are back pain and stiffness. Genetic and environmental factors play key roles in the pathogenesis of all the spondyloarthropathies, including AS.

Classification criteria have been developed for AS (Table 39-1). These are employed in epidemiologic studies in an attempt to standardize AS diagnosis.

ETIOPATHOGENESIS

I. GENETIC ASPECTS

   A. Human leukocyte antigen (HLA)-B27 association. In 1973, Schlosstein and Brewer independently reported a strong association of HLA-B27 with AS. The prevalence of AS has been shown to vary in populations based on the frequency of HLA-B27 in those populations. Recent estimates suggest that HLA-B27 contributes only 16% to 50% of the total genetic risk for AS, which probably helps explain why only a small percentage of individuals with the HLA-B27 allele develop AS.

   B. Family history. A positive family history of AS is found in approximately 15% to 20% of cases. The risk of development of AS in an HLA-B27 relative of an index case is approximately 20%.

   C. Sex distribution. AS is identified more commonly in men than in women by a ratio of 3:1. However, the diagnosis in women may be overlooked or missed for various reasons, such as attribution of symptoms to other causes, or reluctance to perform a radiologic examination of the pelvis in young women.

   D. Environmental aspects. When the HLA-B27 gene and human β-2-microglobulin are introduced into rats, a Reiter's-like syndrome develops. However, if the same molecules are introduced into rats in a germfree environment, disease does not occur. These experiments suggest a role for "pathogens" in the pathogenesis of AS and other spondyloarthropathies.

   However, to date, there is no clear evidence for a specific environmental trigger for AS.

II. THEORIES OF PATHOGENESIS. How does the HLA-B27 gene contribute risk for AS? The answer is not yet known, but structural features of the B27 molecule may offer some clues (see Chapter 6). A leading theory is that the HLA-B27 molecule may present antigenic peptides to T cells, triggering an inflammatory response.

III. PATHOLOGY

   A. Skeletal sites of inflammation in AS include: **sacroiliac joints, intervertebral disc spaces,** and **apophyseal joints; anterior central joints** such as the manubriosternal joint, sternoclavicular joints, symphysis pubis; and large proximal joints **(hips and shoulders).** The presence of peripheral joint inflammation such as in the hands or feet should cause the diagnosis of AS to be questioned and raise the possibility of psoriatic arthritis or reactive arthritis.

   B. Extraskeletal sites of inflammation include the uveal tract, aortic root wall, lung apices, and the heart valves.

   C. Pathologic findings. In AS, inflammation occurs in the annulus fibrosis of the intervertebral disc, subchondral bone (osteitis), the entheses (the insertion areas of tendons and ligaments into bone), and synovium (synovitis). Inflammation of subchondral bone leads to erosion and sclerosis, which later becomes replaced by fibrocartilage and then becomes ossified.

 PREVALENCE

I. **In white Americans, the HLA-B27 gene occurs in approximately 8% of the population** and the prevalence of AS is estimated to be approximately 0.1% to 0.2%. The risk of AS is much higher in native American populations such as the Haida who have a 50% prevalence of HLA-B27, and is very low in native South American and Bantu populations of Africa who have very low HLA-B27 prevalence.

II. **AS typically affects young adults in their 2nd through 4th decades.** The risk of developing AS in a random population of HLA-B27–positive persons is approximately 2%.

 CLINICAL MANIFESTATIONS

I. **The classic presentation** occurs in a young adult who experiences the insidious onset of persistent, dull low back pain and stiffness that is **worse in the morning hours and after prolonged rest.**

II. **The low back pain is typically relieved by physical activity and gets better as the day progresses.** Pain is usually centered in the lumbar region, but may also be present in the buttocks and hips. Over time, pain and stiffness may spread to the upper back and neck. Involvement of the sternocostal joints can cause anterior chest pain that might mimic angina pectoris.

III. **Peripheral arthritis** occurs in half the patients during the course of AS. Involved joints are usually large and proximal, such as the hips and shoulders. Hip involvement is recognized as a major predictor of severe disease and disability.

IV. **Heel, pubic, and ischial pain** is due to local enthesopathy. Achilles tendinitis is also common.

V. **EXTRASKELETAL MANIFESTATIONS**

   A. Acute anterior uveitis, usually unilateral, occurs in approximately 25% of patients with AS. Some patients experience recurrent episodes that can lead to secondary glaucoma.

   B. Aortic valve regurgitation and aortitis occur in small numbers of patients and occasionally may progress to congestive heart failure.

   C. Pulmonary involvement. Restriction of the thoracic cage during respiration, caused by fusion of costovertebral joints, can result in reduced lung volumes, but rarely leads to impaired gas exchange. Fibrocystic involvement can occur at the apices.

VI. **SUBSETS OF AS**

   A. Juvenile AS. In childhood, AS usually presents in older boys as an asymmetric **oligoarticular arthritis** of the lower extremities, often predating back symptoms. **Heel pain** is a common complaint. Over time, the child acquires features more typical of adult AS.

   B. Asymptomatic sacroiliitis. Among asymptomatic HLA-B27–positive relatives of probands with AS and among random asymptomatic persons who are HLA-B27–positive, 20% may be found to have radiographic sacroiliitis. Also, about one-fourth of HLA-B27–positive patients with acute anterior uveitis will have subtle clinical or radiographic evidence of sacroiliitis. Some of these individuals will progress to overt clinical AS.

VII. COMPLICATIONS

   A. Spinal fracture is the most serious complication of AS, which may occur after even minor trauma to the rigid, ankylosed spine, especially in the cervical region.

   B. Cauda equina syndrome due to nerve root traction by bony overgrowth or arachnoiditis occurs rarely.

   C. Osteoporosis of the vertebral bodies is very common in AS and contributes to fracture risk.

   D. Early predictors of severe disease include hip involvement, erythrocyte sedimentation rate (ESR) greater than 30 mm, limitation of lumbar spine movement, unresponsiveness to nonsteroidal anti-inflammatory drugs (NSAIDs), and age of onset less than 16 years.

   E. Premature atherosclerosis occurs in AS and is related to the systemic inflammatory process.

 PHYSICAL EXAMINATION

I. **The major physical findings in AS** are pain and tenderness in the spine and affected areas of the axial skeleton and loss of spinal mobility.

II. **SACROILIAC JOINTS.** Early signs include local tenderness over the sacroiliac joints and tenderness with paraspinal muscle spasm at the lumbosacral vertebral levels. Several maneuvers to detect sacroiliitis have been described.

III. **SPINE.** Loss of spinal motion (lateral motion, flexion, and extension) occurs early in most cases. With progression of disease, typically there is loss of the normal lordosis, progressive kyphosis of the thoracic spine, fixed flexion of the neck, and ultimately a stooped posture with fixed flexion contractures of the hips and knees. Severe kyphosis can be exacerbated by advanced hip flexion contractures.

   A. The Schober's test is useful for assessing restricted forward flexion of the spine. The patient stands erect. The examiner makes marks at two points along the spine, at the lumbosacral junction and a point 10 cm cephalad. The distance between the marks is measured in maximum forward flexion. **Less than 5 cm of distraction** is abnormal.

   B. Costovertebral involvement, which causes reduced chest expansion, can be measured at the 4th intercostal space in men and under the breasts in women. **Less than 5 cm of chest expansion during deep inspiration** in the adult is considered reduced.

   C. Finger to floor measurement. Measuring the distance between the fingertips and the floor or the place along the tibia that is reached during spinal flexion can be used as a guide to the extent of spinal flexion and/or response to treatment or physical therapy.

IV. **OTHER SIGNS AND SYMPTOMS.** Aortic insufficiency may be detected by a systolic regurgitant murmur. Eye inflammation due to acute uveitis may be associated with unilateral ocular pain, erythema, photophobia, and visual blurring.

 DIAGNOSTIC INVESTIGATIONS

The diagnosis of AS requires a combination of clinical features, laboratory tests, and radiographic evidence of sacroiliitis. Clinical suspicion prompting testing should be aroused when patients complain of back pain that suggests inflammation (i.e., worse in the morning and better as the day goes on).

I. **LABORATORY STUDIES**

   A. HLA-B27 is present in 95% of white patients with spondylitis. Rheumatologists perform this test only in rare clinical situations in which the presentation is atypical or complex.

   B. ESR and C-reactive protein are elevated in many cases but do not correlate well with disease activity.

   C. Immune studies. No specific immune abnormalities are observed.

   D. Hematologic tests. A mild normocytic anemia and thrombocytosis are seen in more severe cases.

II. **IMAGING STUDIES**
A. **The demonstration of definite unilateral or bilateral sacroiliitis is diagnostic of AS.** X-rays are an appropriate first step in radiologic imaging. Nuclear scanning, computed tomography (CT) scanning, or magnetic resonance imaging (MRI) may be employed if x-rays are negative or equivocal.
B. **X-rays**
1. **Sacroiliac joints.** Typical changes are "punched-out" **erosions; "pseudowidening"** of the joint; **sclerosis** of the joint margins; and **ankylosis** and **obliteration** of the joint.
2. **Spine.** Typical changes are vertebral bodies appearing "squared," due to periostitis; **bony bridging** of adjacent vertebrae by "flowing" **syndesmophytes;** and **"Bamboo spine"** which refers to the ossification process of advanced AS.
3. **Peripheral joints.** Typical changes are articular erosion and proliferative new bone formation in adjacent tissues ("whiskering"); and in the hip, concentric joint space narrowing.
4. **Entheses.** Inflammation and secondary ossification of entheses (such as the plantar fascia and the Achilles tendon) lead to proliferative "spurs."
C. **Nuclear scans.** In some clinical circumstances, technetium stannous pyrophosphate bone scans may detect areas of active inflammation in AS before standard radiographic changes are present. However, changes are often difficult to assess and may be nonspecific.
D. **CT scan and MRI** are valuable tools in identifying distinctive changes in sacroiliac joints and vertebrae. MRI scans are more sensitive than x-rays in detecting early AS. MRI has also been used in assessing response to anti-TNF medications.
E. **Bone mineral density (BMD) testing** with dual energy x-ray absorptiometry (DXA) of the lumbosacral spine and hip or quantitative CT scanning of the spine may be used to assess osteoporosis and fracture risk.

DIFFERENTIAL DIAGNOSIS

I. **Distinguishing AS from the multitude of other causes of low back pain is challenging.** The clinical history may be a sensitive and specific tool in the differential diagnosis. If four or more of the following features are present, the diagnosis of AS should be strongly considered.
A. Age of onset before 40 years.
B. Insidious onset.
C. Low back pain lasting longer than 3 months.
D. Association with morning stiffness.
E. Improvement with exercise.
II. **Conditions that should be distinguished from AS are the following:**
A. **Mechanical back pain** due to lumbosacral disc disease, "lumbar strain," and degenerative joint disease. The clinical feature of pain intensifying with rest and improving on exercise in patients with spondylitis may be useful in distinguishing the condition as that of AS. Older age of patients and the presence of typical osteophytes on radiographs suggest degenerative arthritis. The sacroiliac joints may be affected by osteoarthritis, but radiologic involvement is limited to the lower part of the joints, whereas complete involvement is the rule in AS.
B. **Other spondyloarthropathies.** Usually, the extra-articular manifestations of these disorders allow clinical differentiation. The spondylitis of reactive arthritis and psoriatic arthropathy is usually less severe than that of typical AS, and syndesmophytes tend to be asymmetric.
C. **Diffuse idiopathic skeletal hyperostosis (DISH)** is an idiopathic proliferative enthesopathy seen in elderly persons. It can mimic AS but lacks apophyseal and sacroiliac involvement. The presence of thick anterior spurs on lateral x-rays of the spine help to differentiate this disease from the spinal disease of AS.
D. **Osteitis condensans ilii** refers to sclerosis confined to the iliac subchondral bone of the sacroiliac joints, seen in parous women. This condition is often asymptomatic but occasionally is associated with low back pain.

TREATMENT

I. The **aims of management** in AS are to control pain, maintain optimal skeletal mobility, prevent deformities, and maintain function. There is no cure for AS. Until recently, there was little hope of preventing progression of the disease, but experience with the anti-tumor necrosis factor-α (anti-TNF-α) agents suggests that this may now be realistic. Management requires education of the patient and understanding, and consists of dedicated physical programs of posture control and exercise, and the use of medications and surgical intervention when appropriate.

II. **PHYSICAL THERAPY.** All patients should be enrolled in a physiotherapy program. Maintenance of erect posture is critical in all activities, including sitting, standing, and walking. The patient should sleep in a prone position or supine on a firm mattress with one small pillow or no pillow. Walking and swimming are excellent ways to maintain joint mobility. Heat application, massage, and other techniques may help reduce muscular spasm and pain.

III. **MEDICATIONS.** The role of drugs is to relieve pain and inflammation so that posture can be preserved and exercises performed to maintain function, and hopefully to interrupt progression of the disease from inflammation to ankylosis.

  A. **NSAIDs.** Numerous NSAIDs have been shown to reduce pain and inflammation in AS. **Indomethacin** (25 to 50 mg three to four times daily, or one 75 mg slow-release capsule twice daily) is probably more effective than other NSAIDs. Trials of several agents are probably indicated **(e.g., naproxen, sulindac, piroxicam, tolmetin, celecoxib, and others)** if one agent is not effective or is not tolerated. These medications are not believed to be disease-modifying. Celecoxib has recently been approved by the FDA for use in AS (400 units orally daily).

  B. **Salicylates,** for unknown reasons, seldom provide an adequate therapeutic response in AS.

  C. **Sulfasalazine and methotrexate** and other traditional second-line agents, used in RA and psoriatic arthritis, generally have disappointing results in patients with spinal inflammation associated with AS. They may be of benefit for the peripheral arthritis seen in some patients.

  D. **TNF-α inhibitors. Infliximab** and **etanercept** have shown remarkable efficacy in reducing pain and stiffness and improving function in many patients with AS. Infliximab is generally given in intravenous doses of 5 mg/kg, initially at 2 weeks and 6 weeks, and then every 8 weeks. Etanercept is usually given 25 mg subcutaneously twice a week or 50 mg weekly. Recently, adalimumab 40 mg subcutaneously every other week has been shown to be efficacious as well.

  1. Preliminary evidence suggests that the TNF-α inhibitors may decrease or inhibit the progression of bony ankylosis in AS.

  2. Precautions and adverse events associated with TNF-α inhibitors are reviewed in Chapter 64. TNF-α inhibitors are indicated when individuals have unsatisfactory control of symptoms due to inflammation, despite use of NSAIDs, or if they have poor prognostic markers.

  E. **Systemic corticosteroids** have been relatively ineffective in managing spinal and axial inflammation in AS, in contrast to the benefit seen in the peripheral arthritis in most other inflammatory arthritides.

  F. **Intra-articular corticosteroids** may be helpful in selected individuals with AS who also have peripheral arthritis.

  G. **Pamidronate.** A controlled trial of the bisphosphonate pamidronate, which has some anti-inflammatory activity, suggested benefit in AS. Dosage was 60 mg intravenous monthly for 6 months.

  H. **Antiresorptive agents,** such as **alendronate** or **risedronate,** in doses used for primary osteoporosis, may be indicated if osteoporosis is present or if fracture risk is high.

IV. **SURGERY.** Surgical procedures are usually reserved for patients with far-advanced disease that is causing painful deformities or loss of function. Total hip arthroplasty is the most commonly performed procedure. Cervical and lumbar osteotomies to relieve severe spinal kyphosis, and stabilization of atlanto-axial subluxation may be necessary. Unfortunately, ectopic ossification at the operative site may occur.

PROGNOSIS

The course of AS varies. In some patients, the disease progresses relentlessly (often despite therapy), with fusion of the spine and peripheral joints. In others, bony ankylosis may develop gradually with little pain or discomfort. In still others, skeletal involvement may be limited to only mild sacroiliitis and never progress to serious disease.

I.   **MORTALITY.** Patients with AS have an increased rate of mortality due to premature atherosclerosis, and the overall burden of disease is similar to RA, with impaired social and work functioning.

II. **PROGNOSTIC FACTORS.** Early hip involvement, limitations of spinal mobility, a high ESR, and peripheral arthritis are associated with worse clinical outcomes.

III. **MODIFYING THE COURSE.** Although AS is not curable, rehabilitation yields important results. Most patients who maintain disciplined exercise and posture programs and take anti-inflammatory medications may lead relatively normal and active lives.

Relentless crippling disease develops in fewer than 10% of patients. The advent of the TNF-α inhibitors heralds a new era in AS treatment, because of the prospect that prolonged use may interrupt the inflammatory process and delay or prevent ankylosis.

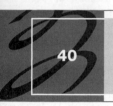

40	**ARTHRITIS ASSOCIATED WITH ULCERATIVE COLITIS AND CROHN'S DISEASE**
	Kyriakos A. Kirou and Allan Gibofsky

■ KEY POINTS

■ Intestinal inflammation is closely linked to the spondyloarthropathies (SpA).

■ Among extraintestinal manifestations of inflammatory bowel disease (IBD), the musculoskeletal ones are most common and include peripheral arthritis (PeA) type I and II, asymptomatic sacroiliitis, ankylosing spondylitis (AS), and enthesitis.

■ Type I PeA resembles reactive arthritis (ReA), may precede enteritis, usually parallels bowel disease activity, and is mostly benign with regard to joint damage.

■ Type II PeA may resemble rheumatoid arthritis and causes more persistent symptoms independent of bowel disease activity.

■ IBD-associated AS has the same course and prognosis as idiopathic AS.

■ Therapy that is targeted at the intestinal inflammation, such as with sulfasalazine, 6-mercaptopurine, and/or azathioprine, is also effective against type I PeA.

■ Nonsteroidal anti-inflammatory drugs (NSAIDs) should be used with caution because they may sometimes exacerbate intestinal disease.

■ Anti-tumor necrosis factor (anti-TNF) agents appear to be very effective for all musculoskeletal symptoms of IBD, but only the anti-TNF monoclonal antibodies may ameliorate intestinal inflammation. These agents should be reserved for more severe cases and those refractory to other treatments.

Ulcerative colitis (UC) and Crohn's disease (CD), the two major forms of inflammatory bowel disease (IBD), share several extraintestinal manifestations among which musculoskeletal involvement is the most common and arguably the most important. Enteritis has been pathogenetically linked to arthritis in IBD and therefore such arthritis is also called enteropathic.

IBD-associated arthritis is one of the spondyloarthropathies (SpA) that are characterized by axial and/or peripheral joint involvement, enthesitis, anterior uveitis, mucocutaneous inflammation, occasional aortitis and heart block, seronegativity for rheumatoid factor, and familial aggregation with a strong association with human leukocyte antigen (HLA)-B27 (see Chapter 5).

Notably, subclinical gut inflammation has been documented in all SpA forms, including ankylosing spondylitis (AS), their prototypic disorder.

 ETIOPATHOGENESIS

I. **INFECTIOUS TRIGGERS**
   A. **Bacteria** have been thought to play a significant role in these diseases, either because of increased exposure to normal intestinal flora (as occurs with increased intestinal permeability in IBD), or because of enteric infection with certain arthritogenic bacteria [in reactive arthritis (ReA)].
   B. Synovial fluid cultures, however, are characteristically negative, and septic arthritides are excluded from the group.

II. **Genetic factors** determine whether patients with IBD will develop arthritis.
   A. **Although patients with IBD have normal incidence of HLA-B27,** patients with IBD-related type I peripheral arthritis (PeA) and IBD-associated AS (IBD-AS) demonstrate increased incidence of this allele.
   B. **Loss-of-function mutations of CARD 15 (NOD2; chromosome 16)** are associated with an increased risk for CD. Gut inflammation may occur through defective mucosal defenses against luminal bacteria.
   C. **Among patients with CD, those with sacroiliitis** have an increased prevalence of CARD 15 mutations.

 PREVALENCE

I. The prevalence of IBD is between 50 and 100/100,000.

II. PeA occurs in 5% to 20% of patients with IBD and is slightly more common in patients with CD. It is seen mainly in the setting of IBD colonic involvement.

III. Axial involvement in the form of inflammatory spinal pain occurs in 6% to 18% depending on the study. However, AS occurs in 1% to 9% of patients with IBD (IBD-AS). IBD-AS is more common in patients with CD, and not associated with any particular intestinal localization.

 CLINICAL MANIFESTATIONS

The European Spondyloarthropathy Study Group (ESSG) classification criterion has greater than 85% sensitivity and specificity for the SpA (Table 40-1).

I. **PeA**
   A. **Men and women are equally affected,** and peak age of onset is between 25 and 44 years.
   B. **Recently PeA has been classified as type I** PeA, which resembles ReA both clinically (asymmetric, large joint, lower extremity, and pauciarticular) and genetically (26% prevalence of HLA-B27), and **type II** PeA that clinically appears to resemble seronegative rheumatoid arthritis (RA) (Table 40-2).
   C. **Resection of affected colon in UC** usually induces remission of type I PeA.

II. **AXIAL ARTHRITIS**
   A. Unlike primary AS, in IBD-associated AS there is no male predominance, it can occur after 40 years of age, and only 50% to 70% of patients are HLA-B27–positive. In fact, AS in HLA-B27–negative patients should predict IBD or psoriatic arthritis.

	The European Spondyloarthropathy Study Group (ESSG) Classification Criteria

TABLE 40-1

Criterion	Definition
1. Inflammatory spinal pain with at least four of the following components: a. Three-months duration b. Age of onset <45 y c. Insidious (gradual) onset d. Improved by exercise e. Associated with morning stiffness	History of past symptoms or current symptoms of spinal pain (low, middle, and upper back or neck region)
2. Synovitis	Past or present asymmetric arthritis, or arthritis predominantly in the lower limbs
3. One or more of the following:	1. Family history: first- or second-degree relatives with AS, psoriasis, acute uveitis, reactive arthritis, or inflammatory bowel disease 2. Psoriasis (past or present) diagnosed by a physician 3. Inflammatory bowel disease (past or present) diagnosed by a physician and confirmed by radiography or endoscopy 4. Nongonococcal urethritis, or cervicitis occurring within 1 month before onset of arthritis 5. Episode of diarrhea occurring within 1 month before the onset of arthritis 6. Enthesopathy: past or present spontaneous pain or tenderness at examination of the insertion site (enthesis) of Achilles tendon or plantar fascia 7. Buttock pain (past or present) alternating between right and left gluteal regions 8. Sacroiliitis: either bilateral grade 2–4, or unilateral grade 3–4[a]

Spondyloarthropathy is diagnosed when criterion 1 or 2 is present together with one or more of the eight conditions in criterion 3

[a]Grades are—0, normal; 1, possible; 2, minimal; 3, moderate; 4, ankylosed (completely fused).
AS, ankylosing spondylitis.
Adapted from Dougados et al. The ESSG preliminary criteria for the classification of spondylarthropathy. *Arthritis Rheum* 1991;34:1218–27.

TABLE 40-2 Peripheral Arthritis in Inflammatory Bowel Disease (IBD)

Type I PeA (~4% of patients with IBD)	Type II PeA (~3% of patients with IBD)
Pauciarticular, including a large joint	Symmetric polyarticular, usually affecting the small joints of the hands (MCP and PIP)
May precede (up to 3 y) or present at the same time as the IBD	Usually follows IBD diagnosis
Acute self-limiting attacks (<10 wk)	Usually persistent symptoms (months to years)
Parallels GI flares	Usually the course is independent of GI flares
Associated with erythema nodosum and uveitis	Associated with uveitis only
Relatively high HLA-B27 prevalence (26%)	HLA-B27 prevalence not increased (4%)

Both types are seronegative for rheumatoid factor.
GI, gastrointestinal; HLA, human leukocyte antigen; IBD, inflammatory bowel disease; MCP, metacarpophalangeal; PIP, proximal interphalangeal.

B. IBD-AS occurs independently of bowel disease activity, and sometimes precedes it by several years. As many as 8% of patients with AS may develop clinically obvious CD.

C. Patients with IBD-AS may also have PeA in up to 50% of cases.

III. **Hypertrophic osteoarthropathy with clubbing** can occur in patients with CD.

IV. **Osteoporosis** can occur as a complication of glucocorticoid usage, intestinal malabsorption, or the systemic impact of the inflammatory process.

V. **Other extraintestinal manifestations include the following:**

  A. **Acute anterior uveitis** (3% to 4% of patients with IBD) that is associated with all types of IBD arthritis (17% to 27%).

  B. **Erythema nodosum** (EN) (in 3% of patients with IBD) that is associated with type I PeA (16%).

  C. Psoriasis, pyoderma gangrenosum (PG), aphthous mouth ulcerations, and urethritis/cervicitis are additional mucocutaneous manifestations of IBD.

PHYSICAL EXAMINATION

I. **A comprehensive examination** is needed, given the multitude of disease manifestations.

II. **MUSCULOSKELETAL EXAMINATION.** Effusions are commonly present in the large joints (mainly knees and ankles) affected in type I PeA. In type II PeA, symmetric synovitis of metacarpophalangeals (MCPs), proximal interphalangeals (PIPs), and wrists is common. In IBD-AS, the typical signs of spine movement restriction (i.e., the Schober's test) are seen as in primary AS.

III. **Physical examination should also focus on the following:**

  A. **Integument:** aphthous oral ulcers, psoriatic skin lesions, EN, PG, urethritis, and cervicitis.

  B. **Heart:** murmur of aortic insufficiency (AI) [AI often occurs with atrioventricular (AV) block and has a high prevalence of HLA-B27].

  C. **Eyes:** signs of uveitis.

DIAGNOSTIC INVESTIGATIONS

I. **LABORATORY TESTS**

  A. Iron deficiency anemia, high erythrocyte sedimentation rate (ESR) and C-reactive protein (CRP) are common with flares of enteritis and type I PeA arthritis. In contrast, axial pain and enthesitis often have low levels of laboratory inflammatory markers. Rheumatoid factor is absent.

  B. Synovial fluid analysis is consistent with inflammatory arthritis: 4,000 to 40,000 leukocytes/mm^3 (70% to 90% polymorphs). Cultures are negative.

  C. HLA-B27 testing is not recommended as a routine diagnostic test.

II. **IMAGING STUDIES**

  A. Radiographic findings of PeA are nonspecific, with soft tissue swelling and perhaps juxta-articular osteoporosis. Rarely, erosions and reactive bone formation may be seen.

  B. Asymptomatic sacroiliitis on plain radiography can occur in 2% to 11% of patients, and often HLA-B27 is absent. Computed tomography (CT) scan may detect earlier changes or clarify questionable involvement.

  C. In symptomatic patients, both sacroiliitis and spondylitis with symmetric syndesmophytes may be seen.

  D. Enthesitis-related bone erosion and bone formation can be seen, typically at the heels.

  E. Ultrasonography and magnetic resonance imaging (MRI) can also be used in assessing arthritis and enthesitis and can detect pathology earlier.

  F. Bone mineral density tests should be done to assess for the presence of osteoporosis.

  G. In cases where type I PeA and IBD-AS precede or coincide with intestinal disease presentation, radiographic and endoscopic studies of the intestine will help establish the IBD diagnosis.

DIFFERENTIAL DIAGNOSIS

I. **TYPE I PeA**
    A. Acute monarthritis can closely resemble septic arthritis, gout, or pseudogout.
    B. PeA in other SpA, such as ReA, is clinically very similar.
    C. Differential diagnosis of above disorders may be more difficult when type I PeA precedes intestinal inflammation.
    D. Glucocorticoid-induced osteonecrosis of a large joint such as the hip may occur and should be differentiated from PeA.

II. **TYPE II PeA.** Symmetric chronic involvement of the small joints of the hands can mimic seronegative rheumatoid arthritis and calcium pyrophosphate dihydrate (CPPD) disease.

III. **AXIAL INVOLVEMENT**
    A. **In the case of IBD-AS,** axial arthritis can be indistinguishable from that of AS. However, in 25% of cases, sacroiliitis can be asymmetric.
    B. **Sacroiliitis involvement** could rarely be caused by infection because of adjacent fistulae or bacteremia.
    C. **Inflammatory spine pain** should be differentiated from other causes of low back pain (LBP) (see Chapter 20).

IV. **Subclinical enteropathy** has been observed at high rates in all SpA, and usually affects the ileum. Histologically, both acute (as in infectious enterocolitis) and chronic (as in CD) intestinal lesions can be seen. In AS, chronic lesions and HLA-B27 negativity may predict development of overt CD in 2 to 9 years.

V. **Nonsteroidal anti-inflammatory drug (NSAID)-induced enteropathy** may occur in patients with SpA taking NSAIDs and, although usually asymptomatic, it may present with bleeding, protein loss, ulcers, and obstruction. This should be differentiated from IBD. A pathognomonic sign of NSAID-enteropathy is jejunal diaphragmatic strictures. NSAID cessation usually suffices to resolve the lesions except for severe strictures where endoscopic dilatation or surgery may be needed. It must be noted that NSAIDs of all types may cause IBD to flare.

TREATMENT

I. **In type I PeA,** therapy should be directed primarily at the intestinal inflammation, because its control will usually lead to control of the acute PeA. In fact, most patients will be already on sulfasalazine, azathioprine, 6-mercaptopurine, and/or glucocorticoids for their bowel inflammation at the time of the onset of PeA. In contrast, type II PeA and IBD-AS have independent clinical courses in relation to gut inflammation and therefore require independent therapy.

II. **Simple analgesics** may suffice for mild forms of arthritis and arthralgias.

III. **NSAIDs and COX-2 inhibitor** provide symptomatic relief from all musculoskeletal manifestations of the SpA, including those of IBD. However, they should be used with caution because they may exacerbate intestinal inflammation in patients with IBD.

IV. **Sulfasalazine** is used for mild to moderately active UC and Crohn's colitis, as well as in maintaining remission in patients with UC. Notably, the drug is reduced in the colon by bacteria to its two active moieties: 5-aminosalicylic acid (5-ASA) (responsible for the effect on the colon) and sulfapyridine (responsible for the drug's effect in RA). It is beneficial primarily for the peripheral and not the axial arthritis.

V. **Azathioprine and 6-mercaptopurine** are effective in controlling both intestinal and peripheral joint inflammation.

VI. **Methotrexate,** in weekly doses of 7.5 to 25 mg with concomitant folic acid therapy, as in RA, can also be used for peripheral but not axial disease.

VII. **The chronic systemic use of glucocorticoids** should be avoided for arthritis alone. Acute flares of joint and intestinal inflammation will be helped by short courses of steroids. Injections into inflamed joints or entheses are helpful.

VIII. **Tumor necrosis factor (TNF) inhibitors** are highly efficacious for all musculoskeletal manifestations of IBD. However, only infliximab and adalimumab, but not etanercept, have shown benefit in the intestinal inflammation of CD. In the largest TNF study in patients with CD and active and severe SpA, 24 patients were treated with infliximab for 12 to 18 months and 12 patients with conventional therapy for CD (including azathioprine, topical and systemic glucocorticoids/salicylates, and metronidazole). Although both groups showed similar improvement in bowel disease, ESR/CRP, and eventually PeA, only the infliximab group showed a dramatic improvement in axial and enthesitis symptoms.

IX.   **Other potential treatments** include pamidronate, thalidomide, statins, and perhaps ω-3 fatty acids.

X.   **The importance of physical therapy,** with emphasis on range of motion, muscle strengthening, and maintenance of good posture, cannot be overemphasized.

PROGNOSIS

I.   The natural history of type I PeA is that of episodic self-limiting arthritis during bowel flares (see Table 40-2). In one study, only 17% of patients with IBD had persistent symptoms. Erosive disease is quite rare.

II.   In contrast, 88% of patients with type II PeA tend to have persistent symptoms with a median duration of 3 years. Despite persistent symptoms, erosive disease is rare.

III.   The prognosis of axial disease is similar to that of AS.

OTHER ENTEROPATHIC ARTHRITIDES

I.   **WHIPPLE'S DISEASE** (see Chapter 50)

II.   **INTESTINAL BYPASS ARTHRITIS (ARTHRITIS-DERMATITIS SYNDROME).** Jejunoileostomy or jejunocolostomy, performed for morbid obesity, often results (after 2 to 30 months) in a symmetric and migratory nondeforming polyarthritis, sometimes associated with tenosynovitis, in 20% to 80% of patients and may become chronic in 25%. The syndrome has been attributed to bacterial overgrowth in the blind loop with alteration of bowel permeability and formation of bacterial antigen-containing immune complexes.

   NSAIDs are effective against arthritis, but courses of oral antibiotics may offer additional help. Nevertheless, only surgical reanastomosis of the bypassed intestinal segment provides a cure.

III.   **CELIAC DISEASE**
Celiac disease or gluten-induced enteropathy is characterized by mucosal abnormalities of the small intestine and malabsorption. Association with many autoimmune disorders, colon cancer, and lymphoma has been noted, and arthritis rarely occurs.

   A.   **Arthritis** is usually polyarticular and often involves hand and wrist joints. Half the patients have no intestinal symptoms. In that clinical scenario, presence of malaise, weight loss, and low serum folate levels can be very helpful in diagnosis. Bone pain due to osteomalacia may also occur.

   B.   **Arthritis usually responds well to a glutenfree diet.**

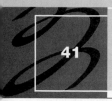

41 | PSORIATIC ARTHRITIS

Petros Efthimiou and Joseph A. Markenson

■ KEY POINTS

■ Psoriatic arthritis (PsA) is a chronic inflammatory arthropathy of the peripheral joints and axial skeleton, occurring in a subset of patients with psoriasis.

■ Arthritis might precede skin psoriatic lesion in 13% to 17% of cases.

■ The extent of skin disease does not generally parallel the arthritic activity.

■ Radiographic findings considered "classic" for PsA include asymmetric distal interphalangeal (DIP) joint erosion and ankylosis, "pencil-in-cup" deformity and resorption of the phalangeal tufts, and "fluffy" periostitis.

■ PsA follows a moderate course, affecting few joints. However, in 20% of cases it evolves into a destructive debilitating arthritis.

■ The modern treatment paradigm is early aggressive treatment with disease-modifying antirheumatic drugs (DMARDs), aiming at a status of no evidence of disease, to avoid joint damage.

Psoriatic arthritis (PsA) is a chronic inflammatory arthropathy of the peripheral joints and axial skeleton, occurring in 7% to 42% of patients with psoriasis. Psoriasis affects 1% to 3% of the general population.

I. **Psoriasis** usually appears in the second to third decades, but the onset of associated arthritis is usually delayed by two decades. However, 13% to 17% of patients with PsA will present with joint symptoms before the appearance of skin lesions, making diagnosis difficult. Although skin disease is a useful diagnostic marker for PsA, its extent does not parallel the activity of arthritis.

II. **Enthesopathy** or inflammation at the sites where tendons and ligaments attach to the bone is a hallmark feature of PsA. The enthesis, composed of fibrocartilage and collagen type II, is a highly vascular structure aimed to absorb and dissipate mechanical stress and appears to be the primary target in PsA.

ETIOPATHOGENESIS

I. **The pathogenesis of PsA** remains unknown. There is evidence of distinct immunologic processes causing persistent skin and synovial inflammation that are not shared with the pathogenesis of rheumatoid arthritis (RA). A predominance of clonally expanded CD8+ T lymphocytes in both skin and synovial tissue suggests the presence of a triggering antigen.

A. **The pattern of proinflammatory cytokines** [tumor necrosis factor-α (TNF-α), interleukin (IL)-1, IL-6, and IL-8], expressed in PsA synovial fluid and surgical explants, is similar to RA, with cytokines expressed at even higher levels. Elevated levels of TNF-α are found in psoriasis in the psoriatic plaques and the uninvolved skin alike.

B. **Angiogenesis** is believed to play a pivotal role in the pathophysiology of PsA synovitis and is controlled by growth factors such as vascular endothelial growth factor (VEGF) and angiopoietin (Ang)-1 and Ang-2, which in turn may be controlled by cytokines such as TNF-α.

    C. Osteoclast precursors are found in large amounts in the blood of patients with PsA and their participation in the development of joint damage is likely. Furthermore, marked upregulation of the osteoclastogenesis enhancer receptor activator of NF-κB ligand (RANKL) and low expression of its natural antagonist osteoprotegerin (OPG) were detected in psoriatic synovial tissues.

II. **GENETIC FACTORS PLAY AN IMPORTANT ROLE.** First-degree relatives of patients with PsA have a 40% to 50% risk of developing the disease. Concordance between monozygotic twins is high (70%) when compared to RA (30%). Human leukocyte antigen (HLA)-B27 has clearly been associated with axial disease, and HLA-DR4 with peripheral polyarticular involvement in PsA. **CARD 15** is the first non-MHC gene that has been recently associated with PsA.

III. **Infectious agents** have long been suspected to act as disease triggers.

IV. **Psoriasis and PsA tend to take a more aggressive form in** patients infected with **human immunodeficiency virus (HIV),** although the incidence of psoriasis in these patients is not greater than in the general population. HLA-associated genes **(HLA-BW38, BW39, AND CW6)** are found in patients with PsA who are HIV infected in a frequency similar to that seen in patients with PsA who are not HIV infected. This is in contrast to HIV-associated reactive arthritis (ReA), where frequency of HLA-B27 can be higher than 75%.

V. **A history of trauma** often precedes the diagnosis of PsA, suggesting the presence of a possible "internal" Köbner's phenomenon (the appearance of psoriasis at sites of traumatic cutaneous injury).

PREVALENCE

Recent community-based epidemiologic studies have suggested a rate of incidence of approximately 6/100,000/annum and a prevalence of 1/1,000. **The male to female ratio is 1:1,** and the peak incidence occurs between the ages of 45 and 54 years.

CLINICAL MANIFESTATIONS

I. Typically, patients present with pain and stiffness of the affected joints, which tend to be less tender than the affected joints in patients with RA. Morning stiffness lasting for over 30 minutes is seen in more than 50% of patients.

II. **Five distinct patterns** of PsA are recognized and are listed as follows:

    A. Oligoarticular (four or fewer inflamed joints) disease that constitutes 70% of all cases of PsA is characteristically asymmetric and affects a few scattered distal interphalangeal (DIP), proximal interphalangeal (PIP), and metacarpophalangeal (MCP) joints, knees, ankles, and feet. These are often in association with dactylitis, manifested by diffuse swelling of one or more fingers and toes in a sausage digit configuration. This diffuse swelling is due to the intense and diffuse inflammatory changes that occur both in the joints and soft tissues, and is not present in RA.

    B. Asymmetric involvement of DIP joints of the hands and feet is sometimes referred to as "classic" psoriatic arthropathy, but this pattern appears in as few as 10% of cases. Digits affected often have characteristic psoriatic nail changes.

    C. Arthritis mutilans is a particularly disabling form occurring in approximately 5% of all cases of PsA. The deformity, most striking in the fingers and toes, is caused by osteolysis of the affected joints.

    D. Symmetric polyarthritis (resembling RA) is usually rheumatoid factor-negative, and constitutes approximately 15% of all cases of PsA. Constitutional symptoms such as morning stiffness and fatigue are common and tend to parallel the activity of joint disease.

    E. Psoriatic spondyloarthritis occurs in up to 5% of patients with PsA and presents with clinical and radiographic features of axial and sacroiliac inflammation. These may be indistinguishable from those of ReA, and their involvement tends to be asymmetric as opposed to the symmetric spinal and sacroiliac disease of ankylosing spondylitis. The histocompatibility antigen HLA-B27 is found in 40% of this group.

III. **Enthesopathy,** although unusual in RA, is a primary feature of PsA. Common clinical manifestations of enthesopathy in PsA include plantar fasciitis, epicondylitis, Achilles tendinitis, and enthesitis of the ligamentous insertions around the pelvic bones.

IV. **EXTRA-ARTICULAR MANIFESTATIONS.** Conjunctivitis and uveitis occur in up to one-third of patients with PsA. Aortic insufficiency may rarely complicate PsA.

V. **SAPHO syndrome** [synovitis, acne, palmoplantar pustulosis (50% to 60% have this or another form of psoriasis), hyperostosis, and osteitis] is often considered a variant of PsA. Features in common with PsA include asymmetric synovitis, pustulosis, enthesopathy (e.g., anterior chest pain), and involvement of the sacroiliac joint. However, the characteristic constellation of symptoms and the absence of HLA-B27–associated sacroiliitis help differentiate this syndrome.

PHYSICAL EXAMINATION

I. **Musculoskeletal examination** shows all of the cardinal signs of inflammation in the affected peripheral, spine, and sacroiliac joints. The most common form of PsA has the characteristic asymmetric pattern of digit involvement. Interphalangeal joint involvement is often associated with a sausage appearance of the digits (dactylitis). The inflamed joints may have a purplish-red discoloration, a feature rarely seen in RA.

II. **Skin psoriasis** may be obvious or may be represented only as an obscure patch on the scalp, umbilicus, elbows, knees or intergluteal fold, dandruff, or nail pitting (onychodystrophy). PsA usually follows well-established cutaneous or nail lesions, although some patients exhibit characteristic patterns of PsA in the absence of the characteristic skin lesions (see Chapter 16).

III. **Nail changes** alone may not be diagnostic, but greater than 20 pits is suggestive and more than 60 can be diagnostic of PsA. Nail involvement correlates closely with skin and arthritic changes, especially of the DIP joints. Fungal and bacterial infections can also cause hyperkeratosis and onycholysis, and should be ruled out before attributing the nail changes to psoriasis.

DIAGNOSTIC INVESTIGATIONS

I. **LABORATORY TESTS**
   There are no definitive laboratory tests in the diagnosis of PsA.
   A. **The anemia** of chronic disease can occur in PsA, as can thrombocytosis.
   B. **Erythrocyte sedimentation rate (ESR)** and other acute-phase reactants are elevated, and parallel the activity of the arthritis.
   C. **Polyclonal hypergammaglobulinemia and hypercomplementemia** are occasionally present and reflect the inflammatory activity.
   D. **Serum uric acid may be elevated** in 10% to 20% of patients with psoriasis as a result of high skin cell turnover.
   E. **Antinuclear antibodies and rheumatoid factor tests** are usually negative.
   F. **HLA markers are rarely sought.**

II. **RADIOLOGIC STUDIES**
   A. **Radiographic features considered classic** are the erosions involving predominantly the DIP joints of fingers and the interphalangeal joints of the toes. Bony ankylosis of the DIP joints of the hand and toes, along with bony proliferation of the base of the distal phalanx, and resorption of the tufts of the distal phalanges of hands and feet are also commonly seen. These are quite distinct from the changes seen in RA.
   B. **Fluffy periostitis of large joints, "pencil-in-cup"** appearance of DIP joints, absence of symmetry, and gross destruction of isolated small joints can also be seen. Changes in the spine and sacroiliac joints may be similar to those seen in

ankylosing spondylitis, but sacroiliac joint and spine changes in PsA are often unilateral.

C. Magnetic resonance imaging (MRI) may be more sensitive than plain radiographs in detecting enthesitis and early articular and periarticular involvement. Sacroiliitis detected by MRI correlates with restricted spinal movement and longer duration of PsA. MRI evidence of increased water content in the bone marrow, known as "bone edema," is frequently found in PsA (and other inflammatory spondyloarthropathies) and is thought to be a "forerunner" of erosions. These abnormalities do improve after therapy with anti-TNF medications.

 DIFFERENTIAL DIAGNOSIS

I. **The cutaneous lesions of ReA** often resemble pustular psoriasis. ReA usually affects large joints and infrequently involves the DIP joints or produces sausage digits. The incidence of HLA-B27 is higher in ReA. In radiographs, ReA may demonstrate periostitis of the plantar surfaces of the calcaneus, metatarsal bones, or ankles. In PsA, periostitis is usually limited to the long bones.

II. **PsA should be differentiated from gout** by the absence of monosodium urate crystals in the synovial fluid. Hyperuricemia may occur in up to 20% of patients with skin psoriasis, but is uncommon during acute flares of PsA. In contrast to monarticular PsA, acute gouty arthritis usually resolves completely in 1 to 2 weeks, even if left untreated. Occasionally, the two conditions may coexist.

III. **Frequently confused with RA,** PsA can be differentiated on the basis of distinct clinical (dactylitis, onycholysis, spondylitis, sacroiliitis, asymmetrical joint involvement, DIP involvement, and psoriatic skin plaques), serologic (usual absence of rheumatoid factor elevation), and radiologic characteristics, including bony proliferation and osteolysis at tendon, ligament, and capsular insertions (entheses). Because both RA and psoriasis are common, they can coexist. At times, it is difficult to differentiate RA from PsA and that does not lead to therapeutic problems because their treatment is quite similar (Table 41-1).

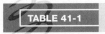**TABLE 41-1**	**Comparison between Psoriatic Arthritis and Rheumatoid Arthritis**	
Disease characteristics	**PsA**	**RA**
Female preponderance	−	++
DIP joint involvement	++	−
Symmetric joint involvement	+/−	++
Erythema over affected joint	++	−
Sacroiliitis	++	−
Spondylitis	+	−
Enthesopathy	++	−
Skin lesions	++	−
Nail lesions	++	−
Dactylitis	++	−
Rheumatoid factor	−	++
Osteopenia	+	++
Osteolysis	++	−
Ankylosis	++	−

−, not seen; +/−, uncommon; +, common; ++, very common.
DIP, distal interphalangeal; PsA, psoriatic arthritis; RA, rheumatoid arthritis.
Adapted from Gladman D. Psoriatic Arthritis. In: Maddison PJ, Isenberg DA, Woo P, et al., eds. *Oxford Textbook of Rheumatology.* 3rd ed. New York: Oxford University Press; 2004.

TREATMENT

I. **The treatment of PsA** includes therapies that often work for both the skin condition and the joint disease. Rheumatologists and dermatologists need to approach the disease as a team with close collaboration for optimal results. This has been especially true after the introduction of biologic medications that have the capacity to induce remission in both psoriasis and PsA and the new paradigm of early aggressive therapy in order to arrest radiographic progression and functional limitation.

II. **The skin lesions** are treated by topical medications including tar, anthralin, vitamin D ointment, and topical corticosteroids, and aimed at controlling the inflammation and skin proliferation. In refractory cases, systemic medications such as methotrexate (MTX), psoralen and ultraviolet A light, retinoic acid derivatives, cyclosporin, and more recently biologic agents (TNF inhibitors and costimulation blockers) are employed.

III. **Nonsteroidal anti-inflammatory drugs (NSAIDS)** [and the selective cyclooxygenase-2 (COX-2) inhibitor] are effective in controlling mild inflammation of PsA. However, no systematic trials exist about their use in the treatment of PsA and there are no comparative studies to help the clinician select a specific compound. NSAIDs do not modify the course of the disease, nor do they prevent erosions, although they can be effective in ameliorating symptoms. They are used in conjunction with disease-modifying antirheumatic drugs (DMARDs).

IV. **DMARDs** are used soon after the diagnosis is made. Combining two DMARDs (usually MTX with cyclosporin) can be effective even in patients unresponsive to either drug alone.

    A. MTX is the most widely used DMARD in PsA, because it is effective for skin and arthritic symptoms, fast acting, and well tolerated. Concerns about severe liver disease resulting from MTX therapy, as shown from the early reports of its use in psoriasis, seem to have been alleviated because more judicious use of folic or folinic acid has become commonplace, and the weekly dose schedule is universal. Frequent monitoring of liver function tests and albumin, and a liver biopsy after a cumulative dose of 1.5 g or 4 to 5 years of therapy is still indicated. This is despite the American College of Rheumatology guidelines that do not recommend such a biopsy in patients with RA unless there are persistent abnormalities in the liver tests. This reflects the feeling that the presence of psoriasis changes the liver toxicity equation toward a potentially greater propensity for MTX-related liver damage.

    B. Cyclosporin A works well for skin and joint disease as well, but toxicity limits its usefulness. Careful observation of blood pressure and serum blood urea nitrogen (BUN)/creatinine is essential.

    C. Sulfasalazine, leflunomide, azathioprine, mycophenolate mofetil, antimalarials, and gold have been used with modest effectiveness in PsA; sulfasalazine may be used in patients with HIV and PsA.

V. **Biologic agents** have revolutionized the therapy for skin psoriasis and PsA alike. Advances in the understanding of immune mechanisms that contribute to the pathophysiology of PsA have allowed the targeting of specific components of the immune response. As a result, a new class of therapeutic agents that is highly efficacious in treating symptoms (skin and joint), arresting disease progression, and improving quality of life has emerged. Currently, biologic agents are divided in two broad categories (Table 41-2).

    A. TNF inhibitors (etanercept, infliximab, and adalimumab). Etanercept was the first anti-TNF agent to be approved in the United States for the treatment of both psoriasis and PsA. In psoriasis, it is used in higher doses (50 mg subcutaneous twice weekly) during the first 3 months of therapy before switching to the standard dose of 25 mg twice weekly. Infliximab and adalimumab are currently in advanced clinical trials. The effect of TNF blockade with all of these agents in PsA has been very dramatic, surpassing at times the therapeutic effect in RA.

    B. Costimulation inhibitors (alefacept and efalizumab) have both been approved for the treatment of severe skin disease and are undergoing trials for their use in PsA.

        1. Alefacept, a leukocyte function antigen (LFA)-3/IgG1 fusion protein, blocks the interaction between CD2 on T lymphocytes and LFA-3 on antigen presenting cells (APCs). It also causes apoptosis of T lymphocytes through mediation

F. Gastrointestinal symptoms. Antecedent diarrhea has generally resolved by the time of onset of arthritis, but may persist at a low-grade level for prolonged periods. Even if the diarrhea has cleared, stool cultures may still be positive for the offending organism.

G. Mucocutaneous symptoms

1. **Circinate balanitis** appears as coalescing, superficial genital ulcers.
2. **Keratoderma blennorrhagicum** is characterized by the appearance of psoriasis-like papulosquamous, keratotic skin lesions on the palms and soles.
3. **Mucosal ulcers** can appear on the tongue or buccal mucosa and are generally painless, but not invariably so.
4. **Cardiac features** are rare but may include heart block, pericarditis, or aortic insufficiency.
5. **Neurologic features,** also rare, may include myelopathy and cranial nerve lesions.

DIAGNOSTIC INVESTIGATIONS

I. **HEMATOLOGIC FINDINGS.** An elevated erythrocyte sedimentation rate is usually present in an acute episode. The anemia of chronic disease usually accompanies a more prolonged course.

II. **URINARY FINDINGS.** Pyuria is common while hematuria is less common. Urethral discharge contains abundant neutrophils.

III. **SYNOVIAL FLUID.** An elevated white blood cell count of 10,000 to 50,000/mm^3, with a predominance of neutrophils, is usually seen in active disease. Results of a Gram stain are carefully examined, and a synovial fluid specimen is sent for culture.

IV. **CULTURE.** In general, a careful search for persistent pathogens should be undertaken. The arthritogenic organisms listed in the preceding text (e.g., *Salmonella*) may on occasion be associated with a true septic arthritis; therefore, appropriate cultures of synovial fluid should always be performed. Urethral discharge or persistent diarrhea demand appropriate culture material (for chlamydial infection and gonorrhea in the former and for gram-negative enteric pathogens in the latter). Immunofluorescence studies of urethral swabs are increasingly being used for assessing chlamydial urethritis.

V. **TISSUE TYPING.** The HLA-B27 antigen is present in 70% to 80% of patients with ReA, but is of diagnostic value only in the appropriate clinical setting (i.e., high pretest probability). A negative test result does not exclude the diagnosis, but may alert the clinician to the possibility of alternative diagnoses.

VI. **RADIOGRAPHS.** Generally, radiographic findings are normal in the acute disease, but reactive new bone at entheses may accompany chronic disease. Radiographic sacroiliitis may occur in the course of ReA and is classically asymmetric. Clinical suspicion of sacroiliac disease with normal radiographic findings is an indication for confirmation of sacroiliitis by bone scan. Magnetic resonance imaging (MRI) has been shown to increase the sensitivity of imaging for evaluation of sacroiliac joints, but the specificity of these techniques is not clearly defined in the acute phase. The development of quantitative MRI scoring systems has enabled it to be applied to imaging sacroiliac joints and spine in patients with ankylosing spondylitis, but it has not been applied systematically in ReA to date.

DIFFERENTIAL DIAGNOSIS

I. **SEPTIC ARTHRITIS.** Appropriate cultures of synovial fluid, and of all potential portals of entry, should be performed to exclude septic arthritis. The most common diagnosis to exclude in a young patient is gonococcal arthritis. ReA and disseminated gonococcal infection may both have associated tenosynovitis, urethritis, conjunctivitis, and dermatitis. The concomitant use of antibiotics for gonococci and *Chlamydia* are commonly employed in patients with defined gonococcal septic arthritis.

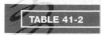

TABLE 41-2	Treatment of Psoriatic Arthritis with Biologic Agents
TNF-α inhibition	**Infliximab:** chimeric (75% human and 25% mouse) mAb-targeting TNF-α, improves both synovitis and skin disease. It is administered as an intravenous infusion in conjunction with oral MTX, initially at weeks 0, 2, 6, and every 4–8 wk thereafter. **Etanercept:** human p75 TNF receptor/IgG1 fusion protein neutralizes both TNF-α and TNF-β (lymphotoxin). Improves both skin psoriasis and PsA. **Adalimumab:** humanized mAb-targeting TNF-α. It is administered as a subcutaneous injection every wk or every alternate wk.
Costimulation inhibition	**Alefacept:** is a human LFA-3/IgG1 fusion protein, which binds to the CD2 receptor on T cells, thereby selectively depleting CD45RO$^+$ memory-effector T cells. Approved for severe skin disease, alefacept has worked for PsA in a small open trial and currently undergoing RCT. **Efalizumab:** humanized mAb disrupts the T-cell costimulatory LFA-1–ICAM-1 interaction. It is approved for severe skin psoriasis and is currently undergoing trials for PsA indication

ICAM, intercellular adhesion molecule; Ig, immunoglobulin; LFA, leukocyte function antigen; mAb, monoclonal antibody; MTX, methotrexate; PsA, psoriatic arthritis; RCT, randomized controlled trial; TNF, tumor necrosis factor.

between natural killer (NK) and T cells. It is administered as an intramuscular injection (15 mg) weekly for 12 weeks with close monitoring of the peripheral blood CD4 count (must be >250 cells/mL).

2. **Efalizumab** is a humanized monoclonal antibody directed against the CD11, a subunit of LFA-1 expressed on T lymphocytes, preventing its interaction with intercellular adhesion molecule (ICAM)-1 (upregulated in psoriasis), expressed on APCs, keratinocytes, endothelial cells, and fibroblasts. Block of costimulation causes loss of leukocyte function.

VI. **SECOND-LINE THERAPIES**

A. **Systemic corticosteroids** have limited application in the management of PsA, but can be effective for the control of acute flares. For patients with oligoarticular disease, in whom disability results from involvement of one or a few joints, intra-articular steroid therapy may be preferred to systemic use.

B. **Retinoic acid derivatives (etretinate)** in open trials showed some benefit, but take longer to act in joint disease (3 to 4 months) than do other therapies. Etretinate cannot be used in women of childbearing age. Side effects include mucocutaneous lesions (dryness) and proximal arthralgias. They should be avoided in axial disease because extraspinal calcifications can develop.

C. **Photochemotherapy** with methoxypsoralen and long-wave ultraviolet-A light may benefit patients who are nonspondylitic and with synchronous joint and skin flares.

VII. **Physical therapy** is used as an adjunct to drug therapy to help preserve joint range of motion and minimize muscle weakness.

VIII. **Reconstructive surgery** is of value in patients with end-stage joint destruction.

PROGNOSIS

The prognosis for patients with PsA generally varies according to the following anatomic pattern:

I. **Most patients have mild localized disease,** affecting only a few joints. For these patients, the prognosis is generally favorable.

II. **Approximately 20% of patients develop severe disabling** and deforming arthritis. Adverse prognostic features during the first visit to the clinic include effusion in more than five joints and high rate of previous DMARD use, although a low ESR seems to be protective.

III. **The axial spondyloarthropathy of PsA** is associated with many of the same extra-articular manifestations seen in idiopathic ankylosing spondylitis (uveitis, conduction defects, and aortitis). These features may significantly contribute to morbidity. Only anti-TNF medications appear to improve the spinal and sacroiliac joint inflammation.

IV. **Complications of therapy,** especially corticosteroids, have been a contributing factor to mortality in several large series. Patients with severe disease may have an increased mortality risk.

V. **The new biologics** utilized in the treatment of PsA are likely to have a profound effect on prognosis in the upcoming years, offering highly efficacious disease management with rare, albeit potentially serious, side effects. Because of the disadvantage of increased cost, criteria should be established for the early identification of patients with severe disease, who will benefit the most from these agents.

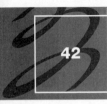

42 REACTIVE ARTHRITIS
Robert D. Inman

■ KEY POINTS

- In arthritis occurring after a recent infection, the first priority is to rule out a septic process in the joint.
- The prognosis is good in most patients and most can be managed with nonsteroidal anti-inflammatory drugs (NSAIDs).
- More refractory cases may need methotrexate, sulfasalazine, or on occasion anti-tumor necrosis factor (anti-TNF) treatment to bring the process under control.
- The efficacy of antibiotics in modifying the natural history of reactive arthritis (ReA) is not resolved.

 INTRODUCTION

I. **Reactive arthritis (ReA)** refers to a nonseptic arthritis that follows an extra-articular infection. The antecedent infection, usually gastrointestinal or genitourinary, can often be identified, but antibiotic treatment does not appear to predictably alter the course of the illness.

II. **ReA has replaced Reiter's syndrome (RS)** as the name of choice for the clinical triad of arthritis, conjunctivitis, and urethritis. The term ReA now encompasses postinfectious seronegative asymmetric arthritis, either alone or in combination with one of the characteristic extra-articular features such as rash, uveitis, or conjunctivitis.

III. **The most common pathogens** implicated in such infections are *Yersinia, Salmonella, Shigella, Campylobacter* (gastrointestinal infections), and *Chlamydia* (genitourinary infections).

IV. **Although ReA occurs in children and the elderly, it is usually seen in young adults,** with a significant male predominance. It is likely that ReA is under-recognized in female patients, because some clinical features (e.g., cervicitis) may be less symptomatic than the extra-articular features in male patients (e.g., balanitis). However, serious, and even refractory, ReA does occur in women, and the clinician should be alert to a typical constellation of symptoms in either of the sexes.

V. **Despite the strong immunogenetic influence on the disease, a positive family history for ReA is uncommon.** However, it has been observed that if there is a positive

family history, it tends to be for ReA, whereas patients with ankylosing spondylitis are more likely to have relatives with that disease than with ReA.

VI. **At present, there are no clinical features that will discriminate** the patients who will develop systemic target organ involvement from those in whom the disease will be limited to the joints, nor are there features that will define a benign, self-limiting course (averaging 3 to 4 months) from a more chronic course.

 ETIOPATHOGENESIS

Despite the strong association with the human leukocyte antigen (HLA-B27), the mechanism whereby this HLA gene might confer disease susceptibility to ReA remains unknown. There are several hypothetical routes by which HLA might interact with a triggering infectious agent.

I. The first is molecular mimicry, whereby an autoimmune response develops after the infection because of cross-reactivity between host and microbial antigens.

II. A second mechanism is a distinctive cellular immune response to the pathogen, determined by unique determinants in the antigen-binding groove of the HLA-B27 molecule, which specifically present "arthritogenic" peptides to a responding CD8+ T-cell population.

III. Another possibility is an altered microbial–host cell interaction, by which certain HLA alleles modulate host response to arthritogenic organisms.

IV. Whatever the mechanism, it is likely that the synovitis that ensues is related to local deposition and persistence of microbial antigens, but definitive proof is lacking to resolve the issue.

 CLINICAL MANIFESTATIONS

I. **HISTORY.** A careful history should be taken to address any recent exposure to an enteric pathogen (e.g., a diarrheal illness after travel abroad) or a sexually transmitted pathogen (e.g., a new sexual contact). The typical interval between the triggering infection and ReA is 1 to 4 weeks, but shorter or longer intervals have been reported. A past history of low back pain or recurrent tendinitis is not uncommon. A history of recent antibiotic therapy may alter culture results. Prior episodes of uveitis may not be mentioned by the patient unless specifically queried.

II. **CONSTITUTIONAL SYMPTOMS.** Fatigue may not be present in the acute phase, but can become significant in chronic ReA.

III. **PHYSICAL EXAMINATION**
A. **Fever** is usually low-grade (<38°C) in most patients. Significant or sustained fever suggests that the original infection may still be active.
B. **Arthritis.** The cardinal feature is an asymmetric arthritis, typically oligoarticular and predominantly in the lower extremities. The most common symptomatic joints are knees, ankles, and metatarsophalangeal joints, but involvement of an upper extremity joint can also be seen. Acute sacroiliitis may present as a diffuse low back pain that is difficult to localize, but may be felt in the deep gluteal area. Low back pain is commonly worse in the morning and gets better as the day progresses, a reflection of its inflammatory character.
C. **Enthesitis.** Plantar fasciitis and Achilles tendinitis are quite specific for ReA and should be sought carefully. Any tendinous insertion into bone can be involved, and tendinitis of hip adductors may be misdiagnosed as arthritis of the hip joint.
D. **Genitourinary symptoms.** Urethritis can be manifested by dysuria and by urethral discharge in male patients. Cervicitis in female patients is usually asymptomatic. Prostatitis and hemorrhagic cystitis may also occur.
E. **Ocular symptoms.** Conjunctivitis, the most common ocular feature, may be mildly or markedly symptomatic, with a burning sensation and local crusting around the eye. Acute anterior uveitis is generally associated with pain and photophobia, and sometimes loss of visual acuity.

II. **ENTEROPATHIC ARTHROPATHY.** Arthritis following diarrhea may represent the rheumatic complication of either Crohn's disease or ulcerative colitis, and gastrointestinal endoscopy and radiology may be required to exclude this possibility. Arthritis may be the presenting manifestation of inflammatory bowel disease and may precede bowel complaints for some period of time.

III. **PSORIATIC ARTHRITIS.** The skin rashes of ReA are quite psoriasislike in appearance and indeed the histopathologic findings of psoriasis and keratoderma are similar. Skin rash that is coincident with arthritis may represent psoriatic arthritis rather than ReA; coexisting urethritis and conjunctivitis, or antecedent diarrhea, would favor a diagnosis of ReA. Pitting of the nails occurs in both conditions, but the nail dystrophy of psoriatic arthritis is generally more severe.

IV. **RHEUMATOID ARTHRITIS.** Development of a chronic polyarthritis may suggest rheumatoid arthritis, but the presence of asymmetry and sacroiliitis, as well as the absence of rheumatoid factor, would favor a diagnosis of ReA. The extra-articular features of rheumatoid arthritis are distinct from those of ReA.

V. **HUMAN IMMUNODEFICIENCY VIRUS (HIV) INFECTION.** There are indications from some series that ReA may occur with higher frequency and severity in patients with HIV infection. The frequency of this clinical overlap is not known. Patients in a high-risk category should be screened for HIV serology. In some patients, the episode of ReA occurs long before clinically overt acquired immune deficiency syndrome (AIDS). This is an important consideration when any immunosuppressive therapy is being considered.

 TREATMENT

I. **ANTIBIOTICS.** It is appropriate to institute appropriate antibiotic therapy if any culture results indicate a persisting infection (e.g., chlamydial urethritis). There has been no consensus on the degree to which antibiotics influence the course of ReA, with two controlled trials finding no benefit of ciprofloxacin or azithromycin. One recent follow-up study suggested that long-term outcome in HLA-B27$^+$ patients with ReA after both gastrointestinal and genitourinary infections might be favorably influenced by a 3-month course of ciprofloxacin, but larger studies will be needed to confirm this. Early treatment of *Chlamydia* genitourinary infection reduces the frequency of subsequent ReA and tetracycline compounds (e.g., lymecycline) may shorten the course of postchlamydial ReA. Antibiotic treatment of *Salmonella* infection may actually prolong the carrier state, a reality that could account for the prolongation of the inflammatory response to the organism.

II. **ARTHRITIS THERAPY**

A. **Anti-inflammatory drugs.** In general, nonsteroidal anti-inflammatory drugs (NSAIDs) form the basis of therapy for ReA. Indomethacin (50 mg three times daily) and diclofenac (50 mg three times daily) are generally well tolerated in the young patients who represent most of the affected patients. Results of a randomized controlled trial suggest that sulfasalazine is superior to placebo in improving the peripheral arthritis of ReA. It is used at a dose of 2 to 3 g/day, and the granulocyte count should be carefully monitored.

B. **Immunosuppressive therapy.** There has been limited, but favorable, experience with methotrexate (15 to 20 mg/week) and azathioprine (50 to 150 mg/day) in cases of chronic disease refractory to other measures. These agents are generally reserved for severe disease. Clinicians are more commonly using methotrexate or sulfasalazine when the response to NSAIDs is unsatisfactory.

C. **Steroid therapy.** Intra-articular steroid injections may be of benefit, but oral steroids are rarely indicated. Local steroid injection in the sacroiliac joint under fluoroscopic guidance has a role, particularly when this is the dominant symptomatic joint.

D. **Anti-tumor necrosis factor (anti-TNF) therapy.** For patients with refractory arthritis and enthesitis not responsive to NSAIDs, sulfasalazine or methotrexate, anti-TNF therapy is effective and safe. The concern about reactivating the triggering infection with such treatment appears to be only theoretical.

III. OCULAR DISEASE. Uveitis should be managed jointly by an ophthalmologist and a rheumatologist. Generally, local steroid drops will suffice, but oral steroids may be required in severe cases. Refractory uveitis can be the indication for intervention with anti-TNF therapy.

PROGNOSIS

In most patients, significant improvement with anti-inflammatory therapy occurs during a 3- to 4-month period. However, a 5-year follow-up study of patients with post-*Salmonella* ReA reported that two-thirds of the patients continued to have subjective complaints at this interval, and that more than a third demonstrated objective changes in the joints.

Long-term functional disability occurs in only a minority of patients. This variability in the clinical course should be mentioned in discussions with the patient.

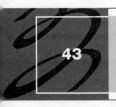

43	**GOUT**
	Theodore R. Fields

■ KEY POINTS

■ Making a crystal diagnosis of gout is always ideal, especially because of the possible need for lifelong therapy. Although "minor criteria" for gout exist, crystal identification is always preferred.

■ Underexcretion of uric acid is the main mechanism of gout, and many medications (such as aspirin and diuretics) worsen this; some medications (such as losartan and fenofibrate) improve the situation.

■ As the understanding of the natural process of ending a gout attack becomes better understood [e.g., related to transforming growth factor (TGF)-β1 production], improved therapies should follow.

■ Gout is especially problematic in patients with renal disease—caution is required with nonsteroidal anti-inflammatory agents, colchicine, and allopurinol; each case is individualized regarding decisions to decrease the dose or consider complete avoidance.

■ The prevalence of gout is increasing and becoming more difficult to treat because of multiple factors, including an aging population, obesity, increased renal disease, and transplantation.

■ Allopurinol has remarkably improved the life of patients with gout, but there are many patients with allopurinol allergy and renal or hepatic disease who are inappropriate or less-than-ideal candidates for this agent.

■ Options in patients with allopurinol allergy include oral or intravenous desensitization, uricosuric agents, and the experimental use of oxypurinol, febuxostat, or pegylated uricase.

■ Patients need clear education about gout and its four stages. Such education will likely improve the recently documented nearly universally poor allopurinol compliance.

*G*out is defined as an inflammatory arthritis caused by the deposition of uric acid crystals, which can also be associated with soft tissue urate deposits (tophi) and kidney stones. Gout often accompanies renal disease, hypertension, and coronary artery disease, but the causative role of uric acid in these conditions remains under active investigation. Modern treatment has remarkably reduced the suffering and complications of gout, but there are still many patients who need new agents for the management of this very painful and disabling disorder.

ETIOPATHOGENESIS

I. **Primary gout** (Table 43-1) is due to genetically determined hyperuricemia, which is caused by urate overproduction or underexcretion. Enzyme defects causing urate overproduction, in a small percentage of patients with gout, have been well worked out. Underexcretion, found in most cases, has recently been tracked to hereditary defects in renal anion transporters of uric acid.

II. **Secondary gout** (see Table 43-1) can be due to intake of medications that decrease urate excretion or cause renal insufficiency, increased purine intake in the diet, and treatments or conditions that lead to cell breakdown and consequent purine production. Uric acid is the end product of purine degradation.

III. **Uric acid crystals induce a classical inflammatory response** via an activation of the innate immune system. Toll-like receptors are involved in recognizing urate crystals; complement, including the membrane attack complex, is activated; neutrophils and then macrophages are recruited into the joint via chemotactic factors; and cytokines [e.g., tumor necrosis factor-α (TNF-α), interleukin (IL)-1, and IL-8] are secreted.

IV. **Gouty attacks are self-limited because of the nature of the immune system response to urate.** This is related to the fact that neutrophils eventually stop entering the joint, and as monocytes mature within the joint fluid, they have been found to produce fewer proinflammatory cytokines.

V. **URIC ACID, THE HEART, AND KIDNEY.** It is clear that hyperuricemia correlates with renal disease and atherosclerosis, but it remains unclear as to what extent, if any, hyperuricemia is directly causative of each. Urate level is routinely elevated in the metabolic syndrome (i.e., insulin resistance, hypertension, central obesity, dyslipidemia, and the proinflammatory and prothrombotic state), at least in part because of high insulin levels, which decrease urate excretion. It is presently unclear whether lowering urate levels in the metabolic syndrome will ameliorate any of the clinical features of this syndrome.

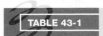 **Causes of Hyperuricemia**

Overproduction (10%)[a]	Underexcretion (90%)
Primary overproduction:	**Primary underexcretion:**
■ Hereditary enzyme defects:	■ Hereditary excretion defects:
–HGPRT deficiency	–URAT1 deficiency
–PRPP synthetase overactivity	
Secondary causes of overproduction:	**Secondary causes of underexcretion:**
■ Ethanol[b]	■ Renal insufficiency
■ Myeloproliferative disorders	■ Drugs and toxins
■ Cytotoxic chemotherapy	–Diuretics
■ Sickle cell anemia	–Ethanol[b]
	–Cyclosporine A
	–Pyrazinamide
	–Lead nephropathy
	–Low-dose aspirin[c]
	■ Ketosis

[a]Underexcretion is essentially universal in gout—present even in overproducers—but overproducers are the patients with hyperuricosuria and worth identifying.
[b]Ethanol both increases urate production and decreases its excretion.
[c]This increase in urate has recently been reported to be transient and of small magnitude.
HGPRT, hypoxanthine-guanine-phosphoribosyltransferase; PRPP, phosphoribosyl pyrophosphate; URAT1, urate transporter.

PREVALENCE

I. **The prevalence of gout is increasing, and there is a trend toward an earlier age of onset.** Gout is the most common inflammatory joint disease in men older than 40 years.
II. **Men continue to outnumber women** in the incidence of gout, but after menopause, women begin to close the gap, possibly related to the loss of the uricosuric effect of estrogen.
III. **Attacks of gout are becoming more severe and difficult to treat.** This likely relates to the aging of the population, with their comorbidities contraindicating many of our therapeutic options. Aging patients have a higher incidence of renal disease and renal failure, which worsens hyperuricemia and limits the use of many of our standard agents. In patients undergoing transplantation, cyclosporine can cause an especially aggressive form of gout, with rapidly forming tophi.

CLINICAL MANIFESTATIONS

I. **Four different stages** are recognized in the clinical evolution of gout.
   A. **Asymptomatic hyperuricemia.** Although no attacks of gout occur in this phase, urate deposits can develop in the joints, and in some patients, their 24-hour urinary urate excretion rate is high enough to increase the risk of kidney stones.
   B. **Acute gouty attacks.** In this stage, the patient develops painful, inflamed joints and almost always seeks treatment.
   C. **Intercritical gout** involves periods between attacks in a patient who has already had at least one attack.
   D. **Advanced and tophaceous gout** is a stage in which patients develop chronic abnormalities, such as chronic arthritis with superimposed flares, x-ray changes in joints, and tophi (visible nodular collections of uric acid) (Fig. 43-1).
II. **Attacks of gout** are generally of very rapid onset, often with systemic features, such as low-grade fever. After a first attack, the second may not occur for 5 to 10 years in some patients, but once the attacks begin to occur frequently, a pattern of closely spaced attacks is almost always established, and long-term spontaneous remission is rare. The classic attack of gout involves only a single joint, but as the disease evolves, it is not rare to see polyarticular attacks and involvement of contiguous joints.

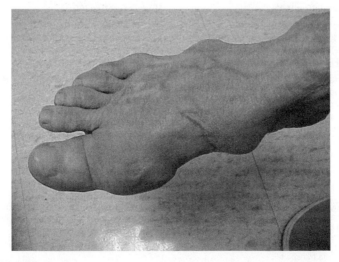

Figure 43-1. Gouty tophi.

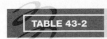

TABLE 43-2	Making the Diagnosis of Gout

One major criterion is sufficient:
- Urate crystals in a joint or a proven tophus

Presence of six of 12 minor criteria:
1. More than one attack of acute arthritis
2. Maximal inflammation developed within 1 d
3. Attack of monarticular arthritis
4. Joint redness observed
5. First metatarsophalangeal joint painful or swollen
6. Unilateral attack involving first metatarsophalangeal joint
7. Unilateral attack involving a tarsal joint
8. Suspected tophus
9. Hyperuricemia
10. Asymmetric swelling within a joint (radiograph)
11. Subcortical cysts without erosions (radiograph)
12. Negative culture result of joint fluid for microorganisms during an attack of joint inflammation

Adapted from Wallace SL, Robinson H, Masi AT, et al. Preliminary criteria for the classification of acute arthritis of primary gout. *Arthritis Rheum* 1977:20;895–900, with permission.

III. **Making the diagnosis of gout** includes clinical features, such as monarticular arthritis and rapid onset of inflammation, as well as laboratory and x-ray criteria (Table 43-2). The criteria described in Table 43-2 were developed to separate gout from rheumatoid arthritis, pseudogout, and septic arthritis and to assure diagnostic uniformity in the setting of epidemiologic studies. Note that they emphasize that it remains optimal to make a crystal diagnosis whenever possible.

IV. **Predisposing factors** to the development of a gout attack can include the immediate postoperative period after major surgery; an acute myocardial infarction or stroke; fasting; alcohol abuse; large intake of food with high purine content, such as red meat or shellfish; rapid weight reduction; and local infection of a joint. Not rarely, infected joints in patients with gout contain urate crystals that have been leached from the joint by the infection (i.e., strip mining) (so that finding gout crystals does not preclude concomitant infection).

 PHYSICAL EXAMINATION

I. **During an attack,** an involved joint is red, hot, swollen, extremely tender, and has significant pain on motion. The peak intensity is generally reached within 24 hours (see Table 43-2).

II. **The joint localization of gout** is characteristic. The first metatarsophalangeal joint is the most commonly affected, followed by the ankle, the olecranon bursa, and the knee. Elderly women, especially, have been noted to develop attacks in distal interphalangeal joints in the site of Heberden's nodes of osteoarthritis. Gout can also involve the wrist and midfoot.

III. **Tophi** (see Fig. 43-1) are firm nodules, which have a propensity to appear in the olecranon bursa, over the Achilles tendon, on the hands and in the finger pads. They may appear as whitish flakes on the external ear. They may exude a white pasty material spontaneously or upon needling.

 DIAGNOSTIC INVESTIGATIONS

To make the diagnosis of gout, laboratory features are as important as clinical features, particularly in the form of demonstrating urate crystals in the synovial fluid polymorphonuclear leukocytes.

I. LABORATORY TESTS

A. **Joint fluid or suspected tophus analysis for urate crystals** is critical to make the definitive diagnosis of gout (see Table 43-2) and is always advised whenever possible. Intra- and extracellular needle-shaped negatively birefringent crystals can be seen with a polarizing microscope or a polarizing attachment on a standard microscope. Urate crystals can often be seen even with ordinary light microscopy, although the birefringence cannot be determined.

Between attacks, asymptomatic joints have been found to have urate crystals. This demonstrates that factors in addition to the presence of crystals are needed for an attack and provides a way to make a diagnosis, when needed, between acute episodes.

B. **Other joint fluid studies** that are helpful are white blood cell (WBC) count (usually 5,000 to 50,000/mm^3 and largely neutrophils) and culture to rule out infection, which masquerades as or coexists with gout.

C. **Uric acid and other blood testing** are useful. Urate level can at times drop during an attack and should therefore be repeated after resolution of the attack. Complete blood count (CBC) can show an elevated WBC count during an attack, usually not higher than 15,000/mm^3. Blood chemistry can reveal secondary causes of gout, such as renal insufficiency.

D. **Urine testing** can detect microhematuria in a patient with gout and a kidney stone and protein in a patient with gout and underlying renal disease. Twenty-four–hour urine testing for uric acid and creatinine can detect overproduction of uric acid in a patient who is at risk for kidney stone, as well as for gout. However, 24-hour urinary urate excretion rate should not be tested during an acute attack, when it may transiently drop. Urate excretion rate has been shown to be variable over time but may be especially nonrepresentative during attacks.

II. IMAGING STUDIES

A. **X-rays,** early in the evolution of a patient's gout, usually show only soft tissue swelling. In case of recurrent or chronic disease, tophi and periarticular erosions with overhanging edges can be seen in the affected joints. As opposed to the periarticular bony thinning seen in rheumatoid arthritis, there is no local osteopenia in gouty lesions on the x-ray.

B. **Urate kidney stones** are radiolucent and are therefore invisible on the x-ray. Urate can also serve as a nidus for calcium phosphate stone formation, in which case the stones will be visible on the x-ray.

DIFFERENTIAL DIAGNOSIS

I. **The degree of inflammation** helps in separating gout from other types of arthritis, such as rheumatoid arthritis. The degree of erythema, heat, and pain in a gouty joint is generally matched only by that found in other crystal diseases—for example, pseudogout, or in very active infection. Fever and chills at onset also fit with crystal disease or infection but are quite unusual in other forms of arthritis. It is uncommon for gout attacks to be associated with body temperature more than 39°C or peripheral WBC count more than 15,000/mm^3.

II. **Podagra** (first metatarsophalangeal joint pain) is characteristic of gout but does have other causes. Pseudogout, hydroxyapatite crystal arthritis, reactive arthritis, psoriatic arthritis, and local infection are some of the pseudopodagra conditions to be considered.

III. **Polyarticular gout,** especially in later phases when arthritis becomes chronic, needs to be distinguished from rheumatoid arthritis, osteoarthritis, psoriatic arthritis, and reactive arthritis. Chronic gouty arthritis lacks the symmetry of rheumatoid arthritis, is more inflammatory than osteoarthritis, and often has associated tophi. Crystal identification is critical and definitive in cases that are difficult to diagnose.

IV. **Gout and rheumatoid arthritis** are reported to coexist less frequently than would be expected from their relative frequencies. This is of some statistical help in determining the etiology of a particular joint flare in a patient with rheumatoid arthritis—the likelihood of coexisting gout is less. Also, joint involvement in the shoulder and hip, common in rheumatoid arthritis, are very rare in gout.

V. **Tophi** must be distinguished from other nodular subcutaneous lesions. On pulling the skin over a tophus, one can commonly see the characteristic whitish color and very firm consistency, but aspiration and crystal identification are the ideal option in separating these from rheumatoid nodules.

VI. **Septic arthritis** must be considered at every attack of gout, in that the two conditions can coexist and their presentation can be similar. When there is any doubt, a culture **and** crystal analysis of the joint will resolve the issue of whether the condition is gout, infection, or a combination of the two. Joint infections can leach gouty crystals off the joint surfaces, and this type of "strip mining" can cause diagnostic problems.

 TREATMENT

I. **Patient education** is critical for successful management of gout. Patients must understand the four stages of gout and their implications to follow the stages of therapy. Dr. Robert Wortmann tells his patients that urate crystals are like matches, and allopurinol removes these crystals, whereas colchicine or indomethacin "makes them damp." This explanation can help patients understand why allopurinol is not for acute attacks and why colchicine will not protect against kidney stones or tophi.

II. **Evidence-based guidelines for gout management** focus on urate level lowering, behavioral modifications, and use of anti-inflammatory medications. Many current gout treatment strategies, however, remain "expert-driven" and "experience-driven" because of lack of adequately controlled published data. The recommendations in the subsequent text incorporate most of these guidelines.

III. **Asymptomatic hyperuricemia** is generally not treated. In very young patients, those with extremely high serum urate concentration, for example, greater than 12 mg/dL, or with a history of kidney stone, the 24-hour urinary urate excretion rate is tested. If the rate is greater than 800 mg/24 hour, allopurinol can be considered for reducing the urate production (and therefore excretion). Provocative recent data questions whether uric acid accelerates cardiovascular disease, but the present evidence is insufficient to justify the administration of allopurinol on this basis.

IV. **ACUTE ATTACK**

A. Treatment is usually satisfactory but requires careful assessment of **individual risk factors** in choosing therapy. Quick institution of therapy has been shown to lead to very rapidly diminished disease activity, whereas delayed therapy often results in a much slower resolution. For this reason, patients are advised to carry medication when they travel and to institute therapy immediately upon the onset of an attack.

B. For all patients, options for treatment of the acute attack include **joint rest and local ice** application. In patients without any contraindications, **nonsteroidal anti-inflammatory agents** such as naproxen (500 mg orally twice daily), indomethacin (50 mg orally three times daily), or ibuprofen (800 mg orally three times daily) are the drugs of choice. The risk profile of some patients best suits the use of **systemic corticosteroids;** for example, prednisone 40 mg the first day and then decreasing by 5 to 10 mg/day, depending on the rapidity of resolution of the attack.

C. **Adrenocorticotropic hormone (ACTH),** given parenterally, is effective and appears to work by binding melatonin receptor 3, in addition to stimulation of cortisol secretion.

D. **Local steroid injection,** when the attack is monarticular, is often an optimal solution (betamethasone is a reasonable choice because this short-acting depot preparation is efficacious in the treatment of gout, and no local reactions have been reported with this agent).

E. **Oral colchicine,** 0.6 mg orally once an hour until resolution of acute attack or until diarrhea develops, is an option that is presently only occasionally used. High-dose oral colchicine should not be given to patients who are already treated with colchicine as a prophylactic measure or to patients with renal or hepatic disease.

F. **Intravenous colchicine** is used rarely, and some avoid it completely. Doses start at 2 mg intravenous, then 0.5 mg every 8 hours to a total dose of 4 mg. This dose is halved or the drug is not used in patients with renal and hepatic dysfunction and is never used if the patient has low marrow reserve. Fatal marrow suppression, especially in patients with renal insufficiency, is the most serious complication. No oral colchicine is given for a week after an intravenous dose, and intravenous colchicine is avoided in patients already treated with colchicine as a prophylactic measure.

V. INTERCRITICAL GOUT (BETWEEN ATTACKS)

  A. **Diet** plays a role in that red meat and shellfish increase gout risk, vegetable protein does not increase gout risk, and dairy protein may be protective.

  B. **Weight loss** is advised to all patients with gout.

  C. **Alcohol** should be used in moderation. Moderate use of wine (e.g., two glasses a day) may be less of a risk than beer or hard alcohol.

  D. **Colchicine prophylaxis** can be used alone, without a urate-lowering agent, at 0.6 mg twice daily (once a day for patients older than 70 years). The dose is markedly reduced in patients with renal insufficiency and not used if the renal insufficiency is severe. Diarrhea can occur with low-dose colchicine, and creatine phosphokinase (CPK) should be followed up at 6-month intervals to detect a rare but serious neuromyopathy.

  E. **Urate-lowering treatment,** using allopurinol or probenecid, is indicated when patients have two attacks in the same year. If patients have kidney stones or tophi, allopurinol would be the drug of choice. The goal is to decrease serum urate level below 6 mg/dL, and in refractory patients it may need to be maintained below 5 mg/dL. Urate-lowering treatment is not started for 2 to 3 weeks after an acute attack.

  F. **Probenecid, the most commonly used uricosuric agent** (i.e., works by increasing urate excretion), is usually well tolerated.

    1. It can be used if the patient has no history of kidney stone, no tophi, normal creatinine clearance, and a 24-hour urinary uric acid excretion rate of less than 500 mg/24 hour.

    2. Generally reserved for patients younger than 50 years.

    3. Dosing starts at 250 mg twice daily and is gradually increased, following the 24-hour urinary urate to be sure that it does not exceed 800 mg during therapy. Dosage can increase to 500 mg twice or three times daily.

  G. **Other uricosuric agents,** which are in common use for other indications, have too mild an effect to be of much use in patients with gout but can be used as an adjunct in some cases. These drugs include losartan and fenofibrate.

  H. **Allopurinol** is the most commonly used agent to lower uric acid.

    1. As a xanthine oxidase inhibitor, allopurinol lowers both serum and urinary uric acid concentration. This effect of allopurinol explains its indication in patients with or at high risk for urate kidney stones.

    2. It is also the indicated agent for patients with tophi because the large urate shifts during treatment may increase the risk for renal stone formation.

    3. Allopurinol dosing starts at 100 mg/day, increasing toward 300 mg/day, and doses as high as 600 to 800 mg/day are needed on occasion.

    4. Allopurinol dosage in renal insufficiency must be individualized, and the usual goal of uric acid less than 6 mg/dL may not always be attainable. In some patients with renal insufficiency, the uric acid level is controlled with allopurinol at 100 mg every other day. Allopurinol is dialyzable and is given after dialysis treatments.

    5. Individualizing allopurinol dose in the patient with renal insufficiency requires considering the degree of renal insufficiency, the severity and frequency of gout attacks, the presence and size of tophi, and the presence of joint damage on the x-ray. Patients with mild cases of gout, who are at higher risk for complications from allopurinol, for example, patients with renal insufficiency, may be dosed less aggressively.

    6. Colchicine prophylaxis should be used during the first 6 months of allopurinol therapy to reduce the tendency of allopurinol to increase gout attacks early in therapy.

    7. Allopurinol drug interactions require a major decrease in azathioprine dose (by 50% to 75% or complete avoidance), a need to lower warfarin (Coumadin) dose in some patients, and an awareness that allopurinol increases the risk of ampicillin skin rash.

8. Allopurinol adverse effects include rash, hepatotoxicity, and a severe hyper-sensitivity reaction with vasculitis, and the risk of these effects is higher in pa-tients with renal insufficiency. Allopurinol is dialyzable and, therefore, is given after dialysis.

9. Compliance with allopurinol therapy has been shown to be poor. Patient educa-tion is critical. Patients especially need to know that allopurinol has a slow onset of action and that it may worsen gout early in therapy. They should not stop taking allopurinol if an acute attack develops.

10. Allopurinol desensitization, in patients with non-life–threatening allopurinol reactions, can permit a return to this therapy (Table 43-3).

11. Patients who cannot tolerate allopurinol, and need it, are currently in a very difficult situation. Options (see Table 43-3) are, at present, fairly lim-ited and imperfect, although new and exciting therapies are under active investigation.

I. **Urine alkalinization** is used to increase urate solubility and reduce kidney stone formation in patients with high urate excretion rate (alkalinization should be gen-erally given along with allopurinol). A urinary pH of at least 6 is aimed for using agents such as potassium citrate (20 mL four times daily). Patients with a history or a high risk of renal stone should drink at least 2 L of fluid a day.

J. **Investigational agents** in development provide hope for patients unable to take allopurinol (see Table 43-3). Febuxostat may allow us to treat patients with gout and allopurinol allergy and/or renal dysfunction. Uricase, an enzyme lacking in humans and apes, but present in almost all other animals, is a logical treatment consideration but as yet limited by issues of half-life and route of administration.

VI. **CHRONIC AND TOPHACEOUS GOUT**

A. **Allopurinol** is the preferred agent in patients with advanced, usually tophaceous gout, with chronic arthritis.

B. **Tophi** are at times very troublesome for patients and can break through the skin and cause infection. In cases where the tophi are too problematic to wait for

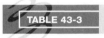

TABLE 43-3	Options in the Patient with Allergy or Intolerance of Allopurinol

Option	Comment
Oral desensitization	Works ~50% of the time, takes a month; this requires a cooperative pharmacist to make up the appropriate dilutions and a rheumatologist committed to very close communication with the patient
Intravenous desensitization	Needs close in-hospital, monitored observation by an allergist, rheumatologist, or intensivist; can be done in 12 h
Probenecid	Only for patients with normal renal function and with normal to low 24-h urinary urate excretion
Oxypurinol (investigational)	Active metabolic breakdown product of allopurinol, 50% allergic cross-reactivity, only for mild allergy.
Febuxostat (investigational)	Oral xanthine oxidase inhibitor; at least as effective as allopurinol with no cross-allergenicity; not renally cleared so can use in renal insufficiency
Pegylated uricase (investigational)	Parenteral: present formulation lasts ~1 mo; anaphylaxis can occur; only nonpegylated form presently approved, for perichemotherapeutic use

allopurinol to work, or where allopurinol is contraindicated, surgical tophus removal can be effective.
   C. Cyclosporine can cause a rapidly accelerating tophaceous gout. Allopurinol is generally required, with the caveats in **v.h.4** (under section Treatment) if renal insufficiency is present. On occasion, chronic gout arthritis in this setting is severe enough to require chronic low-dose prednisone.

PROGNOSIS

I.   The prognosis of properly managed gout is excellent. Chronic deforming arthritis and periarthritis can occur in longstanding untreated cases. Tophi, when untreated, can drain onto the skin or can lead to cellulitis and osteomyelitis.
II. Renal stones can result from chronically elevated uric acid excretion and can be complicated by pain, infection, and renal damage.
III. The direct cardiovascular toxicity of uric acid remains unclear. At this time, the data is not sufficiently compelling to justify treating hyperuricemia purely for this indication, but it does suggest an aggressive application of standard cardiac prophylactic principles (e.g., weight loss and lipid control) in patients with hyperuricemia.

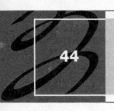

44

PSEUDOGOUT (CALCIUM PYROPHOSPHATE DIHYDRATE CRYSTAL ARTHROPATHY)
Theodore R. Fields

■ KEY POINTS

- Crystal analysis is the gold standard for the diagnosis of pseudogout and should be sought whenever possible; chondrocalcinosis on x-ray, by itself, does not diagnose pseudogout.

- Although most patients will not have metabolic secondary causes that can be identified, it is worth looking for these, especially checking serum calcium, magnesium, alkaline phosphatase, and iron saturation.

- Removal of calcium deposits from joints is not possible, but prophylaxis of recurring attacks of pseudogout, most commonly with colchicine, is often worthwhile.

- The coexistence of pseudogout and septic arthritis is not rare, and the infection may stimulate crystal shedding. Culture of the joint fluid must always be done, even when acute pseudogout has been documented.

- Consider pseudogout when the femoropatellar joint is more involved than the other two knee compartments on x-ray, or when osteoarthritis is especially severe or occurs in unusual locations, such as the elbow or metacarpophalangeal joints.

- When you are considering a diagnosis of gout, but inflammation is present in unusual locations, such as the shoulder or hip, consider pseudogout.

- When an elderly individual presents with a single acutely inflamed joint, always consider pseudogout.

seudogout is an inflammatory arthritis, with acute and chronic forms, caused by the deposition of calcium pyrophosphate dihydrate (CPPD) crystals within a joint. **Chondrocalcinosis,** calcified cartilage seen on radiographs, is found in most patients with pseudogout. The presence of CPPD crystals tends to be associated with more aggressive and destructive osteoarthritis.

ETIOPATHOGENESIS

I.   **Systemic conditions predisposing to pseudogout** include aging, hyperparathyroidism, hemochromatosis, hypophosphatasia (very rare), and hypomagnesemia. Pseudogout attack may follow parathyroidectomy, thought to be related to the flux in calcium level after the procedure.

II. **Local factors predisposing to pseudogout** include trauma, infection of the joint, osteoarthritis and other structural derangements of the joint, and the presence of urate crystals (gout and pseudogout may coexist). Injection of hyaluronic acid preparations for treatment of osteoarthritis has been reported to cause pseudogout attack, presumably by the same "strip-mining" effect wherein crystals within the cartilage are leached off due to a septic process.

III. **Local ion concentrations and inorganic pyrophosphate levels** help determine when joint calcification will occur. Calcium and iron levels play a role. When there is matrix supersaturation with inorganic pyrophosphate, it stimulates chondrocalcinosis, and the level rises with age.

IV. **CPPD crystals induce an inflammatory response** as the crystals re-shed into the joint and undergo phagocytosis by leukocytes. The chronic presence of CPPD crystals in a joint predisposes to joint damage and progressive osteoarthritis.

V.   **The genetics of pseudogout** include an autosomal dominant pattern that has been described in some populations in which disease begins in early adulthood, progresses rapidly, and is polyarticular. A mutation in the human ANK gene has been shown to lead to a leakage of inorganic pyrophosphate from the chondrocyte to the extracellular matrix, which can eventually lead to articular cartilage calcification.

PREVALENCE

Osteoarthritis and chondrocalcinosis are both common disorders, and their exact relation has not been fully established. Eight percent of individuals older than 60 years have radiographic evidence of chondrocalcinosis, although most are asymptomatic. The prevalence of chondrocalcinosis increases with age to involve as many as 28% of the population in the ninth decade.

CLINICAL MANIFESTATIONS

I.   **Four different stages** are recognized in the clinical evolution of CPPD and pseudogout.

   A. **Asymptomatic chondrocalcinosis** refers to the radiographic finding of calcified cartilage in patients, without joint complaints. It is very common in the eighth decade and later. Although no attacks of pseudogout occur in this phase, CPPD deposits in joints can lead to cartilage damage and acceleration of osteoarthritis.

   B. **Acute pseudogout.** In acute pseudogout, there are inflamed joints, often intensely painful. Acute monarthritis occurs in approximately 25% of patients with CPPD. Elderly women are afflicted more often than men. The knee is the most commonly involved joint. Ankle, wrist, and shoulder involvement is also common, and acromioclavicular pseudogout has been described. Attacks are usually self-limiting, lasting several days to several weeks. Surgical procedures, especially parathyroidectomy, and severe medical illness may precipitate acute pseudogout attacks.

   C. **Chronic pseudogout** can present as pseudo-osteoarthritis or pseudorheumatoid arthritis.

      1. **Pseudo-osteoarthritis** is the most common pattern of chronic CPPD arthropathy, and is distinguished from primary osteoarthritis by the pattern of involvement of the wrist and metacarpophalangeal joints, and by atypical knee osteoarthritis (Fig. 44-1). CPPD crystals are clearly associated with more severe osteoarthritis and have been found in 60% of knee joints at the time of knee replacement.

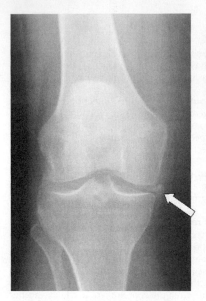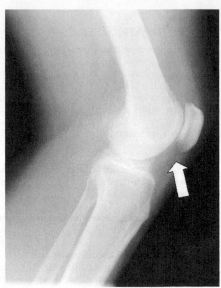

Figure 44-1. Pseudogout of the knee. Note calcification of the meniscus (*thin arrow*) and marked femoropatellar osteoarthritic changes and anterior calcification (*thick arrow*). (Courtesy of the Hospital for Special Surgery Radiology teaching file.)

     2. Pseudorheumatoid arthritis can present with chronic polyarticular inflammation occurring in up to 5% of patients with CPPD deposition. In some patients, prominent symptoms of fatigue, malaise, and morning stiffness may also develop, making the distinction from rheumatoid arthritis difficult.

    D. Pseudoneuropathic joints can result from the deposition of CPPD crystals in the presence of destructive arthropathy, as seen in Charcot joints. This is usually a chronic relapsing arthropathy with a female predominance of 14:1 and associated with tendon ruptures, especially at the shoulder joints.

II. **Making the diagnosis of pseudogout** (Table 44-1) involves the use of history, clinical examination, joint fluid analysis, and x-ray.

PHYSICAL EXAMINATION

I. **Articular features** include inflammatory signs of heat, swelling, and at times, erythema, especially in the knees, wrists, and ankles. The hips and shoulders may likewise have significant inflammation, but the swelling, heat, and erythema may be less obvious. Pain in these joints on motion will often be the major clue. Involvement of the small joints of the hands and feet is less common.

II. **Extra-articular features** include signs of other diseases associated with CPPD arthropathy. Skin pigmentation and the hepatomegaly of hemochromatosis, or the band keratopathy and muscle weakness of hyperparathyroidism may be clues.

DIAGNOSTIC INVESTIGATIONS

I. **Laboratory tests** are done to detect abnormalities in the blood and synovial fluid.

    A. Blood abnormalities reflect the findings in other diseases associated with the development of pseudogout. A reasonable workup in pseudogout includes calcium,

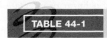

TABLE 44-1	Diagnosis of Pseudogout

Definite pseudogout:
Arthritis and presence of both the cardinal manifestations of pseudogout
   A. Crystals (weak-positive birefringence)
   B. Calcifications on x-ray of joint
Probable pseudogout:
Arthritis and presence of either A or B above
Possible pseudogout:
One of the following two criteria, if other characteristic features are present
   A. Acute arthritis, especially of the knees or other large joints
   B. Chronic arthritis especially of the knees, hips, wrists, elbows, shoulders, metacarpophalangeal joint especially if with acute exacerbations
Characteristic features of pseudogout:
   A. Unusual site for osteoarthritis (e.g., wrist, MCP joint, elbow, or shoulder)
   B. Severe femoropatellar narrowing on x-ray, especially if the rest of knee joint is not as severely involved
   C. Subchondral cyst formation
   D. Loose bodies within the joint or calcified tendons

MCP, metacarpophalangeal.
Modified from Ryan LM, McCarty DJ. In: McCarty DJ, ed. *Arthritis and Allied Conditions*. 10th ed. Philadelphia, PA: Lea & Febiger; 1985:1522, with permission.

uric acid, magnesium, iron saturation, and liver function tests. When indicated, other studies may include parathyroid hormone, and ferritin (Table 44-2).

   B. Synovial fluid examination is the definitive diagnostic study. The white blood cell count ranges from 3,000 to 50,000/mm^3 or more, with 70% or more neutrophils. No organisms are present on Gram stain, with negative cultures.

   C. Synovial fluid CPPD crystals can be identified with compensated polarized microscopy, and are rhomboid-shaped and exhibit weakly positive birefringence. These crystals can also be seen on light microscopy with use of alizarin red S stain. A study of how various laboratories handled specimens for crystal identification found that CPPD crystals were often missed by laboratories.

II. Radiologic studies (see Fig. 44-1) can demonstrate chondrocalcinosis in approximately 75% of patients with pseudogout. Fibrocartilaginous sites that are most likely to demonstrate chondrocalcinosis include the knee menisci, the symphysis pubis, and

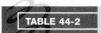

TABLE 44-2	Evaluation of Patients with Pseudogout

History:
Family history regarding hereditary chondrocalcinosis or hemochromatosis
Laboratory:
   A. Do **not** need to screen for diabetes mellitus or hypothyroidism on the basis of chondrocalcinosis alone
   B. Metabolic associations: hyperparathyroidism (most common), hypomagnesemia (rare), hypophosphatasia (rare), and hemochromatosis (almost always with other features first, e.g., liver function test abnormalities or diabetes mellitus)
   C. Reasonable to check: calcium, phosphate, albumin, alkaline phosphatase, magnesium, and iron saturation. If there is a history of acute arthritis, check uric acid looking for associated gout

the triangular cartilage of the wrist. Chondrocalcinosis appears as linear or punctate radiographic densities within cartilage. Subchondral bone cysts and hooklike osteophytes of metacarpophalangeal joints may also be observed. Osteoarthritic changes may be atypical, and include patellofemoral changes more prominent than medial or lateral compartment changes, as seen in Fig. 44-1.

DIFFERENTIAL DIAGNOSIS

I. **The degree of inflammation** helps in separating pseudogout from other types of arthritis, such as rheumatoid arthritis. The degree of erythema, heat, and pain in a joint with pseudogout is generally matched only by that in other diseases involving crystal deposition, for example, gout, or in active infection.

II. **Gout** is differentiated definitively from pseudogout only by joint fluid analysis, but many other clues can help. Involvement of the first metatarsophalangeal joint is very characteristic of gout, although occasionally seen in pseudogout and other disorders such as rheumatoid arthritis and psoriatic arthritis (so-called pseudopodagra). Shoulder or hip inflammation is extremely rare in gout, but often seen in pseudogout. Gout and pseudogout can coexist.

III. **Rheumatoid arthritis,** in the relatively unusual situation of chronic pseudogout presenting as a "pseudorheumatoid arthritis," can be difficult at times to differentiate from pseudogout. X-rays with chondrocalcinosis are helpful in identifying the condition, and the very rapid acceleration of inflammation in a particular joint also points toward pseudogout. Joint fluid analysis is definitive for diagnosis, although rheumatoid arthritis and pseudogout can coexist.

IV. **Septic arthritis** must be considered in every attack of pseudogout, because the two can coexist and their presentation can be quite similar. Infection can "strip-mine" pseudogout crystals from the cartilage into the joint fluid. When there is any doubt, a culture **and** crystal analysis of the joint fluid will resolve the issue of whether this is pseudogout, infection or both.

V. **Hydroxyapatite crystal deposition disease** may produce synovitis or tendinitis, and without crystal analysis, it may be hard to separate these symptoms from pseudogout. Hydroxyapatite crystals may be seen with electron microscopy, but not with routine polarizing microscopy. This disorder can be associated with shoulder calcifications seen on x-ray, and can be seen in patients on hemodialysis. Young women may develop first metatarsophalangeal joint inflammation due to hydroxyapatite crystals.

VI. **Osteoarthritis** needs to be differentiated from the osteoarthritis associated with pseudogout. Chondrocalcinosis may not always be visible on x-ray, so crystal identification is definitive. Features suggesting the presence of pseudogout include acute attacks, as well as atypical sites of severe osteoarthritis such as shoulders, elbows, wrists, and metacarpophalangeal joints. Subchondral bony collapse and tendon calcification are also clues to the diagnosis of pseudogout.

VII. **Single joint involvement** (monarthritis) is the most common pseudogout presentation. The causes of monarthritis are quite numerous, and include reactive arthritis, trauma, osteonecrosis, osteoarthritis, and pigmented villonodular synovitis, along with the conditions given earlier in section **II** to **V** of differential diagnosis. The approach to monarthritis is discussed in Chapter 14.

TREATMENT

I. **Treatment of the acute attack** of pseudogout is generally quite successful, but prophylactic treatment is less so. Unlike gout, the offending crystals cannot generally be removed. As with gout, the therapeutic approach depends on the stage of pseudogout in which the patient presents.

II. **Asymptomatic chondrocalcinosis** is not treated. Note that as many as 20% of elderly patients have chondrocalcinosis on x-ray, with no history of pseudogout.

III. **Acute attacks of pseudogout** are often approached through a combination of joint aspiration and drug therapy. This treatment is generally successful.

A. **Joint aspiration** alone removes a significant quantity of inciting crystals and chemical mediators, thereby allowing the synovitis to subside. In those with a protracted course, intra-articular injection of a long-acting corticosteroid preparation is usually beneficial. Single joint attacks can often be treated with aspiration and injection, without medication.

B. **Anti-inflammatory medication** can be effective, such as indomethacin (50 mg every 8 hours with tapering doses after every 5 days; a medication that may not be well-tolerated in the elderly) or naproxen 500 mg every 12 hours.

C. **Oral colchicine,** 0.6 mg every hour until resolution of acute attack, or until diarrhea develops. This is an option that is presently only occasionally used. High-dose oral colchicine should not be given to patients already on colchicine prophylaxis.

D. **Intravenous colchicine** is used rarely, and some avoid it completely. Doses start at 2 mg intravenous initially, then 0.5 mg every 8 hours to a total dose of 4 mg. This dose is halved or the drug avoided in patients with renal and hepatic dysfunction, and totally avoided if the patient has low marrow reserve. Fatal marrow suppression, especially in patients with renal insufficiency, is a most feared toxic side effect. No oral colchicine is given for a week after an intravenous dose, and intravenous colchicine is avoided in patients already on colchicine prophylaxis.

IV. **Chronic pseudogout** can be managed with anti-inflammatory medication and periodic intra-articular corticosteroid injections. Any associated diseases such as hemochromatosis and hyperparathyroidism should be managed appropriately, but treatment of the underlying disease may not prevent the recurrent attacks of arthritis, and does not remove the joint calcification.

A. **Colchicine prophylaxis** is not as effective as in gout, but worthwhile in many patients. There is evidence favoring long-term prophylaxis with oral colchicine (0.6 mg orally twice daily; once a day for patients older than 70 years) for patients with recurrent acute attacks.

B. **Chronic management of accelerated osteoarthritis** includes physical therapy, chronic analgesics, and, when indicated, joint replacement.

 PROGNOSIS

I. **Associated diseases,** such as hyperparathyroidism or hemochromatosis, even if treated adequately, often leave the patient with continuing episodes of pseudogout.

II. **Chronic joint damage** with accelerated osteoarthritis can result from pseudogout, and this may require joint replacement.

III. **Acute attacks** are usually well controlled with the present regimens, and some decrease in attack frequency and severity can often be attained with colchicine prophylaxis. Some patients fail prophylactic measures, and require recurrent acute therapy.

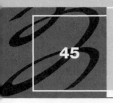

45 HUMAN IMMUNODEFICIENCY VIRUS
Edward Parrish

 INTRODUCTION

I. **A number of musculoskeletal complaints and inflammatory phenomena** develop in individuals infected with the human immunodeficiency virus (HIV). These patients are exposed to a vast array of pathogens and have marked degrees of immune dysregulation, cytokine production, cell growth abnormalities, and a propensity to anaplasia.

II. **Although a clear picture of the epidemiology of rheumatic disease is not available,** studies in small populations and anecdotal evidence suggest an increased occurrence of the manifestations listed in Table 45-1. Highly active antiretroviral therapy (HAART) has decreased the frequency in populations with access to these life-extending agents.

III. **Highly active antiretroviral therapy (HAART) has changed the natural history of HIV infection** and also modified the frequency and expression of some HIV-related musculoskeletal syndromes. In a study of 75 HIV positive patients who presented at one center with musculoskeletal symptoms, septic complications were the most common (41%) and the frequency of spondyloarthropathy was lower compared to the studies pre-HAART.

IV. **The immune reconstitution inflammatory syndrome (IRIS)** that occurs in 25% of patients treated with HAART may result in the aggravation of pre-existing conditions (i.e., sarcoidosis, SLE) or the development of new ones (i.e., Grave's disease, Sjögren's syndrome, reactive arthritis, or SLE).

V. **The general approach to the individual infected with HIV** and rheumatic complaints includes the same principles of sound medical practice as those for uninfected individuals.

VI. **Suspicion of infection or neoplasia** should be paramount. Many clinical phenomena are the direct result of these two underlying processes or will be unmasked by their presence. The clinical expression of infectious agents can be decidedly different in the immunosuppressed patient. Complicating factors include the following:
   A. High incidence of neuropathy, which may coexist with or mimic a number of rheumatic diseases.

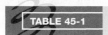 **Rheumatologic Manifestations in Human Immunodeficiency Virus (HIV)-infected Individuals**

Arthralgias	Vasculitis
Painful articular syndromes	Necrotizing
Osteonecrosis	Eosinophilic
Enthesopathy/periosteal syndromes	Leukocytoclastic
Hypertrophic osteoarthropathy	Angiitis of the central nervous system
Arthritis	**Sicca syndrome**
Reactive	Diffuse infiltrative lymphocytosis syndrome
Psoriatic	**Bone disorders**
HIV-associated arthropathy	Osteoporosis
Septic	Osteonecrosis
Myopathy	Osteomyelitis

HIV, Human immunodeficiency virus.

B. Drug regimens that are used to treat individuals infected with HIV may cause both rheumatic and neurologic complaints.

C. Use of illicit drugs that can lead to confounding signs and symptoms.

D. The extensive use of "alternative" pharmaceuticals, megavitamins, herbs, and "health foods" by individuals with HIV can complicate the clinical picture.

E. The frequency of autoantibodies is increased in this population, reflecting the presence of chronic infections, immune dysregulation, and the use of medication.

    1. Antinuclear antibodies, rheumatoid factor, antiplatelet antibodies, and direct antiglobulin (Coombs') antibodies can be seen in patients who are HIV positive; however, a few have clinical significance, including those associated with the development of anemia and thrombocytopenia. While antiphospholipid antibodies occur in 85% of individuals infected with HIV, they do not appear to be associated with as high a frequency of thrombotic events as in uninfected patients with the antiphospholipid syndrome.

    2. Patients with collagen vascular disease often have cross-reacting antibodies against constituents of the HIV or cells infected with HIV, which leads to false-positive results of assays for HIV antibodies.

MYOPATHY

I. ETIOPATHOGENESIS (Table 45-2)

A. HIV infects CD4+ T cells, macrophages, and dendritic cells, which are often found in the affected muscle. HIV also infects cardiac muscle and there is some evidence of direct skeletal myocyte infection.

B. The range of histologic findings in muscle from individuals infected with HIV is broad. Variable fiber fallout consistent with neuropathy is present in many. Others have features indistinguishable from those of idiopathic autoimmune polymyositis—that is, variation in fiber size, often with an inflammatory mononuclear cell infiltrate. Frank necrosis may be present and may be associated with polymorphonuclear cell infiltration. Nemaline rods may be present, usually without inflammation.

C. Red, ragged fibers, also seen in thyroid-associated myopathy, were found in patients treated with azidothymidine (AZT). The defect appears at the mitochondrial level. Other toxins may cause myocyte death or fiber contractility (see Table 45-2).

D. Pyomyositis, a disorder often caused by *Staphylococcus aureus* and previously limited to the tropics, is increased in the HIV population. Nonpyogenic infectious agents may infiltrate the muscle locally or diffusely.

E. Neoplastic infiltration, especially with lymphoma, is not uncommon.

II. PREVALENCE

A. Myopathy is likely the most common rheumatologic problem encountered, yet it is often overlooked because of its highly variable clinical expression.

B. Approximately 92% of patients with untreated HIV have histologic evidence of muscle disease. Of these, half show features of an inflammatory infiltrate similar to polymyositis and half are consistent with neuropathic myopathy.

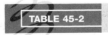	Contributing Factors to Myopathy in Human Immunodeficiency Virus (HIV) Infection		
Infection	**Metabolic**		**Drug/toxic**
HIV	Thyroid disorders		Alcohol
HTLV-I	Adrenal insufficiency		Cocaine
Hepatitis C			AZT
Pyomyositis			Sulfonamides
Mycobacteria			Penicillin
Microsporidia			Rifampin
Toxoplasma			Phenytoin

AZT, azidothymidine; HTLV-1, human T lymphotropic virus type 1; HIV, human immunodeficiency virus.

    C. Myalgia has been reported in 10% to 35% of patients. One study reported the incidence of muscle atrophy at 6%.

III. CLINICAL MANIFESTATIONS

    A. Most cases are silent and uncovered incidentally as transient increases in muscle enzymes. Typically, symptoms and findings will wax and wane with little persistent clinical consequence. Pain is often absent, although sometimes patients are "achy."

    B. Although usually proximal, as in idiopathic polymyositis, it can be distal, and in this distal form, is frequently confused with neuropathy. Indeed, superimposed neurogenic complaints and findings are common.

    C. For clinically significant disease to develop, additional insults such as intercurrent infection, drugs, or metabolic abnormalities contribute, as listed in Table 45-2.

    D. Atrophy may gradually develop in the muscle groups involved, with consequent motor weakness, leading to falls.

    E. HIV wasting illness, more prevalent in the pre-HAART era, may present as diffuse muscle atrophy and weakness. The cause is likely to be multifactorial.

IV. PHYSICAL EXAMINATION

    A. Inspection may reveal diffuse or localized atrophy.

    B. It must be determined if the patient is truly weak or if the apparent weakness is related to pain.

    C. Tenderness elicited by palpation or movement is more indicative of an inflammatory process, although hyperesthesia from a neuropathy can occur.

    D. Distal wasting or weakness is more likely in neuropathic and paraneoplastic disease.

    E. In HIV-wasting disease, there is diffuse atrophy of both muscle and adipose tissues.

    F. Fever likely indicates intercurrent infection or malignancy.

V. DIAGNOSTIC INVESTIGATION

    A. Electrolyte abnormalities. Weakness or frank myonecrosis can occur from alterations in potassium, phosphorus, calcium, or magnesium levels. Nutritional deficiencies may also lead to or exacerbate such findings.

    B. Thyroid function tests and cortisol levels are indicated to rule out endocrinologic etiologies of myopathy.

    C. Muscle enzymes. Creatine kinase (CK) and aldolase are the most sensitive indicators of muscle damage. In general, the CK level should be checked first and aldolase measured as needed if the CK level is not elevated and clinical suspicion remains high. In the face of intercurrent infection, trauma, fever, or use of cocaine or alcohol, the CK level may become dramatically elevated. Typically, after this insult to muscle tissue has been eliminated, CK will return to the normal range within a few days.

    D. Muscle biopsy should be considered whenever infection is suspected or when clinical deterioration continues in the face of therapy. Additionally, muscle biopsy should be considered before the patient is committed to long-term immunosuppressive medications.

    E. Ultrasonography and magnetic resonance imaging (MRI) have been shown to be particularly sensitive in the definition of inflammatory and infiltrative muscle disease. Radionuclide imaging with gallium or technetium pyrophosphate can be helpful.

VI. DIFFERENTIAL DIAGNOSIS

    A. Differentiation between neuropathic and non-neuropathic causes is important. They often coexist.

    B. Focus on the temporal relation between the onset of muscle disease and the introduction of new medications or other clinical changes is also important. If there is no obvious antecedent event and especially when the onset is abrupt, the presence of occult infection or malignancy should be suspected, whether fever is present or not.

    C. Recreational drug use is common in some individuals infected with HIV. A detailed history of medications and alternative medications may reveal possible toxins.

    D. Enthesopathy and periostitis, especially in the distal femur, may produce a confusing picture.

    E. Adrenal insufficiency is common in individuals infected with HIV. Although it does not cause muscle disease itself, one of the most common complaints of the steroid-deficient individual is myalgia.

F. Bursitis and arthritis, especially of the shoulder and pelvic girdle, can mimic muscle disease. Rarely, soft-tissue processes such as erythema nodosum or phlegmon may lead some to consider a localized infectious myositis.

VII. TREATMENT

A. Treatment is indicated for pain and weakness. Due to the waxing and waning nature of muscle disease in this population, the fortuitous finding of myopathy by laboratory criteria does not in itself require intervention. Asymptomatic CK elevations alone do not warrant treatment, and CK improvement is not used as the sole criterion for treatment efficacy.

B. Discontinuation of any offending agents, particularly alcohol, illicit drugs, and any medications that are not absolutely necessary is mandatory. Discontinuing AZT is helpful in resolving myopathy in only 50% of the cases in which it is suspected of being a factor. AZT-induced cardiomyopathy is the most serious complication of AZT therapy and warrants discontinuation of the drug.

C. Symptomatic relief of pain is often required, particularly when disuse leads to atrophy. Mild analgesics may be sufficient, or nonsteroidal anti-inflammatory drugs (NSAIDs) can help.

D. Physical and occupational therapy should be started early to prevent wasting and contractures.

E. Antiretroviral therapy (HAART) is indicated for those patients with HIV-related myositis who are not presently on a medication regimen.

F. Intravenous immunoglobulin works quickly and may be administered at necessary intervals, with months between treatments often being possible in some patients.

G. Corticosteroids. When the above measures have failed to improve the muscle disorder, steroid therapy at moderate doses produces dramatic results and is well tolerated. **Prednisone** (30 mg/day, tapered to 10 mg/day during a 10-day period) is satisfactory for most patients, switching to an alternate-day therapeutic schedule with further tapering, depending on the patient's tolerance. The toxicity of low-level steroid maintenance therapy for several months is not yet known. Within days, however, exacerbation of mucocutaneous candidiasis and reactivation of herpes simplex are common if the patient is not on prophylactic therapy.

H. Rarely cytotoxic therapy is indicated.

HUMAN IMMUNODEFICIENCY VIRUS-ASSOCIATED PAINFUL ARTICULAR SYNDROMES

I.   INTRODUCTION. The term HIV-associated painful articular syndromes was coined in the pre-HAART era to describe a group of patients with exceptional, localized joint pain of unknown cause, with a paucity of anatomic findings. It is convenient to distinguish them from HIV-associated arthropathy by the absence of joint effusions.

II. ETIOPATHOGENESIS. Little is known about the etiology of these syndromes, but recurrent ischemia may be an underlying factor. This idea is supported by the following evidence:

A. The acute form is most reminiscent of the musculoskeletal pain of a sickle cell crisis in its rapidity of onset and resolution, and in the poor correlation between the severity of complaints and the physical findings.

B. Necropsy specimens of knee synovium show effacement consistent with recurrent ischemic insults.

C. Osteonecrosis is increased in the individuals infected with HIV.

III. PREVALENCE. Although reports indicate arthralgias in over 50% of individuals infected with HIV, the prevalence of these specific painful articular syndromes is unknown.

IV. CLINICAL MANIFESTATIONS AND PHYSICAL EXAMINATION. One may discern two types on clinical grounds:

A. Acute painful articular syndrome is dramatic, typically with rapid onset of symmetric pain in the knees or ankles. The physical findings are unimpressive except that the patient may not be able to stand. The symptoms abate within 2 to 24 hours, although they may last for a few days. The recovery is with minimal residuum.

B. Subacute painful articular syndrome typically has a gradual onset over a few weeks. It too has a predilection for knees and ankles. Often, direct palpation of the area of complaint will elicit tenderness of muscle, tendons, and bone, suggesting myositis, enthesitis, or periostitis. Most cases gradually resolve in weeks or months. Some are progressive and lead to significant debility.

V. **DIFFERENTIAL DIAGNOSIS**
   A. The clinical presentations require differentiation from enthesopathy, periostitis, myositis, and neuropathy, although these may coexist.
   B. Classic patellofemoral syndrome should be obvious from the complaint and physical examination.
   C. Hypertrophic pulmonary osteoarthropathy (HPO) presents similarly in the distal long bones and is often associated with pulmonary infections or neoplasia.

VI. **DIAGNOSTIC INVESTIGATION**
   A. There are no diagnostic studies for these syndromes.
   B. Plain x-ray films consistent with patellofemoral disease should correlate with clinical findings and complaints.
   C. Scintigraphy and plain x-ray films are helpful with HPO and periostitis.

VII. **TREATMENT**
   A. In the **acute syndrome,** response to NSAIDs is poor, although the use of intramuscular ketorolac may hold promise. Alternatively, narcotic analgesia usually suffices until the episode abates.
   B. In the **subacute** variety, NSAIDs are variably helpful; usually indomethacin is required for sufficient control. At times, the level of disability is so severe that a trial of systemic steroid is warranted. Usually, this produces dramatic relief. Steroids often may be tapered rapidly and discontinued over 1 week.
   C. Treatment of intercurrent infection or malignancy may lead to resolution of the complaints.

HUMAN IMMUNODEFICIENCY VIRUS-ASSOCIATED ARTHROPATHY

I. **INTRODUCTION.** HIV-associated arthropathy resembles the subacute form of the painful articular syndrome, but a **joint effusion is present.**

II. **ETIOPATHOGENESIS.** Although the joint fluid is not inflammatory, synovial biopsy in these patients usually shows some degree of mononuclear and plasma cell infiltrate, which is usually mild and is seldom of the severity seen in other forms of inflammatory arthropathy. It is tempting to view this syndrome as part of a continuum of periarticular ischemia that produces the acute painful articular syndromes.

III. **CLINICAL PRESENTATION AND PHYSICAL EXAMINATION**
   A. **Symptoms develop during a period of weeks and abate, usually within a month.** The pain may be quite severe. There is a predilection for the lower extremities often with bilateral knee or ankle swelling and direct distal long bone tenderness. It is prudent to exclude intercurrent infection, especially of a pulmonary source, in these patients.
   B. **There are usually no findings consistent with a spondylarthropathy.**

IV. **DIFFERENTIAL DIAGNOSIS.** It is important to distinguish this syndrome from classic presentations of infectious or reactive arthritis, spondyloarthropathy, HPO, or crystalline disease, as well as from less common causes of inflammatory arthropathy.

V. **DIAGNOSTIC INVESTIGATION**
   A. **The joint fluid is typically not inflammatory ($<10^3$ cells/mL).**
   B. **Periosteal reaction** may be found on radiographs, and these patients may have hypertrophic osteoarthropathy. Chest x-ray may reveal pathology.
   C. **Human leukocyte antigen (HLA)-B27 is not increased in this population.**

VI. **TREATMENT. The patient may respond dramatically to intra-articular steroids.** It is important to treat intercurrent pulmonary disease.

HUMAN IMMUNODEFICIENCY VIRUS-RELATED REACTIVE ARTHRITIS, PSORIATIC ARTHRITIS, AND SPONDYLOARTHROPATHY

I. **INTRODUCTION.** These disorders appear to be increased in both frequency and severity in patients with HIV. HIV-related–immune dysfunction has an impact upon the disease presentation and its treatment.

II. **ETIOPATHOGENESIS AND PREVALENCE**

   A. The increased incidence of these disorders is thought to be related either to a direct effect of the HIV on the immune system or on the basis of exposure to the same pathogens (*Chlamydia* and enteric pathogens) known to elicit reactive arthritis in individuals who are not infected with HIV.

   B. Evidence that gonococcal and chlamydial products may persist in joint fluids in individuals with non-HIV arthritis suggests that inadequate therapy or other host factors lead to incomplete eradication. It is unclear whether HIV infection is associated with persistence of these agents or their products.

   C. While no excess of HLAs associated with classic psoriasis has been found in individuals with HIV, spondyloarthropathy-related HLA-B27 appears increased.

III. **CLINICAL PRESENTATION AND PHYSICAL EXAMINATION**

   A. **Joint findings range from frank synovitis to enthesitis and axial skeletal involvement.**

   B. **Extra-articular manifestations** include dermal (psoriasiform, keratoderma blennorrhagicum, and circinate balanitis), ocular (conjunctivitis and uveitis), mucosal (palatine and buccal ulcerations), genital (urethritis, cervicitis, and prostatitis), and intestinal involvement. Any combination of findings may coexist.

   C. **Infection** with an array of enteric pathogens is common in HIV disease. Chronic or recurrent diarrhea is virtually the norm in advanced non-HAART treated patients and the causes are legion.

   D. The high incidence of **sexually transmitted diseases** in the individuals infected with HIV is mirrored in the increased frequency of gonococcal and chlamydial infection.

   E. **Psoriasiform lesions are increased** in both frequency and severity in individuals infected with HIV. These include the vulgaris, pustular, and erythroderma forms.

IV. **TREATMENT**

   A. **NSAIDs** are often sufficient to control both joint and extra-articular manifestations of the disease. Long-term use is usually required. Many cases will respond only to indomethacin.

   B. **Sulfasalazine** has been shown to be helpful in achieving disease control in patients unresponsive to NSAID therapy alone. Dosages of 1 to 2 g/day are often adequate. **Dapsone** has been used with success as well.

   C. **Etretinate** was incidentally found to relieve joint symptoms in patients with psoriasis. It appears to be helpful in those without overt skin disease but with enthesopathy. The use of etretinate must be weighed against possible hepatic and hematologic toxicity.

   D. **Antibiotics** help eradicate gonococci and *Chlamydia*. Long-term treatment with tetracycline derivatives in the form of doxycycline may help, perhaps due to their anti-inflammatory properties.

   E. **Immunosuppressive, cytotoxic, and biologic therapies.** Reports of the onset of acquired immunodeficiency syndrome (AIDS), opportunistic infection, Kaposi's sarcoma, and death in some patients soon after the use of methotrexate or azathioprine for the treatment of arthritis has led to the widespread notion that these agents are contraindicated in patients infected with HIV. With the advent of HAART, many have tolerated these medications. Prudence would require, however, that other less immune-suppressing treatments be used initially, and if found to be ineffective, a course of therapy with either methotrexate or azathioprine is undertaken. There have been numerous anecdotes of anti-tumor necrosis factor (anti-TNF) biologics in patients resistant to the above measures. Most patients have responded, and long-term complications are unknown.

SICCA SYNDROME AND DIFFUSE INFILTRATIVE LYMPHOCYTOSIS SYNDROME

I. **INTRODUCTION. Xerostomia and xerophthalmia** are common in patients infected with HIV and impact their health by decreasing caloric intake.

II. **ETIOPATHOGENESIS. CD8+ lymphocytes, rather than the CD4+ cells of classic autoimmune Sjögren's syndrome, infiltrate the parotids and lacrimal glands.** There is a notable absence of the autoantibodies (anti-Ro and anti-La) classically found in the idiopathic syndrome. A subset of patients manifest far more extensive visceral involvement by CD8+ lymphocytes, especially of the lungs, gastrointestinal system, and central nervous system. This visceral involvement has been designated diffuse infiltrative lymphocytosis syndrome (DILS).

III. **CLINICAL MANIFESTATIONS AND PHYSICAL EXAMINATION**
   A. **Decreased tearing and saliva are most common.** Patients may develop associated corneal abrasion due to dryness. Swallowing is difficult without copious fluid.
   B. **Parotid and submandibular gland enlargement may occur,** sometimes dramatically. This condition is usually nontender.
   C. **CNS involvement** may present as photophobia.

IV. **DIAGNOSTIC INVESTIGATION**
   A. **Serum transaminases** may be elevated in DILS with hepatic involvement.
   B. **Biopsy** of affected glands should reveal CD8+ lymphocytic infiltrate and will help distinguish from lymphomatous invasion.
   C. **Lumbar puncture** would be indicated if there is suspicion of CNS involvement.

V. **DIFFERENTIAL DIAGNOSIS**
   A. Other causes of Sicca symptoms include medications and infection (e.g., *Candida*).
   B. The possibility of lymphoma is the most common concern. The lymphoma is characteristically a B-cell lymphoma, similar to that seen in the autoimmune Sjögren's syndrome and in HIV in general.

VI. **TREATMENT**
   A. Avoidance of medications that exacerbate xerostomia and xerophthalmia is important. In particular, substitution for, or elimination of antihistamines, decongestants, NSAIDs, antihypertensives, tricyclic antidepressants, and other anticholinergic agents must be sought.
   B. Lubricant oral sprays may help.
   C. Aggressive treatment of candidiasis is important.
   D. Use of topical methylcellulose lacrimal substitutes will often prevent corneal abrasion.

 VASCULITIS

I. Vasculitides of various types have been documented in patients with HIV. The presence of necrotizing vasculitides such as polyarteritis nodosa is often a harbinger of rapid demise. Leukocytoclastic angiitis and eosinophilic vasculitides of small and medium vessels are seen more frequently. Isolated angiitis of the central nervous system may play a role in the development of stroke or dementia in these patients (see Chapter 37).

II. Hepatitis B and C viruses are implicated in the development of necrotizing and cryoglobulinemic vasculitides, respectively. Modalities directed at control of viral replication in both these entities have led to disappointing results to date in the patient infected with HIV.

 BONE DISEASE

I. **Osteoporosis** is increased in individuals infected with HIV. Alendronate has demonstrated therapeutic benefit.

II. **Osteonecrosis** is increased in the individuals infected with HIV beyond what could be explained by the use of steroids or other predisposing agents.

III. **Osteomyelitis** is increased in the individuals infected with HIV with advanced disease, consistent with immunosuppression.

 ADDITIONAL OBSERVATIONS

I. **Cytomegalovirus** produces a vasculitis by direct infection and necrosis of the vascular endothelium and may mimic noninfectious vasculitis.

II. **Endocarditis** is well known for its array of immune clinical syndromes, including arthritis, leukocytoclastic vasculitis, stroke, and glomerulonephritis. In patients using intravenous drugs, endocarditis remains a common cause of morbidity and mortality.

III. **Syphilis** continues to live up to its "accolade" as the great imitator. In the presence of HIV, reactivation of the syphilitic infection can occur and the clinical presentation may be quite atypical. The secondary stage of syphilis may have an associated arthropathy.

IV. **Interferon-α,** used in the treatment of Kaposi's sarcoma, appears to predispose the patient to autoimmune disease and serologic phenomena, particularly thyroid abnormalities.

V. **Primary B-cell lymphoma** often takes atypical forms in patients with HIV infection. In particular, destructive bony or joint lesions often mimic infectious or inflammatory lesions. Localized infiltration of muscle may cause a mass lesion, pain, or weakness.

VI. **Erythema nodosum** may be confused with a phlegmon, infiltrative mass lesions, or arthritis, depending on its location and appearance. Postinfectious, intercurrent mycobacterial, or paraneoplastic stimuli for erythema nodosum are common in the individuals infected with HIV. Lipodystrophy syndromes associated with the use of HAART can give the appearance of muscle wasting as well as of acute panniculitis.

VII. **Mycobacteria, tuberculous and atypical forms,** may cause joint infection by direct extension or hematogenous spread. Atypical forms may be isolated from blood or joint fluid. Tubercle bacilli are somewhat more difficult to isolate; if their presence is strongly suspected, synovial membrane biopsy with culture, histologic assessment, and polymerase chain reaction (PCR) may be required. Unlike the clinical picture in individuals not infected with HIV, osteomyelitis caused by atypical mycobacteria may lead to rapid destruction of bone.

INFECTIOUS ARTHRITIS
Barry D. Brause and Juliet Aizer

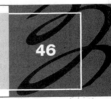 46

■ KEY POINTS

■ Septic arthritis should be diagnosed and appropriately treated with urgency to reduce the risk of permanent loss of joint function.

■ The microbial etiology of septic arthritis is not predictable; therefore, cultures of synovial fluid and any appropriate extra-articular site should be obtained before starting antibiotic therapy.

■ Septic arthritis of the hip joint (or any other joint which cannot be drained effectively by percutaneous aspiration) should be treated with surgical drainage as soon as possible.

■ When evaluating patients with acute polyarticular arthritis, bacteremic or viremic etiologies should be considered.

■ When evaluating patients with acute synovitis and negative routine bacterial cultures, (a) possible interference with cultures from prior antibiotic therapy, (b) the presence of a fastidious microorganism [including *Borrelia* (Lyme disease), anaerobic bacteria, viruses, mycobacteria, and fungi], or (c) a noninfectious etiology, should be considered.

■ Septic bursitis is associated with pain only on extreme flexion or extreme extension, as opposed to septic arthritis in which pain is elicited even with small degrees of joint motion.

I **nfectious arthritis (septic arthritis or pyogenic arthritis) represents the invasion of articular synovium by any microorganism.** The clinical presentation, course, and prognosis in patients with septic arthritis are determined by the interaction of specific pathogens and host inflammatory responses with the involved synovial tissue, cartilage, and bone. **Early recognition of the pathologic process,** along with timely, appropriate medical and surgical intervention, can neutralize potentially disabling tissue destruction and can provide a favorable functional outcome.

ETIOPATHOGENESIS

I. **ROUTES OF INFECTION.** The pathogen arrives at the synovium by one of three routes of infection: hematogenous seeding, contiguous extension from sepsis in adjacent tissue, and direct introduction.

   A. Hematogenous seeding. Infections of the skin and soft tissues, genitourinary tract, respiratory tract, and gastrointestinal tract can spread to the synovial membrane through the bloodstream.

   B. Contiguous spread. Local septic processes in tissue contiguous to the joint, such as cellulitis, infected skin ulcerations, paronychia, infected synovial cysts, and osteomyelitis, can invade synovial membranes by direct extension.

   C. Direct introduction. Microorganisms can be introduced into articular tissue by traumatic injury, arthrocentesis, intra-articular injections, and orthopedic surgery.

II. **ESTABLISHMENT OF INFECTION AND JOINT DAMAGE.** Invasion of the synovial membrane by microorganisms is the initial event in all pyogenic arthritides involving native (nonprosthetic) articulations. Subsequently, the infection extends into the joint space, where a paucity of phagocytes, antibodies, and complement permits a closed-space infection to be established. As the pathologic process continues, the avascular cartilage is degraded by bacterial and leukocyte enzymes.

   A. The infection progresses at a rate determined by the virulence of the pathogen, the nature and extent of the inflammatory reaction, and the vulnerability of the underlying host tissue. Polymorphonuclear leukocytes, recruited by microbial chemotactic factors, appear to be essential for tissue destruction. Inflamed hypertrophic synovium becomes an aggressive form of granulation tissue (pannus), which expands throughout the entire articulation.

   B. Irreversible loss of joint function is related to the extent of cartilaginous dissolution, which may occur over a very short period, and to the subsequent overgrowth of adjacent osseous tissue in the form of secondary osteoarthritis.

III. **MICROBIOLOGY.** *Staphylococcus aureus* is the most frequent cause of septic arthritis, responsible for up to 65% of infections, particularly in patients with rheumatoid arthritis, diabetes mellitus, or intravenous drug use. Streptococci are isolated in 20% to 30% of cases, often associated with autoimmune diseases, chronic skin infections, and trauma. Gram-negative bacilli are seen in 5% to 20% of patients, including neonates, aging adults, intravenous drug users, and immunocompromised hosts.

   A. *Haemophilus influenzae* had been the cause of 30% to 60% of septic joints in children younger than 2 years but is now rarely seen because of the magnificent effect of *H. influenzae* type b vaccination.

   B. Gonococci had earlier accounted for 75% of bacterial joint infections in patients older than 15 years but now accounts for less than 5% as a result of the increased use of safer sex techniques and the marked decrease in the incidence of mucosal gonorrhea.

   C. Coagulase-negative staphylococci are the most common cause of prosthetic joint sepsis, but they do not have a major role in native joint infections.

PREVALENCE

I. **Patients are generally prone to joint infections because of either local factors at their articulations or systemic factors that increase the risk of bacteremia.** Therefore, while the annual incidence of septic arthritis is two to five cases/100,000 in the general population, the annual incidence is 28 to 38/100,000 among patients with rheumatoid arthritis.

II. **Predisposing factors, often occurring together,** include the following (approximate frequencies given in parentheses):
    A. Extra-articular infection (25% to 50%).
    B. Previous damage to joint (27%), resulting from rheumatoid arthritis, osteoarthritis, crystal-induced arthritis, psoriatic arthritis, systemic lupus erythematosus, neuropathic arthropathy, trauma, or surgery.
    C. Serious underlying chronic illness (19%), usually associated with immunologic defenses, including malignancy, diabetes mellitus, hepatic cirrhosis, renal disease, and parenteral drug abuse.
    D. Immunosuppressive or corticosteroid therapy (50%).

CLINICAL MANIFESTATIONS

I. **ARTICULAR**
    A. **Synovitis.** The acute onset of joint pain is the most characteristic symptom, with increasing severity on flexion, extension, or weight-bearing (joint pain is subacute or chronic in fungal and mycobacterial infection; see specific entities and problems discussed later in this chapter). Articular pain is induced by even minimal degrees of joint motion. Arthralgia produced only by extreme flexion or extreme extension is suggestive of periarticular inflammation, as seen in septic bursitis. Local soft tissue swelling, tenderness, erythema, and warmth accompany a restricted range of motion in the involved articulation. Synovial effusions are present in 90% of cases.
    B. **Distribution of the joint involvement.** Bacterial arthritis usually affects only one joint; however, polyarticular infection is seen in 10% of patients and frequently reflects bacteremia or viremia. Knees and hips are the most commonly infected joints, but septic arthritis in parenteral drug abusers often affects the sternoclavicular, sacroiliac, or shoulder articulations. Sepsis within the hip joint can be difficult to diagnose because focal symptoms may be minimal and effusions difficult to demonstrate.

II. **EXTRA-ARTICULAR**
    A. **Systemic.** Fever is an almost constant feature of pyarthrosis (90% of cases). Systemic sepsis with septic shock can occur with particularly virulent pathogens in vulnerable patients.
    B. **Dermatitis-arthritis syndromes.** Certain pyarthroses are accompanied by dermatologic manifestations, along with articular involvement. This presentation is most commonly recognized with *Neisseria gonorrhoeae* and *H. influenzae.*
        1. Gonococcal arthritis is often associated with prodromal or concomitant tenosynovitis and erythematous papular, vesiculopustular, or petechial skin rashes characteristic of the disseminated stage of gonococcemia.
        2. *H. influenzae* pyarthrosis can be associated with tenosynovitis and erysipeloid, pustular, or petechial rashes. Similar presentations have been described for bacterial arthritis associated with *Neisseria meningitidis* and *Streptobacillus moniliformis* (rat bite fever).
        3. The pathognomonic appearance of erythema chronicum migrans can be essential for the diagnosis of early *Borrelia burgdorferi* arthritis [Lyme disease (see Chapter 47)].
        4. Exanthems are important features in the presentation of viral arthritis associated with rubella (infection or vaccination), acute hepatitis B, and parvovirus B19.
    C. **Tenosynovitis** manifesting as tenderness, erythema, and slight swelling at periarticular tendons can be seen in infectious arthritis due to gonococcus, *H. influenzae,* atypical mycobacteria, and sporotrichosis.

DIAGNOSTIC INVESTIGATIONS

I.   LABORATORY TESTS

A. **The peripheral blood white blood cell (WBC) count** is normal in 30% of patients.

B. All possible foci of infection (sputum, urine, skin lesions, oropharynx, urethra, uterine cervix, and rectum) should be cultured, and at least two blood cultures should be obtained. Specific culture media for gonococci (Thayer-Martin or chocolate agars) should be employed in addition to aerobic and anaerobic media for specimens from mucosal surfaces and skin lesions. Nucleic acid amplification or hybridization tests can be used on endocervical or intraurethral swab specimens as alternatives to gonococcal cultures. In 49% of cases, the same organism is cultured from an extra-articular site and the joint.

II. IMAGING STUDIES

A. **Radiograph** of the joint should be obtained to document the extent of previous damage, observe for evidence of osteomyelitis, and provide a baseline for follow-up studies.

1. The earliest radiographic sign of joint infection is periarticular soft tissue swelling, with displacement of the adjacent fat pads by synovial edema or an articular effusion during the first week of pyarthrosis. After this period, periarticular osteopenia (subchondral bone rarefaction) develops because of local hyperemia and proinflammatory cytokines in addition to bone atrophy secondary to relative immobility.

2. With more fulminant infection, uniform joint space narrowing becomes visible by radiography because of articular cartilage dissolution.

3. Subsequently, osseous erosions, induced by pannus, can be seen in subchondral sites or in peripheral areas between the joint capsule insertion and the joint cartilage, where the synovium is in direct contact with bone.

4. Eventually, fibrous or bony ankylosis may develop in chronic infections. Radiologic evaluation of the infected joint is helpful but not diagnostic because these anatomic changes are not specific for septic processes.

B. **Radioisotope bone scans** may be of value in diagnostic problems involving deep-seated joints such as hip, shoulder, or spine. However, the findings are not specific, and the scan usually has little role in the initial evaluation of acute infectious arthritis.

C. **Ultrasonography** can be of value by identifying and monitoring small and deep joint effusions, providing needle guidance for difficult arthrocenteses, and evaluating periarticular tissues.

III. ARTHROCENTESIS. Aspiration of synovial fluid is mandatory for any joint inflammation in which infection is a possibility. Initial aspiration is by closed-needle technique, with a needle large enough (16- to 18-gauge) to permit recovery of thick, purulent material (see Chapter 8). Hip joint sepsis represents an exception to this approach. In this situation, a radiographically guided aspiration may be more appropriate, and assessment should include an orthopedic surgical evaluation because arthroscopic or open surgical drainage may be necessary. Synovial fluid analysis is the basis for initiating therapy and for confirming the specific microbiologic diagnosis (Table 46-1). The following studies are ranked in order of importance; if the size of the synovial fluid sample is small, culture and Gram stain receive priority.

A. **Culture.** Optimally, fluid should be inoculated onto media promptly at the bedside, or the sample should be promptly delivered to the laboratory for immediate incubation. Media selection is defined by the clinical picture and should be focused on gram-positive and gram-negative aerobes (blood agar and MacConkey's agar), *Neisseria gonorrhoeae* and *H. influenzae* (chocolate agar or Thayer-Martin agar), anaerobes (thioglycolate broth), and, if indicated, fungi and mycobacteria.

Cultures of synovial fluid confirm the presence of specific etiologic microorganisms in all bacterial arthritides, except in gonococcal infection, in which only 50% positivity is found, and the diagnosis is then made on the basis of urethral, cervical, pharyngeal, and rectal cultures or on the basis of the presence of tenosynovitis and the characteristic skin lesions of disseminated gonococcemia.

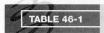

TABLE 46-1	Synovial Fluid Analysis		
	Normal	**Inflammation**	**Bacterial infection**
Color	Colorless, pale yellow	Yellow	Yellow
Turbidity	Slight	Turbid	Turbid, purulent
Leukocyte count	<1,000	1,000 to 25,000	10,000 to >100,000
Cell type	Mononuclear	Neutrophils	Neutrophils
Synovial fluid/blood glucose	0.8–1.0	0.5–0.8	<0.5
Gram stain	Negative	Negative	Positive (in 65% of cases)
Culture	Negative	Negative	Positive

Culture results may remain negative in 10% to 20% of cases of infectious arthritis. In cases in which the culture results are negative, it is important to consider the following: possible use of antibiotics before taking cultures, infectious arthritis due to organisms that do not grow on routine media (anaerobes, *Borrelia*, viruses, fungi, and mycobacteria), and noninfectious etiologies (see section Differential Diagnosis).

B. Gram stain. Pending the results of cultures, the Gram stain is the cornerstone of initial antibiotic selection (see Table 46-1). However, it may be positive in only 65% of cases in which cultures will eventually be positive.

C. Cell count and differential count. Synovial fluid leukocytosis with predominance of neutrophils is common, but the range of WBC counts is wide (6,800 to 250,000/mm^3 cells). The probability of infection increases with higher WBC counts; 40% of patients with bacterial arthritis have synovial fluid WBC counts greater than 100,000/mm^3, whereas patients with rheumatoid arthritis and crystal-induced arthritis rarely produce these counts. (Note: Gout and pseudogout crystals may be found in the synovial fluids of patients with septic arthritis, a finding thought to be related to the "strip mining" effects of infection upon pre-existing crystals lodged throughout the joint.)

D. Synovial fluid glucose. In septic joints, the synovial fluid glucose level is usually less than 50% of the simultaneous serum glucose levels; however, this relation holds only for fasting specimens because postprandial blood glucose may not equilibrate promptly with the synovial fluid glucose level. The synovial fluid glucose level is reduced in only 50% of infected patients, and reductions can be seen in uninfected, inflamed joints in patients with rheumatoid arthritis.

 DIFFERENTIAL DIAGNOSIS

A list of diseases that should be considered in the differential diagnosis is as follows: crystal-induced arthritis, reactive arthritis, acute flare of a noninfectious inflammatory arthritis (rheumatoid arthritis, psoriatic arthritis, inflammatory osteoarthritis, and other connective tissue diseases), traumatic arthritis, rheumatic fever, subacute bacterial endocarditis, and periarticular inflammation with or without infection (including septic bursitis).

 TREATMENT

I.   INITIAL TREATMENT

A. Antibiotic therapy, empirically based on Gram stain results, is summarized in Table 46-2. Administration should be initiated promptly and parenterally to ensure reliable serum levels. Most antimicrobial agents achieve effective synovial fluid levels with parenteral dosing; therefore, an intra-articular instillation or irrigation is not indicated and may be hazardous. Antibiotics injected directly into the joint

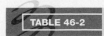

TABLE 46-2	Initial Antibiotic Therapy for Pyogenic Arthritis, Based on Gram Stain of Synovial Fluid	
Gram stain finding	**Initial antibiotic therapy**	**Alternative antibiotic therapy**
Gram-positive cocci	Nafcillin[a]	Vancomycin
Gram-negative cocci	Ceftriaxone, cefotaxime, or ceftizoxime[b]	Spectinomycin[b] or ciprofloxacin (additional coverage needed if *Neisseria meningitidis* suspected)
Gram-negative bacilli	Gentamicin	Ceftazidime[c]
Septic clinical picture—no organism seen	Ampicillin/sulbactam[a] plus gentamicin	Vancomycin plus ceftizoxime[a]

[a]Vancomycin should be used if methicillin-resistant *Staphylococcus aureus* is prevalent.
[b]Ceftizoxime and spectinomycin should not be used if *Neisseria meningitidis* is a possible pathogen.
[c]Gentamicin should be used if patient is a compromised host (e.g., hepatic cirrhosis, diabetes mellitus, intravenous drug abuse, neoplastic disease, or immunosuppression).

space can cause a chemical synovitis and can be absorbed systemically, resulting in potentially toxic serum levels.

B. Joint immobilization (usually in extension) should be employed only initially when joint pain is incapacitating. A range of motion exercises (without weight-bearing) should be started as soon as possible because this technique may enhance nutritional diffusion to cartilage and may assist in restoring natural cartilage repair mechanisms inhibited by immobilization. Such exercises also prevent the development of contractures. Weight-bearing should be avoided until joint inflammation has resolved substantially to reduce the risk for damage to articular cartilage.

C. Analgesics, such as codeine (30 mg every 4 hours), that do not affect fever should be used. Anti-inflammatory drugs (e.g., aspirin and indomethacin) should not be used initially so that the response to treatment can be assessed (in addition, these agents are antipyretics).

II. SUBSEQUENT TREATMENT

A. General measures. The daily assessment of patient status includes assessment of temperature, strength and appetite, change in range of motion in the joint, peripheral blood WBC count, and resolution of any extra-articular foci of infection.

B. The definitive antibiotic therapy can be selected when the culture results become available. Antibiotic guidelines for specific pathogens are set forth in Table 46-3.

C. Duration of antibiotic therapy varies with different types of bacterial arthritis. Gonococcal arthritis can be treated with 7 days of parenteral therapy, whereas other bacterial pathogens require 2 to 4 weeks of antibiotic therapy, depending on the microorganism, response to therapy, and condition of the underlying articular tissues. Treatment of infections in prosthetic total joint arthroplasty is discussed in the subsequent text.

D. Serial joint aspiration. Because septic arthritis is a closed-space infection, drainage procedures are essential to decrease intra-articular pressure and to reduce leukocyte enzyme activity. Simple arthrocentesis is commonly adequate to accomplish this aspect of therapy, and serial aspirations are necessary, as prompted by reaccumulation of inflammatory effusions, often on a daily basis and occasionally twice daily. The response to therapy can be monitored by serial synovial fluid leukocyte counts. After 5 to 7 days of effective treatment, the joint fluid WBC count should decline by 50% to 75%. Failure to achieve such a reduction should be viewed as an indication of inadequate therapy, and surgical drainage should be considered.

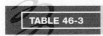

TABLE 46-3	Antibiotic Therapy Based on Culture Identification of Organism	
Organism	**Antibiotic**	**Alternative agent**
Staphylococcus aureus	Nafcillin	Vancomycin
Methicillin-resistant *S. aureus*	Vancomycin	Linezolid, quinupristin/dalfopristin, or daptomycin
Streptococci (nonenterococcal)	Penicillin	Cefazolin, ceftriaxone, or vancomycin
Enterococci	Penicillin plus aminoglycoside[a]	Vancomycin plus aminoglycoside[a]
Neisseria gonorrhoeae[c]	Third-generation cephalosporin[b]	Spectinomycin or ciprofloxacin (If patient not pregnant)
Enterobacteriaceae	Third-generation cephalosporin	Aminoglycoside[a], ciprofloxacin, or aztreonam
Haemophilus influenzae	Third-generation cephalosporin	Trimethoprim/sulfamethoxazole a ciprofloxacin or chloramphenicol
Pseudomonas	Aminoglycoside[a]	Ceftazidime, or an antipseudomonas penicillin

[a]Gentamicin, tobramycin, or amikacin.
[b]Ceftriaxone, ceftizoxime, or cefotaxime.
[c]Patients with disseminated gonococcal infection should be treated presumptively for concurrent *Chlamydia trachomatis* infection, unless appropriate testing excludes this infection.

E. **Surgical drainage** by arthroscopy is also used routinely as an alternative to serial aspiration at centers where this procedure is routinely performed.
  1. Surgical drainage, often with synovectomy, is indicated in the treatment of hip infections (particularly with *S. aureus* or gram-negative bacilli) because of the mechanical difficulty encountered in percutaneous needle aspiration of this deep articulation.
  2. Operative debridement is essential when pyarthrosis is inadequately responsive to arthrocentesis because of loculation of infection by intra-articular adhesions or underlying joint disease. Arthroscopic techniques have often been employed instead of open arthrotomy for debridement in these situations, especially when the knee is involved. Arthroscopy provides for more complete visualization of the tissue (by magnification and access to posterior compartments), decreases morbidity (lower complication rate), increases joint mobility (earlier postoperative motion because of decreased incision size and associated pain), and is more economical (shorter hospitalization period).
  3. **The indications for surgical drainage include the following:**
    a. **Hip infection.**
    b. **Failure of needle aspiration to drain the joint adequately** (widely varying WBC counts in repeated aspirates suggest loculated pockets of purulence).
    c. **Lack of local or systemic response to therapy** (e.g., joint fluid cultures remain positive; patient remains febrile after 3 to 6 days of what appears by sensitivity testing to be appropriate antibiotic therapy). A low threshold for early exploratory arthrotomy or arthroscopy should be maintained in the compromised host with gram-negative bacillary arthritis.
    d. **Recrudescent or recurrent infection** should prompt consideration of surgical drainage and debridement with histopathologic examination of synovial tissue and cultures for fastidious bacteria, mycobacteria, and fungi if appropriate.

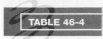

TABLE 46-4	Prognosis for Recovery of Baseline Joint Function Related to Specific Pathogens Causing Joint Infection

Microorganism	Patients recovering baseline articular function after appropriate therapy
Neisseria gonorrhoeae	>94%
Streptococcus pneumoniae	94%
Streptococcus pyogenes (group A)	85%
Staphylococcus aureus	73%
Gram-negative bacilli	21%

PROGNOSIS

I. **Mortality associated with infectious arthritis ranges from 5% to 20% of cases, often related to associated comorbidities.** Overall, an average of 40% (range up to 73%) of patients with infectious arthritis develop a permanent reduction in joint function.

II. **Prognosis varies according to the pathogen involved** (Table 46-4) and with the timing of initiation of appropriate therapy. When appropriate therapy is initiated within 7 days, two-thirds of patients recover full joint function. However, when appropriate therapy is delayed for more than 7 days, only one-third of patients recover full joint function.

III. Inability to sterilize the joint fluid within 6 days can be a predictor of a poor functional recovery. Similarly, if the synovial fluid WBC count is not reduced by 50% after 5 to 7 days of therapy, a poor prognosis is more likely.

SPECIFIC ENTITIES AND PROBLEMS

I. **GONOCOCCAL ARTHRITIS**
   A. **Diagnostic features**
      1. **Polyarthritis and monoarthritis** occur in approximately equal proportions at presentation. Commonly, migratory asymmetric joint pain is followed by mono- or polyarticular infection in distal joints.
      2. **Pustulovesicular skin lesions,** often with central necrosis, occur in 44% of cases.
      3. **Tenosynovitis** occurs in 68% of cases.
      4. **Positive results of cultures** are obtained from urethra (81%), synovial fluid (60%), blood (24%), pharynx (17%), and rectum (13%). Mucosal symptoms are frequently absent.
   B. **Treatment.** Drug therapy (as recommended by the Centers for Disease Control and Prevention).
      1. Ceftriaxone (1 g intramuscular or intravenous every 24 hours), ceftizoxime (1 g intravenous every 8 hours), or cefotaxime (1 g intravenous every 8 hours for 7 days).
      2. Ciprofloxacin (400 mg intravenous every 12 hours), ofloxacin (400 mg intravenous every 12 hours), or spectinomycin (2 g intramuscular every 12 hours) should be administered for individuals allergic to β-lactam drugs. Quinolones should not be used during pregnancy or in patients likely to have acquired infection in Asia, where resistance has been demonstrated. In certain geographic areas (e.g., California and Cleveland, Ohio), where strains with decreased susceptibility to quinolones are endemic, quinolones should not be used to treat gonorrhea. Reliable patients with uncomplicated disease in whom all symptoms resolve within 24 to 48 hours may be treated for a total of 7 days of treatment with oral cefixime (400 mg twice daily); if not pregnant, with oral

ciprofloxacin (500 mg twice daily); or oral ofloxacin (400 mg twice daily). Patients treated for gonococcal arthritis should be treated presumptively for concurrent *Chlamydia* infection (unless appropriate testing has excluded this infection) with azithromycin (1 g orally in a single dose), doxycycline (100 mg orally, twice daily for 7 days), ofloxacin (300 mg orally twice daily for 7 days), or levalbuterol hydrochloride (Levaquin) (500 mg orally for 7 days).

   3. Indications for hospitalization include inability of patient to follow or tolerate an outpatient regimen, uncertain diagnosis, and presence of a purulent joint effusion.

II. TUBERCULOUS ARTHRITIS

   A. Diagnostic features. Tuberculous arthritis typically presents as chronic monarthritis or spondylitis. Skeletal tuberculosis is usually combined osteomyelitis and arthritis because infective lesions in epiphyseal bone invade the adjacent joint. The chest radiographic findings are often normal, and constitutional symptoms may not be present. The tuberculin skin test result is almost always positive. Synovial fluid analysis reveals an elevated WBC count (usually 10,000 to 20,000/mm^3) with neutrophil predominance (80% of cases). Acid-fast stains of joint effusions are positive in only 27% of patients, and although joint fluid culture is positive in 83%, cultivation requires 4 to 6 weeks of incubation. Synovial biopsy is the procedure of choice for immediate diagnosis; histopathology demonstrates granuloma formation in 95% of cases, caseation in 55% of cases, and the presence of tubercle bacillus in 10% of cases.

   B. Treatment consists of isoniazid (300 mg/day) and rifampin (300 mg twice daily) for at least 12 months, with pyrazinamide (25 mg/kg/day maximum of 2.5 g/day) for the initial 2 months.

III. ATYPICAL MYCOBACTERIAL ARTHRITIS

   A. Diagnostic features. *Mycobacterium marinum* is the most common cause of atypical tuberculous arthritis. Presentation is usually a subacute or chronic interphalangeal or metacarpophalangeal monarthritis or tenosynovitis. Symptoms commonly develop several weeks after local traumatic contact with marine life (i.e., fish, fishing equipment, and fish tanks). Diagnosis is assisted by synovial biopsy revealing granulomas or acid-fast bacilli. Mycobacterial cultures of synovial tissue are diagnostic; however, the microbiology laboratory should be alerted to incubate specimens at 30°C for optimal results.

   B. Treatment consists of rifampin (300 mg twice daily) and ethambutol (15 mg/kg/day for 6 weeks) or minocycline (100 mg twice daily) for 16 weeks.

IV. FUNGAL ARTHRITIS

   A. Diagnostic features. Fungal arthritis usually presents as a chronic monoarticular infection, but acute polyarticular disease with or without erythema nodosum can be seen. Diagnosis depends on synovial tissue histopathology and mycotic cultures. Key features of specific types of fungal arthritis follow:

   1. **Candidiasis** causes hematogenous septic arthritis in immunosuppressed hosts. Approximately 70% of patients present acutely, 40% have multiple joint involvement, and 65% have evidence of osteomyelitis.

   2. **Coccidioidomycosis and histoplasmosis** both exhibit an acute, self-limited, hypersensitivity-type polyarthritis with erythema nodosum. Subsequently, a chronic granulomatous infectious synovitis may develop.

   3. **Blastomycosis** primarily involves the lungs, with spread to skin and bone; knee, ankle, and elbow are the most commonly affected joints. Synovial fluid culture result is positive for the organisms in 90% of cases.

   4. **Sporotrichosis** affects joints rarely by extension of infection from the usual cutaneous and lymphatic or osseous sites of involvement. More frequently, a slowly progressive polyarticular infection develops as a result of hematogenous seeding of the synovium.

   B. Treatment of coccidioidomycosis, histoplasmosis, blastomycosis, and sporotrichosis can be successful with oral imidazoles. Candidiasis is treated with intravenous amphotericin B. Surgical debridement is often necessary to eradicate fungal infection.

V. VIRAL ARTHRITIS. Rubella virus, hepatitis B virus, and parvovirus are the most common identifiable viral pathogens, although arthritis can be a manifestation of mumps,

infectious mononucleosis (Epstein-Barr virus), herpes simplex, or infection with arbovirus, enterovirus, varicella-zoster, or adenovirus.

A. Diagnostic features. Viral arthritides commonly involve multiple joints, particularly in the hands and wrists. Rubella is accompanied by polyarthritis after appearance of the exanthem and usually resolves within 2 weeks. Polyarthritis may also develop following rubella vaccination. Prodromal hepatitis B is associated with polyarthritis and skin eruptions such as urticaria, maculopapular rashes, petechiae, purpura, and angioneurotic edema. Joint symptoms usually resolve after 1 to 3 weeks, which is coincident with the onset of jaundice. Recurrent arthritis can be seen with chronic active hepatitis or persistent antigenemia. Parvovirus can produce symmetrical polyarthritis that can resemble rheumatoid arthritis in distribution, typically resolving within 2 weeks.

B. Treatment consists of nonsteroidal anti-inflammatory drugs.

VI. Lyme disease is discussed in Chapter 47.

VII. SEPTIC BURSITIS

A. Diagnostic features. Because of their superficial location, the prepatellar and olecranon bursae are most frequently infected directly through the skin (not through bacteremia), usually following local trauma. The antecedent trauma may be direct or repetitive, or, simply, constant pressure. Patients present with the acute (2 days) or subacute (12 days) onset of local pain and inflammation, with cellulitis in 75% and regional lymphadenopathy in 25% of cases. Pain is evident on palpation of the bursa and on extreme flexion and extreme extension of the adjacent joint but not on limited motion, as seen in septic arthritis. Bland (nonseptic) bursitis is far more common than septic bursitis. Fever, tenderness, peribursal cellulitis, and local skin lesions that may serve as portals of entry are also more common in septic than in nonseptic cases. Infection of the prepatellar or olecranon bursa does not imply involvement of the deeper joints because there is normally no communication between the two spaces. However, infection of a synovial cyst (e.g., Baker's cyst) does imply the presence of septic arthritis. Bursal fluid analysis reveals abnormalities similar to those of infected joint fluid. The etiologic pathogen is *S. aureus* in more than 90% of cases.

B. Treatment involves drainage by percutaneous aspiration (repeated as indicated by reaccumulation of bursal fluid) and antibiotic therapy. Clinically mild infections can be treated with oral antibiotics for 3 to 4 weeks. If the condition of such patients worsens or if the patients fail to improve within 1 to 2 days, parenteral or high potency oral therapy should be considered for more severe infections. In these cases, intravenous or high-potency oral treatment should be continued for 10 to 14 days followed by additional oral therapy, as clinically appropriate, but there has been no consensus on treatment duration. Surgical bursectomy is indicated for persistent infection or chronic inflammation.

VIII. PROSTHETIC JOINT INFECTION

A. Diagnostic features. Total joint replacement infections can present as acute, fulminant illness with fever, joint pain, local swelling, and erythema when caused by relatively virulent organisms (e.g., *S. aureus*). Subacute presentations with gradually progressive joint pain and no fever suggest indolent infection with a relatively avirulent organism (e.g., *S. epidermidis*). A painful prosthetic joint can be caused by both infectious and noninfectious, mechanical loosening. Radiography, bone scan, leukocyte scans, WBC counts, and sedimentation rate are not diagnostic for infection. Therefore, the diagnosis of prosthetic joint infection rests on isolation of the pathogen by arthrocentesis or, occasionally, by exploratory arthrotomy. Staphylococci are the predominant organisms (*S. epidermidis*, 22%; *S. aureus*, 22%), with streptococci in 21%, gram-negative bacilli in 25%, and anaerobes in 10% of cases.

B. Treatment. Eradication of the pathogen in prosthetic joint infection requires removal of the prosthesis. Metallic joint excision followed by 6 weeks of bactericidal parenteral antimicrobial therapy and subsequent reimplantation is successful in 90% to 97% of cases. Prosthetic joint removal with reimplantation in a one-stage procedure employing antibiotic-impregnated cement is successful in 70% to 80% of patients. Success with long courses (3 to 6 months) of antibiotic therapy, using rifampin, in combination with other antimicrobial agents, has been reported in select patients with retained orthopedic implants. Occasionally, protracted oral antibiotic therapy is given to suppress prosthetic joint infection when the prosthesis cannot be removed, the pathogen is relatively avirulent, or the prosthesis is not loose.

C. Prevention. Because prosthetic joint infection is a catastrophic event for the patient, prevention is of considerable importance. The hematogenous route is responsible for 20% to 40% of these infections. The use of prophylactic antibiotics, in patients with prosthetic joints, for events or procedures associated with anticipated bacteremia is controversial at present, and the adequacy and cost-effectiveness of such measures have not been determined. The American Dental Association and the American Academy of Orthopedic Surgeons have jointly advised that prophylactic antibiotics be given to select patients undergoing dental procedures associated with significant bleeding (including periodontal scaling). The select patient population includes individuals with inflammatory arthropathies (including rheumatoid arthritis and systemic lupus erythematosus), immunosuppression, diabetes mellitus, malnutrition, hemophilia, previous prosthetic joint infection, and all those who have undergone joint replacement within the last 2 years. The American Urologic Association and the American Academy of Orthopedic Surgeons have also jointly advised that prophylactic antibiotics be considered in similar select patient populations undergoing urologic procedures with higher bacteremic risk. Clinical decisions about prophylactic antibiotics for expected bacteremias in patients with prosthetic joints should be made on an individual basis. The following schedules are for consideration by physicians who wish to employ prophylactic antibiotics in some settings for certain patients.

  1. Dental procedures (associated with gingival hemorrhage)
      a. Amoxicillin, cephalexin, or cephradine (2 g orally 1 hour before a procedure).
      b. Clindamycin (600 mg orally 1 hour before procedure).
  2. Certain urologic procedures
      a. Ciprofloxacin (500 mg), levofloxacin (500 mg), or ofloxacin (400 mg) orally, 1 to 2 hours preoperatively.
      b. Ampicillin (2 g intravenous) or vancomycin (1 g intravenous) if patient is allergic to ampicillin, over 1 to 2 hours preoperatively.
      c. Plus gentamicin 1.5 mg/kg intravenous, 30 to 60 minutes preoperatively.

LYME DISEASE

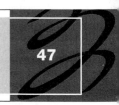

Anne R. Bass and Steven K. Magid

47

▨ KEY POINTS

▪ Lyme disease is caused by the spirochete *Borrelia burgdorferi*.

▪ In endemic areas, *B. burgdorferi* is transmitted by the bite of an *Ixodes* tick. This generally occurs in the late spring or early summer.

▪ Early Lyme disease is characterized by the rash, erythema migrans (EM). Early dissemination of *B. burgdorferi* can result in fever, headache, myalgias, disseminated skin lesions, cranial neuropathy, radiculitis, meningitis, carditis, and/or arthritis. Manifestations of late, untreated Lyme disease include monoarthritis or oligoarthritis, peripheral neuropathy, or encephalopathy.

▪ Early Lyme disease is diagnosed clinically. There is generally no role for serologic testing in this setting.

▪ In late Lyme disease, serologic testing is virtually always positive.

- Lyme disease should never be diagnosed based on a positive serology alone. The diagnosis of late Lyme disease can be made when symptoms specific for Lyme disease are present, and serology is positive.

- The most common cause of "seronegative Lyme disease" is misdiagnosis.

- A positive result for Lyme disease on enzyme-linked immunosorbent assay (ELISA) must be confirmed by Western blot test before using it to confirm a diagnosis of Lyme disease.

- Lyme disease is treatable with antibiotics.

- A small number of patients with a history of Lyme disease continue to have symptoms after completing a full course of intravenous antibiotics. Studies have shown that additional antibiotic treatment does not relieve these symptoms.

*L*yme disease was first detected in the United States in 1977, when clusters of an illness, first thought to be juvenile idiopathic arthritis, were noted in three small communities in Connecticut. Although the earliest cases of Lyme disease were thought to have occurred 25 years ago in Cape Cod and in Connecticut, the spirochete has been identified in ticks collected more than 50 years ago.

Lyme disease is now the most common vector-borne illness in the United States. Although it is most prevalent in the Northeast Coast of the United States, the disease is also seen in Wisconsin and Minnesota, some West Coast states, and in Europe.

 ETIOPATHOGENESIS

I. **SPIROCHETE. Lyme disease is caused by the spirochete *Borrelia burgdorferi.*** The *B. burgdorferi* that is found in the United States belongs to the subspecies *B. burgdorferi sensu stricto*, whereas in Europe, *B. burgdorferi garinii* and *B. burgdorferi afzelii* predominate. This may account for some of the differences in the clinical presentation of Lyme disease that is found in Europe from that found in the United States.

  A. More than 30 *B. burgdorferi* proteins have been identified. There are three major outer surface proteins (Osp): Osp A (30 kDa), Osp B (34 kDa), and Osp C (23 kDa). Strain-specific differences in Osp C influence the ability of *B. burgdorferi* to disseminate from the skin.

  B. There is also a 41-kDa flagellar (Fla) antigen that is shared by other spirochetes. Basic membrane protein A (Bmp A) (39 kDa) appears to be highly specific for *B. burgdorferi*. In contrast, the 58-, 60-, 66-, and 72-kDa antigens are heat shock proteins, which are widely conserved in all cells and have strong homology with other organisms.

II. **VECTOR. *B. burgdorferi* is transmitted by ticks of the *Ixodes* family.** On the East Coast of the United States, *Ixodes scapularis* is the most important vector. In the western United States, *I. pacificus* is responsible. *I. ricinus* is the main vector in western and central Europe, and *I. persulcatus* is found in eastern Russia, China, and Japan.

  A. The life cycle of *I. scapularis* spans 2 years and includes three stages of development: larva, nymph, and adult. Ticks eat once at each stage of life and can acquire *B. burgdorferi* during the process of eating. There is no vertical transmission from adult tick to larva.

  B. In the endemic areas of the Northeast, 30% to 50% of nymphal and adult ticks may be infected with *B. burgdorferi*. In the north central United States, infection rates of 10% to 20% are reported, while on the Pacific Coast the rate of tick infection is approximately 1% to 2%.

  C. White-footed mice (plus the occasional bird, small mammal, or human) are the preferred host for larval and nymphal ticks, and serve as a reservoir for *B. burgdorferi*. Adult ticks feed on deer by attaching to its body (hence the term "deer tick") or, rarely, by attaching to humans.

  D. *B. burgdorferi*, acquired by larva, can be passed on to humans when those larvae become nymphs, and feed again. Nymphs feed during the late spring and early summer, which accounts for the peak time of onset of early Lyme disease. The small size (1 mm) of the nymphs, and the light clothing worn by humans at this time of year contribute to the ease of disease transmission. Although adult ticks can also transmit *B. burgdorferi* when they feed in the fall, their large size makes them easy to see and remove before transmission of disease can occur. In practice, human contact of *B. burgdorferi* from the bite of an adult deer tick is rare.

III. **TRANSMISSION.** *B. burgdorferi* are present in low numbers in the midgut of the tick, where they express Osp A. When the tick attaches and feeds on a host, the spirochete multiplies, but remains in the gut of the tick for at least 15 hours. After 48 hours, when the temperature in the gut reaches 37°C, the spirochete disseminates to the salivary glands of the tick from where it can be transmitted to the host (Osp C is up-regulated and Osp A is down-regulated at this time). The implication of this is that the risk of disease transmission is low if a tick has been attached for less than 36 hours (i.e., is not engorged with blood).

IV. **INFECTIOUS OR REACTIVE DISEASE?** Polymerase chain reaction (PCR) testing, culture, and staining of human tissues and tissues of experimental animals suggest that *B. burgdorferi* is present at sites of pathology, albeit in small numbers. This, and the response of the disease to antibiotics, suggest that it is an infectious, rather than a "reactive" process.

Nonetheless, host factors play a role in disease expression, and a subset of patients with the human leukocyte antigen (HLA)-DR4 haplotype may develop an antibiotic-resistant chronic arthritis, which may be reactive in nature. It has been hypothesized that cross-reactivity between *Borrelia* Osp A, and the human leukocyte antigen, leukocyte function antigen-1 (LFA-1), may lead to autoimmunity in these immunologically susceptible hosts.

VI. **IMMUNITY.** Prior infection with *B. burgdorferi* results in serologic immunity, but in most cases does not seem to confer protection from repeated infection.

PREVALENCE

The incidence of Lyme disease has been increasing in the northeastern United States over the last 25 years. This is likely due to the replacement of farmland by suburbs, and an associated increase in forestation. Forested areas, adjacent to "meadows" (lawns) serve as ideal habitats for white-footed mice, and deer. After 1982, more than 157,000 cases of Lyme disease have been reported in the United States and 23,763 cases were reported in 2002 to the various Centers for Disease Control and Prevention.

I. The overall incidence in the United States is approximately 7/100,000 individuals/year, but in endemic areas it may be as high as 1 to 3/100 individuals.

II. As of 2001, cases of Lyme disease have been reported in all states except Montana. Eight states (Connecticut, Rhode Island, Massachusetts, New York, New Jersey, Pennsylvania, Maryland, and Wisconsin) accounted for 90% (15,385) of the 17,029 cases reported. New York State and Connecticut reported 45% (7,680) of all cases.

III. Cases of Lyme disease have been reported from most European countries, in addition to Russia, China, Japan, and Australia. Lyme disease occurs in all age groups, but is seen most often in children aged 0 to 14 years, and in adults aged 30 to 49 years.

CLINICAL MANIFESTATIONS

The clinical manifestations are as follows (Table 47-1):

I. **EARLY LOCALIZED DISEASE (STAGE 1).** Erythema migrans (EM), the characteristic rash of Lyme disease, develops in 80% of patients, 3 to 32 days (mean 7 days) after transmission of *B. burgdorferi* through the bite of an infected tick. Only one-third of patients will remember a tick bite.

    A. EM may be seen anywhere, but it frequently occurs behind the knee, in the groin, or the axilla. In children, the crease of the earlobe is a common site.

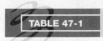

TABLE 47-1	Clinical Manifestations of Lyme Disease

Early localized:
Erythema migrans
Early disseminated:
Fever, headache, myalgias, fatigue, malaise, mild liver test abnormalities
Disseminated erythema migrans skin lesions
Carditis: atrioventricular block, rarely myocarditis or pericarditis
Migratory arthralgias, brief episodes of oligoarthritis
Meningitis
Painful demyelinating radiculoneuropathy
Encephalomyelitis (more common in Europe)
Late persistent:
Intermittent monoarthritis or oligoarthritis
Chronic monoarthritis
Peripheral axonal neuropathy (more common in Europe)
Chronic encephalopathy (more common in the United States)
Acrodermatitis chronica atrophicans (more common in Europe)

B. The rash is generally macular, erythematous, nonpainful, and nonpruritic, although some patients may describe burning or pruritus. Occasionally the rash will be vesicular or necrotic, particularly at its center. Its borders are characteristically regular (not blotchy), and it is typically circular or oval in shape. The rash gradually increases in size (up to 1 to 2 cm/day) to 3 to 70 cm (mean 15 cm). As it expands, a bright red outer border may develop. There can be central or other areas of clearing producing a ringlike, or "bullseye" appearance.

C. Even if antibiotics are **not** given, the lesions usually clear within a month. If antibiotics are used, the lesions clear in several days.

II. EARLY DISSEMINATED DISEASE (STAGE 2). Within days to weeks of the tick bite, the spirochete can disseminate systemically through the blood or lymph. Symptoms at this time can include fever, headache, myalgia, arthralgia, and fatigue; the most common clinical manifestations of early disseminated Lyme disease relate to the heart, joints, and neurologic system.

A. Constitutional symptoms at this stage, among those affected by the disease, are common in the United States, but much rarer in Europe.

B. Arthritis can develop as early as a few weeks after the onset of disease and occurs in 80% of untreated patients. It is usually asymmetrical and oligoarticular (involving four or fewer joints). Large joints are preferentially involved, especially the knee. Initially, these attacks are brief and may last days or weeks and then remit without antibiotic therapy. Although some patients have continuous inflammation, most do not.

C. Carditis develops in 1% of patients and 4% to 8% of untreated patients 2 to 8 weeks after infection. Atrioventricular block (first, second, or third degree) is the most common finding. The duration is usually brief (3 days to 6 weeks). Complete heart block is rare, and when present, usually lasts less than a week. Temporary pacing is occasionally needed. Ventricular tachycardia is uncommon but has been reported. Other uncommon manifestations include mild left ventricular dysfunction, electrocardiographic abnormalities, acute myopericarditis, and rarely pancarditis. Valvular lesions are not seen.

D. Neurologic manifestations develop in 15% of untreated patients 2 to 8 weeks after infection.

1. Cranial neuropathy. Bell's palsy is the most common cranial neuropathy seen in Lyme disease. One-third of cases are bilateral. Other cranial neuropathies are less common and may occur with or without Bell's palsy. Some patients with cranial neuropathy will also have evidence of meningitis on testing of cerebrospinal fluid (CSF) even in the absence of headache or meningeal signs. This has important implications for therapy (see under Treatment in subsequent text).

2. **Radiculoneuropathy.** A painful radiculoneuropathy can develop, often in the same dermatome as the tick bite. It is usually unilateral, but can be sequential or bilateral. Physical examination does not demonstrate impingement. Nerve conduction studies reveal conduction block (demyelination).

3. **Meningitis.** Recurrent attacks of severe headache may occur and are often associated with stiff neck, photophobia, nausea, and vomiting. Patients are frequently afebrile. Such severe attacks may last weeks and alternate with periods of milder headache. Spinal fluid shows a lymphocytic pleocytosis with increased production of immunoglobulin G (IgG). Evidence of local antibody to B. burgdorferi may be found. Oligoclonal bands may also be seen.

E. **Meningoencephalitis** is a rare but severe acute manifestation of Lyme disease seen more commonly among patients in Europe than in the United States. It can be manifested by symptoms such as confusion, cerebellar ataxia, or myelitis.

F. **Secondary EM lesions** can also develop at distant sites on the skin.

G. **Laboratory testing** may reveal a mild hepatitis.

H. **Spirochetes have been found in pathologic specimens** from the heart, retina, muscle, bone, synovium, spleen, liver, meninges, and brain.

III. **LATE PERSISTENT INFECTION (STAGE 3).** Late disease is manifested by neurologic disease, skin disease, or arthritis.

A. **Chronic peripheral neuropathy.** Patients can present months to years after infection with an axonal neuropathy, manifested by numbness and tingling in a stocking-glove distribution. This neuropathy is not a later manifestation of early radiculoneuropathy (see Early Disseminated Disease) but a distinct process. It is seen most commonly in European female patients with acrodermatitis atrophicans (see in the subsequent text).

B. **Encephalopathy.** This rare, late manifestation of Lyme disease is seen primarily among patients in the United States. Patients complain of difficulty with memory and concentration. Hypersomnolence, depression, irritability, and marked memory loss are noted.

C. **Arthritis.** Intermittent arthritis develops in 50% of untreated patients. It is usually an asymmetric oligoarthritis or monoarthritis of the large joints, and most patients have knee involvement at some point of time in their illness. Less commonly, arthritis of the ankle, wrist, and temporomandibular joint can develop, and occasionally the elbow and hand can also be involved.

1. **Joint swelling is often dramatic and is usually out of proportion to pain.** Baker's cysts can be seen.

2. **Synovial fluid** leukocyte counts range from 500 to 110,000/mm^3. Polymorphonuclear leukocytes predominate.

3. **Ten percent of untreated patients will develop a chronic monoarthritis.** The transition from episodic attacks to chronic arthritis has been associated with the development of antibodies to Osp A. The presence of the HLA-DR4 haplotype places a patient at greater risk for the development of chronic arthritis.

IV. **ACRODERMATITIS CHRONICA ATROPHICANS.** This chronic skin lesion is seen only among patients in Europe, where it is associated with the *Borrelia* subspecies *B. burdorferi afzelii*. Localized primarily to the extensor surfaces of the extremities, the early lesion consists of erythematous plaques. These then coalesce to form a thickened reddish-brown area. With time, the skin can atrophy and ulcerations can develop.

 DIAGNOSTIC INVESTIGATIONS

I. **The diagnosis of Lyme disease is a clinical one** based on epidemiologic data, a characteristic clinical presentation, and the exclusion of other disorders in which articular, cardiac, and neurologic phenomena occur. Lyme disease can be diagnosed in any patient with EM, or in a patient with a manifestation of early disseminated or late persistent Lyme disease, who also has a positive Lyme serology.

II. **Enzyme-linked immunosorbent assay (ELISA)** is the preferred serologic screening method. Sonicated, whole-*B. burgdorferi* extracts are used as the antigens. IgM antibodies appear 2 to 4 weeks after the EM rash (2 to 6 weeks after infection). They peak after 8 weeks and usually normalize by 4 to 6 months. IgG antibodies occur within 6 to 8 weeks after appearance of the the EM rash, peak after 4 to 6 months, and may remain elevated indefinitely. IgG antibodies remain positive even after successful treatment of Lyme disease. Early antibiotic treatment (i.e., within 2 weeks of infection) may abrogate an antibody response.

III. **Antibody testing has no role in stage 1 disease (EM), because it will generally be negative and early treatment with antibiotics may abrogate an antibody response. Serologic testing in late Lyme disease, on the other hand, is virtually universally positive.**

IV. **A positive ELISA must be confirmed by Western blot testing** as false-positive ELISAs, because of antibodies to flagellar or heat shock proteins, are common. False-positive ELISAs can also be due to cross-reactivity with other nonpathogenic spirochetes such as those that cause gingivitis, or less commonly, pathogenic spirochetes such as *Treponema pallidum*.

   A. Cross-reactive antibodies are commonly seen in the context of polyclonal B-cell activation, particularly in patients whose sera contain rheumatoid factor, antinuclear antibodies, or antithyroid antibodies. They can also be seen in patients with malaria, Epstein-Barr virus infection, or Rocky Mountain spotted fever.

   B. Patients who have received the Lyme vaccine may have a positive Lyme ELISA, but Western blot testing will be negative for Lyme disease. Serologies remain positive even after successful treatment of Lyme disease, so follow-up testing is not necessary.

V. **WESTERN BLOT.** This technique separates the major *B. burgdorferi* proteins on an agar gel by molecular weight. By overlaying a patient's sera, it is possible to determine which *B. burgdorferi* proteins (if any) are the targets of an antibody response. Characteristic patterns of antibody formation after infection with *B. burgdorferi* have been used by the Centers for Disease Control and Prevention to develop the following criteria for a positive Western blot:

   A. **IgM.** At least two of three positive bands: 24 (Osp C), 39 (Bmp A), and 41 (Fla) kDa.

   B. **IgG.** At least 5 of 10 bands: 18, 21, 28, 35, 39, 41, 45, 58, 66, and 93 kDa.

   C. A positive IgM Western blot is diagnostically useful in patients suspected of having early disseminated disease, while a positive IgG Western blot can support a diagnosis of either early disseminated or late persistent disease.

VI. **Cultures** of biopsies of the leading edge of EM lesions will be positive in 88% of patients, but cultures of blood, joint fluid, and CSF are almost invariably negative.

VII. **PCR** is a technique that "amplifies" a single copy of *B. burgdorferi* DNA into many millions of copies, allowing the detection of even a single *B. burgdorferi* genome. It is most useful in testing inflammatory fluids such as cerebrospinal and joint fluid rather than blood (blood PCR is generally only positive at the time of early dissemination of *B. burgdorferi* from the skin).

   A. Sensitivity of PCR is 60% to 85% in the synovium, 40% to 60% in the CSF, and 60% to 80% in the skin. Some commercial labs offer PCR on urine specimens, but their reliability is poor.

   B. The PCR technique is limited by the fact that it cannot distinguish between the DNA from living *Borrelia* and the DNA from nonviable organisms. In addition, special laboratory techniques are required to avoid false-positive results. Finally, the Osp A primers used for PCR testing in the United States may not detect European strains of *B. burgdorferi*.

 TREATMENT

I. **PREVENTION**

   A. **Protection from tick bites** is an important method of combating Lyme disease. This is accomplished by wearing protective, light-colored clothing tucked in at the ankles and wrists, using insect repellent on clothing, inspecting for ticks, and modifying residential landscapes (such as clearing leaf litter, brush, and tall grass, removing stone walls and wood piles, and erecting deer barriers). Area application of acaricides is effective, but raises safety concerns.

B. Proper tick removal minimizes the risk of inoculating the contents of the tick into the body in the process of removal. Tweezers should be used to grasp the tick behind its head and pull it out slowly and gently.

C. Vaccination. A recombinant Osp A vaccine was available for use until 2002. Human antibodies to Osp A, induced by the vaccine, were shown to cause antibody-mediated death of *B. burgdorferi* inside the feeding tick, before it could be transmitted to the vaccinated host. The vaccine was taken off the market amid concerns that immunity to Osp A might provoke chronic arthritis in HLA-DR4 positive individuals.

Vaccine-induced protection from Lyme disease lasts only 2 years. Vaccinated individuals may have a positive result on testing by ELISA for Lyme disease, but will have a negative result on testing by Western blot.

II. PROPHYLAXIS. The risk of acquiring Lyme disease from the bite of a tick depends on the infection rate of *B. burgdorferi* on the local tick. Anywhere from 0% to 50% of nymphal ticks, depending on the geographic area, will be infected. In endemic areas, the risk of EM after the bite of a deer tick is 1.2% to 3.2%. The risk of infection after the bite of an **infected** tick is 8%.

A. Transmission rates vary with the duration of time the tick remains attached to the body. Because transmission of *B. burgdorferi* generally does not occur until after 36 hours of attachment of the tick to the body, nonengorged ticks are virtually never found to have transmitted Lyme disease. Engorged deer ticks carry a 9.9% risk of transmitting Lyme disease in endemic areas. A single dose of doxycycline 200 mg will reduce this risk to 1.3%.

B. Because the risk of *B. burgdorferi* transmission is so low after removal of a nonengorged tick, we do not recommend prophylactic antibiotics in this setting.

C. When an engorged tick is removed, the patient can be given the choice of either taking a single 200 mg dose of doxycycline or monitoring symptoms for Lyme disease by observing the site of the bite for the next 4 weeks. Doxycycline should not be given to children, nor to pregnant women. Other antibiotics have not been studied for prophylactic use.

III. TREATMENT. *B. burgdorferi* is sensitive, in animal studies and *in vitro*, to tetracycline, ampicillin, cefuroxime, ceftriaxone, and imipenem. *B. burgdorferi* is also sensitive to erythromycin, but macrolide antibiotics are less effective *in vivo* than tetracyclines, penicillins, or cephalosporins, and should never be the first antibiotic of choice. The advantages of doxycycline over tetracycline are better gastrointestinal absorption, better central nervous system (CNS) penetration, and the convenience of twice-daily dosing. They should not be given to pregnant women or children. They can both cause photosensitive rashes, which limit their use during the summer months.

A. In general, an oral dose of antibiotics is adequate for the treatment of Lyme disease, but refractory arthritis and many neurologic manifestations of Lyme disease require intravenous antibiotics. Treatment recommendations for Lyme disease are summarized in Table 47-2.

B. Early localized disease. A ten- to 21-day course of oral doxycycline, amoxicillin, or cefuroxime is recommended to treat EM. Macrolide antibiotics are less effective, but may be used if necessary. A recent study suggested that a 10-day course of doxycycline was as good as either a 20-day course of doxycycline, or a single dose of ceftriaxone intravenous followed by 10 days of doxycycline, even if patients had constitutional symptoms.

C. Early disseminated disease

1. Carditis. First- and second-degree heart block can be treated with oral antibiotics for 14 to 21 days. Third-degree heart block should be treated with intravenous ceftriaxone for 14 to 21 days.

2. Meningitis or radiculoneuropathy. Intravenous ceftriaxone 2 g/day for 14 to 28 days is recommended.

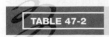

TABLE 47-2	Recommendations for Antibiotic Treatment

Erythema migrans with or without flulike illness:
Doxycycline, 100 mg b.i.d. for 10–21 d
Amoxicillin, 500 mg b.i.d. for 10–21 d
Cefuroxime, 500 mg b.i.d. for 10–21 d
If there is no alternative, use azithromycin 500 mg q.d. for 5–10 d, or erythromycin 500 mg q.i.d.
 for 10–21 d
Early disseminated:
Cardiac disease:
 First- or second-degree atrioventricular block: oral antibiotics as above, for 14–21 d
 Third-degree atrioventricular block: ceftriaxone 2 g intravenous daily for 14–21 d
 (may require a temporary pacer)
Meningitis or radiculopathy: Ceftriaxone 2 g intravenous daily for 14–28 d
Cranial nerve palsy:
 Normal CSF: oral antibiotics for 14–21 d
 Abnormal CSF: ceftriaxone 2 g intravenous for 14–28 d
Late persistent:
Arthritis (without neurologic disease): Oral antibiotics for 28 d
Recurrent arthritis after oral regimen: Repeat oral antibiotics for 28 d or Ceftriaxone 2 g
 intravenous daily for 14–28 d
CNS or peripheral nervous system disease: Ceftriaxone 2 g intravenous daily for 14–28 d

b.i.d., twice daily; CNS, central nervous system; CSF, cerebrospinal fluid; q.d., daily;
q.i.d., four times daily.

3. **Cranial nerve palsy.** Treatment is based on the presence or absence of CSF abnormalities. All patients should undergo a lumbar puncture. If the CSF is normal, oral antibiotics can be given for 14 to 21 days. If the CSF is abnormal, then intravenous ceftriaxone 2 g/day should be administered for 14 to 28 days.

D. **Late persistent disease**
   1. **Arthritis.** Most patients who have chronic or intermittent arthritis can be successfully treated by administering a course of oral antibiotics for 28 days. Complete resolution of symptoms may be delayed after completion of antibiotics administration.
   2. **Patients who have recurrent arthritis after completion of an oral regimen,** or whose symptoms have not completely resolved several months after completion, can either be treated with another 28-day course of oral antibiotics, or with intravenous ceftriaxone 2 g/day for 14 to 28 days.
   3. **Intra-articular steroids should be avoided** before the institution of antibiotic therapy because they have been associated with an increased risk for antibiotic failure. Lyme arthritis is not typically erosive, and does not require therapeutic aspiration or surgical debridement. Arthroscopic synovectomy can, however, be beneficial in treating the rare case of chronic Lyme arthritis that is refractory to other modalities.
   4. **CNS disease or peripheral neuropathy.** Late Lyme disease of the central or peripheral nervous system should be treated with intravenous antibiotics for 14 to 28 days.
IV. **ANTIBIOTIC-REFRACTORY LYME DISEASE.** The most common explanation for "refractory" Lyme disease is misdiagnosis. Some patients, however, may have symptoms resulting from tissue damage from prior *B. burgdorferi* infection, even if the organism has been successfully eradicated. This can be seen, for example, in the rare patient with a history of **erosive** arthritis, or encephalitis from Lyme disease. Joint fluid and CSF in these instances will be normal, and PCR for *B. burgdorferi* will be negative.

PROGNOSIS

I.   Although antibiotic therapy is generally very effective for manifestations of even late persistent Lyme disease, a small number of patients do complain of chronic symptoms such as cognitive impairment, radicular pain, paresthesias, fatigue, or musculoskeletal pain after a full course of intravenous antibiotics.

II. Persistent symptoms may correlate with a longer duration of disease before commencing antibiotic treatment. A recent study demonstrated that an additional 1-month course of intravenous ceftriaxone followed by 2 months of oral doxycycline was no better than placebo in alleviating these symptoms. Recommendations, therefore, are simply to treat these patients symptomatically.

III. Individuals who are HLA-DR4 positive and with truly antibiotic-refractory arthritis may be treated with synovectomy and/or anti-inflammatory agents.

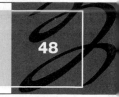

OSTEOMYELITIS
Juliet Aizer and Barry D. Brause

48

■ KEY POINTS

■ The diagnosis of osteomyelitis is dependent upon understanding the pathogenetic mechanisms involved in the three routes of infection: hematogenous osteomyelitis, introduced infection, and contiguous infection.

■ The three routes of bone infection are associated with different and distinct clinical presentations.

■ X-ray is the most specific and least expensive imaging technique for diagnosing osteomyelitis (with the exception of childhood acute hematogenous infection).

■ Bone biopsies should be sought, percutaneously or by operative debridement, when there is no overlying skin ulcer and the microbiologic etiology has not been otherwise determined.

■ Sinus tract and sinus drainage cultures often reflect colonizing flora and cannot be relied upon to identify the actual cause of deep osseous infection.

■ Designing a therapeutic regimen for osteomyelitis depends substantially on the sensitivity of the isolated pathogen to specific antimicrobial agents, which underscores the essential importance of delineating the pathogen in these infections.

■ When acute osteomyelitis is complicated by abscess formation or extensive necrosis, surgical debridement is an important adjunct to antibiotics.

■ In chronic osteomyelitis microorganisms persist in foci of gross or microscopic necrotic bone (sequestra) and intermittently invade surrounding tissues, causing acute exacerbations.

Osteomyelitis represents the invasion of bone by microorganisms. A useful classification for bone infection, based on the pathogenetic route of infection, divides cases into three types: (a) hematogenous osteomyelitis; (b) introduced infection, which results from contamination accompanying surgical and nonsurgical trauma; and (c) contiguous infection, which results from the spread of microorganisms from adjacent infected tissue and includes osteomyelitis associated with peripheral vascular disease.

ETIOPATHOGENESIS AND PREVALENCE

I. **HEMATOGENOUS OSTEOMYELITIS.** The etiologic pathogens in hematogenous osteomyelitis reflect the microorganisms associated with bacteremia in specific patient populations (Table 48-1). The osseous site of involvement in hematogenous infection is age-dependent.

   A. **Childhood hematogenous osteomyelitis.** From birth through puberty, the metaphyseal regions in the long bones of the extremities (tibia, femur, humerus) are most frequently involved owing to their large blood flow during the developmental years.

   B. **Adult hematogenous osteomyelitis.** In adults, blood-borne pathogens preferentially infect the spine (lumbosacral, thoracic) because vertebrae receive relatively more blood flow with maturation. In bacteremia, the more vascular anterior end plates are seeded, and osteomyelitis commonly involves two adjacent vertebral bodies and the intervertebral disc space. The septic process compromises the nutrient supply to the intervertebral disc, resulting in disc necrosis and disc space narrowing.

II. **INTRODUCED OSTEOMYELITIS.** Patients are at risk for the introduced form of osteomyelitis whenever the skin and soft tissues overlying and protecting bone are breached by trauma or surgery. Approximately 70% of compound fractures are contaminated by skin and soil microflora, but thanks to effective debridement and perioperative antibiotic therapy, infection develops in only 2% to 9%. Prophylactic antibiotics and extensive antiseptic operative techniques allow large foreign bodies to be inserted into bones during reparative and reconstructive orthopedic surgery with infection rates less than 2%. Indwelling foreign bodies decrease the magnitude of bacterial inoculum necessary to establish infection in bone, and they permit pathogens to persist on the surface of avascular material, often within host- or microbe-derived biofilms, sequestered from circulating immune factors and systemic antibiotics.

III. **OSTEOMYELITIS BY CONTIGUOUS SPREAD (INCLUDING VASCULAR INSUFFICIENCY).** Osteomyelitis develops by contiguous spread in one-third to two-thirds of patients with diabetes who have longstanding foot ulcers. More hospital days are utilized to treat foot infection than any other complication of diabetes mellitus. Osseous involvement reflects unsuccessful reversal of or compensation for underlying severe neuropathy and vascular insufficiency. These neuropathic and vasculopathic processes prevent a skin ulcer from healing, so that progressively deeper microbial invasion culminates in spread to contiguous bone. This clinical scenario is also seen in patients with chronic skin ulcerations resulting from other conditions associated with severe sensory neuropathy (e.g., meningomyelocele) or vascular insufficiency (e.g., decubitus ulcers, vasculitis, atherosclerosis, and arteriosclerosis). The most common pathogens are staphylococci, streptococci, gram-negative bacilli, and anaerobes. Multiple organisms are isolated in more than 60% of cases.

IV. **THE PATHOLOGIC PROCESS.** In all three forms of osteomyelitis, the microorganisms induce local metabolic changes and inflammatory reactions that produce osseous edema. As infection spreads within the bone, local thrombophlebitis develops, increasing edema and intraosseous pressure, that can result in ischemic necrosis of large areas of bone, called sequestra. If the osseous cortex is breached, subperiosteal abscesses can develop, with periosteal inflammation and periosteal formation of new bone in adjacent soft tissue, called an involucrum.

V. **MICROBIOLOGY.** Virtually all microbes can infect bone. Bacteria are the usual pathogens, and staphylococci are the most common etiologic agents in all three types of osseous infection. *Staphylococcus aureus* causes approximately 60% of cases of hematogenous and introduced osteomyelitis and is the most prominent pathogen when osseous infection develops from sepsis in contiguous tissue. *Staphylococcus epidermidis* and the other coagulase-negative staphylococci have become the major

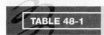 TABLE 48-1	Predispositions, Anatomic Sites, and Prominent Pathogens in Forms of Osteomyelitis		
Form of osteomyelitis	**Predisposing condition**	**Site**	**Prominent pathogens**
I. Hematogenous			
a. Childhood	None	Long bones	*Staphylococcus aureus*
		Multiple	Streptococci
			Haemophilus
	Sickle cell hemoglobinopathy		*Salmonella*
b. Adult	Urinary tract infection or instrumentation	Vertebrae	*S. aureus*
			GNB
			Streptococci
	Skin infection	Vertebrae	*S. aureus*
			Streptococci
	Respiratory infection	Vertebrae	Streptococci
			Mycobacterium tuberculosis
	Intravenous drug abuse or vascular catheters	Vertebrae	GNB
			Staphylococcus
			Candida
	AIDS	Multiple	Fungi
			Mycobacteria
	Endocarditis	Vertebral	Streptococci
			Staphylococcus
II. Introduced type	Fractures	Fracture site	*S. aureus*
			Staphylococcus epidermidis
			GNB
	Prosthetic joint	Prosthesis	*S. epidermidis*
			S. aureus
	Puncture wounds	Foot	*Pseudomonas aeruginosa,*
			S. aureus, anaerobes
III. Contiguous spread	Skin ulcer (e.g., diabetic, decubitus, stasis, and vasculitic)	Foot, leg	Polymicrobial
			–Staphylococci
			–Streptococci
			–GNB
			–Anaerobes
	Sinusitis	Skull	Streptococci
			Anaerobes
	Dental abscess	Mandible	Streptococci
		Maxilla	Anaerobes
	Human or animal bites	Hand	Streptococci
			Anaerobes
			Pasteurella multocida
	Felon	Finger	*S. aureus*
	Gardening	Hand	*Sporothrix*

AIDS, acquired immunodeficiency syndrome; GNB, gram-negative bacilli.
From Brause BD. Osteomyelitis. In: Bennett JC, Plum F. *Cecil-Loeb Textbook of Medicine.* 20th ed. Philadelphia, PA: WB Saunders; 1996:1625, with permission.

pathogens in bone infections associated with indwelling prosthetic materials and foreign bodies, such as joint replacement implants and fracture fixation devices, which are responsible for 30% of these cases. Streptococci, gram-negative bacilli, anaerobes, mycobacteria, and fungi are causative agents in a variety of clinical situations (see Table 48-1).

VI. CHRONIC OSTEOMYELITIS. Unsuccessful therapy for acute osteomyelitis results in relapse or chronic infection. Microorganisms persist in foci of gross or microscopic necrotic bone (sequestra) and intermittently invade surrounding tissues, causing the acute exacerbations of chronic osteomyelitis. Because of the avascular nature of sequestra, persistent pathogens are not eradicated by systemic antibiotics; however, local immune responses may control or eliminate the septic process. Recrudescent infection usually involves not only local tissue but may spread through the overlying soft tissue to produce a drainage tract or sinus that eventually reaches the skin surface, creating a cutaneous draining sinus orifice. The sinus commonly drains sporadically from an osseous origin (often at a site of necrotic bone, or sequestrum) and reflects the degree of active infection and inflammation in the bone. Rare complications of chronic osteomyelitis include squamous cell carcinoma in overlying draining sinus tracts and secondary amyloidosis.

CLINICAL MANIFESTATIONS

I. ACUTE HEMATOGENOUS OSTEOMYELITIS IN CHILDHOOD. Most children with acute hematogenous osteomyelitis show evidence of systemic illness—fever, chills, malaise, leukocytosis, and elevated erythrocyte sedimentation rate—along with local symptoms. Focal bone pain is a characteristic feature, with overlying erythema, warmth, and swelling variably seen. Limb motion may be limited by local pain (pseudoparalysis) when the infection is near an articulation. Adjacent joint effusions can occur but are usually sterile when the epiphyseal cartilage is intact.

II. ADULT HEMATOGENOUS OSTEOMYELITIS (INCLUDING VERTEBRAL OSTEOMYELITIS). Vertebral osteomyelitis most often presents subacutely with prominent back pain and spinal tenderness following urinary tract instrumentation or infection (30%), skin infection (13%), or respiratory infection (11%). In one-third of cases, the source of the bacteremia is unidentifiable. Fever is present in less than 50% of patients and is commonly low-grade. The infection can extend beyond the vertebral column and produce suppuration at the particular spinal level of involvement, such as a retropharyngeal abscess, mediastinitis, empyema, or subdiaphragmatic and iliopsoas abscesses, in addition to meningitis. **If paresis, sensory deficits, or bowel or bladder dysfunction develop, spinal epidural abscess, the most feared complication of vertebral osteomyelitis, should be considered and evaluated immediately.** Tuberculous infection should be considered in relatively indolent infections of the spine, hip, and knee.

III. INTRODUCED OSTEOMYELITIS. Osteomyelitis following trauma or bone surgery commonly presents with persistent or recurrent fever, increasing pain at the operative site, and poor wound healing. Incisional healing difficulties include protracted drainage, cellulitis, suture abscesses, wound hematomas or seromas, and dehiscence. Bone infection should also be considered as a potential cause of fracture nonunion and failed arthrodesis. Prosthetic joint infection is associated with joint pain (95%), fever (43%), or cutaneous sinus drainage (32%).

IV. OSTEOMYELITIS BY CONTIGUOUS SPREAD. Osseous involvement by spread of infection from an overlying chronic ischemic or neuropathic foot ulcer typically presents in patients with longstanding insulin-dependent diabetes mellitus or other vascular or neuropathic disease and involves the metatarsals (44%) or the proximal phalanges (32%). It is characterized by erythema (86%), swelling (75%), cellulitis, and necrosis, but pain is variable because of the frequent presence of sensory neuropathy (94%). Features correlated with the development of osteomyelitis in patients with such ulcers include the duration of unhealed ulceration (mean, 4 months), size of the ulcer (area ≥ 2 cm^2 and depth >3 mm), and the presence of exposed bone. Additional presentations of osteomyelitis caused by contiguous spread of infection are listed in Table 48-1.

V. CHRONIC OSTEOMYELITIS. Acute exacerbations of chronic osteomyelitis present with local bone pain and tenderness in the area of previous osseous involvement. Fever with focal swelling, erythema, and increased warmth may also occur. Purulent drainage through an old or new cutaneous sinus frequently develops and usually is accompanied by defervescence as the inflammatory process is decompressed.

DIAGNOSTIC INVESTIGATIONS

The diagnosis of osteomyelitis is based on the compilation of clinical observations (history and physical examination) and findings from well-chosen imaging studies, exercising sound clinical judgment to give appropriate weight to the data collected. It is essential to be mindful of the pathogenesis attributed to the specific clinical situation being evaluated. Establishing the presence of osteomyelitis includes both confirming the site of bone involvement and identifying the causative microorganism(s). Anatomic delineation of bone infection depends substantially on imaging techniques.

I.   IMAGING STUDIES

  A. Plain radiographs

   1. X-rays are the most specific and least expensive imaging technique for diagnosing osteomyelitis. The earliest osseous x-ray changes in hematogenous infection are medullary areas of lucency, which require 30% to 50% decalcification to be seen and take 2 to 4 weeks to develop. As sepsis progresses, periosteal elevation, thickening, and new bone formation may be seen, with sequestra and sclerosis occurring in chronic cases. Vertebral osteomyelitis appears initially as disc space narrowing with subsequent cortical degradation at the adjacent end plates. With the introduced form of osteomyelitis, bone resorption is evident at the site of the fracture, fixation device, or bone-cement interface of a joint prosthesis. When bone infection develops by spread from contiguous tissue, subperiosteal bone lucencies and cortical erosions are demonstrable and followed by lytic medullary lesions. When chronic deep ulcerations are overlying the bone, periosteal reaction reflects periosteal inflammation but is not diagnostic of bone infection.

   2. In patients with very acute, fulminant infection (such as childhood hematogenous osteomyelitis), x-rays may not be sufficiently sensitive to reveal diagnostic abnormalities at the time of presentation, and additional studies are needed. However, most cases of bone infection present subacutely, with adequate duration of infection for demineralization to occur, and can be well evaluated by radiologic techniques.

   3. There is commonly a delay in radiographic improvement during the healing phase of bone infection, and 30% of patients have worsening x-ray findings while they are improving clinically on therapy.

  B. Computed tomography (CT) scan can be useful in demonstrating small osseous changes, sequestra, and extraosseous extension of infection. It can be particularly helpful in evaluating the small bones of the foot in the presence of subluxation and other deformities.

  C. Magnetic resonance imaging (MRI) can detect osteomyelitis earlier and with a sensitivity equal to or greater than that of radiography, and its spatial resolution is much better than that of scintigraphy. Negative MRI findings are strong evidence against the presence of osteomyelitis. However, this technique is too nonspecific to be the optimal determinant for the presence of bone infection. An increased MRI signal represents small increases in tissue water content. Gadolinium is deposited in the extracellular fluid compartment in areas of increased vascular permeability and thereby increases the sensitivity of MRI for inflammation of all etiologies. MRI detects the bone edema of osteomyelitis; however, differentiation of nonspecific reactive marrow edema from the adjacent foci of infection or other causes of soft-tissue edema is often not possible. The specificity of MRI for osteomyelitis is significantly diminished because of false-positive results related to sterile inflammation, edema in tissues adjacent to bone, bone infarction, recent trauma, diabetic osteoarthropathy, heterotopic bone formation, neoplasm, and local radiation therapy (Table 48-2). A recently developed technique that uses fat suppression with MRI scans has increased the specificity, but not yet to the level needed for confidence.

  D. Radionuclide scans. Technetium diphosphonate bone scans, gallium citrate scans, and indium-labeled leukocyte scintigraphy are much more sensitive than plain

TABLE 48-2	Estimated Relative Value of Different Imaging Techniques for the Diagnosis of Osteomyelitis in Complicated Cases	
Imaging technique	**Sensitivity (%)**	**Specificity (%)**
X-ray	69	82
Technetium bone scan	77	36
Gallium scan	95	38
Indium-labeled WBC scan	74	69
Sequential indium and technetium scans	86	72
Magnetic resonance imaging	83	75

Complicated cases include patients with diabetes, neuropathic osteoarthropathy, cellulitis, and recent trauma (orthopedic surgery, fractures).
WBC, white blood cell.

x-rays and CT scans and usually demonstrate increased radionuclide uptake at the onset of symptoms. However, these imaging methods are plagued by inadequate specificity and spatial resolution, so they cannot be relied on to be definitively diagnostic. Inflammatory and degenerative processes in surrounding soft tissues, areas recently subjected to orthopedic surgery or trauma, bone fractures, and neoplasms produce abnormal findings on nuclide scans in the absence of osteomyelitis. Table 48-2 lists the approximate sensitivity and specificity of various imaging techniques in clinical situations in which the diagnosis is ambiguous because of the presence of a pathologic process in adjacent tissues (e.g., cellulitis and edema) or a comorbid state in the osseous tissue (e.g., diabetic osteoarthropathy, bone infarction, and recent trauma).

II. **MICROBIOLOGIC STUDIES.** The specific etiologic pathogen in osteomyelitis should be identified because the microbe that is assumed to be the causative infectious agent is never sufficiently predictable to allow routine presumptive therapy (see Table 48-1). Moreover, knowledge of the antimicrobial sensitivity of the isolated causative bacterium is essential to design optimal therapy. Blood cultures are positive in 25% to 50% of children with acute hematogenous osteomyelitis but in less than 10% of children with other forms of bone infection. If septic arthritis or soft-tissue abscess accompanies the osseous infection, arthrocentesis or abscess aspiration cultures can be diagnostic. However, superficial cultures of open wounds, wound drainage, or skin ulcerations and cultures of cutaneous sinus tracts do not delineate the true bone pathogen(s). Sinus tract and sinus drainage cultures often reflect colonizing flora and cannot be relied upon to identify the actual cause of the deep osseous infection. In patients with deep, chronic skin ulcers from which infection has spread to the bone, curettage cultures from the base of the ulcer have a 75% correlation with osseous tissue cultures. Bone aspirate cultures are positive in 50% to 60% of patients, whereas bone biopsy cultures are positive in 70% to 93% of cases. Bone biopsies should be sought (percutaneously or by operative debridement) when there is no overlying skin ulcer and the microbiologic etiology has not been otherwise determined. Specific cultures for mycobacteria, fungi, and anaerobes should be considered when routine bacterial cultures are negative.

III. **GUIDELINES FOR DIAGNOSING OSTEOMYELITIS (BASED ON PATHOGENESIS)**
  A. **Childhood acute hematogenous osteomyelitis**
   1. Plain x-rays of the suspect bone. CT scans if additional detail is needed.
   2. Technetium bone scan, if the radiographs are not diagnostic.
   3. MRI with gadolinium if radiographs and technetium bone scan are not diagnostic but clinical suspicion is strong.
   4. Blood cultures.
   5. Bone biopsy for cultures and histopathology.

B. Adult acute hematogenous osteomyelitis (vertebral osteomyelitis)
1. Plain x-rays of the suspect bones. CT scans if additional detail is needed.
2. MRI with gadolinium if radiographs are not diagnostic.
3. Blood cultures.
4. Bone biopsy for cultures and histopathology.

C. Introduced form of osteomyelitis
1. Plain x-rays of the suspect bones. CT scans if additional detail is needed. Serial x-rays or CT scans at intervals during a 4-week period to observe any meaningful osseous changes.
2. Arthrocentesis (if a prosthetic joint is present) for cultures.
3. Bone biopsy, usually with debridement surgery, for cultures.

D. Osteomyelitis caused by contiguous spread of infection
1. Plain x-rays of the suspect bones. CT scans if additional detail is needed. Serial x-rays or CT scans at intervals during a 4-week period to observe any meaningful osseous changes.
2. Indium-labeled–leukocyte scan (or sequential indium or technetium scan) if suspicion for osteomyelitis is low, specifically for the negative predictive value of the scan. A positive scan result is not as diagnostic or as meaningful as osseous changes on serial x-rays.
3. MRI with gadolinium and fat suppression if clinical suspicion is strong.
4. The base of soft-tissue ulcer is cultured before starting antibiotic therapy. The ulcer base is prepared with iodine, then alcohol (allowing alcohol to evaporate). The ulcer base is abraded with a culture swab or a curettage to obtain culture material.
5. Percutaneous bone biopsy is avoided if possible because (a) this trauma may induce bone necrosis and infection, (b) the histopathology of neuropathic osteopathy may resemble that of osteomyelitis, and (c) the bone biopsy specimen can be contaminated with organisms from the contiguous infected soft tissue.
6. If soft-tissue infection is present, it is treated with antibiotics and serial radiographs are obtained with the patient off antibiotic therapy at intervals during a 4-week period to determine subsequently the presence or absence of osteomyelitis.

E. Chronic osteomyelitis
1. Plain x-rays of the suspect bone.
2. CT scan or MRI to delineate sequestra.
3. Sinogram (radiographs with dye inserted into a cutaneous sinus tract) to demonstrate the osseous site of sinus tract origin, which often is the site of sequestrum. (Note: Sinus tract cultures are not reliable for delineating the true etiologic pathogen.)
4. Bone biopsy (percutaneously or at debridement surgery) for cultures and histopathology.

DIFFERENTIAL DIAGNOSIS

Osseous infection should be differentiated from septic arthritis and bursitis, cellulitis, soft-tissue abscesses, SAPHO (synovitis, acne, plantar pustulosis, hyperostosis, and osteitis), bone fractures, neoplasms, and from bone infarcts seen with sickle cell hemoglobinopathy and Gaucher's disease.

TREATMENT

I. ANTIBIOTICS
A. Acute osteomyelitis is curable with adequate antimicrobial therapy accompanied by surgical debridement when necessary. Intravenous antibiotics are commonly used, but oral agents are also effective when the quantitative susceptibility of the pathogen is sufficient and when gastrointestinal absorption and compliance are

ensured. The exact potency and duration of treatment necessary to eradicate bone infections are not known. Antimicrobial agents that produce trough serum bactericidal activity at a 1:2 titer have been associated with highly successful outcomes. Therapy should be administered for at least 4 to 6 weeks. Designing a therapeutic regimen for osteomyelitis depends substantially on the sensitivity of the isolated pathogen to specific antimicrobial agents, which underscores the essential importance of identifying the pathogen in these infections.

B. Chronic osteomyelitis is treatable but not curable with systemic antibiotics. Acute exacerbations of these persistent infections can be suppressed successfully by debridement of identifiable sequestra followed by protracted courses of parenteral or oral antimicrobial agents. Theoretically, depot administration of appropriate antibiotics by diffusion into the site of infected, avascular bone via antibiotic-loaded polymethylmethacrylate beads could eradicate the persistent bacteria unreachable by systemic (blood vessel–dependent) therapy.

II. **SURGERY.** When acute osteomyelitis is complicated by abscess formation or extensive necrosis, surgical debridement is an important adjunct to antibiotics. In cases associated with prosthetic joints or internal fixation devices, the foreign body usually needs to be removed to effect a cure. In chronic osteomyelitis, surgery is often the primary therapeutic treatment. Necrotic tissue and sequestra should be removed when possible, and dead spaces should be eliminated with packing, bone grafts, muscle pedicles, or skin grafts. Surgery is also important when neurologic structures are threatened (e.g., cord compression in vertebral osteomyelitis). In osteomyelitis associated with peripheral vascular disease, revascularization should be considered. Amputation of the affected area is frequently required if the infection does not respond to parenteral antibiotics.

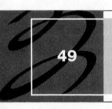

RHEUMATIC FEVER
49
Allan Gibofsky and John B. Zabriskie

■ KEY POINTS

■ Acute rheumatic fever (ARF) is a systemic rheumatic disease that occurs in a genetically susceptible individual following streptococcal pharyngitis.

■ The streptococcal pharyngitis that causes acute rheumatic fever may be so mild that it is not recalled by the patient or parent.

■ The recent reports of ARF in the United States suggest that the Jones's Criteria should now be used more widely to prevent the underdiagnosis of this condition.

*A*cute rheumatic fever (ARF) is the term used to describe a systemic rheumatic disease manifested clinically by a constellation of inflammatory tissue responses following pharyngeal streptococcal infection.

ETIOPATHOGENESIS

I. **The disease occurs as a sequela to streptococcal pharyngitis,** and the latent period between the period of infection and the onset of disease varies from 2 to 6 weeks or longer. ARF is almost exclusively associated with the group A strains that cause pharyngitis, and rarely, if ever, follows infections that cause impetigo or kidney disease.

II. **The available evidence suggests that the abnormal immune response** of the host to streptococcal antigens cross-reactive with target mammalian antigens, at both cellular and humoral level, is responsible for the pathologic damage. These cross-reactive antigens include the hyaluronic capsule of the streptococcus and a number of streptococcal antigens, including M proteins that share antigenic determinants with cardiac tropomyosin and myosin. Similar molecular mimicry appears to play a role in the pathology found in the kidney, central nervous system, and skin.

III. **A genetic basis for the disease has been suggested** for more than 100 years, and family studies indicate that gene inheritance is either autosomal recessive or dominant with limited penetrance.

PREVALENCE

I. **Both the prevalence and severity of rheumatic fever have declined dramatically** during the last six decades in the United States and other developed countries; however, a resurgence in new and recurrent cases deserves renewed attention. Changes in living conditions, nutrition, and virulence of the organism, in addition to antibiotic therapy for streptococcal pharyngitis, have all been suggested as reasons for the decreased incidence.

II. **The overall incidence of rheumatic fever in the United States is currently estimated to be less than 1 in 100,000 children of school age/year,** but groups with poor standards of living have a much higher incidence. In some developing nations, the incidence of rheumatic fever remains high: 60 in 100,000 children (aged between 5 and 14 years)/year or more.

III. **Rheumatic heart disease,** a chronic sequela of rheumatic fever, is the most common cause of heart disease in individuals younger than 40 years in these countries. Rheumatic fever therefore represents a significant worldwide health problem.

CLINICAL MANIFESTATIONS

I. **Antecedent streptococcal pharyngitis** most commonly occurs 2 to 3 weeks before the onset of the symptoms of rheumatic fever. It may be mild, however, and a history of fever and sore throat cannot be elicited in all patients.

II. **Fever,** which has no specific pattern, is almost always present at the onset of an acute attack and fades away in days to weeks without anti-inflammatory treatment. Fever resolves promptly with salicylate therapy.

III. **Arthritis** with fever is the most common manifestation of ARF, occurring in 50% to 75% of cases. It usually involves the large peripheral joints, especially the knees and ankles, but any joint may be affected. Arthritis, which occurs within 5 weeks of the streptococcal infection (when antistreptococcal antibody titers are usually high), subsides without treatment in a few weeks and very rarely causes joint deformity. Carditis occurs less frequently in cases with severe arthritis.

IV. **Arthralgia** without objective evidence of joint inflammation may precede the development of synovitis. Severe arthralgia, especially if migratory, is an important diagnostic feature.

V. **Carditis** is the most important manifestation of ARF because it frequently leads to chronic valvular damage. In rare cases, it is a cause of death from cardiac failure or arrhythmias associated with myocarditis during an acute episode. Carditis occurs in 40% to 50% of attacks of ARF in some series, but this incidence seems to be decreasing.

   A. **Chest pain or dyspnea** may occur with ARF, but these complaints are often non-specific and are thought to be musculoskeletal in origin.

   B. **Major signs**

   1. **Significant new or changing murmurs,** described in the subsequent text, are characteristic of acute valvulitis and differ from the murmurs of valvular stenosis or regurgitation that may be heard later. They often disappear with resolution of acute inflammation.

      a. **Mitral valvulitis murmur** is blowing, high-pitched, holosystolic, and apical and transmits to the axilla. It must be distinguished from the click/murmur of the mitral valve prolapse syndrome, which has a mid-systolic click and late systolic murmur.

     b. Carey Coombs' murmur is mid-diastolic, low-pitched, and apical and often associated with the mitral valvulitis. It is best heard with the patient in the left lateral recumbent position and should be distinguished from the murmur of mitral stenosis.

     c. Aortic valvulitis murmur is a soft, high-pitched, decrescendo blow, heard immediately after the second heart sound, along the left sternal border, auscultated with the patient leaning forward. It must be distinguished from the murmur of a congenital bicuspid aortic valve.

  2. Cardiomegaly should be carefully monitored by physical examination and serial chest x-rays.

  3. Congestive heart failure occurs more commonly in children younger than 6 years and in patients without severe arthritis.

  4. Pericarditis, when present, usually occurs in association with other features of rheumatic carditis. Pericarditis may be manifested as chest pain, friction rub, effusions, and electrocardiographic changes. Large effusions are rare.

  5. Other cardiac findings may include tachycardia at rest (out of proportion to fever) and a soft, dull, variable first heart sound secondary to a prolonged PR interval. Atrioventricular block is commonly seen in cases of ARF without other evidence of carditis or subsequent idiopathic heart disease. It is thought to be a toxic manifestation of ARF and is not specifically indicative of carditis.

VI. Erythema marginatum, a rare manifestation of ARF, is a nonpruritic rash that begins as a pink macule and spreads outward in a sharp ring with central clearing or as serpiginous coalescing lines. The rash is evanescent and rarely raised, blanches with pressure, is brought out by application of heat, and is distributed over the trunk and proximal extremities, never on the face, and rarely on the distal extremities. The rash may appear at any time in the course of ARF. Its appearance and resolution are unrelated to the course of other manifestations or to treatment. Rash secondary to drug reaction or systemic juvenile idiopathic arthritis can usually be differentiated by the characteristics just mentioned and other associated clinical manifestations.

VII. Subcutaneous nodules are firm, nontender, nonpruritic, freely movable swellings located in crops of variable numbers over bony prominences and tendons, without overlying skin discoloration. They are smaller and less persistent than those of rheumatoid arthritis. Nodules are a late and infrequent manifestation associated with severe carditis.

VIII. Sydenham's chorea is a late manifestation of ARF and may follow other manifestations of ARF or may appear alone. It is characterized by involuntary, purposeless, abrupt, and nonrepetitive movements, muscular weakness, and emotional lability. The abnormal movements subside during sleep.

  A. When subtle, chorea is demonstrated in the following instances: squeezing the examiner's hand reveals an erratic "milkmaid's grip"; raising the hand straight ahead causes pronation of one or both arms; extending the hands straight ahead causes spooning of the hand with wrist flexion and extension of fingers; and protruding the tongue produces snakelike darting movements.

  B. Because the latent period from streptococcal infection to chorea is 1 to 6 months, antistreptolysin O (ASO) titers and levels of acute-phase reactants may be normal. Investigation of other streptococcal antigens usually will reveal antibodies to one or more with rising titers in all but those patients with isolated chorea.

  C. The duration of chorea ranges from 1 week to 1 year, with an average of 3 months. Some patients with Sydenham's chorea have an antibody that reacts with basal ganglia and cross-reacts with streptococcal cell membranes. Sydenham's chorea must be distinguished from other neurologic entities, including Huntington's chorea, central nervous system lupus, Wilson's disease, and toxic drug reactions (especially to the phenothiazine).

IX. Poststreptococcal reactive arthritis. Cases have been reported of adults who develop a migratory polyarthritis following a documented streptococcal infection, sometimes followed by carditis. There is some controversy as to whether these patients have true rheumatic fever or an incomplete form or its variant.

TABLE 49-1	Jones's Criteria (Revised) for Guidance in the Diagnosis of Rheumatic Fever

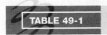

Major criteria	Minor criteria
Carditis	Clinical
Polyarthritis	Fever
Chorea	Arthralgia
Erythema marginatum	Previous rheumatic fever
Subcutaneous nodules	Previous rheumatic fever with heart disease
	Laboratory
	Increased ESR or CRP levels
	Prolonged PR interval

Supporting evidence of preceding streptococcal infection: increased ASO or other streptococcal antibodies, positive throat culture for group A streptococci, or recent scarlet fever.
ASO, antistreptolysin O; CRP, C-reactive protein; ESR, erythrocyte sedimentation rate.
Adapted from special report: Jones's criteria (revised) for guidance in the diagnosis of rheumatic fever. *Circulation* 1984;69:204A.

 DIAGNOSTIC INVESTIGATIONS

The revised Jones's criteria (Table 49-1) indicates a high probability of ARF when evidence of a preceding streptococcal infection is found simultaneously with the presence of two major criteria; a diagnosis of ARF based on the presence of one major criterion and two minor criteria is less definitive. The Jones's criteria were developed to provide uniformity and to minimize the overdiagnosis of ARF.

 LABORATORY TESTS

I. **Evidence of preceding streptococcal infection** may be obtained by throat cultures (positive in approximately 25% of cases), and it is recommended that **at least two** cultures be taken to confirm the infection. ASO antibodies are elevated in approximately 80% of cases, and serial serum samples should be drawn during the acute stage and 2 weeks later. Testing for antihyaluronidase, deoxyribonuclease B, and streptozyme titers increases the precision of the documentation of a preceding streptococcal infection to 97%.

II. **Acute-phase reactants,** such as C-reactive protein, and the erythrocyte sedimentation rate (ESR) reflect ongoing inflammation and are useful in monitoring response to therapy. It would be quite uncommon for a patient with ARF to have a normal ESR study.

III. **Antiheart antibodies** that cross-react with streptococcal cell membranes are found in sera of patients with ARF, but the test has not been standardized for routine use.

IV. **Serial chest x-rays** are important to reveal cardiomegaly as a sign of carditis.

V. **Serial electrocardiograms** may reveal the nonspecific atrioventricular block or changes of myocarditis and pericarditis.

VI. **Echocardiography** is useful in differentiating patients with bicuspid aortic valves or mitral prolapse syndrome from those with rheumatic heart disease. It may also be used to evaluate pericardial effusion and myocardial function.

 DIFFERENTIAL DIAGNOSIS

I. **Bacterial infections,** including septic arthritis, osteomyelitis, and subacute bacterial endocarditis, should be ruled out by appropriate culture. Lyme disease should be considered, especially in areas where it is endemic.

II. **Viral infections,** particularly rubella arthritis, arthritis associated with hepatitis B infection, arthritis associated with parvovirus B19, and infectious mononucleosis should be considered.

III. **Collagen vascular disease,** including rheumatoid arthritis, systemic lupus erythematosus, and vasculitis such as Henoch-Schönlein purpura may be differentiated on clinical and laboratory grounds.

IV. **Immune complex disease** induced by an allergic reaction to drugs may be suggested by history and by clinical features such as pruritic or urticarial rash.

V. **Sickle cell hemoglobinopathies** may superficially resemble ARF but are not difficult to differentiate.

VI. **Malignancies,** especially leukemias and lymphomas, can present with fever and acute polyarthritis.

VII. **Mucocutaneous lymph node syndrome (Kawasaki's disease)** may initially resemble ARF, but the desquamating rash and absence of rising ASO titers should make differentiation possible.

 TREATMENT

I. **Antibiotic treatment** with penicillin, or erythromycin in case of penicillin allergy, is recommended for all patients in a standard 10-day course for streptococcal pharyngitis, to eradicate residual organisms. There is, however, no evidence that such therapy significantly alters the acute or chronic phase of the disease. Penicillin prophylaxis is begun after the 10-day course of treatment to reduce the risk for recurrence of the disease.

II. **Prophylaxis** with penicillin G (250,000 U orally twice daily) or penicillin benzathine (1.2 million U intramuscular every 4 weeks) clearly reduces the chance of recurrent rheumatic fever and progressive cardiac damage.

    A. In areas where high exposure to streptococci is expected and in all cases of valvular damage, the injections should be given every 3 weeks. Alternatively, the injection is given every 4 weeks with supplemental oral penicillin dosing during the last 10 days of each month. With penicillin VK (250 mg orally twice daily) in the place of penicillin G, absorption from the intestinal tract is improved and is more reliable.

    B. Penicillin benzathine prophylaxis has the advantage of ensured compliance, but cases of recurrent rheumatic fever have occasionally been reported, probably as a consequence of individual variations in the pharmacokinetics of the drug.

    C. Patients who are allergic to penicillin may be treated with 250 mg of erythromycin twice daily. The minimum recommended duration of prophylaxis is 5 years from the last recurrence because recurrences are most common during this period. Recurrent attacks in adulthood have been reported, however, and as long-term prophylaxis appears to be benign, it is advisable to continue prophylaxis indefinitely. All patients with evidence of chronic rheumatic heart disease, regardless of age, should be on continuous prophylaxis because recurrent disease usually includes carditis.

III. **Anti-inflammatory** treatment provides symptomatic relief but does not appear to alter the duration of the attack or cardiac sequelae.

    A. **Analgesics** for the management of joint pains are helpful, especially while diagnostic evaluation is in progress and before anti-inflammatory treatment is started.

    B. **Salicylates** are highly effective in controlling fever and arthritis but should not be used before an adequate period of observation allows a firm diagnosis to be established. A dosage of about 80 mg/kg/day in four divided doses, with a resultant blood level of 20 to 30 mg/dL, is usually effective in controlling fever, arthritis, and mild carditis when given for 2 weeks, followed by a dosage of approximately 60 mg/kg/day for 6 subsequent weeks.

    C. **Corticosteroids** have not been shown to be more effective than aspirin in reducing long-term cardiac damage. Nevertheless, they are often used to treat carditis, especially when congestive failure is present. Prednisone (1 to 2 mg/kg/day in divided doses) is used for 2 to 4 weeks. Salicylates are often added for an additional 4 to 8 weeks.

IV. **CARDIAC MEDICATIONS.** Sodium restriction, digitalis, and diuretics for heart failure may be helpful. Digitalis should be used with caution, as myocarditis is almost invariably present.

V. **Treatment of chorea** includes keeping the patient in a quiet, protective environment and sedating with phenobarbital, diazepam, or chlorpromazine as indicated. Valproic acid and haloperidol appear to be useful in reducing the severity of choreiform movements.

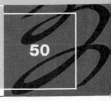

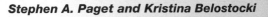

■ KEY POINTS

■ Whipple's disease (WD) is a rare multisystem syndrome caused by the gram-positive actinomycete *Tropheryma whippelii*.

■ The clinical manifestations of WD include insidious onset of fever, arthritis, malabsorption, generalized lymphadenopathy, skin hyperpigmentation, uveitis, or progressive encephalopathy and symmetric, transient, and nondeforming polyarthritis.

■ Diagnosis is based on recognition of the characteristic clinical picture in addition to typical histologic findings on duodenal or jejunal biopsy and perhaps by polymerase chain reaction (PCR) analysis of tissue or fluid.

■ Treatment with parenteral antibiotics (penicillin G and streptomycin) followed by oral trimethoprim/sulfamethoxazole is recommended.

■ Relapses commonly occur months to years after the initial presentation and usually respond to the same antibiotic that initially induced remission.

$\mathcal{W}$hipple's disease (WD) is a rare multisystem syndrome caused by the gram-positive actinomycete *Tropheryma whippelii*. It was first described in 1907 when George Whipple reported the case of a 36-year-old physician who died after hospitalization for weakness, fever, cough, abdominal pain, diarrhea, weight loss, arthralgias, hypotension, hyperpigmentation, and anemia. At autopsy, enlarged mesenteric and retroperitoneal lymph nodes with cystic fatty changes were found, and Whipple called the disease intestinal lipodystrophy.

The diverse clinical manifestations of WD reflect the systemic nature of the infection caused by *T. whippelii*. Nearly every organ system can be involved and WD can march through many different clinical phases, with multiple misdiagnoses and their attendant inappropriate therapies.

ETIOPATHOGENESIS

I. **The bacterium *T. whippelii*,** a member of the actinomycetes group, has been found in a variety of cell types and organs in patients with WD and shown to be the causative organism. It has also been detected in various body fluids including cerebrospinal fluid.

II. **The pathogenesis** of WD is not well understood.
    A. Immune defects involving T cells and macrophages have been described.
    B. Reduced levels of interleukin-12 and interferon-γ production have been detected in patients with WD. These cytokines may be important because of their ability to contain and clear intracellular bacteria, and could explain the longstanding infection and the presence of the organism in macrophages for years in patients with WD.

PREVALENCE

WD is rare, with the frequency of the disease less than 0.1% in postmortem studies. It is seen primarily in white men (male to female ratio is 10 to 1).

T. whippelii may be an environmental agent present in water, with a possible oral infectious route of the bacillus. It could therefore be present in a larger portion of the population in the absence of clinical WD, possibly as an oral commensal organism. Studies utilizing polymerase chain reaction (PCR) technology have demonstrated the presence of *T. whippelii* in 5% to 35% of diseasefree individuals.

CLINICAL MANIFESTATIONS

I. The course of WD often includes a **prodromal or collagen vascular/immune phase** in which the cardinal features are intermittent and can occur over many years: arthritis, abdominal pain and bloating, diarrhea, cough, weight loss, and asthenia. The arthritis can occur 10 to 20 years **before** the telltale malabsorption diarrhea occurs. Lymphadenopathy and hyperpigmentation are frequently found on physical examination.

    A. Musculoskeletal. The joint manifestations of WD may precede the diagnosis by many years. Migratory and nondeforming arthralgias and arthritis can be accompanied by sacroiliitis and spondylitis. A rheumatoid arthritislike symmetrical presentation can also be seen. Synovial fluid is inflammatory, at times showing periodic acid-Schiff's (PAS) positive macrophages, with a negative culture for routine bacteria. Synovial biopsies reveal a mild, nonspecific synovitis with hyperplasia of the synovial lining cells and increased vascularity.

    B. Neurologic. Neurologic manifestations can vary over time and may dominate the disorder in some patients. Up to 5% of patients with WD can have a neurologic presentation with the disease confined to the nervous system for the bulk of the disease course. Abnormalities include: headaches, personality disorders, alteration in consciousness, encephalopathy, disturbances of ocular movements, clonic movements, spastic paresis, dementia, posterior column disease, and microinfarcts in the brain.

II. The next phase is the **period of decline or the gastrointestinal phase** in which the evolving and cumulative manifestations lead to progressive organ dysfunction. Patients present with an addisonian-type disorder, severe gastrointestinal problems, cardiac abnormalities, pleuropulmonary signs and symptoms, fevers, or even sudden death.

    A. Up to 15% of patients do not have gastrointestinal symptoms throughout their illness.

    B. Cardiovascular manifestations are reported in 20% to 55% of patients with WD. Pericarditis, endocarditis, myocarditis, coronary arteritis, congestive heart failure, and sudden death have been reported.

    C. Less common (atypical) clinical features include: granulomatous disease of the liver, pulmonary artery involvement with pulmonary hypertension, inflammatory eye disease, gastrointestinal hemorrhage, and testicular and prostatic inflammation and pain.

DIAGNOSTIC INVESTIGATIONS

I. **Nonspecific laboratory findings** include elevated acute phase reactants (erythrocyte sedimentation rate and C-reactive protein), anemia, leukocytosis or leukopenia, and occasionally eosinophilia.

II. **BIOPSY.** Confirmation of clinically suspected WD is based on the presence of characteristic histology on biopsy.

    A. In classic WD, endoscopic duodenal or jejunal biopsy demonstrates PAS-positive macrophages.

    B. These PAS-positive cells have also been detected in colon, stomach, esophagus, gall bladder, liver, pancreas, spleen, heart, lungs, kidneys, central nervous system (CNS), blood vessels, and joints.

III. **PCR.** A specific diagnosis can now be made from tissue or peripheral blood with use of PCR to verify the presence of the causative microorganism.

    This technology can be particularly helpful in confirming the diagnosis and perhaps to define disease activity or response to treatment. Although highly sensitive, an important limit of PCR is its specificity. Caution is advised in interpreting PCR results without histologic confirmation.

IV. **CULTURE.** *T. whippelii* can be cultured from tissue of affected individuals. Specific antibodies can also be used in the immunodetection of microorganisms in tissue.

DIFFERENTIAL DIAGNOSIS

The protean clinical manifestations of WD can cause diagnostic confusion as signs and symptoms of WD frequently overlap with those of other disorders.

WD may be confused with malignancy, collagen vascular disease, sarcoidosis, Addison's disease, tuberculosis, viral infections (such as human immunodeficiency virus, hepatitis B virus, hepatitis C virus, and parvovirus B19), or Crohn's disease.

TREATMENT

I.   **Parenteral antibiotic therapy with penicillin G** (1.2 million U/day) and streptomycin (1 g/day) is recommended for the first 2 weeks, followed by oral trimethoprim/sulfamethoxazole (160/800 mg twice daily) for 1 to 2 years.

II. **Agents that do not cross the blood-brain barrier should be avoided** because organisms sequestered in the CNS may lead to disease relapse.

III. **It takes approximately 3 to 4 weeks for a clinical response** as well as eradication of the organism from the affected tissues.

IV. **PCR may be helpful in monitoring treatment response,** thereby providing a more rational approach to treatment decisions such as antibiotic selection and duration of treatment. Clinical signs and symptoms of active disease are useful guides to defining the length of antibiotic treatment.

V.   **With the ability to culture** *T. whippelii*, tests for antimicrobial susceptibility will ultimately allow for a more tailored therapeutic approach.

PROGNOSIS

I.   **Relapses can occur months to years after the initial presentation** and usually respond to the same antibiotic that initially induced remission.

II. **Some patients, particularly those with CNS disease, may be refractory to a broad range of antibiotics.** In such situations, alternative treatments such as interferon-γ have been employed.

III. **A persistently positive PCR for *T. whippelii* despite appropriate therapy** is thought to be predictive of a poor clinical outcome.

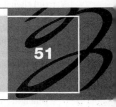

OSTEOARTHRITIS

51

John F. Beary, III and Michael E. Luggen

▮ KEY POINTS

▪ Osteoarthritis (OA) is the most common musculoskeletal problem in patients older than 50 years, and affects 21 million Americans.

▪ OA is a disease that involves all tissues of the joint organ, and is characterized by focal degeneration of joint cartilage and by new bone formation/osteophytes.

▪ Risk factors for OA include aging, increased joint loading from obesity, muscle weakness (e.g., quadriceps weakness in knee OA), and lower limb alignment abnormalities (e.g., varus/valgus deformities).

- Most subjects older than 55 years will have radiographic signs of OA at some locations in their skeletal system. However, many of these radiographic OA sites are asymptomatic, and some of them are only intermittently symptomatic.

- There are no commonly available clinical laboratory tests useful in the diagnosis or routine management of OA. If an elevated C-reactive protein (CRP), abnormal hematology profile, high titer rheumatoid factor (RF), or abnormal clinical chemistry tests are obtained, consideration should be given to diagnoses other than OA.

- Treatment of OA is symptomatic using nonpharmacologic modalities and analgesics/anti-inflammatories. There are currently no structure-modifying OA drugs (SMOADs) approved by the Food and Drug Administration (FDA).

- When a knee joint or hip joint fails due to OA disease, total joint prosthetic surgery is very successful when performed by an experienced surgeon who does a high volume of procedures. A prosthetic knee or hip joint can be expected to last 20 years or so as long as the patient uses it sensibly.

O**steoarthritis (OA) is the most common musculoskeletal problem in individuals older than 50 years.** It is characterized by **focal degeneration** of joint cartilage and **formation of new bone** in the form of osteophytes at the base of the cartilage lesion in the subchondral bone and at the joint margins. **During the past two decades, OA has come to be viewed as a disease involving the entire joint organ** (bone, cartilage, and supporting elements) rather than as primarily a problem of the cartilage alone. Although it may be initiated by multiple factors, including genetic, developmental, metabolic, and traumatic causes, OA involves all tissues of the diarthrodial joint.

OA is the result of both mechanical and biologic events that destabilize the normal coupling of degradation and synthesis of articular cartilage and subchondral bone. Ultimately, OA is manifested by morphologic, biochemical, molecular, and biomechanical changes of both cells and matrix.

 ## PREVALENCE

I. **Primary OA is the most common form of arthritis in North America and Western Europe and affects 21 million Americans.** The natural history of the disease takes approximately 20 years to be expressed; therefore, most patients are older than 60 years. OA results in 68 million lost workdays/year and 4 million hospitalizations/year. Approximately 100,000 patients in the United States are unable to walk from their bed to the bathroom because of OA. OA of the knee is the second leading cause of disability, following heart disease, in older individuals.

II. **Radiographic surveys reveal that most subjects older than 55 years have radiographically defined disease.** It must be emphasized, however, that most radiographically defined OA is not symptomatic.

III. **Women older than 55 years are affected by OA more than are men.** From the ages of 40 to 55, there is little difference in the prevalence of OA between men and women. Studies of ethnic groups in the United States reveal that African American women are more likely to get knee OA than are whites.

 ## ETIOPATHOGENESIS

I. **PRIMARY OA.** The forces exerted on the normal joint by motion and weight-bearing are dissipated by joint cartilage, subchondral bone, and surrounding structures (joint capsule and muscle). Joint cartilage has unique properties of compressibility and elasticity, attributable to the presence of an intertwined mesh of both collagen and proteoglycan (PG). Cartilage collagen is type II collagen and forms a three-dimensional network of cross-linked fibers that create the structural framework for cartilage. PGs are large molecules that individually consist of a protein core with negatively charged glycosaminoglycan side chains composed of keratan sulfate and chondroitin sulfate.

PGs exist mostly as aggregates and are attached as side chains by a link protein to a core of hyaluronic acid. The PGs bind large amounts of water molecules, which are released when the cartilage is compressed, and recaptured when compression is removed. The primary PG of articular cartilage is termed aggrecan and gives cartilage the ability to undergo reversible deformations.

Primary OA is a multifactorial disease process that involves the joint constituents (chondrocytes, collagen, PGs, subchondral bone, and synovial membrane) in various ways. Although a precise pathogenesis has not been elucidated, the following factors are germane to the development of primary OA:

A. Aging bone and cartilage. The ability of articular cartilage to withstand fatigue testing diminishes progressively with age. No specific biochemical defect of aging cartilage has yet been identified. However, abnormalities of aging human chondrocytes include decreased cell division and decreased mean telomere length, consistent with chondrocyte senescence.

B. Mechanical factors (wear and tear)
1. **Accumulated microtrauma** causes changes in subchondral bone, which is likely to affect the ability of a joint to absorb the forces associated with constant loading, thereby leading to degeneration of cartilage. This factor may account for occupational OA, such as that seen in the metacarpophalangeal (MCP) and shoulder joints of boxers, elbows of jackhammer operators, knees of basketball players, ankles of ballet dancers, and spines of coal miners.
2. **Lower limb alignment.** Varus knee deformities have been shown to be a risk factor for the development of OA in the medial compartment of the knee. Abnormal joint stresses lead to activation of cartilage-damaging enzymes. This has important therapeutic significance, because the re-establishment of joint alignment and mechanics to as near normal as possible, along with decreased trauma to the weight-bearing joints due to decrease in body weight, can have profound positive effects.

C. Genetic factors. It is known that factors such as the collagen content of cartilage and the ability of chondrocytes to synthesize PGs are genetically determined. Polymorphisms of the type II collagen gene have been identified in several families affected with premature OA. It is likely that changes in the amino acid composition of type II collagen make the collagen less able to handle mechanical stresses, and more susceptible to proteolytic degradation that is set up by abnormal joint stresses.

D. Biochemical factors. The principal early change in cartilage affected by OA is a decreased content of PGs, with collagen content remaining normal. The loss of PGs causes biomechanical problems, such as a loss of compressive stiffness in the cartilage, decreased elasticity, and an increase in hydraulic permeability. Later, collagen unravels and is lost because of increased enzyme activity in the form of matrix metalloproteinase.

II. SECONDARY OA: PATHOGENESIS. Disorders that damage joint surfaces and cause cartilage changes characteristic of OA include the following:

A. Mechanical incongruity of the joint
1. **Congenital, genetic, and developmental disorders** such as hip dysplasia, slipped femoral capital epiphysis, multiple epiphyseal dysplasia, Marfan's syndrome, and Ehlers-Danlos syndrome.
2. **Prior joint trauma.**
3. **Prior joint surgery,** such as meniscectomy.

B. Prior joint-damaging, inflammatory joint disease such as rheumatoid arthritis (RA) or infectious arthritis.

C. Prior bone disease, such as Paget's disease or osteonecrosis.

D. Bleeding dyscrasias. Hemarthrosis affects 90% of patients with hemophilia, most commonly in the knee, ankle, and elbow. With recurrent hemarthrosis, a proliferative synovitis occurs, which promotes development of secondary OA.

E. Neuropathic joint disease. Loss of pain or proprioceptive sensation leads to decreased joint protection and subsequent secondary OA. Examples of diseases responsible for the development of neuropathic arthropathy include diabetes, syphilis, pernicious anemia, spinal cord trauma, and peripheral nerve injury. Radiographic findings reveal the most severe and extensive forms of OA changes with loss of cartilage, exuberant osteophyte formation, bizarre bony overgrowth, fragmentation of subchondral bone with pathologic fractures, and eventual disintegration of the joint structure.

F. Excessive intra-articular steroid injections. Judicious use of steroid injections is helpful in the management of OA. However, injecting a joint more than four times in 1 year could lead to damage. For example, although intra-articular injection relieves knee pain in football players, it could also mask pain that has a protective function and lead to overuse of an already damaged joint, thereby leading to premature knee OA.

G. Endocrinopathies and metabolic disorders (see Chapters 43, 44, and 55)
  1. **Acromegaly.**
  2. **Cushing's disease** and long-term corticosteroid therapy through the mechanism of osteonecrosis. Corticosteroids inhibit osteoblast function and may also cause a secondary hyperparathyroidism, which activates osteoclasts and so accelerates subchondral bone damage.
  3. **Crystal arthropathies.** Calcium pyrophosphate dihydrate deposition (CPPD) disease is strongly associated with OA. Basic calcium phosphate crystals play a key role in the destructive arthropathy of large joints, known as the Milwaukee's shoulder syndrome.
  4. **Gout.**
  5. **Ochronosis.** These patients lack homogentisic acid oxidase, which results in increased urinary excretion of homogentisic acid and increased binding of homogentisic acid to connective tissue. The latter presumably is responsible for the secondary OA seen in this disorder. The pigment is deposited in cartilage, skin, and sclera. Degenerative disease of the spine with calcification of the intervertebral discs is characteristic.
  6. **Wilson's disease.** Premature OA, pseudogout, and chondromalacia patellae are articular manifestations of this disorder involving copper metabolism.
  7. **Hemochromatosis.** Hemosiderin granules are deposited in cartilage. CPPD crystals are also associated with this disease. The arthropathy of hemochromatosis characteristically involves the second and third MCP joints.

PATHOLOGY OF OSTEOARTHRITIS

Various features are seen in cartilage, bone, and other tissues as the disease progresses and include the following:

I. **STRUCTURAL BREAKDOWN OF CARTILAGE.** In the order of progression, this process consists of the following: (a) superficial fibrillation and fissuring; (b) focal and diffuse erosions of the cartilage surface; and (c) thinning and complete denudation of cartilage.

II. **Changes in subchondral bone** include subchondral bony sclerosis, cyst formation, and bone thickening with eburnation.

III. **Reactive proliferation of new bone and cartilage** at the joint periphery produces osteophytes. It has been previously shown that the bony changes of subchondral cortical sclerosis and osteophytosis precede changes in articular cartilage thickness, measured radiographically. In addition, there are local osteoporosislike changes in the cancellous bone of the proximal tibia of patients with OA.

IV. **OTHER TISSUE CHANGES.** Some mild degree of synovitis can be expected, perhaps as a contributor to joint damage and/or as a consequence of attempts to remove degenerative bone and cartilage debris from the synovial space. Additional pathologic changes in the joint organ include degeneration of menisci and periarticular muscle atrophy.

CLINICAL MANIFESTATIONS

I. **PRIMARY OA**
  A. **Localized OA.** Heberden's nodes [bony protuberances arising from distal interphalangeal (DIP) joints] without other joint involvement represent the most common form of primary OA. Family studies reveal that genetic factors are

important in the development of Heberden's nodes. These nodes are ten times more common in women than in men and tend to be seen in both mothers and their daughters.

B. Generalized OA is determined by involvement of three or more joints. Joint features of generalized OA include a predilection for postmenopausal women and episodic joint inflammation. A familial pattern, associated with Heberden's nodes, has been reported in a subset of patients with generalized OA.

C. Erosive OA, also known as inflammatory OA, may be a distinct disease. However, there is also a possibility that erosive OA merely represents the end of the OA spectrum and is characterized by severe disease. DIP and proximal interphalangeal (PIP) joints of the hands are affected. Joint radiographs reveal both osteophytes and erosions.

II. SECONDARY OA. The preceding text lists causes.

A. Symptoms

1. Symptomatic patients are usually **older than 40 years.**

2. Patients complain of **pain** of insidious onset in **one or a few joints.** The pain is often dull and persistent and is poorly localized.

3. The pain initially occurs after normal joint use and is **relieved by rest.** As the disease progresses, pain develops even during periods of rest. Joint stiffness lasts less than half an hour in the morning. Knee OA is commonly associated with a "theater sign" in which prolonged sitting leads to stiffness that lasts for a few paces while walking before normal gait returns.

4. Degenerative changes in the menisci may cause a feeling of "giving way," and pieces of osteophytes that get broken off can cause locking of the knee.

5. **Systemic symptoms are absent.**

B. Most common sites of involvement are the DIP, PIP, and first carpometacarpal (CMC) joints of the hand and the first metatarsophalangeal (MTP) joint in the foot. Other common areas include the hips, knees, and the lumbar and cervical spine. OA rarely involves the MCP joints, wrists, elbows, and shoulders or ankles, unless secondary OA is present. In general, correlation between joint symptoms and radiographic changes in early OA is poor. However, as the disease progresses, pain resulting from the pathology in bone, which is richly innervated, is more common. Later-stage disease is characterized by osteophytes and radiographic narrowing of joint space, particularly in large, weight-bearing joints such as the knee and hip.

III. PHYSICAL EXAMINATION

A. Joints may be **tender** even in the absence of overt inflammation, which does occur on occasion in patients with OA. Pain may occur with weight-bearing, but may be absent on passive range-of-motion testing. Joint **enlargement** may result from the presence of effusion, synovial hyperplasia, or osteophytes.

B. In the later stages of disease, there may be a crackling sound called **crepitus** on movement of the affected joint, gross deformity and subluxation caused by cartilage loss, collapse of subchondral bone, bone cysts, and gross bony overgrowth. However, crepitus alone can be seen in some forms of early OA such as patellofemoral disease in older individuals.

C. Limitation of motion increases as disease progresses, perhaps caused by joint surface incongruity, muscle spasms and contracture, capsule contracture, or mechanical blockage by osteophytes or loose bodies.

IV. RADIOGRAPHIC FINDINGS. Radiographs are not needed in most clinical situations and can be reserved for situations of persistent unexplained joint symptoms. However, when a radiographic film is obtained, one must be aware that OA is very common and should not overlook any evidence of other arthritides or fractures when evaluating a painful joint. A plain anteroposterior, weight-bearing, standing x-ray of the knee is still the best screening test for OA. Magnetic resonance imaging (MRI) is **not** a routine test in OA. **Radiographic criteria** for OA are as follows:

A. Joint space narrowing secondary to degeneration and disappearance of articular cartilage can be detected in more advanced disease.

B. Osteophyte (spur) formation at joint margins or sites of ligamentous attachment.

C. Subchondral bone sclerosis (increased bone density).

D. **Subchondral bone cysts.**

E. **Altered shape of the end of a bone caused by bone remodeling.**

V. **OTHER IMAGING MODALITIES.** Scintigraphy has been shown to predict the progression of OA in some studies but is rarely used in routine practice. It is difficult to view the bone component of the joint organ with MRI, but MRI can help to define ligamentous or meniscal abnormalities.

VI. **LABORATORY STUDIES**

A. **No specific or diagnostic abnormalities are seen in primary OA.** No cartilage or bone markers of OA disease progression have yet been validated.

B. **Blood and urine.** Because of the localized nature of OA and the absence of systemic manifestations, clinical laboratory testing is usually not necessary to manage the patient. Erythrocyte sedimentation rate (ESR), complete blood cell count, rheumatoid factor (RF), blood biochemistry studies, and urinalysis are generally normal. These laboratory tests are helpful in evaluating associated conditions and causes of secondary OA and in excluding other causes of arthritis. It should be kept in mind that low titers of RF are not an uncommon false-positive finding in the older individuals.

C. **Synovial fluid,** when present, is usually noninflammatory, with fewer than 2,000 (mainly mononuclear) white blood cells/mm^3.

SPECIFIC PATTERNS OF OA JOINT DISEASE

I. **HANDS**

A. **History.** DIP joints are the most frequent site of hand involvement in OA, and PIP joints are also commonly affected along with the DIP joints. The first CMC joint may be involved and be quite symptomatic, especially in patients whose occupations require repetitive use of this joint.

B. **Physical examination.** In patients with Heberden's (DIP) or Bouchard's (PIP) nodes, swellings over the joint are present, and the range of motion is decreased. The nodes are usually not tender. In some patients, small gelatinous cysts occur on the dorsal aspect of the DIP joints; they seem to be attached to tendon sheaths, resemble ganglia, and usually precede the development of Heberden's nodes. When the first CMC joint is affected, range of motion becomes limited, and a tender prominence develops at the base of the first metacarpal bone, which may lead to a "squared-off" appearance of the hand.

C. **Radiographs.** Because the physical signs of OA in hands are so characteristic, hand radiographs are rarely needed. Patients with mild radiographic changes usually have no symptoms. Images of Heberden's nodes show irregular joint space narrowing, subchondral sclerosis, cysts, and spurs. Although nodes may feel hard and bonelike, they may not be radiodense. When the first CMC joint is involved, subluxation of the base of the first metacarpal bone may be noted.

II. **HIPS**

A. **History.** Because of the key role of the hip in locomotion, patients with OA of the hip may be significantly disabled. Patients are usually older than those with hand involvement. Men are more often affected than women. In 20% of patients with unilateral disease, contralateral disease will develop within 8 years. Patients often complain of pain that increases with motion and weight-bearing, and decreases with rest. They may also complain of stiffness and a limp.

Hip pain is usually felt on the outer aspect of the groin or inner thigh. Pain that originates in the hip may sometimes be perceived as originating in the medial knee or distal thigh (20% of patients), buttocks, or sciatic region. Patients may walk with an antalgic (pain-avoiding) gait, which may alter the gait pattern and cause pain in other joints of the lower extremities or the back. Sitting or rising may be especially difficult for these patients. It is important to distinguish true hip pain from pain caused by a lumbar radiculopathy, femoral hernia, or vascular insufficiency.

B. **Physical examination.** Decreased range of motion and pain on motion are the primary findings. Internal rotation is affected first. As deterioration progresses, there is further loss of rotation, extension, abduction, and flexion. Joint contractures may develop. In the early stages of OA, flexion may not cause pain; however, extension and rotation will do so. In cases where the radiation of pain is atypical (to the knee), symptoms attributed to the hip can be reproduced by moving the hip through the extremes of motion while fixing all motion of the knee. Shortening of the limb caused by contracture or progressive lateral and upward subluxation of the femoral head may be observed. Compensatory lumbar lordosis of the spine may also be observed secondary to flexion contracture of the hip.

C. **Radiographs.** Compared with OA symptoms in other joints, hip joint OA symptoms correlate better with radiographic findings. Virtually all patients with severe radiographic findings will have complaints affecting the hip. Anteroposterior views of the **pelvis** should be obtained routinely when OA of the hips is suspected; these will provide information about the hips, sacroiliac joints, and pelvic bones. Advanced cases of hip OA may show protrusion of the femoral head into and through the cup-shaped acetabular component of the hip joint.

D. **Associated and predisposing conditions.** Some authors feel that OA of the hip is usually secondary to a developmental abnormality.

1. **Congenital dysplasia of the hip** may account for 25% of cases of OA in older white patients. The **acetabulum** does not develop properly and is shallow, which often results in femoral head subluxation and secondary degenerative changes. Patients may present with a limp in childhood or with premature OA in adulthood.

2. **Slipped capital femoral epiphysis.** Just before the femoral epiphysis closes (between ages 16 and 19), the **femoral head** may be displaced posteromedially. These patients may present with a painful limp in adolescence or early adulthood.

3. **Legg-Calvé-Perthes disease** is idiopathic osteonecrosis of the proximal femoral capital epiphysis, which occurs in young (3 to 8 years old) boys. The osteonecrosis often results in an abnormally large, flat femoral head with a wide, short neck.

III. **KNEES**

A. **History.** The knee is frequently affected by OA. Even during normal walking, about four times the body weight is transmitted through the knee joint. Patients complain of trouble with kneeling, climbing stairs, and getting in and out of chairs. Locking of the knee may result from loose joint bodies. Morning stiffness is common but usually lasts less than 30 minutes.

B. **Physical examination.** Tenderness may be present along the joint line. Osteophytes may be palpated as irregular bony masses. Crepitus may be felt with the examiner's hand held over the patella during knee motion. Quadriceps atrophy may be present.

1. **Medial and lateral compartment disease.** The medial compartment is the most frequently affected of the three knee compartments. Genu varus (a bowed-leg deformity) commonly occurs with the loss of cartilage in the medial compartment. Genu valgus (a knock-knee deformity) due to loss of cartilage in the lateral compartment is less common.

   The knee may be unstable because of cartilage loss and secondary lengthening of the collateral ligaments. It is important to compare the degrees of varus or valgus deformity (of the extended knee) with and without weightbearing. If a change into varus alignment or an increase in the degree of deformity occurs with weight-bearing, it is evidence of cartilage loss and compartment deformity rather than of ligamentous laxity alone.

2. **Patellofemoral disease.** With patellofemoral OA, the patella loses side-to-side mobility, which results in a loss of approximately 10% of extension and flexion. Pain and tenderness are most marked anteriorly. Pain may be elicited if the patella is held firmly against the femur and the quadriceps is isometrically contracted. Patellofemoral disease alone may occur without medial or lateral compartment disease.

C. Radiographs

1. **Standard views** are the anteroposterior and lateral for most clinical situations. It is important to obtain these films of the patient during weight-bearing to assess the degree of varus or valgus deformity and joint space narrowing. Films of the patient in the **standing** position, with approximately 6 degrees of knee flexion, show the femoral cartilage and tibial plateau cartilage in direct contact and demonstrate joint space narrowing more reliably than films of the patient in non–weight-bearing positions. Osteophytes, subchondral bone sclerosis, and cyst formation are observed as OA progresses.

2. **A tunnel view** is obtained with the knee in slight flexion to expose the intercondylar notch. This view allows evaluation of loose bodies, intra-articular spurs, and changes in the tibial intracondylar spines.

3. The orientation of a **sunrise view** is tangential to the flexed knee; this view allows evaluation of the patellofemoral articulation.

D. Associated and predisposing conditions for knee OA

1. Fractures of the tibial plateau or femoral condyles with mechanical incongruence.
2. Ligamentous injuries causing instability.
3. Chronic patellar dislocation.
4. Severe varus and valgus deformities.
5. Internal derangement. Torn menisci predispose to OA, as do absent menisci after meniscectomy.
6. Osteonecrosis (see Chapter 52).
7. RA and other inflammatory arthropathies.
8. Chondromalacia patellae is a degeneration of the patellar cartilage most prominent in the age group of 15 to 30 years. There is pain during activity, especially descending stairs. Pain is elicited when the patella is pressed into the femoral groove as the patient tightens the quadriceps muscle.

IV. **SPINE.** Degenerative disease of the spine may be categorized as **OA** or **spondylosis.** Because the posterior apophyseal joints are true diarthrodial joints, they may undergo the usual changes of OA, including joint space narrowing, sclerosis, and spur formation. The degenerative changes that affect the discs and vertebral bodies are properly referred to as spondylosis. Discs may herniate and compress the spinal cord or nerve roots. Degenerative changes of the vertebral bodies result in osteophytes that may cause mechanical compression of vital structures (spinal cord, nerve root, esophagus, and rarely, vessels). Stenosis of the central canal can occur alone or in the company of foraminal stenosis in both the cervical and lumbosacral spines. Lumbar stenosis is often due to a combination of disc protrusion, thickening of the ligamentum flavum, and impingement by osteophytes.

A. History

1. **Local pain and stiffness** may be caused by paraspinal ligament involvement or paraspinal muscle spasm.

2. **Radicular symptoms** occur at all spinal levels, but are more common in the lumbar area and in the C5-6 and C6-7 roots.

   a. Involvement of the **cervical spine** is usually seen at a neural foramen, secondary to impingement by osteophytes. Radicular symptoms tend to occur in the cervical spine because neural foramina and the spinal canal are relatively small in this area. Symptoms include neck pain that often radiates to the shoulder, upper back, and more distal aspects of the upper extremity. Weakness and paresthesias of the hand and arm may also occur.

   b. **Lumbar spine.** Patients complain of low back pain that often radiates down the buttocks and may extend to the legs and feet. The pain may increase with coughing and straining. With severe lesions, motor and sensory abnormalities may be present. A cauda equina syndrome with sphincter dysfunction can also develop (see Chapter 20). Lumbar spinal stenosis can present in the setting of a long history of lumbosacral pain and/or radicular symptoms and heaviness of the legs or neurogenic claudication.

3. **Cord compression** by intervertebral ridges at cervical and thoracic levels may result in progressive myelopathy with minimal or no radicular pain. This can present with leg weakness, gait abnormality, or balance problems.

4. Mechanical compression of vital structures also occurs mostly at the level of the cervical spine. Large anterior spurs may cause **dysphagia,** hoarseness, or cough. Compression of vertebral arteries may produce symptoms of **vertebrobasilar insufficiency** with vertigo, double vision, scotomas, headache, or ataxia. These symptoms often vary with head and neck position. Compression of the anterior spinal artery may produce a central cord syndrome.

B. Physical examination. The spinal examination may reveal decreased range of motion and local tenderness. A careful neurologic evaluation to detect absent reflexes, long-tract signs, and a radicular pattern of weakness and sensory abnormalities is important.

C. Radiographs. Severe degenerative changes may be present on radiographs in the setting of few symptoms. In contrast, a small spur that is critically placed may cause significant morbidity. **Oblique films** must be obtained to evaluate neural foramina. Standard anteroposterior and lateral views will not demonstrate impingement by a bone spur or a subluxation of an apophyseal joint. Osteophytes usually arise from the anterior and anterolateral aspects of vertebral bodies and are best seen on lateral films. A decrease in the intervertebral disc space that occurs secondary to disc degeneration is seen most often in the lower cervical and lumbar spine. A **vacuum phenomenon** (a linear band of air density within the disc) is indicative of disintegration of the nucleus pulposus of the disc. Anterior vertebral wedging may be seen. Specialized imaging methods such as computed tomography (CT) scan and MRI are useful for further selective investigations. CT scan may be of value in defining any bony cause for neurologic compression symptoms. MRI is useful to study soft-tissue structures of the neck, such as discs, when clinical examination and plain radiographs do not yield the diagnosis.

In summary, advanced imaging techniques are best reserved for those clinical situations in which standard initial therapy has failed, or in which neurologic signs or symptoms are progressive.

V. FEET

A. History. The first MTP joint is one of the most common sites of OA involvement. Acute swelling and pain may be caused by bursal inflammation at the medial side of the metatarsal head (bunion). Patients often have a history of using improper footwear. In contrast, OA of the ankle or tarsal joints is rare and, when present, is usually secondary to trauma or to a systemic disease such as hemochromatosis.

B. Physical examination may reveal tenderness over the first MTP joint and a hallux valgus deformity. The great toe is unable to bear weight normally, and added stress is placed on the metatarsal heads.

C. Radiographs. Typical changes of OA, such as sclerosis, joint space narrowing, and osteophyte formation, may be seen at the first MTP joint. Subluxation of the great toe with hallux valgus deformity may be noted. Radiographic changes in the midtarsal joints are common; however, they are infrequently associated with symptoms.

VI. TEMPOROMANDIBULAR JOINT. Crepitus, tenderness, and pain (often referred to the ear) are common problems that are sometimes attributed to dental malocclusion. Radiographic characterization of this joint is difficult. MRI can be utilized when more extensive imaging is indicated.

 DIFFERENTIAL DIAGNOSIS

Primary OA can be confused with other forms of arthritis because it may occasionally present as an inflammatory polyarthritis of the hands or as monarticular arthritis. In addition, radiographic evidence of OA is so common that its presence may be unrelated to the true etiology of the patient's complaints.

I. RA

A. Monarticular RA. When RA presents early in its course as monarticular arthritis of a large joint, differentiation from OA may be difficult and is based on the following:

1. The eventual development over 3 to 6 months of the typical symmetrical polyarthritis of the small joints of hands and feet.

2. **Synovial fluid analysis.** RA fluid contains more white blood cells (>5,000) with a higher percentage of neutrophils, and has poorer viscosity than OA fluid.
3. **Radiographs** in patients with advanced RA usually show erosions and juxta-articular osteoporosis, although the findings are often normal in early RA. Osteophytes, subchondral bone cysts, and sclerosis suggest OA. However, Heberden's nodes and other degenerative abnormalities may coexist with RA.
4. **Blood studies.** The ESR is often elevated, and rheumatoid factor (RF) is usually present in RA.
5. **Follow-up observations** may eventually reveal a pattern of erosive joint destruction typical of RA. It may take as long as 2 years before the clinical picture is clear.

B. **Polyarticular RA**
1. **Distribution of joint involvement** is important when differentiating RA from inflammatory erosive OA.
   a. **RA.** MCP, PIP, and wrist involvement is seen.
   b. **OA.** DIP, PIP, and first CMC joints are characteristically affected.
2. **Radiographic features.** See the preceding section.

C. **Distinguishing clinical features of RA**
1. More inflammation with greater loss of joint function.
2. Involvement of a greater number of joints involved in a symmetric fashion.
3. Quicker progression.
4. Less involvement of the knee.
5. More involvement of the hand.
6. Morning stiffness lasting longer than 30 minutes.
7. Significant systemic symptoms such as fatigue.
8. The presence of anemia, elevated ESR and C-reactive protein (CRP), and the presence of RF and anticyclic citrullinated peptide (anti-CCP) in the serum.

II. **SPONDYLOARTHROPATHIES.** These inflammatory diseases frequently present in large, lower extremity joints in an asymmetric fashion, often with associated low back stiffness in the morning due to sacroiliitis and spondylitis. In addition to the joints being strikingly more inflammatory than is the case in OA, other key differentiating features are the following:
A. **Psoriatic arthritis.** Skin and nail lesions and typical patterns of psoriatic arthropathy affecting distal interphalangeal and other joints in an asymmetrical distribution.
B. **Reactive arthritis.** Presence of conjunctivitis, urethritis, and characteristic skin lesions.
C. **Inflammatory bowel disease.** Complaints that are referable to large or small intestine.
D. **Ankylosing spondylitis.** Sacroiliitis, uveitis, and fine, symmetric, marginal syndesmophytes.

III. **CRYSTAL-INDUCED ARTHRITIS**
A. **Gout** primarily affects the first MTP joint in addition to other joints of the foot and lower extremity. Tophaceous deposits over the small joints of the hand may be confused with osteophytes. The diagnosis of gout is confirmed by the identification of urate crystals in polymorphonuclear leukocytes (PMNs) in the joint fluid.
B. **Calcium pyrophosphate dihydrate arthritis (pseudogout)** may coexist with OA. The wrist, shoulder, knee, and ankle joints are commonly involved. Radiographs reveal chondrocalcinosis in most patients with pseudogout. The diagnosis is confirmed by identifying positively birefringent, rhomboidal CPPD crystals in the joint fluid PMNs. Another type of crystal, basic calcium phosphate, is implicated in the pathogenesis of the destructive OA variant known as Milwaukee's shoulder syndrome.

IV. **Other disorders** that may coexist with OA but are important to identify and treat include the following:
A. **Occasionally seen but requires urgent treatment.** Infectious arthritis.
B. **Somewhat common.** Periarticular tendinitis or bursitis in the vicinity of an OA joint.

C. Rare conditions
1. **Neoplastic synovitis.** Lymphoma or leukemia may be identified with synovial fluid cytology.
2. **Pigmented villonodular synovitis.** The joint effusion is usually bloody and the diagnosis is confirmed by synovial biopsy.
3. **Neoplastic metastasis to juxta-articular bone** wherein bone scan confirms the diagnosis.

 TREATMENT

The American College of Rheumatology (ACR) has published guidelines for the management of hip and knee OA that are available on their Website, www.rheumatology.org. Therapy directed at other joints follows similar principles.

I. **NONPHARMACOLOGIC THERAPY.** Correction of predisposing factors should optimally take place before anatomic changes occur. Weight reduction in the obese patient is a particularly important intervention. Valgus or varus knee deformity and eversion or inversion ankle deformity may benefit from custom braces and optimal exercises that reduce the load on the affected joint compartment. Those patients who fail to respond may eventually require surgical correction.

A. **Patient education** and self-management programs. Participation in Arthritis Foundation activities (Telephone: 1-800-283-7800) provides patients with a reliable flow of practical information.

B. **Joint rest.** Excessive use of an involved joint may increase symptoms and accelerate degenerative changes. It is important to protect joints. Weight-bearing joints may be unloaded by use of a cane (held in the hand opposite to the involved extremity and extended in tandem with it), crutches, or a walker. A neck collar may be useful for cervical OA. A first CMC joint splint can be quite helpful in a flare of CMC joint pain.

C. **Physical therapy** helps to relieve pain and stiffness, recover and maintain joint mobility, aid in optimal joint alignment, and strengthen supporting muscles. It is particularly helpful in patients with hip, knee, low back, and neck disease.

1. **Therapeutic exercise.** The goal is to preserve range of motion and muscle strength.

2. **Heat therapy** generally relieves pain and muscle spasm. Many methods are available, including diathermy and ultrasonography (for deep pain), infrared, hot packs, warm bath or shower, and paraffin bath (for hands) (see Chapter 61 for regimens).

D. **Occupational therapy** helps patients to adapt to their disabilities and helps minimize the stress placed on involved joints during activities of daily living (see Chapter 62).

II. **PHARMACOLOGIC THERAPY**

A. **Analgesics**

1. **Oral.** Acetaminophen is a standard baseline therapy. If sufficient analgesic effect is obtained, it avoids the gastric side effects of nonsteroidal anti-inflammatory drugs (NSAIDs). The dosage of acetaminophen is 500 to 1,000 mg every 6 hours as required. Concurrent alcohol use should be avoided, and liver disease is a contraindication to its use.

2. **Topical.** Capsaicin cream (available in 0.025% and 0.075% strengths) is derived from the pepper plant and relieves pain by local reductions of substance P. It is applied three or four times a day to the affected area. Care must be taken to avoid contact with the eyes. It may take 2 weeks to obtain a therapeutic effect, so it is customary to use an oral medication during this period. The analgesic effects of acetaminophen and topical capsaicin are synergistic, and this can be a useful combination in the older individuals. Finally, some patients will get symptomatic relief from topical analgesic products such as methyl salicylate 30% (BenGay), which can be applied three times a day.

B. **NSAIDs.** The choice of an NSAID should take into account such factors as efficacy, cost, adverse reactions, compliance, comorbidities, and past treatment. If NSAIDs are indicated after failure of the treatment modalities described in the preceding text, they should be first used at low doses and on an as-needed basis to minimize adverse events, especially in older individuals. Older individuals are especially prone to peptic ulceration and unpredictable bleeding. These adverse events are clinically more serious in them than in young patients, who tend to have more physiologic reserve and are less likely to have multiple diseases and also less likely to be taking multiple medications that can further exacerbate gastrointestinal insults. In addition, the aging process leads to a slow decrease in renal function and that in turn makes elderly patients more susceptible to the adverse renal actions of NSAIDs, as detailed in the subsequent text.

   1. **Adverse reactions** to the NSAIDs include peptic ulcer in approximately 2%, appearance of rash in 2%, central nervous system effects such as tinnitus, and idiosyncratic hepatitis (rare). Dyspepsia is a frequent reason for discontinuation of NSAID. Renal reactions, listed in order of decreasing frequency, are edema, transient acute renal insufficiency, tubulointerstitial nephropathy, hyperkalemia, and renal papillary necrosis.
   2. **Choice of nonsteroidal anti-inflammatory drug.** There is no evidence that any one class of NSAIDs is superior in analgesic efficacy to another class. The first cyclooxygenase-2 (COX-2) inhibitor drugs entered the U.S. market in 1999, on the basis of causing less gastrointestinal injury compared to standard NSAIDs. Recently, concerns were raised about the long-term cardiovascular safety of the COX-2 class, that is presently composed of celecoxib alone, and all other NSAIDs. Until this issue is resolved, those prescribing drugs should carefully assess the risk:benefit ratio of these medications in the individual patient, taking into account all potential concomitant patient-specific factors (see Chapter 64). High-risk patients for coronary artery disease should be considered for the concomitant use of 8 mg aspirin. It is reasonable to try an NSAID for 3 to 4 weeks, stop it if there is no therapeutic benefit, and then select another NSAID from a different structural class. Gastroprotection can be provided by prescribing proton pump inhibitors for those patients who are on chronic NSAID therapy. A more complete discussion of NSAIDs can be found in Chapter 64.

C. **Corticosteroids, joint injections, and hyaluronate**
   1. **Systemic.** Oral corticosteroids have no role in the treatment of OA.
   2. **Intra-articular injections of corticosteroid** may be of benefit if used judiciously in patients with one or two persistently inflamed joints. Typically, injections three or four times a year for a particular joint will be sufficient. However, occasional patients may need more than this number of injections. It is important to observe appropriate sterile technique in order to avoid infectious complications. Patients should be advised not to overuse the joint so that recovery is not prolonged or the joint is not damaged further. Dosages for specific joints and precautions are listed in Chapter 8.
   3. **Intra-articular hyaluronic acid products** are available and can provide modest symptomatic relief lasting for several months when given as a series of injections. They are indicated for OA of the knee. These hyaluronate polymer drugs (Synvisc, Hyalgan, and others) may be useful in patients who cannot tolerate NSAIDs or in whom NSAIDs have failed. Synvisc can be given in a series of three injections 1 week apart and Hyalgan can be given in a series of five injections.

D. **Glucosamine and chondroitin sulfate.** It should be noted that glucosamine sulfate has been reported in several papers to provide a moderate improvement in the symptoms of OA. However, no data suggesting a claim on its effect on any disease have been provided by sponsors of the study to the United States Food and Drug Administration (FDA) for review. Glucosamine is regulated and sold in the United States under the 1994 Dietary Supplement Act as a food, in contrast to being regulated as a medicine by the FDA. The National Institutes of Health (NIH) data will likely provide authoritative guidance on the scientific questions related to glucosamine and are expected soon.

Finally, there is no substantial evidence to indicate that glucosamine or chondroitin sulfate has any structure-modifying effect.

SURGICAL TREATMENT

In addition to traditional surgical procedures and prosthetic joint replacement, a relatively recent advancement is transplantation of cartilage in younger patients who have focal chondral defects (often from trauma) that are suitable for repair. Although it is not a routine procedure and is quite costly, cartilage transplantation adds to the tools available to preserve joint function.

I. INDICATIONS
  A. Relief of pain or severe disability after failure of conservative measures to halt or alleviate the pathologic process.
  B. Correction of a mechanical derangement that may lead to OA.

II. CONTRAINDICATIONS FOR SURGERY
  A. Infection.
  B. Poor vascular supply.
  C. Emotional instability or occupational factors that make surgical rehabilitation unlikely to succeed.
  D. Obesity (relative contraindication).
  E. Serious medical illness (relative contraindication).
  F. Movement disorders, such as Parkinson's disease, and other neurologic diseases, such as Charcot joint.

III. KNEE AND HIP PROCEDURES. See Chapter 59 for a discussion of surgical therapy, including prosthetic joint replacement. Experienced surgeons obtain excellent functional results with hip and knee replacement surgery. Prostheses can be expected to last 20 years or so. Arthroscopic examination and removal of large loose articular bodies can relieve pain and improve function. However, arthroscopic debridement and irrigation have been shown to perform no better than sham arthroscopic surgery.

PROGNOSIS

The prognosis of OA is highly variable and is site-dependent. With DIP involvement of the hand, there is moderate pain and stiffness but little limitation of overall function. Disease of weight-bearing joints is more likely to cause disability. The time between the onset of hip pain and the development of serious disability averages 8 years. OA of the knee carries a worse prognosis than OA of the hip. Varus knee deformity and early onset of pain are poor prognostic signs.

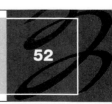

OSTEONECROSIS

John H. Healey and Andrea Piccioli

52

Osteonecrosis (ON) is defined as the death *in situ* of a segment of bone. Avascular necrosis (AVN), aseptic necrosis, and bone infarction are terms often used synonymously. All elements of the bone succumb: osteocytes, osteoblasts, osteoclasts, vascular elements, stroma, hematopoietic marrow, and fatty marrow. Deficient circulation is the typical cause. This can be spontaneous or post-traumatic.

EPIDEMIOLOGY

I. **Spontaneous ON** usually affects middle-aged adults. Any bone can be affected, but the femoral head is the most frequently involved. Other common sites are the distal femur, proximal humerus, tibial plateau, and talus. It may be bilateral in as many as 25% of cases.

II. **Secondary ON** affects patients of ages commensurate with the underlying primary disease process: for example, 16 to 30 years for patients with sickle cell anemia and systemic lupus erythematosus (SLE); and 60 to 80 years for patients with osteoarthritis of the knee. It may occur in 25% of patients with osteoarthritis of the hip.

III. **Post-traumatic cases** follow site-specific fracture epidemiology. Fractures of the scaphoid, radial head, and femoral head/neck commonly cause ON.

PATHOPHYSIOLOGY

Bone normally has a rich blood supply, but it varies widely. Certain sites such as the femoral head have an end-capillary circulation that is vulnerable to interruption. This accounts for it being the most common location for ON.

I. **Three mechanisms** of circulatory compromise of bone are recognized and one or more may play a significant role in a given patient.
A. **Mechanical disruption** (e.g., traumatic fracture/dislocation or stress fracture).
B. **Arterial (inflow) failure**
1. **Intrinsic vascular** (e.g., vasculitis, radiation injury, and vasospasm).
2. **Extrinsic** (e.g., compression by fat hypertrophy or Gaucher's cells).
3. **Embolic** (e.g., fat embolism, sickle cells, or nitrogen—"Caisson's disease").
C. **Venous outflow failure** (e.g., when venous pressure exceeds arterial pressure by any mechanism or by thrombosis). This mechanism may, in fact, be the final common pathway of the other two mechanisms.

II. **ETIOLOGY**
A. **Idiopathic.** This is most common and accounts for approximately 50% of cases.
B. **Secondary**
1. **Corticosteroid.** The exact cause is unclear, although fat embolism and local clotting are implicated in corticosteroid-related ON (Fig. 52-1). This is a significant cause of ON because of the use of steroids for many diseases, including SLE, rheumatoid arthritis, inflammatory bowel disease, nephrotic syndrome, lymphoma, and other myelogenous diseases, respiratory disease,

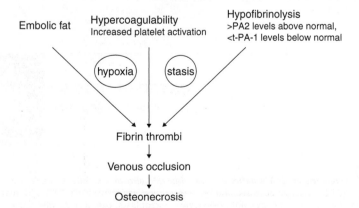

Figure 52-1. Mechanisms of ischemic necrosis of bone.
t-PA-1, tissue plasminogen activator-1; PA2, plasminogen activator.

and central nervous system disorders. In SLE, a high average daily dose (more than 16.6 mg) and pulse therapy are considered important predictors for the development of ON.

2. **Alcohol.** There is a clear dose–response relation: consumption of more than 400 mL weekly results in a tenfold greater risk for ON. Fat emboli from alcohol-induced fatty liver, increased blood cortisol levels, and altered lipid metabolism are all proposed mechanisms of ON in alcoholics.

3. **Hypercoagulability.** A high incidence of coagulopathy exists in patients with ON. Factor V Leiden mutation is associated with a 4.5-fold increased risk of ON. Twenty-two percent of patients with ON have thrombophilia (compared to 7% in control populations).

4. **Other**
   a. **Radiation.**
   b. **Dysbarism.**
   c. **Smoking.** Smokers have a fourfold to fivefold greater risk for ON.
   d. **Pregnancy.** Possible mechanisms include venous congestion and the well-known phenomenon of hypercoagulability of pregnancy.

5. **Metabolic bone disease.** High-turnover osteoporosis or even osteomalacia may coexist with ON.

 DIAGNOSIS

ON is diagnosed on the basis of history, physical examination, and radiologic studies.

I. **PATIENT HISTORY.** The presence of the risk factors discussed previously should be investigated. Night pain or recumbent pain reflects venous hypertension. Pain with weight-bearing is mechanical and suggests the presence of a subchondral fracture or osteoarthritis.

II. **PHYSICAL EXAMINATION.** There are no specific findings. Joint capsular tenderness and restricted motion reflect synovitis, but they may be absent. Late changes of degenerative arthritis may occur (e.g., stiff hip and coxalgic gait).

III. **IMAGING.** Plain radiographs, bone scan, and magnetic resonance imaging (MRI) are indicated, and each can be helpful depending on the stage of evolution of ON.

IV. **STAGING.** Two modern staging systems have been validated and are in common use.
   A. **The University of Pennsylvania System** (Table 52-1). The importance of this system is that it incorporates the type and extent of radiologic and pathologic changes.
   B. **The Japanese Investigation Committee for AVN of the femoral head.** This classification system is based on plain anteroposterior radiographic findings. It is the most predictive of prognosis and, therefore, a valuable guide to treatment.

V. **HISTOLOGY.** It is the standard for the definitive diagnosis of ON.
   A. **Necrosis.** Initially after vascular compromise, no histologic changes occur. Then examination of the marrow reveals death of hematopoietic cells, capillary endothelial cells, and lipocytes. Osteocytes shrink and produce the empty lacunae that are characteristic of dead bone. These early necrotic changes are associated with increased interstitial water, which produces a marrow abnormality detectable on MRI.
   B. **Osseous repair.** Appositional bone is deposited on existing dead trabeculae, which creates an osteosclerotic area radiographically. Initially, reactive hyperemia and fibrous repair occur in the adjacent bone. Revascularization occurs at the leading edge of necrotic bone. Creeping substitution is a secondary process. Necrotic tissue is removed and is coupled with new bone formation. In the cortex, these "cutting cones" remodel the bone.
   C. **Temporal sequence.** The bone is a composite of both necrotizing and reparative processes. When resorption progresses faster than formation of new bone, the bone becomes weak. Standard mechanical forces can fracture the vulnerable bone. Radiographically, the subchondral radiolucent line representing collapsed cancellous trabeculae, beneath an intact articular cartilage surface, is known as the crescent sign.
   D. **End stage.** Segmental collapse of the articular surface, femoral head deformity, and joint incongruity lead to the development of secondary osteoarthritis.

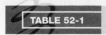 **TABLE 52-1**	Steinberg-University of Pennsylvania Staging System of Osteonecrosis of the Hip
Stage 0	Normal or nondiagnostic radiograph, bone scan, and MRI

Stage 1	Normal radiograph; abnormal bone scan and MRI
	  A. Mild
	  B. Moderate
	  C. Severe

Stage 2	Lucent and sclerotic changes in femoral head
	  A. Mild
	  B. Moderate
	  C. Severe

Stage 3	Subchondral collapse (crescent sign) without flattening
	  A. Mild
	  B. Moderate
	  C. Severe

Stage 4	Flattening of femoral head
	  A. Mild
	  B. Moderate
	  C. Severe

Stage 5	Joint narrowing, acetabular changes
	  A. Mild (average of femoral head involvement)
	  B. Moderate (as determined in stage 4 and estimated)
	  C. Severe (acetabular involvement)

Stage 6	Advanced degenerative changes

Mild: <15% of the surface of femoral head or <2 mm depression; moderate: 15% to 30% or 2 to 4 mm depression; severe: >30% or >4 mm depression.
MRI, magnetic resorance imaging.

 TREATMENT

The treatment of ON depends on the etiology, stage, and extent of the lesion.

I. **STOP THE INSULT.** Contributing factors such as steroid therapy, alcohol, and smoking must be avoided. Even if there is degenerative arthritis in the affected joint, it is important to prevent new sites of necrosis. Some advocate the use of anticoagulants for procoagulant disorders.

II. **MINIMIZE MECHANICAL FORCES.** Crutches, or whatever necessary, are used to relieve pain and prevent bone collapse.

III. **TREAT THE SYNOVITIS.** Nonsteroidal anti-inflammatory medications and rest are recommended.

IV. **ADDRESS THE METABOLIC BONE DISEASE**
  A. Osteoporosis. Bone density should be preserved or augmented. Physiologic doses of calcium and vitamin D are recommended for all.
  B. High turnover osteoporosis. High levels of N-telopeptides confirm this patient subset of high turnover osteoporosis. This process may be quenched with antiresorptive therapy (e.g., bisphosphonates or calcitonin).

V. **EARLY SURGERY.** For patients in an early stage of disease (i.e., before subchondral collapse has occurred), **core decompression** represents the best option for pain relief and prevention of progression, to collapse and total hip arthroplasty. This procedure removes a core of bone from the necrotic bone segment. It involves taking a sample for histologic diagnosis, relieves venous hypertension in the bone, and promotes revascularization and healing of the necrotic area. Core decompression can help delay total hip arthroplasty significantly—on average, almost 10 years for patients with symptoms and normal radiographic findings, almost 5 years for patients with early radiographic changes (cystic and sclerotic lesions), and even 3 years for patients with structural failure of the femoral head (subchondral radiolucency with fracture or deformity of the femoral head). **Vascularized bone grafting** (fibula for femoral head ON) may lend early mechanical support and promote revascularization and healing.

VI. **LATE SURGERY. Osteotomy** is a less popular treatment, but sometimes it is indicated to rotate the necrotic bone out of the weight-bearing axis and transfer the load to healthy joint surfaces. For advanced stages of ON, total hip arthroplasty is the standard treatment. Hemiarthroplasty may be considered in very young patients with intact cartilage on the opposite side of the joint (e.g., conserving the acetabulum).

VII. Joint replacement is the procedure for advanced disease with severe secondary osteoarthritis and profound functional limitation and pain.

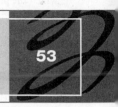

OSTEOPOROSIS

Alexander Krawiecki, Joseph M. Lane,
and Joseph L. Barker

53

■ KEY POINTS

- Osteoporosis (OP) is often undertreated and underrecognized.
- The best way to avoid the complications of OP is to take early action to resist the development of OP.
- Investigating underlying causes of OP is important.
- Healthy diet and calcium/vitamin D supplementation should be combined with appropriate medical treatment, such as bisphosphonate, for the optimal management of OP.
- Physical therapy and conditioning prevent falls.

 INTRODUCTION

I. **Osteoporosis (OP)** is a common metabolic bone disease, characterized by a decrease in bone density, deterioration of bony matrix microarchitecture, diminished material properties, and susceptibility to low-energy "fragility" fractures. OP is a silent disease often underrecognized and undertreated. Fracture may be the first and only manifestation, making OP a major contributor to morbidity and mortality worldwide.

A. **The World Health Organization (WHO)** has defined OP on the basis of bone mineral density (BMD) measurements obtained on dual energy x-ray absorptiometry (DEXA) as a T-score equal to or greater than 2.5 standard deviations (SD) below ideal bone mass.

B. **Fracture** is the result of an unfavorable combination of bone mass, bone geometry, material properties, and vector of trauma. A low BMD is associated with an increased risk of fracture.

C. **Low bone density** may be secondary to failure to achieve optimal bone mass, bone loss caused by increased bone resorption, or inadequate replacement of lost bone as a result of decreased bone formation.

D. **Primary OP (80%)**
   1. **Type I,** idiopathic OP, is seen in postmenopausal women. Peak bone mass is reached at the age of 25 to 30 years in women with accelerated loss during the perimenopausal period. Estrogen maintains bone density, leaving postmenopausal women at increased risk of fracture.
   2. **Type II,** senile OP, affects men and women older than 70 years.

E. **Secondary OP (20%)** is a result of some underlying disease state and may be corrected by treatment of the primary disease.

II. **Osteopenia** refers to radiographic finding of decreased bone density, classically a T-score between 1.0 to 2.5 SD below ideal. Osteopenia may coexist with OP, osteomalacia (OM), or other conditions.

III. **OM** is characterized by delayed or altered mineralization of normal matrix, independent of the amount of bone mass. The same disease, affecting growing bones in children, is called rickets.

 ETIOPATHOGENESIS

I. **Bone strength** is a result of many factors including mineralization, turnover, and microarchitecture. Low initial levels of adult bone mass or acceleration in bone loss can reduce bone mass and strength to below the fracture threshold (the bone mass below which the propensity to fracture is increased).

II. **Bone density** is by far the greatest measurable predictor of fracture risk, accounting for 70% of bone strength. Genetics may account for 70% to 85% of the variation in peak bone mass.

III. **Areas rich in trabecular bone** (e.g., the vertebral bodies, the intertrochanter of the hip, and the distal radius) have the greatest turnover and therefore the greatest propensity to fracture.

IV. **GENERAL ETIOLOGY**
 A. Advanced age.
 B. Female gender.
 C. White race and/or northwest European extraction; first-generation Chinese.
 D. Family history (one-third have strong inheritance).
 E. Fall risk (impaired vision and dementia).
 F. History of fragility fracture (a major risk factor). **Prior fracture is the strongest predictor of future fracture.**
 G. Collagen disorders (e.g., osteogenesis imperfecta, Ehlers-Danlos syndrome, and Marfan's syndrome) and unspecified hypermobility variants.
 H. Rheumatologic diseases such as rheumatoid arthritis and ankylosing spondylitis.
 I. Multiple myeloma.

V. **NUTRITION AND SOCIAL PRACTICE**
 A. Inadequate calcium intake.
 B. Malabsorption including celiac sprue (4.7% of patients with OP), inflammatory bowel disease (e.g., Crohn's or ulcerative colitis), irritable bowel syndrome (IBS), lactose intolerance, and gastric bypass surgery.
 C. Alcoholism/smoking.
 D. Vitamin D deficiency (20% to 40% of the population).
 E. Low body weight or body mass index (BMI).

VI. **ENDOCRINE CONDITIONS**
 A. Estrogen deficiency
  1. Menopause. Inadequate calcium intake and postmenopausal estrogen deficiency account for 90% of OP cases.
  2. Amenorrhea/oligomenorrhea (e.g., the female athlete).
  3. Lactation. Contributes to negative calcium balance if calcium supplementation is inadequate.
 B. Androgen deficiency.
 C. Hyperthyroidism.
 D. Hyperparathyroidism.
 E. Cushing's disease.
 F. Type I diabetes mellitus.

VII. **IMMOBILIZATION**
 A. Neuromuscular diseases.
 B. Illness.
 C. Sedentary lifestyle/weightlessness.

VIII. **IATROGENIC CAUSES**
 A. Corticosteroids (most common iatrogenic cause).
 B. Heparin.

C. Anticonvulsants (e.g., phenytoin and barbiturates).
D. Neuroleptics.
E. Lithium.
F. Methotrexate/cyclosporine and other immunosuppressants.
G. Excessive thyroid hormone [suppresses thyroid stimulating hormone (TSH)].
H. Castration (e.g., oophorectomy, radiation, and chemotherapy).

PREVALENCE

I. **OP is the most common metabolic bone disorder,** affecting 44 million Americans.
   A. In the United States, there are 1.5 million osteoporotic fractures. Of these, 700,000 fractures are located in the spine, 300,000 in the hip, and 200,000 in the wrist.
   B. Lifetime risk of fracture is 40%; mortality equal to that of breast cancer.
   C. Ninety percent of all fractures in the elderly can be attributed to OP.
II. **Up to 20% of vertebral fractures and 30% of hip fractures occur in men.**
III. **More common in whites, Asians, and Hispanics than in African Americans.** Fifty percent of white women have OP or osteopenia 10 years after menopause.

CLINICAL MANIFESTATIONS

I. **Medical history** often reveals additional manifestations of collagen defects.
   A. Fractures (low energy, e.g., wrist and rib).
   B. Hernias (e.g., inguinal).
   C. Mitral valve prolapse.
   D. Easy bruising.
   E. Other risk factors (noted in the preceding text).
II. **Physical examination** often reveals the manifestations of many of the risk factors:
   A. Low body weight is often present; a decrease in body fat correlates with a decrease in estrogen production (<127 lbs in 5′5″ women; or BMI <21).
   B. Kyphosis and height loss are often the result of one or more vertebral body fractures. Other findings include: scoliosis, degenerative spondylolisthesis.
   C. Skeletal deformity may lead to gait abnormalities, difficulty in balancing, decreased size of the thoracic and abdominal cavities, and iliocostal friction.
   D. Increased flexibility, hyperextensible joints, flat or pronated feet, short fifth digit, bluish sclera, and poor dentition may all be manifestations of collagen defects.
   E. Focal neurologic findings may be a result of central cord or root compression.
   F. Pain may lead to a diminished quality of life.

DIAGNOSTIC INVESTIGATIONS

I. **Criteria** for diagnosis are set by the WHO as mentioned in the preceding text.
II. **Laboratory tests** to rule out underlying causes. In primary OP, all lab values should be normal. Abnormal values imply an underlying problem:
   A. Serum calcium/phosphate.
   B. 25-hydroxy vitamin D (abnormal <30; OM).
   C. Parathyroid hormone (PTH) (intact PTH).
   D. Bone alkaline phosphatase.
   E. Urinary calcium (24-hour) (abnormal <100 mg/L; OM).
   F. TSH.
   G. Complete blood count/sedimentation rate.
   H. Albumin (abnormal <3.5; malnutrition and liver disease).
   I. Urine and serum protein and immunoelectrophoresis (for multiple myeloma).
   J. Liver function tests.
   K. Urine Type I collagen–cross-linked N telopeptide (NTX). NTX is a useful marker for bone turnover. High turnover results from increased bone resorption while low turnover is caused by decreased osteoblastic activity.

III. IMAGING STUDIES

A. DEXA of the lumbar spine, femoral neck, and sometimes the distal radius is the gold standard for evaluation of OP. It is accurate and consistent, making it a useful tool both for diagnosis and for follow-up. T-score relates bone mass to young normals and Z-score relates to age matured peers. Postmenopausal women with a T-score of 0 to -1 SD are considered normal, -1 to -2.5 SD below normal represents osteopenia and less than -2.5 SD below normal represents OP. Severe OP is defined as less than -2.5 SD below normal and a fracture. Premenopausal women should be evaluated by T-score and risk factors. The patient is classified by the lowest score of the anteroposterior spine, femoral neck, intertrochanteric area, and total femur. Greater than 3% change in T-score after 1 year is considered significant. Errors in technique can result in some discrepancy and are a common cause of significant BMD changes. Therefore, DEXA studies should be done on the same machine, if at all possible.

B. Indications for obtaining a DEXA BMD have been set forth by the National Osteoporosis Foundation to include white women 65 years or older not receiving antiosteoporotic therapy, postmenopausal women 50 to 65 years with a risk factor for OP, patients on steroids, and individuals who have sustained a low-energy fracture.

C. Other findings on radiographic studies such as plain radiographs, CT scanning, or magnetic resonance imaging (MRI) may aid in the diagnosis because OP is clinically silent and often manifests only in the form of a fracture. These studies, however, should not be used as screening tools for OP.

    1. Fractures of the wrist (Colles's fracture), hip (femoral neck and intertrochanteric), and pelvis are common.

    2. Osteopenia may be apparent as a loss of horizontal vertebral trabeculation.

    3. Compression fractures of the vertebral bodies may include wedge, crush, or biconcave injury with intact posterior elements and most commonly occur in T-11–L-2 distribution. MRI shows marrow edema with new fractures.

    4. There are no lytic or blastic lesions.

 DIFFERENTIAL DIAGNOSIS

Treatable causes of secondary OP should be identified.

I.   MULTIPLE MYELOMA. An elevated erythrocyte sedimentation rate, anemia, proteinuria, monoclonal gammopathy (urine/blood), bone pain or fracture, and radiographic lytic lesions on x-ray but with a normal bone scan.

II.   OM. Low serum calcium and phosphorus levels, high levels of alkaline phosphatase, low levels of 25(OH)-vitamin D, elevated intact PTH, and radiographic pseudofractures. Bone biopsy showing wide osteoid seams and delayed mineralization.

III. HYPERTHYROIDISM. Suggested by weight loss, heat intolerance, palpitations, elevated serum thyroxine, low TSH, and elevated urinary calcium and hydroxyproline.

IV.   HYPERPARATHYROIDISM. Elevated serum calcium, low or normal phosphorus, and elevated serum intact PTH. Radiographic evidence of endosteal and periosteal resorption. Biopsy showing osteitis fibrosa cystica and tunneling resorption.

V.   RENAL OSTEODYSTROPHY. Uremia, elevated phosphorus, low calcium, and ectopic calcification being the diagnostic clues.

VI.   GASTROINTESTINAL (GI) DISEASE. Symptoms of malabsorption or a history of previous GI surgery suggests a cause for OP or OM. Lactose intolerance, IBS, and celiac sprue should be considered.

 TREATMENT

I.   PREVENTION. The best way to avoid the complications of OP is to take early action to resist the development of OP.

A. Calcium and vitamin D_3 supplementation or increased dietary intake started at a young age can increase peak bone mass and prevent or delay the onset of OP.

B. **Exercise,** especially weight-bearing exercise, will increase the quality and quantity of bone. Balance enhancing programs are especially useful for elderly patients.

C. **Healthy diet and lifestyle.** Foods high in vitamins and minerals and the avoidance of smoking and a sedentary lifestyle help build stronger bones.

II. **MEDICAL.** Because of the high morbidity and mortality of fractures (i.e., 10% to 20% mortality within one year after a fracture), especially in the elderly, treatment is largely focused on fracture prevention. Medical treatment should be initiated in all patients who meet the criteria for OP.

A. **Risk assessment**
   1. **Careful review** of pharmaceutical agents, vision, walking devices, and household conditions can greatly reduce fall risk.
   2. **Hip protectors** have been shown to reduce hip fractures by 60% in the frail elderly population but compliance is uncertain.
   3. **Balance and exercise training** such as thai chi can reduce falls by 47% as well as increase strength and mobility.

B. **Calcium and vitamin D₃** have been shown to raise BMD by 2% to 10% and lower fracture rates by 35% to 50%. The National Institutes of Health (NIH) recommends that postmenopausal women consume 1,000 to 1,500 mg of elemental calcium and 400 to 800 IU of vitamin D_3 a day. These values are best met with a combination of a diet high in calcium as well as calcium supplements. Calcium carbonate requires a very acidic pH and commonly causes gas. Calcium citrate is more easily absorbed and helps prevent kidney stones. Magnesium helps to relieve constipation caused by calcium supplementation.

C. **Bisphosphonates** are first-line pharmaceutical treatment for OP. They have been shown to increase BMD and decrease the incidence of both vertebral and hip fractures. Bisphosphonates inhibit osteoclast function and bone resorption and therefore are most useful for high-turnover OP. Both oral preparations have to be taken before eating. Common side effects include GI upset and can lead to esophageal and gastric ulcers (patients cannot lie down after swallowing a pill). Flulike symptoms may occur with the intravenous preparations. Bisphosphonates delay maturation of fracture callus. Lowering the dose should be considered if bone markers are markedly depressed.
   1. **Alendronate** (Fosamax) 70 mg/week orally. A drug with a 10-year half-life.
   2. **Risedronate** (Actonel) 35 mg/week orally. Equal efficacy, 3-year half-life.
   3. **Ibandronate** (Boniva) 150 mg/month orally.
   4. **Pamidronate** (Aredia) 30 mg intravenous infusion every 3 months or 60 mg every 6 weeks.
   5. **Zoledronate** (Zometa) 4 mg intravenous infusion once a year only with normal kidney function.

D. **Parathormone** (Forteo) is an anabolic agent resulting in the formation of new bone. It is useful for low-turnover OP and enhances healing of new fractures. PTH is a subcutaneous 40 µg/day injection used for a 2-year period followed by a course of bisphosphonates. Side effects include cramps and orthostatic hypotension. This is preferred in premenopausal women with low bone turnover, or in patients who have not responded to or developed fractures while on bisphosphonate.

E. **Calcitonin** (Miacalcin) nasal spray, 200 IU/day, provides slight protection from spine fractures but does not protect from nonvertebral fractures. It seems to have some analgesic effects and is frequently used for bone pain and healing fractures. Side effects are minimal and include nosebleeds.

F. **Estrogen** used in OP has been a long debated topic. Although there is solid evidence that estrogen is beneficial for the skeleton, various risks such as venous thromboembolism, stroke, and breast cancer outweigh the benefits, especially in the light of other safe and effective treatment. It is generally accepted that hormone replacement therapy may be used for a short period of time to treat perimenopausal symptoms but not as a first-line treatment of OP.

G. **Selective estrogen receptor modifiers** enhance bone mass and decrease spinal fractures. There is no protection for nonvertebral fractures. They are possibly protective against breast cancer, but can cause increased postmenopausal symptoms and phlebitis.

III.   ORTHOPEDIC. In the event that a fracture is sustained, appropriate treatment is imperative for optimal recovery. A fracture is a sentinel event in a patient's life. It should stimulate the performance of a bone density assessment and optimal institution of calcium and vitamin D_3 supplements and bisphosphonates. In the acute fracture setting, PTH enhances healing while bisphosphonates may delay maturation of fracture callus.

   A. Limb fractures are treated routinely and followed by bone mass assessment and optimal and aggressive treatment of bone density abnormalities.

   B. Spine fractures are very common and often asymptomatic. However, back pain is also very common and can last several weeks. Bed rest and analgesics are recommended until the patient is comfortable, and then activity as tolerated with no heavy lifting or high-impact activities. Spine fractures can be treated surgically if the pain is ongoing and severe.

   1. Vertebroplasty. Stabilization of a fractured vertebral body with cement.

   2. Kyphoplasty. An attempt to reduce the vertebral fracture to regain height and decrease kyphosis, similar to a vertebroplasty.

PROGNOSIS

I.   OP is a clinically silent disease. Pain, dysfunction, and disability are secondary to subsequent fractures. If fractures can be avoided, the prognosis is good and the loss of BMD can be arrested or even reversed with appropriate treatment. However, hip fractures are a major cause of morbidity and mortality in the elderly population. Fifteen percent of women and 30% of men die within 1 year of fracturing their hip.

II.   Secondary OP can be treated effectively by managing the underlying disease. Bone mass will often return to normal; however, medication such as corticosteroids or radiation therapy can have permanent effects on the skeleton.

III.   Fractures will heal in the setting of OP. However, a low-turnover state such as with bisphosphonate therapy may delay healing. PTH may quicken healing.

IV.   Functional compromise can be well managed with regular physical therapy, strength training, extension exercises, balance training, and fall prevention.

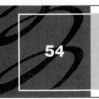

54   PAGET'S DISEASE OF BONE
John H. Healey and Andrea Piccioli

O riginally called **osteitis deformans,** Paget's disease of bone (PDB) is a disease characterized clinically by inflammatory and mechanical bone/joint pain and bony deformity. Microscopically, it is characterized by metabolic overactivity of the affected bone. Increased bone resorption is followed by excessive production of woven bone. This enlarges and weakens bones. The disease may be monostotic or polyostotic (asymmetric).

EPIDEMIOLOGY

The disease is present radiographically in 3% of the population. Symptomatic Paget's disease is much less common. Individuals of white origin are most commonly affected, but no clear inheritance pattern has been identified. There is a slight male predominance. Paget's disease is rare in patients younger than 40 years (<6% of cases). Analysis of 1,487 patients with PDB over three decades shows that there may be a continued secular trend for PDB to present in older subjects with less extensive skeletal involvement, and a declining prevalence of Paget's disease.

ETIOPATHOGENESIS

I.   ETIOLOGY. The etiology is unknown. Evidence is accumulating, however, that PDB may be a "slow-virus" infection since the first report in 1974. Mutations in the ubiquinone sequestosome 1 gene (SQSTM1; also known as p62) have recently been identified as the cause of 5q35-linked PDB. Osteoclasts and osteoclast precursors from patients with Paget's disease contain paramyxoviral transcripts and appear hyperresponsive to 1,25-dihydroxy vitamin D and receptor activator of NF-κB ligand (RANKL). A common polymorphism of the osteoprotegerin protein predisposes to the development of sporadic PDB and familial PDB that is not caused by SQSTM1 mutations.

II. GENETICS. There is probably a significant genetic component. The disease is rare in Scandinavia and Japan. Giant cell tumors are frequent among PDB families from Avellino, Italy.

III. HISTOLOGY. Increased bone turnover is evident. Osteoclast resorption may dominate. New bone is woven and has a mosaic pattern. Cement lines (reversal lines) are conspicuous. Changes consistent with hyperparathyroidism and marrow fibrosis are seen in 15% of the cases.

IV. PATHOPHYSIOLOGY. Hyperemia can produce aches and pain. It can also create a steal syndrome that causes neurologic compromise or congestive heart failure due to high output mechanisms. Hearing loss develops through a cochlear mechanism that is closely related to loss of bone mineral density in the cochlear capsule. This mechanism accounts well for both the high-frequency–sensorineural hearing loss and the air-bone gap.

 CLINICAL PRESENTATION

Most patients with Paget's disease are asymptomatic. The disease is usually recognized fortuitously when a radiograph is obtained for another purpose, or an elevated alkaline phosphatase is found and assessed. Symptomatic patients present with pain, deformity, or pathologic fracture. Hearing loss is also common. Clinically important secondary degenerative arthritis, neural compression, changes in skin temperature, high-output heart failure, and bone sarcoma (1%) can be related to or occur in an area of Paget's disease (Table 54-1).

I.   SITES OF INVOLVEMENT
   A. Sacrum (56%).
   B. Spine (50%), lumbar most frequently.
   C. Right femur (31%).
   D. Cranium (28%).
   E. Sternum (23%).
   F. Pelvis (21%).
   G. Left femur (21%).

II. ASSOCIATED CONDITIONS
   A. Hyperparathyroidism.
   B. Hyperuricemia (40%).
   C. Heart disease—congestive failure or valvular disease in most extensive cases.
   D. Hearing loss.
   E. Hypercalcemia in severe untreated cases, immobilization, or fracture.
   F. Osteoporosis resulting from both disuse and concomitant hyperparathyroidism.

 DIAGNOSTIC STUDIES

I.   LABORATORY STUDIES
   A. Elevated serum alkaline phosphatase indicates increased bone formation.
   B. Elevated collagen breakdown products, such as N- and C-terminal telopeptides, N-pyridinolines, and hydroxyproline (less sensitive and slower to respond to therapy) correspond to bone resorption and turnover.
   C. Chemical and hematologic tests are normal, including calcium and phosphorus levels.

TABLE 54-1	Radiographic and Clinical Manifestations of Paget's Disease of Bone

Location	Radiographic findings	Clinical symptoms
Skull	Osteoporosis circumscripta	None
	Cranial enlargement	Occasionally painful
	Basilar invagination	Occipital neuralgia; lower cranial nerve impingement; medullary compression; ventricular obstruction and increased intracranial pressure; vertebro-basilar artery insufficiency
	Temporal bone involvement	Hearing loss
	Auditory ossicle involvement	Hearing loss
Face, jawbones	Unilateral changes	Proptosis; trigeminal neuralgia; displacement of teeth
Spine	"Window frame" vertebra(e)	Nerve root compression; spinal stenosis
Pelvis, hip	Acetabular and femoral head disease with degenerative arthritis; protrusio acetabuli; sacroiliac joint ankylosis	Pain; end-stage arthritis
Knee joint	Bone and joint deformity	Pain; arthritis; fracture
Tibia, femur, humerus	Bowing, with or without fracture	Pain; arthritis; fracture

II. IMAGING STUDIES

A. Features. Paget's disease begins at one epiphysis and progresses to the other epiphysis of bone. A resorptive "lytic flame" is seen early at the leading edge of the lesion. Reactive bone formation enlarges the overall bone. The inflamed, weakened long bones bow. The areas of cortex thicken (e.g., iliopectineal line of pelvis), and trabeculae coarsen. Circumscribed skull lucency (osteitis circumscripta) may occur. Paget's sarcoma is suggested by the appearance of lytic areas within sclerotic pagetic bone or the development of an associated soft-tissue mass.

B. Imaging work-up

1. Radiographs. Anteroposterior and lateral views of the entire involved bone are identified by plain radiography.

2. Scintigraphy. Survey for sites of involvement. Differential nuclear scans, for example gallium scan, is hot in cancer but cool in the surrounding pagetic bone.

3. Magnetic resonance imaging or computerized topography. Evaluate the degree of spinal stenosis in patients with back pain or neurologic findings.

4. Positron-emission tomography. Look for sarcoma in a suspicious lesion.

DIFFERENTIAL DIAGNOSIS

I. METASTATIC CARCINOMA. Prostate and breast carcinoma in bone may resemble Paget's disease, but bony expansion is lacking and cortical destruction is more frequent. In any site, if destruction of bone, extracortical extension, or a possible soft-tissue mass is present, neoplasia must be ruled out, especially if pain is increasing.

II. Hemangioma of bone (especially of vertebrae) may be sclerotic and resemble monostotic Paget's disease.

III. CAFFEY'S DISEASE. Infantile cortical hyperostosis affects individuals in the young age group, may be more widespread, and predominantly affects cortical bone, although radiographic and histologic findings closely resemble those of juvenile Paget's disease.

IV. HYPERPARATHYROIDISM. Histology may be similar, and the conditions can coexist (7% to 14%). Biochemical and radiographic findings, however, differ.

MEDICAL TREATMENT

I. ASYMPTOMATIC PATIENTS. Treat if a major joint, nerve, or weight-bearing bone is affected.

II. SYMPTOMATIC PATIENTS. Symptoms usually respond to treatment in 1 to 3 months, and improvement in biochemical parameters usually parallels improvement in symptoms. All agents now used inhibit osteoclast activity and block the initial resorptive phase of Paget's disease.

A. Bisphosphonates block osteoclast function and recruitment. However, they inhibit mineralization and osteoblast function to a variable degree. In a randomized trial of patients with previously untreated PDB, alendronate and pamidronate have similar efficacy in achieving biochemical remission.

   1. Dosage
   a. Alendronate—10 to 40 mg/day orally.
   b. Pamidronate—30 to 90 mg weekly to monthly intravenous for 3 months.
   c. Risedronate—30 mg/day orally for 2 months.
   d. Etidronate—5 to 20 mg/kg/day orally for 3 to 6 months. Lower dosages are preferred except in severe cases. A 6-month interval should elapse before a course is repeated.

   2. Response. Rapid improvement in symptoms and biochemical parameters is usually seen. A paradoxical increase in pain is observed in 15% of patients.

   3. Side effects. Increased pain, diarrhea, osteomalacic fractures, and delayed fracture healing.

B. Calcitonin is a polypeptide hormone with receptors on osteoclasts that decrease bone resorption. May be used in conjunction with bisphosphonate in refractory cases.

   1. Dosage. Salmon calcitonin is the preferred agent because of its high activity and low antigenicity, and cost. Initial dosages of 50 to 150 U/day subcutaneously for 1 to 3 months may be used, then tapered to a maintenance dosage of 50 U three times weekly for 3 to 6 months.

   2. Response. In two-thirds of patients, symptomatic relief and biochemical improvement may last 6 to 12 months after a therapeutic course is completed. Antibody formation does not preclude a good response but may require a switch to human calcitonin.

   3. Side effects include nausea, flushing, local reactions at injection sites, and urticaria; these respond to antiemetics and antihistamines.

C. Combination calcitonin and bisphosphonates (low dose) may produce a faster, longer-lasting response and may be more cost-effective.

D. Gallium nitrate blocks osteoclasts and may promote activity of osteoblasts. It is also a very effective treatment of hypercalcemia.

E. Mithramycin, a DNA inhibitor, has been successful in treating hypercalcemia of malignancy. Toxicity restricts its use to cases of acute neurologic compression syndromes in Paget's disease.

III. FOLLOW-UP. Treatment benefit is seen within 6 months of treatment. Biochemical deterioration occurs after 12 to 24 months. Therefore follow-up, every 6 to 12 months for alkaline phosphatase and annually for radiographs, is recommended.

ORTHOPEDIC TREATMENT

I. SURGERY. General considerations: It may be successful, but deformity, poor bone quality, and soft-tissue hyperemia make surgery difficult. Calcitonin treatment for at least 6 weeks before procedures is recommended. Etidronate should be avoided if an osteotomy is to be performed. The effect of pamidronate or other bisphosphonates on osteotomy healing is unknown.

II. **FRACTURES**
  A. Pseudofractures may persist for 6 to 12 months and should not be overtreated once symptoms subside.
  B. Completed fractures usually heal with closed methods, but healing may be delayed.
  C. Bisphosphonates should be avoided if possible.
  D. Biopsy occasionally is necessary to exclude sarcoma.
III. **IMMOBILIZATION.** Intravenous bisphosphonates, gallium nitrate, calcitonin, and occasionally mithramycin (now called plicamycin) will be necessary to treat hypercalcemia.
IV. **JOINT REPLACEMENT.** Results of total hip arthroplasty using uncemented components in patients with Paget's disease are excellent during the first decade after implantation. These patients may be at higher risk for heterotopic bone formation and increased perioperative blood loss because of hypervascularity of the bone. Therefore, disease control preoperatively is necessary.
V. **SPINE DECOMPRESSION.** Neural compression may require surgery.
VI. **COCHLEAR IMPLANTS.**

 PROGNOSIS

Bone sarcomas occur in less than 1% of patients and are almost always fatal. Benign giant cell tumors also occur and may respond to corticosteroid therapy.

Uncomplicated Paget's disease generally responds to medical management and becomes quiescent. Degenerative arthritis and deformity usually require surgery. Medical management may prevent disease progression and is usually warranted.

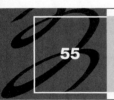

55 ENDOCRINE ARTHROPATHIES
Michael D. Lockshin

■ **KEY POINTS**

■ The musculoskeletal manifestations of endocrine diseases include muscle dysfunction, disorders of bone metabolism, and cartilage deformation.

■ Endocrinopathic musculoskeletal disease tends to be diffuse and poorly described.

■ The most important diagnostic step is to consider the possibility of endocrinopathy.

■ Routine clinical laboratory tests are usually not helpful; radiographs often first suggest the possibility of an endocrinopathy.

■ Treatment of the underlying endocrinopathy relieves the musculoskeletal manifestations; however, the rate of remission varies with the endocrinopathy.

*T*he **musculoskeletal manifestations of endocrine diseases** include muscle dysfunction, disorders of bone metabolism, and cartilage deformation.

Tendons, ligaments, and tendon attachment sites are regularly symptomatic, for example; symptoms are more often periarticular than articular. Crystal arthropathies and calcific tendinitis may be symptoms of endocrine disease.

CLINICAL MANIFESTATIONS

Endocrinopathic musculoskeletal disease tends to be diffuse and poorly described.
Except for crystal arthritis, it is more often periarticular than articular. Table 55-1 lists the
rheumatic manifestations of common endocrinopathies.

| TABLE 55-1 | Rheumatic Manifestations of Common Endocrinopathies |

Endocrine abnormality	Rheumatic manifestation	Putative pathogenesis
Thyroid—hyper	Proximal myopathy	Muscle/protein metabolism
	Thyroid acropachy	Growth hormone
	Myalgia (during changing thyroid states)	Unknown
Thyroid—hypo	High creatine kinase	Muscle membrane abnormality
	Bland joint effusion	Abnormal cartilage metabolism
	Chondrocalcinosis	Unknown
	Hyperuricemia	Renal tubular dysfunction
	Myalgia (during changing thyroid states)	Unknown
	Osteonecrosis-type joint damage that may necessitate joint replacement	Unknown
Parathyroid—hyper	Osteopenia, bone resorption, fractures, cysts, myopathy, and pseudogout	Hypercalcemia increased osteoclast activity
Parathyroid—hypo	Osteopenia	Decreased osteoblast activity
Parathyroid—hypo (congenital)	Short stature and short metacarpals	Unknown
Pituitary—hyper	Increased cartilage growth, accelerated osteoarthritis, and osteopenia	Growth hormone excess and abnormal joint mechanics
Pituitary—hypo	Short stature and osteopenia	Lack of growth hormone
Adrenal—hyper	Osteopenia	Effect on calcium metabolism and osteoblasts and osteoclasts
	Proximal myopathy	Muscle protein catabolism and hypokalemia
Gonads—hyper	Short stature	Premature closure of epiphyses
Gonads—hypo	Osteopenia	Unopposed osteoclast activity
Pancreas (diabetes)	Charcot joints	Neuropathy
	Eheiroarthropathy	Unknown
	Dupuytren's contracture	Unknown
	Palmar fasciitis	Unknown
	Carpal tunnel syndrome	Unknown
	Septic arthritis or osteomyelitis	Increased infection risk in DM
	Scleredema	Unknown
Hemochromatosis	Pyrophosphate arthropathy	Iron deposition in cartilage
	Hooks on metacarpophalangeal joints	Unknown

DM, diabetes mellitus.

DIAGNOSTIC INVESTIGATIONS

I. **The most important diagnostic step is to consider the possibility of endocrinopathy** and then to evaluate whether the patient's symptoms might be explained by that abnormality. History, physical examination, and often radiology define the rheumatologic problem, and directed laboratory studies define the associated endocrinopathy.

II. **Myalgias, proximal myopathy, and, on occasion, high levels of creatine kinase** suggest thyroid disorders. Less commonly, acromegaly and disorders causing hyperkalemia or hypokalemia cause muscle weakness. **Carpal tunnel syndrome** occurs in hypothyroidism, acromegaly, and diabetes. **Scleredema,** a thickening of the skin of the upper back, is characteristic of advanced diabetes.

III. **Osteopenia** is characteristic of hyperparathyroidism and hyperadrenalism, but it also occurs in patients with thyroid and pituitary dysfunction.

IV. **Characteristic syndromes** may be diagnostic; the **cheiroarthropathy** (flexion contractures of the hands) of advanced diabetes and **thyroid acropathy** (periostitis accompanied by clubbing and pretibial myxedema) in Grave's disease are examples. **Chondrocalcinosis** and characteristic metacarpophalangeal disease ("hooked" metacarpals) are diagnostic of hemochromatosis.

V. **Routine clinical laboratory tests** such as complete blood count or erythrocyte sedimentation rate are routinely performed but are usually not helpful, except for being negative in assessment for systemic autoimmune rheumatic disease, such as rheumatoid factor or antinuclear antibody. It is necessary to confirm the suspected endocrinopathy with appropriately directed tests.

VI. **Radiographs** often first suggest the possibility of an endocrinopathy. Parathyroid disorders, acromegaly, most heritable disorders such as Marfan's syndrome, pseudohypoparathyroidism, ochronosis, and advanced diabetes show characteristic radiologic abnormalities. In the heritable disorders, these abnormalities include scoliosis and long thin bones, short metacarpals, especially the fourth metacarpal, and cartilage calcification, respectively.

DIFFERENTIAL DIAGNOSIS

I. Rheumatoid arthritis and osteoarthritis, gout, pseudogout, lupus, dermatomyositis, and scleroderma may each be suggested by some manifestation of an endocrinopathy. Normal levels of antinuclear antibody, rheumatoid factor, and muscle enzymes, and a normal erythrocyte sedimentation rate help exclude these diagnoses, but abnormal test results do not positively confirm them. Hypothyroidism due to Hashimoto's thyroiditis can commonly coexist with other autoimmune disorders.

II. A noninflammatory **synovial fluid analysis** (except in pseudogout associated with diabetes, hyperparathyroidism, or hemochromatosis) is most characteristic of endocrinopathy. In myxedema, synovial fluid is often very viscous and colorless.

TREATMENT AND PROGNOSIS

I. **Treatment of the underlying endocrinopathy** relieves myalgia, myopathy, tendinitis, and, to some extent, osteopenia and skin manifestations, but it will not reverse established bone and cartilage deformity. The **rate of remission** varies with the endocrinopathy.
    A. In **thyroid** disease, myalgias remit within weeks to months, myopathy within months, and acropachy in years, if at all.
    B. In **parathyroid** disease, bone pain abates in months, and bone remineralization occurs within years. Normal bone structure may not be completely restored, particularly if bone trabeculae have become discontinuous.
    C. **Adrenal** myopathy improves in months.

D. The skeletal changes of **pituitary, gonadal, and congenital** endocrinopathies usually do not regress. Estrogen replacement retards bone loss, but remineralization of osteoporotic bone requires calcium, calcitonin, bisphosphonate, or teriparatide therapy.

E. The skeletal and soft-tissue abnormalities of **diabetes and hemochromatosis** do not improve.

II. Medical treatment (other than treatment of the endocrinopathy) is nonspecific and symptomatic. Nonsteroidal anti-inflammatory drugs (NSAIDs) and analgesics are commonly used. There is no role for corticosteroid preparations, antimalarial agents, disease-modifying antirheumatic drugs (DMARDs), or immunosuppressive drugs. The following **specific precautions** are necessary:

A. Patients with **hyperthyroidism** metabolize drugs rapidly; standard doses may be ineffective.

B. Patients with **hypothyroidism** metabolize drugs slowly; standard doses may be toxic.

C. In **diabetes and hyperparathyroidism,** renal dysfunction should be anticipated.

D. In **hemochromatosis,** hepatic dysfunction should be anticipated.

III. Surgical treatment is useful for **carpal tunnel syndrome** and, on occasion, for orthopedic repair, but specific concerns are as follows:

A. Osteopenic bones heal and hold prostheses poorly.

B. Charcot joints heal poorly and tend to refracture. Fusions may be indicated. Joint replacements may be problematic owing to the constant trauma imposed upon them by the neurologic dysfunction.

C. Diabetic cheiroarthropathy responds very poorly to attempts at surgical correction.

FIBROMYALGIA AND CHRONIC PAIN

Daniel J. Clauw and John F. Beary, III

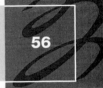

56

▓ KEY POINTS

▪ Fibromyalgia (FM) is a painful, noninflammatory condition characterized by a history of widespread pain, and diffuse tenderness on examination.

▪ The hallmark of FM appears to be a central disturbance in pain processing that is largely unexplained by psychological factors.

▪ Functional imaging studies have confirmed that when patients with FM are given a low-pressure stimulus (that would not be felt as painful by a control subject), they not only experience pain, but also have activations in the pain-processing regions of the brain.

▪ FM frequently coexists with other conditions. Approximately 25% of patients with rheumatoid arthritis (RA), lupus, osteoarthritis (OA), and hepatitis C also have FM.

▪ Three types of treatment have been demonstrated in randomized, controlled trials to be of benefit for the spectrum of FM illness: symptom-based pharmacotherapy, aerobic exercise, and cognitive behavioral therapy (CBT).

INTRODUCTION

I. **Fibromyalgia (FM) is a painful, noninflammatory condition characterized by a history of widespread pain, and diffuse tenderness on examination.** Although FM is defined on the basis of pain and tenderness, most individuals with FM also display a number of nondefining symptoms, including fatigue, sleep disturbances, headaches, or memory difficulties.

    A. In fact, it has become increasingly clear that there is considerable overlap between FM and "systemic" conditions such as chronic fatigue syndrome, as well as other "organ-specific" syndromes such as migraine headache, tension headache, irritable bowel syndrome, temporomandibular disorders, and mitral valve prolapse.

    B. In 1990, the definition of FM was redefined by a subcommittee of the American College of Rheumatology (ACR). The new definition requires a history of chronic widespread pain (pain lasting for more than 3 months in all four quadrants of the body plus the axial skeleton), and the finding of 11 or more positive results on the 18 tender points examined.

II. **Chronic musculoskeletal pain can result from** a central non-nociceptive mechanism such as in FM, from peripheral nociceptive mechanisms such as in mechanical osteoarthritis (OA) or in inflammatory rheumatoid arthritis (RA), or from neuropathic pain mechanisms such as in diabetic neuropathy.

III. **FM tender points are** discrete regions of the body where a 4-kg pressure is applied with digital palpation, and if the individual experiences pain when this area is pushed, it is considered a "positive" tender point. Even when this definition was originally adopted, it was stated that these criteria were not meant to be strictly applied in clinical practice. Only about half of the patients seen in clinical practice who clearly present with FM will meet these strict criteria; many individuals have pain that is more limited in distribution, or have fewer than 11 tender points.

    A. The usefulness of the "tender points" concept is currently being debated, because it is now clear that the primary problem in FM is a **generalized** disturbance in pain processing. Patients with FM are more tender throughout the entire body, even in control areas such as the thumbnail or forehead. The tenderness is diffuse rather than regional, and not just confined to certain types of tissues (i.e., muscle).

    B. Tender points merely represent regions of the body, such as the lateral epicondylar area, where even normal individuals are more tender. When a patient with FM is stimulated at these tender points, the pain is likely to be amplified as compared to a control subject.

 ETIOPATHOGENESIS

I. **The precise cause for FM remains unclear.** There have been numerous studies suggesting that there is a strong familial aggregation of FM, although no studies have differentiated whether this is due to hereditary or shared environmental influences.

II. **It is also clear that there are a number of environmental "stressors,"** including physical trauma, infections, autoimmune disorders, endocrine conditions, and emotional stress, that seem to be capable of "triggering" the development of FM.

III. **There have been several types of physiologic abnormalities** that have been identified in individuals with FM and related conditions that may help explain the basis of symptoms. The hallmark of FM appears to be a central disturbance in pain processing that is largely unexplained by psychological factors. The evidence for this comes from numerous studies employing various types of experimental pain testing paradigms, as well as from objective abnormalities of neurotransmitters (e.g., substance P) in the cerebrospinal fluid of patients with FM.

IV. **Most recently, functional imaging studies** have confirmed that when patients with FM are given a low-pressure stimulus (that would not be felt as painful by a control subject), they not only experience pain, but also have activations in the pain-processing regions of the brain, again confirming augmented central processing of pressure, heat, and other stimuli. There have also been a number of abnormalities in both neuroendocrine and autonomic function that have been identified in subgroups of patients with FM.

V. **Although the dualistic notion that any illness is either "organic" or "functional"** should be abandoned, because of the realization that all illnesses likely have a biological basis, this debate still continues with respect to FM and other related conditions. It is likely that in many individuals this illness begins as primarily a neurobiological problem, and in some individuals never progresses past this point because of appropriate treatment, good coping skills, and adequate support systems. But in other individuals, with chronicity of symptoms, concurrent psychological, psychiatric, and behavioral factors either develop or become more prominent.

VI. **Examples of factors that portend a worse prognosis include** ways in which individuals perceive their pain (e.g., catastrophizing or having a very negative view of the pain, and/or having an external locus of control, which means that individuals feel they cannot do anything about their pain), maladaptive illness behaviors (i.e., the bad habits patients get into, as a result of long-term symptoms, that aggravate or amplify symptoms), secondary gain issues (e.g., litigation and compensation), and concurrent mood disorders.

VII. **Although comorbid depression should be treated if it is identified, this rarely leads to a decrease in pain.** This has been demonstrated both with functional imaging studies, and with clinical trials showing that when patients with chronic pain are given drugs that have both antidepressant and analgesic effects, the drug actions and benefits seem to occur independent of one another.

 PREVALENCE

I. **Approximately 2% to 4% of the population in industrialized countries** (e.g., United States, Canada, Israel, and Germany) have FM, as defined by the ACR criteria. However, these population-based studies suggest that it may be better to consider FM as "the end of a spectrum" rather than as a discrete, unique illness. For example, both the pain and tenderness domains are continuously distributed across a wide range in the population. Approximately 10% of the United States population has chronic widespread pain, and 20% has chronic regional pain; and both symptoms occur approximately 1.5 times more commonly in women than in men. This is in contrast to earlier studies that cite a female to male ratio of 8:2, and a peak prevalence in the age range of 20 to 55 years.

II. **There is a wide continuum of tenderness within the population,** ranging from those who are very tender, to those who are quite nontender. Women are more sensitive to cutaneous pressure than are men, and in fact are ten times more likely to have 11 tender points than are men. Because the ACR definition uses an arbitrary cut-off of 11 tender points to define the subset of patients with chronic widespread pain who are tender enough to meet FM criteria, FM, as defined by these criteria, occurs almost exclusively in women. This is problematic because most men who have chronic widespread pain (but inadequate numbers of tender points to meet ACR criteria), are likely to have the same underlying problem.

III. **Other studies have demonstrated that FM frequently coexists** with other conditions. Approximately 25% of patients with RA, lupus, ankylosing spondylitis, OA, hepatitis C, and a number of other conditions display concurrent FM.

IV. **These data suggest that it may be better to consider FM as a construct** that helps explain chronic pain in the absence of a peripheral inflammatory or mechanical stimulus. This central or "non-nociceptive" pain occurs commonly throughout the entire body (i.e., FM), in a single region of the body (e.g., temporomandibular syndrome and myofascial pain syndrome), or concurrently with other medical conditions (especially those characterized by chronic pain). Table 56-1 shows that FM and other non-nociceptive pain syndromes differ in many ways from classic "nociceptive pain."

 CLINICAL MANIFESTATIONS

I. **SYMPTOMS.** The character of pain in FM is different than in most other musculoskeletal conditions. Although most individuals with FM will have a few areas where they always experience pain, this condition is characterized by wide variation in the location, as well as the intensity, of pain. Patients will frequently report worsening of pain in response to activity, weather changes, menstrual status, and stressors. It is common to have subjective weakness, morning stiffness, swelling (especially of the hands and feet), and nondermatomal dysesthesias or paresthesias that accompany the pain. Additional symptoms that frequently coexist are fatigue and difficulties with short-term memory and concentration.

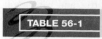

TABLE 56-1	Mechanistic Characterization of Chronic Pain

Peripheral (nociceptive)	Central (non-nociceptive)

■ Primarily due to inflammation or mechanical damage in periphery
■ NSAID, opioid responsive
■ Responds to procedures
■ Behavioral factors minor
■ Examples:
  – Osteoarthritis
  – Rheumatoid arthritis
  – Cancer pain
	■ Primarily due to a central disturbance in pain processing
	■ Tricyclic, neuroactive compounds most effective
	■ Psychological, behavioral factors more prominent
	■ Examples:
	  – Fibromyalgia
	  – Irritable bowel syndrome
	  – Tension and migraine headache
	  – Interstitial cystitis/vulvodynia, noncardiac chest pain and others

NSAID, nonsteroidal anti-inflammatory drug.

II. **The physical examination** in FM is classically normal except for the finding of diffuse tenderness. Occasionally, patients will also display mild muscle weakness, perhaps because of pain and/or disuse.

DIAGNOSTIC INVESTIGATIONS

I. **LABORATORY TESTS.** FM is a diagnosis of exclusion, because there are no laboratory or imaging studies that are predictably abnormal in this entity. Initial testing in a patient suspected of having FM should include routine hematology and chemistry panels, thyroid function tests, and an erythrocyte sedimentation rate or C-reactive protein. Unless there are specific signs and symptoms suggesting illnesses such as RA (e.g., synovitis on examination) or systemic lupus erythematosus, tests such as antinuclear antibodies (ANAs) and rheumatoid factor have a very low predictive value and should be avoided.

A. For example, it has been estimated that for every ANA ordered on a patient with the nonspecific complaints of myalgias, arthralgias, and fatigue, there will be at least 20 false-positive results for every true positive (i.e., a patient with an autoimmune disorder).

B. There seem to be some laboratory abnormalities that occur more commonly in this spectrum of illness than in the general population, such as elevated titers to certain viruses such as Epstein-Barr virus, positive ANAs, and lipid abnormalities. However, these tests are neither sensitive nor specific for FM.

II. **IMAGING STUDIES.** There are no specific imaging tests that have clinical utility. Functional magnetic resonance imaging (fMRI) studies of the brain of patients with FM show distinctive patterns of activity; however, fMRI remains an experimental tool.

DIFFERENTIAL DIAGNOSIS

I. **It is important to rule out treatable medical conditions** that can generate secondary FM symptoms, before settling on the diagnosis of primary FM. More caution is required in this in patients who are older than 50 years. Fever and weight loss do not occur from FM, and must be explained. Polymyalgia rheumatica produces shoulder and hip girdle pain, and is associated with anemia and an elevated sedimentation rate. In overweight men, sleep apnea should be considered as a cause for morning achiness and mental sluggishness.

II. **Common conditions that should be excluded** are thyroid disorders, especially hypothyroidism, anemia, occult infections such as hepatitis C, and depression with somatic symptoms. Lipid-lowering drugs in the statin class can cause muscle aches. Less common conditions include rheumatic diseases that are presenting in an atypical manner. It should be remembered that polymyositis is more likely to present as weakness rather than as muscle pain. Patients who are having their corticosteroids tapered will report increased achiness and malaise.

TREATMENT

I. **There are three types of treatment** that have been best demonstrated in randomized, controlled trials to be of benefit within this spectrum of illness: symptom-based pharmacotherapy, aerobic exercise, and cognitive behavioral therapy (CBT). Perhaps the most important role of the physician is to educate the patient that FM is a chronic condition wherein pain occurs although there is no damage to the body, and that there is no pill or "magic herb" that will "cure" this illness. Patients with this condition rarely improve significantly unless they accept that they need to play an active role in their own treatment, and that this should include daily exercise and appropriate lifestyle modifications.

II. **PHARMACOTHERAPY.** The class of drugs with established efficacy in FM are the tricyclic compounds, with cyclobenzaprine (Flexeril) and amitriptyline (Elavil) being the best studied. These medications are best tolerated if they are given several hours before bedtime (to help prevent the "hungover" feeling that patients often report). They must both be started at low dosages (e.g., half of a 10-mg tablet) and slowly escalated by 5 to 10 mg every 1 to 2 weeks until efficacy is found or a dosage of 50 mg/day is reached.

   A. Because FM is not an inflammatory condition, "anti-inflammatory" dosages of nonsteroidal anti-inflammatory drugs (NSAIDs) are neither necessary nor of much benefit. In addition to tricyclics, analgesics [e.g., low dosages of NSAIDs, acetaminophen, or tramadol (Ultram)] may be helpful. If patients cannot tolerate tricyclics or get incomplete relief, the next class of drugs to consider are the mixed reuptake inhibitors [e.g., venlafaxine (Effexor) and duloxetine (Cymbalta)]. These drugs inhibit the uptake of both serotonin and norepinephrine.

   B. Other drugs that can be of some benefit in reducing the pain caused by FM include high dosages of gabapentin (Neurontin) (approximately 2,000 mg/day with a higher percentage of dosage at night), or tizanidine (Zanaflex). If selective serotonin reuptake inhibitors are used, it is generally felt that those that are least selective [e.g., fluoxetine (Prozac), paroxetine (Paxil), sertraline (Zoloft)] may be the best analgesics, especially if used in higher doses.

III. **Aerobic exercise therapy** can be extremely beneficial in FM and related conditions. Mildly affected individuals can sometimes be adequately managed only with these modalities. A graded, low-impact, aerobic exercise program is extremely beneficial. Patients should be instructed to begin with 5 to 10 minutes of low-impact exercise (e.g., water exercise, stationary bike, treadmill, and walking) three to four times/week and to increase this by 1 to 2 minutes/week. Beginning at high levels of exercise or escalating more rapidly is poorly tolerated, and frequently will make the individual feel worse. The eventual goal should be 20 to 30 minutes of aerobic exercise four to five times weekly.

IV. **CBT** is an education-based program that has been successfully used to treat a number of chronic medical conditions, including chronic pain states, FM, and chronic fatigue syndrome. These programs can be used either in an individual or in a group setting, and focus on teaching the patients the techniques that reduce their symptoms (e.g., biofeedback and relaxation exercises). Maladaptive illness behaviors that the patient (usually unknowingly) displays, and which make the illness worse, are identified and explained. An example is the tendency for patients to "overdo it" on "good days," which will lead to several "bad days."

PROGNOSIS

Although FM is typically a chronic illness lasting for several years, life expectancy is not affected. Most afflicted individuals can expect to lead a relatively normal life with appropriate management.

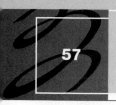

57 PARANEOPLASTIC MUSCULOSKELETAL SYNDROMES AND HYPERTROPHIC OSTEOARTHROPATHY

Alan T. Kaell

INTRODUCTION

I. **If a close temporal relation exists between the discovery of a malignancy and the onset of a rheumatic syndrome, an association is often presumed.** In many cases, the association may be coincidental. In other cases, the response of the rheumatic syndrome to successful management of the malignancy suggests an inter-relation of the two problems. Similarly, the recurrence of a rheumatic syndrome that heralds or follows the relapse of a malignancy is an even stronger indication of a pathogenetic linkage.

II. **The clinical and temporal relation between various rheumatic syndromes and malignant neoplasms takes any one of several forms.**
   A. Rheumatic syndrome as a manifestation of an established or occult malignancy.
   B. Malignancy occurring in the setting of an established rheumatic syndrome.
   C. Malignancy as a complication of antirheumatic therapy.
   D. Rheumatic syndrome as a complication of antineoplastic therapy.

ETIOPATHOGENESIS

I. **The pathogenesis of a rheumatic syndrome in a patient with cancer may be known.**
   A. Cancer may primarily involve joints, bones, muscles, blood vessels, or nerves and thereby mimic rheumatic disease. Examples of this include neuroblastoma and leukemia in children.
   B. Alternatively, cancer may invade adjacent tissues or secondarily metastasize to such tissues. This is seen in both solid neoplasms and hematologic malignancies.
   C. Hyperuricemia from high cellular turnover (e.g., leukemia) may manifest as gout.

II. **The pathogenesis of a rheumatic syndrome in a patient with cancer is often unknown and remains speculative.**
   A. Systemic manifestations of cancer can occur without tissue invasion by the tumor itself. Such remote effects, or **paraneoplastic** phenomena, may present as rheumatic syndromes. A cytokine or immune-mediated pathogenesis is likely. Dermatomyositis (DM) in patients with ovarian carcinoma is an example of this phenomenon.
   B. In **hypertrophic osteoarthropathy** (HOA) (pulmonary), the pathogenesis remains speculative. Humoral factors such as platelet-derived growth factors, cellular, neural, and vascular mechanisms have been suggested.

III. **The pathogenesis of increased lymphoma in certain patients with rheumatic disease is unknown but may reflect underlying immune dysregulation,** abnormalities in apoptosis, genetic predispositions, or a risk associated with certain therapies.

IV. **The pathogenesis of increased malignancy associated with certain therapies is unknown but may reflect alterations in immune surveillance.** The determination of the reasons for excess cases of cancer is confounded by the lack of ideal control groups, an unknown denominator of patients with the illness, and the necessity to utilize historical databases.
   A. An increased incidence of large B-cell non-Hodgkin's lymphoma (NHL), noted with untreated classic rheumatoid arthritis (RA) and Sjögren's syndrome, is perhaps related to abnormalities in apoptosis.

B. Lymphoma and certain solid neoplasms are associated with some immunosuppressive therapies, presumably reflecting alterations in tumor surveillance or apoptosis. Patients with RA and on treatment with methotrexate also develop non-Hodgkin's lymphomas that contain Epstein-Barr virus (EBV), the latter likely acting as a cofactor along with the medication given.

V. **Finally, some therapies for cancer may be associated with rheumatic syndromes.** The pathogenesis remains speculative.

 PREVALENCE

I. **RHEUMATIC SYNDROME AS A MANIFESTATION OF AN ESTABLISHED OR OCCULT MALIGNANCY.** The incidence of malignancy presenting as a rheumatic disease is unclear, but likely ranges between 1% and 10% of all malignancies. The incidence is likely to be higher for HOA and DM. Unclassified rheumatic disorders in hospitalized patients may be associated with an underlying occult neoplasm in up to 24% of cases during a 2-year period. The frequency may be higher in men and patients older than 50 years. The malignancy is usually discovered on routine physical examination.

  A. HOA (Table 57-1)—the incidence of HOA is highest among patients with lung cancer.

  B. DM—may herald underlying malignancy of any type. Overall, malignancy occurs in 5% to 20% of individuals with myositis. DM has a stronger association with cancer than does polymyositis and inclusion body myositis. The association is most apparent in men older than 40 years. Myositis may precede the discovery of a malignancy by several months to a few years. Among the many types of malignancies that present with myositis, lung, breast, and ovarian carcinomas are the most common.

  C. Polyarticular, pauciarticular, or monarticular arthritis as a presenting manifestation of malignancy is less than 1% for solid neoplasms, but is more likely in hematologic neoplasia. An age-appropriate cancer assessment needs to be done in all patients presenting with arthritis.

II. **MALIGNANCY OCCURING IN THE SETTING OF AN ESTABLISHED RHEUMATIC SYNDROME.** The observed number of cases of any particular type of cancer in patients with a rheumatic disease is likely to exceed the expected number of cases of cancer seen in sex- and age-matched general population. If therapy appears to be associated with an observed increase in malignancy, then the expected number of cases of cancer should be determined from a **disease- and age-matched, untreated** population. Unfortunately, such data are sparse.

  A. Patients with RA do not appear to have an overall increased risk of cancer, and the risk of gastrointestinal neoplasms may be decreased compared to the general population.

  B. Patients with RA do have a higher relative risk of Hodgkin's disease, NHL, and leukemia compared to the general population. This increased risk of NHL correlates with the severity and duration of RA and is independent of drug therapy. The copresence of Sjögren's syndrome raises this risk. The risk ranges from two- to 25.8-fold for patients with the most severe RA, and this risk is thought to increase by 2.6 times for every 10 years of increase in age. The mean time between the onset of RA and NHL ranges from 11 to 17 years.

  C. DM is associated with all types of cancer. Incidence varies widely, depending upon the series studied.

  D. Patients with hepatitis C and its rheumatic complications have a higher risk of NHL.

  E. Patients with systemic lupus erythematosus (SLE) exposed to cyclophosphamide are at increased risk for leukemia and bladder cancer.

  F. Clubbing or HOA may signal underlying neoplasia (see Table 57-1).

  G. Progressive systemic sclerosis can be associated with bronchoalveolar cell carcinoma.

  H. Patients with Wegener's granulomatosis exposed to cyclophosphamide are at increased risk for leukemia and bladder cancer.

III. **Malignancy as a complication of antirheumatic therapy** may be associated with an increased risk of malignancy or NHL. The true incidence of these associations is difficult to ascertain and range between 0.1% and 3%. In some cases, the underlying disease may predispose to the malignancy (e.g., RA, Sjögren's syndrome, and hepatitis C). In other

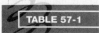

TABLE 57-1	Conditions Associated with Hypertrophic Osteoarthropathy	
Neoplasms	Pulmonary and pleural	Primary lung tumors—squamous cell carcinoma, large- and small-cell carcinoma, lymphoma
		Metastases from soft-tissue, muscle, and bone sarcomas; nasopharyngeal, gastrointestinal, and renal carcinomas
		Mesothelioma of pleura
		Fibromas
	Gastrointestinal	Stomach and colonic mucus-producing carcinomas
		Esophageal carcinoma
		Hepatoma
		Small intestinal carcinoma
		Polyposis of colon, esophagus
	Miscellaneous	Secondary myelofibrosis
		Thymoma
		Neurilemmoma
		Chronic myelogenous leukemia
Chronic suppurative diseases	Pulmonary and pleural	Bronchiectasis
		Cystic fibrosis
		Empyema
		Lung abscess
		Other: tuberculosis, sarcoid, hydatid cyst
	Gastrointestinal	Inflammatory bowel disease (Crohn's disease and ulcerative colitis)
		Other: bacillary and amebic dysentery, ascariasis, subphrenic abscess, tuberculosis
Other conditions	Cardiovascular	Cyanotic congenital heart disease
		Subacute bacterial endocarditis
		Other: pulmonary hemangioma, infected aortic prosthesis, aortic aneurysm, Takayasu's arteritis
	Miscellaneous	Primary biliary cirrhosis, nontropical sprue, blood dyscrasias, myxedema, amyloidosis, syringomyelia, thyroid acropachy
	Familial and idiopathic	

cases, the risk of malignancy is more directly related to drug exposure (e.g., cyclophosphamide) and may correlate with the dose and duration of exposure as well as postexposure duration. There are inherent statistical and epidemiologic problems in defining the actual cancer risk in diseases in which we are unaware of the number of patients with the disease; the screening of all patients with cancer is incomplete; the confirmation of the diagnosis is not certain; and the monitoring systems are poor.

A. Azathioprine (Imuran)—NHL.

B. Methotrexate—NHL, in particular, EBV-associated.

C. Cyclophosphamide (Cytoxan)—bladder carcinoma/leukemia.

D. Anti-tumor necrosis factor-α (anti-TNF-α) biologics. The use of biologics to date is not associated with an increased incidence of observed solid malignancies over that expected in the general population or patients with RA. NHL incidence is elevated in patients with RA treated with TNF-α antagonists, but this has been attributed to the known higher incidence associated with RA itself. Because the experience with these drugs is only for 6 years, longer observation is needed.

E. Anti-interleukin (IL-1) anakinra (Kineret)—no clear and convincing evidence of excess malignancies.

F. Leflunomide (Arava)—no clear and convincing evidence of excess malignancies exists.

IV. RHEUMATIC SYNDROME AS A COMPLICATION OF ANTINEOPLASTIC THERAPY. (See section Clinical manifestations.) The incidence of rheumatic syndromes related to antineoplastic therapies is variable and ranges from 1% to 25% depending upon the agent and the syndrome. The interferon agents and neutrophil growth factors such as granulocyte–colony-stimulating factor (G-CSF) and granulocyte macrophage (GM)-CSF have the highest incidence of nonspecific myalgias and arthralgias.

CLINICAL MANIFESTATIONS

The clinical and temporal relation between various rheumatic syndromes and malignant neoplasms can take any one of several forms.

I. RHEUMATIC SYNDROME AS A MANIFESTATION OF AN ESTABLISHED OR OC-CULT MALIGNANCY

A. Primary bone and joint neoplasms. Primary bone tumors such as chondrosarcoma, giant cell tumor, and osteogenic sarcoma may present as monarticular pain. They can either directly invade the joint capsule and synovium or induce a synovial reaction by involving juxta-articular bone.

B. Tenosynovial sarcomas are rare and usually present as a painless soft-tissue mass near a joint of the lower extremity. Extension directly into the joint is uncommon.

C. Lymphoproliferative disorders

1. **Leukemia.** Leukemic cells may directly infiltrate articular tissues. Polyarthritis occurs more often with hematologic malignancies than with solid neoplasms. In childhood, the metaphyseal portion of bones is occupied by red marrow. Acute lymphocytic leukemia can present as a migratory or symmetric polyarthritis by infiltrating the periosteum, joint capsule, or metaphysis. It may even mimic rheumatic fever or juvenile idiopathic arthritis (JIA). The ankle or knee is usually involved. Characteristically, the joint pain is quite severe, awakens children at night, and is disproportionate to any physical findings. The erythrocyte sedimentation rate (ESR) may be normal. Articular manifestations may develop before the appearance of leukemic cells in the peripheral blood. An elevated serum lactate dehydrogenase or mild leukopenia may help distinguish children with malignant neoplasms who present with musculoskeletal complaints from those who ultimately have JIA. In some cases, immunocytologic analysis can identify leukemic cells in synovial fluid.

   Vasculitis seen in patients with leukemia is usually limited to cutaneous involvement. Recurrent leukemic infiltrations into muscles may mimic localized, tender swelling of polyarteritis. Hairy-cell leukemia has been associated with polyarteritis nodosa. Rheumatic manifestations can precede or follow the clinical onset of leukemic symptoms and diagnosis. Pathogenesis involves either leukemic infiltration or immune-driven inflammation.

2. **Lymphoma.** Monarticular or polyarticular symptoms may be related to lymphomatous involvement of juxta-articular bone. Both Hodgkin's and NHL may present with musculoskeletal symptoms. This is attributed to either induction of a synovial reaction by adjacent osseous lymphoma or direct invasion of the joint capsule or synovium. In patients with T-cell lymphomas, a chronic polyarthritis may also develop.

   Vasculitis associated with lymphoma is usually limited to cutaneous involvement, presumably on an immune basis. In rare patients with intravascular lymphoma, multiorgan involvement may mimic vasculitis and symmetric polyarthritis.

3. **Angioimmunoblastic lymphadenopathy** can be associated with rash, polyarthritis, polyclonal hypergammaglobulinemia, and Coombs'-positive hemolytic anemia. This condition may mimic SLE.

4. **Myelodysplastic disorders** have also been associated with a variety of musculoskeletal symptoms and signs, including polyarthritis, lupuslike conditions, polychondritis, vasculitis, and erythromelalgia.

5. **Gout,** secondary to rapid cell turnover or tumor lysis, is seen mainly in patients with leukemias and lymphomas. Institution of allopurinol helps prevent this complication. The dosage of azathioprine and 6-mercaptopurine must be reduced by 75% or avoided if the patient receives concomitant allopurinol therapy.

D. **Paraproteinemias**

1. **Amyloid arthropathy** is attributed to deposition of amyloid light chain protein and is associated with dysproteinemias, such as multiple myeloma. It occurs in up to 5% of patients with myeloma and is more common in men and those with γ light chains. This arthropathy can mimic RA and is associated with carpal tunnel syndrome, shoulder pad sign, and nodules. Erosions are rarely noted. Additional clinical clues that warrant consideration of amyloidosis are hepatosplenomegaly, congestive heart failure, macroglossia, pinch purpura, raccoon eyes, and nephrosis. Biopsy sites to establish a tissue diagnosis include abdominal fat, rectum, synovium, and bone marrow.

2. **POEMS syndrome** (plasma cell dyscrasia with **p**olyneuropathy, **o**rganomegaly, **e**ndocrinopathy, **m**onoclonal protein, and **s**kin changes) can mimic a systemic, multiorgan rheumatic disorder. The skin changes are similar to those of scleroderma. Raynaud's phenomenon, digital ischemic necrosis, and vasculitis may occur in patients with dysproteinemias. Tendon **xanthomas,** typically seen in familial hypercholesterolemia, have been reported with near-normal lipid levels in patients with dysproteinemias such as multiple myeloma and monoclonal gammopathy of unknown significance (MGUS).

E. **Metastatic carcinomatous arthritis associated with solid neoplasms.** Metastatic deposits of solid neoplasms in bone, synovium, or periarticular tissue can masquerade as monarthritis or polyarthritis. This is a rare occurrence.

In children, neuroblastoma should be considered as a cause of metastatic carcinomatous arthritis. In most instances, the primary neoplasm is evident. If the tumor is occult, tomography, bone scan, or biopsy becomes necessary for accurate diagnosis. In general, therapy is directed toward the underlying neoplasm.

F. **HOA**

1. The clinical presentation is one of periostitis and chronic periosteal reaction. Periostitis occurs predominantly at the distal ends of the long bones. The term periostosis may more accurately describe these radiologic changes without necessarily implying an inflammatory mechanism. If early periostitis is not evident on plain radiographs, bone scan is useful in demonstrating its presence. Patients present with symmetric painful tenderness and swelling near the wrist and ankle regions. The discomfort is typically exacerbated by dependency of the limb, and relieved by its elevation. Periostitis without clubbing does not constitute HOA. Periostitis alone can occur in hypervitaminosis A and retinoic acid toxicity, thyroid acropachy, hyperphosphatemia, and sarcoidosis.

2. **Clubbing of the fingers.** Although finger clubbing is invariably present in HOA, it may develop only after pain in the distal long bones occurs. In synovial hypertrophy, with or without joint effusions, synovitis affects predominantly the knees and ankles but may also involve metacarpophalangeal and proximal interphalangeal joints. Effusions, if present, are typically not inflammatory and may reflect a "sympathetic" reaction to nearby disease.

3. **Underlying disorders** should always be considered in patients with HOA (see Table 57-1). Associated conditions include pleural, pulmonary, cardiovascular, gastrointestinal, hepatic, and miscellaneous diseases. Although clubbing occurs in most patients with cyanotic congenital heart disease and cystic fibrosis, it is seen in fewer than 5% of patients with the other disorders listed in Table 57-1. Overall, pulmonary problems predominate in most series of patients with HOA. Bronchogenic carcinoma and suppurative lung disease are the two most common associated pulmonary conditions. The incidence of HOA in patients with these diseases is 2% and 5%, respectively.

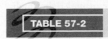

TABLE 57-2	Rheumatic Syndromes and the Cancers They May Herald

Rheumatic syndrome	Cancer type
Established associations	
Hypertrophic osteoarthropathy	Intrathoracic neoplasms, colon and hepatic neoplasms
Dermatomyositis	All tumor types
Secondary gout	Lymphoproliferative disorders, leukemia
Amyloid arthropathy/carpal tunnel syndrome	Plasma cell dyscrasias
Metastatic carcinomatous arthritis	Lung, breast, large intestine tumors predominate
Migratory arthritis	Acute lymphocytic leukemia
Raynaud's phenomenon; digital ulcers	Plasma cell dyscrasias, lymphoma
Palpable purpura	Lymphoproliferative disorders, other
Subcutaneous fat necrosis/polyarthritis	Pancreatic tumors
Possible associations	
Palmar fasciitis/polyarthritis	Ovarian, other
Carcinomatous polyarthritis	Prostate, other
"Lupuslike" syndrome	Hypernephroma, gastric, and cervical; breast carcinoma; gastrointestinal lymphoma; testicular seminoma
Progressive systemic sclerosis	Breast, uterus, prostate, lung
Polyarthritis nodosa	Hodgkin's disease, hairy-cell leukemia
Giant cell arteritis	Malignant histiocytosis, myeloma

G. RA and carcinomatous polyarthritis
   1. **RA.** Classic RA has never been clearly documented as a sign of occult malignancy.
   2. **Carcinomatous polyarthritis.** The concept of a rheumatoidlike arthropathy that heralds a malignancy remains controversial (Table 57-2). In general, an age-appropriate malignancy assessment is appropriate in patients presenting with new-onset arthritis.

H. DM and polymyositis
   In the absence of an easily detectable neoplasm, defined as part of an age-appropriate malignancy assessment, an exhaustive search for an occult malignancy may not be cost-effective (see section Prevalence). However, in patients who develop DM when they are older than 50, some specialists will do a computerized, transaxial tomography examination of the chest, abdomen, and pelvis. Patients with interstitial lung disease and antibodies to Jo-1 appear to be less likely to have an associated malignancy.

I. Subcutaneous fat necrosis, arthritis, and eosinophilia.
   Panniculitis, with or without monarthritis or polyarthritis, may herald pancreatic carcinoma. Painful nodules or periarticular fat necrosis often precedes the onset of abdominal pain. Eosinophilia is variably present. In male patients with subcutaneous fat necrosis and monarthritis or polyarthritis, pancreatic carcinoma should be strongly suspected, especially when eosinophilia is present. Endocrine tumors can mimic a variety of rheumatic disorders. Pituitary tumors causing acromegaly mimic polyarthritis; carcinoid can mimic scleroderma; and pheochromocytoma can mimic vasculitis.

J. Vasculitis
   1. **Palpable purpura.** An unexplained necrotizing cutaneous vasculitis warrants consideration of, or surveillance for, an underlying lymphoreticular or myelodysplastic disorder. The mechanism is likely immune-mediated and not attributable to direct vascular involvement by tumor, except in the rare case of intravascular lymphoma. Cutaneous vasculitis as a paraneoplastic syndrome is unusual. Only

8 of 192 patients (4.2%) with cutaneous vasculitis had an underlying malignancy. Six of the eight were hematologic malignancies.

2. **Raynaud's phenomenon, digital ulcers, purpura, and gangrene.** Serum cryoproteins associated with plasma cell dyscrasias and lymphomas should be considered. Cryofibrinogen, evident in plasma, is associated with metastatic malignancy.

3. **Polyarteritis nodosa** may rarely develop in patients with hairy-cell leukemia or Hodgkin's disease.

4. **Giant cell arteritis.** Giant cell arteritis may occur as the initial manifestation of malignant histiocytosis. Biopsy-proven arteritis has also been associated with follicular small cleaved-cell lymphoma, hairy-cell leukemia, lymphoplasmacytoid lymphoma, multiple myeloma, amyloidosis, and Waldenström's macroglobulinemia.

5. **Polymyalgia rheumatica** should not prompt an extensive workup for occult malignancy more than and beyond an age-appropriate malignancy assessment. Associated neoplasia is usually a chance occurrence and may involve any primary site. When polymyalgia rheumaticalike symptoms predate neoplasia, the latter is usually apparent within 3 months of onset of symptoms.

6. **Mimics of vasculitis** associated with protean, multiorgan symptoms and signs can occur in patients with pheochromocytoma, left atrial myxoma, intravascular lymphoma, tumor emboli, and anticardiolipin antibodies.

K. **SLE**

1. **SLE.** There are no well-documented cases of occult malignancy presenting as SLE. Although antinuclear antibodies (ANAs) can be present in patients with solid neoplasms, lymphomas, or leukemias and who lack other evidence of a rheumatic syndrome, the significance of this is not understood. Lupus erythematosus (LE) cells or ANAs can be seen in patients with lymphoma or **angioimmunoblastic lymphadenopathy with dysproteinemia (AILD).** Diagnostic confusion may arise, because lymphadenopathy and splenomegaly are features that are also common in SLE.

2. **A "lupuslike" syndrome,** manifested by typical SLE serologic and laboratory abnormalities but lacking clinical criteria for SLE, has been associated with certain tumors and myelodysplastic disorders. For example, hypernephroma has been found in a peripartum woman, but this may have been an incidental finding because a similar lupuslike syndrome can occur during pregnancy. Other tumors include gastric, cervical, and breast carcinomas, gastrointestinal lymphoma, AILD, and testicular seminoma.

   In general, a diagnosis of clinical SLE should not prompt a search for occult malignancy. However, lupuslike serology and unexplained Coombs'-positive anemia or thrombocytopenia without clinical features of SLE warrant consideration of an occult neoplasm. In addition, in a patient with a known tumor who presents with pleural effusions, pericarditis, or nondeforming polyarthritis, although the tumor is the most likely culprit, an associated lupuslike illness should be considered.

L. **Scleroderma.** Rarely, hematologic malignancies, bladder cancer, and breast or stomach carcinoma become apparent shortly after the onset of scleroderma. The scleroderma may improve following treatment of these malignancies. Carcinoid tumors are associated with sclerodermalike changes of the lower extremities. POEMS may also be associated with sclerodermalike changes in the skin. Scleroderma may be erroneously diagnosed before these disorders are considered.

M. **Miscellaneous.** Rheumatic syndromes that may be a harbinger of neoplasia include eosinophilic fasciitis and the disorders listed subsequently. Patients should be followed up for development of hematologic disorders (e.g., aplastic anemia and lymphoid malignancies).

1. **Reflex sympathetic dystrophy** may occur secondary to brain tumor, ovarian carcinoma, or Pancoast's lung tumor.

2. **Erythromelalgia** (burning, red, and warm feet) may be associated with myeloproliferative disorders in 10% of cases.

3. **Sweet's syndrome,** or acute neutrophilic dermatosis, is associated with malignancy in at least 15% of cases, most commonly with acute myelogenous leukemia.

4. **Palmar fasciitis.**

5. **Osteomalacia** may develop in patients with a variety of benign or malignant mesenchymal tumors, giant cell tumor, hemangioma, angiosarcoma, hemangiopericytoma, neurilemmoma, and nonossifying fibroma. Epidermal nevus syndrome is also associated with this condition. Patients exhibit hypophosphatemia, normal or slightly decreased serum calcium, and usually normal serum parathyroid hormone concentrations. Abnormalities revert to normal following successful removal of tumor tissue.

6. **Osteoporosis** can be a manifestation of an underlying malignancy such as multiple myeloma, a disorder that presents with bone fractures, anemia, and an elevated sedimentation rate.

7. **Bone and joint infections.** Patients with malignancy, especially those receiving cytotoxic therapy, are predisposed to septic complications such as pyarthrosis and osteomyelitis. Organisms include both common and opportunistic pathogens. Pyogenic arthritis caused by *Streptococcus bovis* or enteric organisms may signal an occult colonic neoplasm.

8. **Referred pain** to the joints, neck, or back. Knee pain, exacerbated by recumbency, has been attributed to diffuse histiocytic lymphoma of the spinal cord. Back pain and radiculitis may be secondary to leukemic meningeal involvement, or may be the initial manifestation of Hodgkin's disease, or could reflect an intra-abdominal and pelvic malignancy. Shoulder pain with normal findings on shoulder examination may be referred pain caused by subdiaphragmatic or intra-abdominal neoplasms. Alternatively, intrathoracic neoplasms (e.g., Pancoast's tumor) may extend into the brachial plexus and cause pain in a shoulder with a normal range of motion but with evidence of muscle atrophy and loss of deep tendon reflexes.

9. **Ectopic adrenocorticotrophic hormone (ACTH),** seen as a paraneoplastic syndrome, can cause myalgia, weakness, and osteoporosis.

10. **Pituitary tumors** can produce rheumatic symptoms attributable to hypothyroid and adrenal insufficiency.

11. **Mimics of vasculitis** such as subacute bacterial endocarditis, cholesterol emboli, and antiphospholipid syndrome may occur in any patient with concomitant neoplasia.

II. **MALIGNANCY OCCURRING IN THE SETTING OF AN ESTABLISHED RHEUMATIC SYNDROME**
The risk for certain types of cancer appears to be increased in patients with some of the rheumatic syndromes. The increased incidence of malignancy does not appear to be related to antirheumatic therapy in the following instances:

A. **Polymyositis and inclusion body myositis** are associated with all types of neoplasms. Although the increased risk for cancer after the diagnosis of polymyositis is consistent with bias in cancer detection, clinical vigilance for associated neoplasia is indicated. Routine urinalysis, complete blood count, examination of stools for occult blood, sigmoidoscopy, mammography, prostate and testicular examinations, chest radiography, and Papanicolaou's smear are recommended screens. A more extensive search for occult malignancy may be indicated in patients at greatest risk, such as older men, or patients with severe and treatment-refractory DM.

B. **RA,** even in the absence of treatment with potentially oncogenic drugs, appears to be associated with an increased risk for hematologic malignancies, including lymphoma and myeloma. There is also an increased risk for leukemia in patients with some cohorts of RA. In certain patients with Felty's syndrome, there is a twofold increase in total cancer incidence and a 12-fold increased risk for NHL. There is also an increased risk for CD16+ large granular lymphocytes and leukemia. Patients with RA and with secondary Sjögren's syndrome are at a 33-fold increased risk for NHL. Paraproteins are an additional marker of increased risk for hematopoietic neoplasms. The overall risk for malignancy is reduced in some cohort studies of

RA. Prospective, longitudinal cohort studies of patients with RA have demonstrated a lower incidence of stomach and colon carcinomas; the latter is possibly related to the use of nonsteroidal anti-inflammatory drugs (NSAIDs).

C. Patients with primary and secondary Sjögren's syndrome are at increased risk for the development of NHL and Waldenström's macroglobulinemia. Women with primary Sjögren's syndrome are at greatest risk. Risk factors such as disappearance of RF are predictive of the evolution of NHL. Development of lymphadenopathy, splenomegaly, and pulmonary infiltrates; monoclonal protein; new-onset leukopenia, and anemia; and a loss of previously present specific autoantibodies [i.e., antinuclear antibodies (ANA) anti-SS-A/B] have all been associated with the development of lymphoma.

D. Patients with systemic sclerosis with pulmonary fibrosis and "honeycomb" lung may be at increased risk for bronchoalveolar cell carcinoma. A 60-fold increase in occurrence of squamous cell carcinoma of the tongue exists.

E. Immunodeficiency states. Patients with X-linked hypogammaglobulinemia, common variable immunodeficiency, ataxia–telangiectasia, and Wiskott-Aldrich syndrome are at increased risk for the development of lymphoreticular malignancy. Leukemia, medulloblastoma, and adenocarcinomas may also occur with increased frequency. Asymptomatic patients with isolated immunoglobulin A deficiency do not appear to have an increased risk for neoplasia.

F. Patients with SLE may be at increased risk for developing NHL and for neoplasia complicating cytotoxic therapy (Table 57-3). **Discoid lupus** erythematosus lesions may develop into epidermoid carcinoma.

G. Mixed cryoglobulinemia associated with vasculitis and hepatitis C is associated with a 7% incidence of NHL. Monitoring for hepatocellular carcinoma should also be considered.

H. Paget's disease. Osteogenic sarcoma may complicate Paget's disease in 1% of patients and present with persistent, severe pain. Bone biopsy may be necessary for accurate diagnosis.

I. Multicentric reticulohistiocytosis may herald a subsequent malignancy.

J. Vasculitis. Malignancy is found in 5% of patients with vasculitis. Many solid and hematopoietic malignancies have been associated. Overall, the incidence may not differ from age-matched healthy population. However, the relation between cutaneous hypersensitivity vasculitis and hematopoietic malignancies is more than coincidental.

K. Chronic osteomyelitis. Squamous cell carcinoma may occur in adjacent cutaneous tissue in up to 2% of cases.

L. Patients with eosinophilic fasciitis are at increased risk for associated aplastic anemia and lymphoproliferative disease.

III. **MALIGNANCY AS A COMPLICATION OF ANTIRHEUMATIC THERAPY**
The influence of immunosuppressive drug therapy in altering the incidence of cancer in the rheumatic population is unclear, but an increased risk for neoplasia is apparent with some regimens.

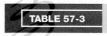

TABLE 57-3   Malignancies Associated with Established Connective Tissue Disorders

Connective tissue disorder	Malignancy
Progressive systemic sclerosis	Possibly bronchoalveolar cell carcinoma
Systemic lupus erythematosus	Non-Hodgkin's lymphoma
Discoid lupus erythematosus	Epidermoid
Sjögren's syndrome	Lymphoma
Polymyositis	All types
Eosinophilic fasciitis	Aplastic anemia, perhaps lymphoproliferative neoplasia
Mixed cryoglobulinemia associated with hepatitis	Lymphoma, hepatoma

A. **Alkylating agents** such as cyclophosphamide and chlorambucil can increase the risk of leukemia and myelodysplastic syndromes. Cytogenetic abnormalities of chromosome 5/7 are associated with therapy-related myelodysplastic syndromes seen in rheumatic disease. In addition, cyclophosphamide is associated with bladder cancers. As the bladder cancer may occur 20 years after exposure, ongoing surveillance should be considered. Sodium-2-mercaptoethane sulfate (Mesna) can bind the toxic cyclophosphamide metabolite acrolein and may diminish the incidence of bladder carcinoma associated with intravenous infusions in the setting of SLE and the vasculitides. Recently, it has been reported that the use of cyclophosphamide in SLE is associated with a threefold increase in cervical cancer at a 3-year follow-up.

B. **Immunosuppressive agents**
   1. **Purine antimetabolites** such as azathioprine are associated with an increased risk for lymphomas and nonmelanoma skin carcinomas in renal transplant recipients. The possibility of a similar increased incidence of malignancy in patients with rheumatic disease treated with azathioprine remains to be firmly established. An increased incidence of NHL and cervical carcinoma in patients with SLE on azathioprine has been suggested. There is no apparent relation between the amount and duration of cytotoxic therapy and the development of malignancy.
   2. **Folic acid antagonists.** Methotrexate may rarely be associated with the development of large B-cell NHL in patients with RA. As many as 30% of these tumors are positive for EBV and some regress on withdrawal of the drug. Here, the medication and virus work as cofactors in a disorder that already has an increased incidence of these tumors.
   3. **Cyclosporine,** although not mutagenic, is associated with lymphoproliferative disorders in up to 3% of patients undergoing renal transplantation treated with concomitant azathioprine and prednisone. Whether patients with rheumatic diseases who are taking cyclosporine, with or without methotrexate, have an increased risk for lymphoma and brain or skin cancers remains to be determined.
   4. **Leflunomide (Arava),** used in RA, is not clearly associated with malignancy, but data on long-term exposure are limited.
   5. **Mycophenolate mofetil (CellCept),** increasingly used in patients with SLE nephritis, may be associated with an increase in the development of lymphoproliferative disorders.

C. **Biologic agents**
   1. **Anti-TNF therapy** [etanercept (Enbrel), adalimumab (Humira), or infliximab (Remicade)]. Compared to the general population, patients with RA on anti-TNF therapy have a twofold increase in NHL. It remains unresolved whether any or all of these agents are associated with a higher risk for NHL compared to patients untreated for RA. It is unknown whether the combination of methotrexate with anti-TNF therapy has a higher risk for NHL compared to the use of anti-TNF alone. Increased surveillance is certainly indicated in patients with RA on these therapies. These drugs should not be used in patients with a history of lymphoma.
   2. **IL-1 receptor antagonist** (IL-1ra) anakinra (Kineret) has not been clearly associated with an increased risk of solid neoplasm or NHL, but vigilance is suggested.

D. **Radiation therapy.** Patients with ankylosing spondylitis treated with spinal irradiation have an increased frequency of leukemia. The risk for myeloproliferative disorders and osseous sarcoma is likely increased in patients with RA treated with total nodal irradiation.

E. **X-ray exposure.** Diagnostic imaging may be associated with a small increased risk of malignancy. The lifetime risk of cancer associated with diagnostic radiation exposure is less than 1% for most countries. This risk is balanced by the benefit of the imaging and prompts us to prescribe only medically necessary diagnostic imaging tests.

F. **Aspirin and NSAID therapy.** The use of aspirin, NSAIDs, and COX-2 selective NSAID therapy is controversial. The hope is that aspirin and/or NSAIDs may decrease the risk of colon cancer. The prospective Nurses Health Study found a surprising increase in the relative risk for pancreatic cancer in women on aspirin for a long term. However, the absolute risk is exceedingly small.

IV. RHEUMATIC SYNDROME AS A COMPLICATION OF ANTINEOPLASTIC THERAPIES

A. Anthracyclines can cause transient polyarthritis. Liposome-encapsulated doxorubicin used to treat human immunodeficiency virus-related Kaposi's sarcoma is associated with a painful hand–foot syndrome. Painful, reddened, swollen hands and feet may ulcerate, fissure, and desquamate.

B. Busulfan can cause a syndrome resembling sicca syndrome.

C. Bleomycin (Blenoxane) can produce sclerodermalike features involving the skin and lungs.

D. Cisplatin (Platinol) has been associated with Raynaud's phenomenon.

E. Cytosine arabinoside (ara-C). Most vascular reactions have been noted after combination chemotherapy, but treatment with ara-C as a single agent has also been associated with necrotizing cutaneous vasculitis.

F. Fluorouracil is associated with a hand–foot syndrome characterized by palmar–plantar erythrodysesthesia.

G. CMF (cyclophosphamide, methotrexate, and 5-fluorouracil) adjuvant therapy for breast cancer has been associated with arthralgia and polyarthritis.

H. Any immunosuppressive therapy may **predispose** a patient to **bone and joint infections.**

I. Hormonal manipulation. Tamoxifen is reported to be associated with cases of cutaneous leukocytoclastic vasculitis and polyarthritis.

J. Luteinizing hormone-releasing hormone (LHRH) agonists, such as leuprolide, buserelin, and nafarelin; and antiandrogens, such as flutamide, may be associated with myalgia and arthralgias.

K. Antibacterial and antiviral agents used in the treatment of opportunistic infections may cause a variety of rheumatic problems.

    1. Zidovudine azidothymidine (AZT) is associated with a syndrome resembling DM and polymyositis.

    2. Ciprofloxacin has been associated with tendon ruptures and flares of SLE.

    3. Cephalosporins are associated with serum sicknesslike reactions.

L. Radiation therapy may be associated with a delayed obliterative radiation arteritis and avascular necrosis.

M. Growth factors and biologic response modifiers

    1. G-CSF and GM-CSF may be associated with Sweet's syndrome, flares of SLE, vasculitis, and arthritis.

    2. ILs and interferons have been associated with the development of signs and symptoms of autoimmune diseases or autoantibodies. Treatment with interferon-α is associated with Raynaud's syndrome and SLE-like illness. The manifestations vary depending on the underlying disease being treated. When used to treat myeloproliferative disorders, interferon-α can induce formation of ANAs and RF, polyarthritis, or polyarthralgia. The incidence for these complications appears to be much lower in patients treated for carcinoid or viral hepatitis. Ongoing clinical trials of IL-4, IL-10, and other biologic response modifiers should continue to monitor for any increase in autoantibodies or autoimmune complications.

N. Bone marrow transplantation may be associated with chronic graft versus host disease that includes sclerodermalike skin changes, alopecia, xerostomia, keratoconjunctivitis sicca, photosensitivity, myositis, and joint contractures.

O. Antithymocyte globulin is associated with a serum sickness reaction that consists of arthralgia/arthritis and a distinctive erythematous, serpiginous rash on the hands and feet at the margins of the palmar and plantar skin ("moccasin" distribution).

P. Intravesical therapy with bacille Calmette-Guérin (BCG) for bladder cancer can be associated with a reactive or RA-like arthritis. The possibility of disseminated BCG exists in patients with RA who have received this therapy for bladder cancer and are placed on anti-TNF therapy.

PHYSICAL EXAMINATION

I. Clubbing of fingers is seen with HOA. The characteristic bulbous deformity or drumstick appearance of the fingertips is easy to recognize. However, before obvious clubbing develops, the only abnormality may be a fingernail that can be rocked or floated upon its nail bed to produce a spongy sensation. Next, the ungual–phalangeal angle (the angle between the nail plate and the proximal digit) increases beyond 160 degrees and becomes obliterated at 180 degrees. Alternatively stated, the normal nail plate forms an angle of 20 degrees or more dorsally with the axis of the digit. The circumference of the nail bed becomes greater than the circumference of the distal interphalangeal joint. The nail may eventually appear convex, like a watch crystal. A very rare, familial form of HOA is pachydermoperiostitis. This is not associated with any underlying disorder and is typically associated with coarse facial features and painless periostitis. Familial clubbing does exist and can be helpful information as one embarks on the search for a malignancy.

II. **Heliotrope rash, Gottron's** papules, and V-neck rash are seen with DM.
III. **Lymphadenopathy,** hepatomegaly, and splenomegaly are seen with RA, Sjögren's syndrome, and malignancy, especially NHL.
IV. **Palpable purpura** is the hallmark of cutaneous vasculitis.
V. **Muscle weakness** and **myopathy** are the hallmarks of DM and polymyositis.

 DIAGNOSTIC INVESTIGATIONS

History and physical examination, supplemented with laboratory and radiologic studies, are the foundation of diagnosing both rheumatic illness and neoplasms. Pathologic tissue biopsy is necessary to diagnose malignancy.

 LABORATORY TESTS

I. **There is no single laboratory test to make a definitive diagnosis of a rheumatic illness in a patient with cancer.**
  A. ANA, RF, and ESR may all be positive or elevated in healthy individuals and patients with rheumatic illness, infection, or neoplasms.
  B. Serum protein electrophoresis and serum analysis are able to evaluate for an associated monoclonal gammopathy.
II. **There is no lab test to confirm or rule out a malignancy in a patient with rheumatic disease.** Tissue biopsy is usually necessary to establish a diagnosis of neoplasia.

 IMAGING STUDIES

I. **Radiographs are important** in diagnosing **underlying bony pathology** in patients with rheumatic symptoms. They may show lytic or blastic metastatic lesions, or periosteal reaction.
II. **Periostitis** may be seen in HOA or leukemic infiltration or primary bone tumors.

 DIFFERENTIAL DIAGNOSIS

I. **Part of the early differential diagnosis of many patients with a rheumatic disease is infection and neoplasm.**
  A. Monarticular arthritis, pauciarticular or polyarticular joint complaints, polymyositis/ DM, HOA, vasculitis, polyarteritis nodosa, or leukocytoclastic vasculitis.
  B. DM and HOA are most likely to signify an associated neoplasia.
II. **Any patient with RA on immunosuppressive therapy** should be evaluated for infectious and neoplastic complications of the disease or therapy.
III. **Vasculitis,** clinically or pathologically confirmed, can be associated with rheumatic, infectious, and neoplastic conditions.

TREATMENT

I. **HOA.** If a neoplasm can be successfully resected, the presenting musculoskeletal symptoms of HOA often resolve within weeks. A patient with inoperable bronchogenic carcinoma may respond to chemotherapy or radiation therapy. In those patients with an untreatable underlying disorder, chemical or surgical vagotomy may be beneficial. NSAIDs can be helpful in the control of local joint symptoms.

II. **DM.** Corticosteroids, with or without cytotoxic agents, and intravenous immunoglobulin (IVIG) remain the mainstay of therapy. Severe, progressive myositis that responds poorly to steroid therapy may improve after successful treatment of the neoplasm. Relapsing or refractory cases of DM warrant a search for and treatment of recurrent, or secondary malignancy.

III. **GOUT.** Institution of allopurinol helps prevent this complication of treatment seen in leukemias and lymphomas. The dosage of azathioprine and 6-mercaptopurine must be reduced by 75% or avoided completely if the patient receives allopurinol therapy. Colchicine therapy should be avoided if leukopenia from bone marrow toxicity is likely, or if renal insufficiency or biliary obstruction precludes its safe use. (see Chapter 43 for treatment of acute gout).

IV. **Treatment of an associated malignancy** may help treat the underlying rheumatic disease.

V. **In general, treatment of a rheumatic disease in a patient with a history of malignancy is standard therapy with surveillance for malignancy recurrence. Anti-TNF therapy should be avoided in patients with prior lymphomas.**

PROGNOSIS

I. **In general,** the **prognosis** of a rheumatic syndrome occurring as a paraneoplastic syndrome or direct result of a malignancy depends upon the course of the underlying malignancy.

II. It is **important to remain alert** to the development of malignancy in any patient with a rheumatic syndrome, either: (a) as a concomitant of the association with immunosuppressive or biologic therapy; or (b) associated with the disease process itself.

III. Patients with the conditions listed below **require special attention or surveillance for malignancy**.
   A. HOA.
   B. DM or polymyositis.
   C. Cytotoxic or immunosuppressive therapy.
   D. Immunodeficiency states (patients with lupuslike serology and unexplained Coombs'-positive anemia, or thrombocytopenia, without clinical features of SLE).
   E. Hepatitis C–associated mixed cryoglobulinemia/vasculitis.

IV. **Refractory DM** in conjunction with malignancy has a poor prognosis.

V. The **safety of anti-TNF therapy in patients with RA and a prior history of malignancy** or who are currently undergoing chemotherapy or radiation for malignancy is not known.
   A. Data from a longitudinal data bank established in 1988 of 20,000 patients with RA suggests that therapy with anti-TNF is not associated with an increased risk of cancer recurrence in those patients with neoplasia who were treated prior to enrollment.

VI. **Pharmacovigilance** is important for monitoring all patients with rheumatic disease who may be at increased risk of malignancy from their underlying disease process or treatment.

   Adverse events related to use of biologics or drugs used should be reported to the U.S. Food and Drug Administration's (FDA) MedWatch program. **Contact options** include: phone at 1-800-FDA-1088; fax at 1-800-FDA-0178; online at http://www.fda.gov/medwatch, or mail to 5600 Fishers Lane, Rockville, MD 20852-9787.

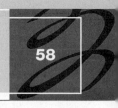

MISCELLANEOUS DISEASES WITH RHEUMATIC MANIFESTATIONS

58

Diana A. Yens, Chiara Baldini, and Stefano Bombardieri

$\mathcal{T}$he disorders listed below in Table 58-1 are miscellaneous only in that they do not fit comfortably in other chapters in this Manual. However, they share many characteristics with the others in that they manifest systemic and profound effects upon organ or patient function, have a genetic basis, masquerade as prototypical autoimmune disorders, or reflect the interconnection between the neurologic and musculoskeletal systems.

 ## AMYLOIDOSIS

I. **INTRODUCTION**
   A. **Amyloidosis** is a disorder in which extracellular deposition of an insoluble fibrous protein in the connective tissues of one or more organs ultimately leads to disruption of tissue structure and function.
   B. There are at least 32 different proteins that result in amyloid disease.
   C. Joint disease is a rare manifestation of amyloidosis.
   D. The amyloidoses may be clinically classified.
      1. **Primary or myeloma-associated** amyloidosis is characterized by the deposition of **light-chain amyloid (AL) protein** that arises from immunoglobulin (Ig) κ or λ light chains.
      2. **Secondary or reactive amyloidosis** is associated with chronic infections (i.e., leprosy, tuberculosis, and osteomyelitis) or inflammatory diseases [i.e., rheumatoid arthritis (RA), ankylosing spondylitis, juvenile idiopathic arthritis, psoriatic arthritis, and familial Mediterranean fever (FMF)] and is characterized by tissue deposition of the acute-phase reactant **serum amyloid A (SAA) protein.**
      3. **Hereditary amyloidoses** are a heterogeneous group of disorders that are characterized by a mutation in the genes that code for the proteins that are precursors of hereditary amyloid. Musculoskeletal involvement is very rare except for transthyretin familial amyloidosis, which is clinically similar to that of AL amyloidosis.
      4. **Hemodialysis-associated amyloidosis** is related to deposition of β_2-microglobulin in patients undergoing long-term dialysis treatment; however, cases among patients who are not on dialysis have also been reported.
      5. **Senile amyloidosis.**
      6. **Localized amyloidosis.**

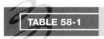 **TABLE 58-1**   Miscellaneous Diseases with Rheumatic Manifestations

Amyloidosis	Sarcoidosis
Hemochromatosis	Pigmented villonodular synovitis
Hemophilic arthropathy	Reflex sympathetic dystrophy
Hemoglobinopathies	Hereditary periodic fevers
Storage disorders	Multicentric reticulohistiocytosis

II. ETIOPATHOGENESIS

A. The amyloid protein is a proteolysis-resistant fibrillar protein with a β-pleated sheet secondary structure. The protein consists of a homogeneous hyaline eosinophilic material, identified pathologically by three features.

   1. Congo red binding with a unique green–yellow (apple-green) birefringence under polarized light.

   2. Characteristic ultrastructure that is distinguished by fine, nonbranching, rigid fibrils of 70 to 100 Å in diameter.

   3. The presence of the serum amyloid P component, which falls under the family of proteins termed pentraxins. All forms of amyloid deposition have been found to contain the P component, apolipoprotein E, and heparan sulfate proteoglycan. The role of these molecules is still unclear. Pentraxins also include the C-reactive protein and have a characteristic structure of paired pentagonal subunits.

B. Each type of amyloid disease is associated with deposition of a specific protein and the resulting organ involvement can be linked to the location, quantity, and ratio of deposition.

III. PREVALENCE

A. Prevalence is highly variable depending upon the type of amyloidosis.

B. Amyloidosis caused by AL protein is one of the most common forms of systemic amyloidosis with an incidence of approximately 1 case/100,000 person years of observation for Western countries.

C. Secondary or reactive amyloidosis is another of the more common forms of systemic amyloidosis. This type is more common in RA patients in Europe than those in the US.

IV. CLINICAL MANIFESTATIONS

A. Primary and myeloma-associated amyloidosis may have amyloid fibrils localized to the synovial membrane and tendon sheaths, in the synovial fluid, and in the articular cartilage in a small percentage of patients with AL deposition.

   1. Patients may have chronic involvement of small or large joints (shoulders, wrists, knees, or fingers) either symmetrically or asymmetrically.

   2. Stiffness (not pain) is characteristic, with effusion, limitation of motion, and subcutaneous nodules.

   3. Shoulder involvement may be striking, with accumulation of amyloid at the joint producing the **"shoulder pad"** sign.

B. Secondary amyloidosis is characterized by renal involvement with proteinuria often accompanied by renal insufficiency.

C. Hemodialysis-related amyloidosis involves the musculoskeletal system with infiltration of the carpal ligaments, formation of periarticular bone cysts, scapulohumeral periarthritis, stiff and painful fingers, and destructive cervical spondyloarthropathy with cyst formation and occasional odontoid fracture.

   1. Cervical disease usually takes the form of vertebral end-plate erosion without osteophyte formation. Rapid joint destruction then usually follows.

   2. Median nerve compression is very common, resulting in carpal tunnel syndrome.

V. DIAGNOSTIC INVESTIGATIONS

A. Primary and myeloma-associated amyloidosis

   1. Synovial fluid analysis or synovial biopsy may demonstrate the fibrils with features of amyloid. The fluid is noninflammatory and yellow or xanthochromic.

   2. Sonogram of the shoulder may help distinguish amyloid from other forms of shoulder disease.

   3. Plain radiographs may show soft-tissue swelling and generalized osteoporosis with or without lytic lesions.

   4. Subcutaneous fat aspiration is a low risk, often high-yield diagnostic study.

   5. Serum and urine immunoelectrophoresis reveals the monoclonal Ig precursor protein in most patients.

B. **Hemodialysis-related amyloidosis**
1. **Wrist sonogram** may identify characteristic thickening of the carpal ligaments.
2. **Radiography** may show subchondral radiolucent bone cysts consisting of amyloid deposits and erosions.
3. **Subcutaneous fat aspiration** is typically nondiagnostic.

VI. **DIFFERENTIAL DIAGNOSIS**
A. **The etiology of the amyloid should be evaluated once diagnosed.** Evaluation for a primary inflammatory disease, such as RA, or for a primary plasma cell dyscrasia should be undertaken.
B. **Patients with chronic renal failure** may also have other conditions that could have an impact upon the musculoskeletal system, such as secondary hyperparathyroidism, aluminum overload, and apatite crystal deposition resulting in arthropathy.

VII. **TREATMENT**
A. Therapy is dependent upon the **primary cause** of the amyloid precursor.
B. **Primary or myeloma-associated disease** should have the goal of reducing the number of cells producing the amyloid precursor via treatment of the primary disease.
C. **Secondary amyloidosis due to RA** can be improved with optimal control of the inflammatory process and the use of daily, oral colchicine 0.6 mg twice daily.
D. **Hemodialysis-related amyloidosis** can be halted by renal transplant, but this will not reverse the symptoms from existing lesions. Modern dialysis filters may also improve the amyloid burden.

VIII. **PROGNOSIS**
Prognosis is dependent primarily upon the outcome of the associated disease. Those clinical manifestations that are already present are difficult to reverse.

 HEMOCHROMATOSIS

I. **INTRODUCTION**
A. **Hemochromatosis is one of the most common genetic disorders.** It is characterized by **excessive body stores of iron and deposition of hemosiderin,** causing tissue damage and organ dysfunction.
B. **Prolonged excessive iron intake,** as the result of repeated blood transfusions for chronic hypoproliferative anemia and thalassemia, may also result in iron deposition. When not associated with tissue damage, this disorder is known as **hemosiderosis;** when organ damage is present, it is called **secondary hemochromatosis.**

II. **ETIOPATHOGENESIS**
A. **Classic hereditary hemochromatosis is an autosomal recessive iron-overload disorder** usually associated with a point mutation of the *HFE* gene located on chromosome 6. The *HFE* gene encodes a 343 amino acid protein expressed on the intestinal cell surface in complex with the transferrin receptor (TfR), thought to facilitate the uptake of iron into the duodenum. The phenotypic expression may vary greatly and, because of this, routine genetic testing has not been as effective in predicting outcome as it had been expected to be.
B. **Duodenal transfer of iron to plasma is inappropriately high** for body iron stores with the rate of absorption being approximately four to five times normal. Absorption of iron generally exceeds iron loss. This, along with other dysregulation of iron management, results in disease.

III. **PREVALENCE**
A. **Approximately one in every 250 to 300 individuals** is homozygous for the most common mutation. This is one of the most common genetic disorders. Prevalence is 30 to 60/10,000 individuals. The incidence is estimated to be two to four/100,000 cases/year.
B. **Men are affected four times more frequently than women,** who are protected by physiologic blood losses.
C. **Arthropathy** is present in 40% to 60% of patients, most commonly in homozygous patients.

IV. CLINICAL MANIFESTATIONS

   A. **Classic hereditary hemochromatosis consists of the triad of hepatic cirrhosis, cardiomyopathy, and "bronze" diabetes mellitus.** Manifestations may also include pituitary dysfunction, sicca syndrome, skin pigmentation, weakness, lethargy, and increased sleep requirement. Liver abnormalities are probably the most constant and common manifestation.

   B. **Chronic progressive destructive arthritis, predominantly affecting the second and third metacarpophalangeal (MCP) and proximal interphalangeal (PIP) joints** is the presenting feature in about half of all cases. Larger joints such as shoulders, hips, knees, and ankles may be affected.

   C. **The joint involvement** presents clinically as stiffness and pain in the hands, often after excessive use, and symmetric, mildly tender joint enlargement without erythema or increased warmth.

   D. **Acute episodes of inflammatory arthritis** may be secondary to calcium pyrophosphate deposition (pseudogout).

   E. *Yersinia* **septic arthritis** is an unusual complication that may arise because of the predilection of this microbe for an iron-rich environment.

V. DIAGNOSTIC INVESTIGATIONS

   A. **Laboratory tests**

   1. **Elevated serum iron, elevated ferritin concentrations, and increased saturation of transferrin characterize the disease.** The test to estimate the saturation of transferrin should be conducted as a morning fasting blood test.

   2. **Synovial fluid analysis** shows good viscosity, with leukocyte counts below $1,000/mm^3$. During acute episodes of pseudogout, synovial fluid leukocytosis and calcium pyrophosphate crystals may be found.

   3. **Synovial biopsy** will show iron deposition in the type B-cell lining of the synovium.

   4. **Needle biopsy of the liver** will confirm the diagnosis.

   5. **ESR** is normal and **rheumatoid factor** is typically absent.

   B. **Imaging studies**

   1. **Plain radiographs show cystic lesions with sclerotic walls,** joint space narrowing, sclerosis, osteophytes, and osteoporosis.

   2. **Chondrocalcinosis as seen on radiographs** occurs in 15% to 30% of patients and involves the cartilages of the knees, wrists, intervertebral discs, and symphysis pubis.

   3. **MRI of the liver** is a very helpful diagnostic test to determine the presence and extent of disease.

   4. **MRI of the joint** may show excessive amounts of iron signal.

VI. DIFFERENTIAL DIAGNOSIS

Hemochromatosis may be confused with RA because of MCP and PIP involvement that is often bilateral, and because of acute inflammation that may be due to acute pseudogout.

VII. TREATMENT

   A. **Arthritic symptoms** may be brought under control by nonsteroidal anti-inflammatory drugs (NSAIDs), although sometimes arthroplasty is required. Close observation of liver function tests is needed in these patients treated with NSAIDs.

   B. **Phlebotomy** removes excess iron but does not usually relieve the arthropathy. Damage to the synovial membrane and cartilage seems to be irreversible.

HEMOPHILIC ARTHROPATHY

I. INTRODUCTION

Hemophilia is an inherited, X-linked recessive disorder of blood coagulation found almost exclusively in males. Female heterozygotes are asymptomatic carriers of the disease. **Recurrent joint hemorrhages** result in a synovial proliferative response, and its attendant chronic inflammation is responsible for the arthropathy associated with hemophilia.

II. **ETIOPATHOGENESIS**
   A. **Hemophilia A** (classic hemophilia) is caused by a factor VIII deficiency.
   B. **Hemophilia B** (Christmas disease) is caused by a factor IX deficiency.
   C. **The pathogenesis of the joint disease is not well understood,** but it may result from excessive iron deposition in the synovial tissue and articular cartilage. The blood in the joint remains liquid due to absence of prothrombin and fibrinogen. The plasma is gradually resorbed and the remaining red cells undergo phagocytosis by the synovial lining cells and macrophages.
   D. **Hemosiderin is found in synovial lining cells** where it may be toxic, causing chronic inflammation with proliferation of the synovium and pannus formation.

III. **PREVALENCE**
   A. **One in 10,000 males** is born with hemophilia A and **one in 100,000 males** is born with hemophilia B.
   B. **Two-thirds of all patients affected by hemophilia have hemarthrosis,** the most common bleeding manifestation.

IV. **CLINICAL MANIFESTATIONS**
   Three stages of hemophilic arthropathy can be distinguished.
   A. **Stage 1: Acute joint** hemarthrosis is usually characterized by the development of an acute effusion with warmth, tenderness, and decreased range of motion. The joints usually affected are the knees, elbows, and ankles.
   B. **Stage 2: Subacute hemophilic arthropathy** often follows repeated episodes of intra-articular hemorrhage. There is persistent synovitis of the joint with thickening of the synovium, moderate effusion, and pain.
   C. **Stage 3: Chronic hemophilic arthropathy** is characterized by joint deformity, fibrous ankylosis, and osteophyte overgrowth. Soft-tissue swelling and joint effusion are less common at this stage, and the pain is fluctuating and variable. Late manifestations include muscle hemorrhage, muscle cysts, contractures, and osseous pseudotumors.

V. **DIAGNOSTIC INVESTIGATIONS**
   A. **Laboratory tests**
      1. **Hemophilia can be detected on the basis of laboratory tests that measure factor VIII and factor IX levels** that are directly correlated with the severity of the hemophilia and the ensuing hemarthrosis.
         a. The complete absence of either of the factors is associated with spontaneous bleeding in the muscles and joints.
         b. A factor level of 1% to 5% of normal is associated with either spontaneous bleeding or bleeding after minor trauma.
         c. A factor level of 5% to 25% may be associated with excessive bleeding after minor surgery.
         d. A factor level of 25% to 50% can result in excessive bleeding after major surgery or injuries.
   B. **Imaging studies**
      1. **Radiographs typically show degenerative arthritis.** In children, radiographic findings include epiphyseal irregularities, squaring of the inferior patella, and enlargement of the proximal radius in the elbow.
      2. **Ultrasonography and magnetic resonance imaging** (MRI) can provide information regarding progression of the articular disease and synovial hypertrophy.

VI. **DIFFERENTIAL DIAGNOSIS**
   In patients with acute hemarthrosis, other diagnoses that must be considered include pigmented villonodular synovitis (PVNS), mechanical derangement, fracture, the use of anticoagulant drugs, and joint trauma.

VII. **TREATMENT**
   A. **Factor replacement therapy** is essential to improve the longevity and prognosis of patients with hemophilia.
   B. **Acute hemarthrosis must be treated promptly** with cold applications, analgesics, and joint immobilization followed by a carefully designed physiotherapy program.
   C. **Aspiration (after factor replacement) is less commonly performed,** unless the joint is very tense or sepsis is suspected.

D. Corticosteroids (oral or intra-articular) do not seem to be effective.

E. Chronic arthropathy may be treated with NSAIDs. Joint replacement can be performed in those patients who have advanced joint destruction. This demands a team approach with optimal factor replacement.

HEMOGLOBINOPATHIES

I. **INTRODUCTION**

A. **Sickle cell disease and β-thalassemia** are two of the most common hemoglobinopathies that produce musculoskeletal complications. Others are the compound heterozygous states including sickle-β-thalassemia, sickle-C disease, and sickle-D disease.

B. **β-thalassemia major** is associated with osteoporosis, pathologic fractures, and epiphyseal deformities. In β-thalassemia minor, recurrent asymmetric arthritis may be seen.

II. **ETIOPATHOGENESIS**

Osteoarticular symptoms may arise as a result of bone and joint involvement secondary to juxta-articular/periarticular bone infarcts or synovial ischemia and infarction. Local bone ischemia resulting from venous occlusion by sickle cells may cause osteonecrosis of the femoral head in up to one-third of patients.

III. **CLINICAL MANIFESTATIONS**

A. **Sickle cell crisis** can produce a painful arthritis of the large joints with a noninflammatory effusion.

B. **Dactylitis secondary to vascular occlusion** in the bones of the hands and feet may represent the first manifestation of the disease in about one-third of infants. This results in acute, painful, nonpitting swelling in the hands and feet, which may lead to premature fusion and shortened digits when necrosis is at the central part of the epiphysis.

C. **Osteomyelitis is increased in patients with sickle cell disease,** with *Salmonella* accounting for approximately 50%.

IV. **DIAGNOSTIC INVESTIGATIONS**

A. **Laboratory tests.** Hemoglobin electrophoresis will reveal the type of hemoglobinopathy.

B. **Imaging studies**

1. Osteonecrosis and synovial hypertrophy can be seen on MRI.

2. Plain radiographic findings are consistent with degenerative arthritis with increased soft-tissue density around joints, or osteonecrosis.

V. **TREATMENT**

Treatment is supportive therapy including intravenous hydration, oxygen, folate supplementation, and analgesics.

VI. **PROGNOSIS**

A. **A high risk of septic arthritis** is associated with the hemoglobinopathies.

B. **Osteonecrosis of the femoral heads occurs in up to 20% of patients.** Other joints may be involved including the humeral head, the knees, and the small joints of the hands and feet.

C. **Gout** may be a rare complication of hemoglobinopathies. Hyperuricemia occurs in more than 40% of patients, but clinical gout is very unusual and typically does not involve the great toe.

STORAGE DISEASES

I. **GAUCHER'S DISEASE**

A. **Introduction and etiopathogenesis**

Gaucher's disease (GD) is an autosomal recessive disease resulting from the accumulation of glucocerebroside in organs and tissues, mainly throughout the reticuloendothelial system, in the form of the characteristic storage cells

(Gaucher's cells). The condition is caused by a deficiency of the lysosomal enzyme glucocerebrosidase. Clinical or radiographic evidence of bone disease occurs in 70% to 100% of patients with GD.

B. Clinical manifestations

1. **Type 1 (neuropathic adult form) and type 3 (juvenile form)** may manifest acute severe pain (bone crisis) accompanied by tenderness, swelling, erythema, and fever (pseudo-osteomyelitis).

2. Osteonecrosis of the hip and talus have been described. Pathologic fractures of the long bones and low back pain also occur.

3. Other manifestations include hepatosplenomegaly, pulmonary hypertension, spasticity, and myoclonic seizures.

C. Diagnostic investigations

1. **Laboratory tests**

    a. Bone marrow biopsy and analysis of the peripheral blood leukocytes for residual β-glucocerebrosidase and β-glucosidase activity establishes the diagnosis.

    b. Erythrocyte sedimentation rate, fibrinogen, and leukocyte adhesion may be increased. Patients often have anemia.

    c. The diagnosis is often made in the setting of a workup of thrombocytopenia found prior to joint replacement surgery.

2. **Imaging studies**

    a. Periosteal elevation (pseudo-osteomyelitis) may be seen on plain radiographs during bone crisis symptoms.

    b. MRI reveals marrow involvement and presence of fibrosis and/or infarction.

    c. Rarefaction, patchy sclerosis, and cortical thickening are common on plain radiographs. Widening of the distal femur appearing as an Erlenmeyer's flask is a frequent finding.

D. Treatment

1. **Enzyme replacement therapy** is the principal treatment. The current protein therapy imiglucerase (recombinant formulation of a human enzyme) is an infusion given over a period of 1 to 2 hours at 2-week intervals.

2. **Splenectomy** treats the thrombocytopenia.

3. **Total joint arthroplasty** is the ultimate treatment of osteonecrosis.

4. **Bone marrow transplantation and organ transplantation** for end-stage disease involving the failure of a single organ are being explored.

E. Prognosis

The disease is progressive, although many months of infusions of replacement enzyme may result in regression of disease. Enzyme therapy results in resolution of bone pain after 2 years of therapy in 50% of patients who are symptomatic. In patients with prior bone crisis, 80% to 90% do not have further bone crisis.

II. HURLER-SCHEIE SYNDROME

A. Introduction

Hurler-Scheie syndrome is an autosomal recessive disorder that is a result of a deficiency of the lysosomal enzyme α-L-iduronidase. This syndrome belongs to a group of disorders designated the mucopolysaccharidosis diseases.

B. Etiopathogenesis

1. The α-L-iduronidase gene has been mapped to chromosome 4 with more than 70 mutations that have been described.

2. The skeletal abnormalities result from lack of skeletal remodeling, disordered endochondral and intramembranous ossification, and the infiltration of the ligaments, tendons, joint capsules, and other soft-tissue structures by glycosaminoglycans.

C. Prevalence

The estimated incidence is 1 in 88,000 live births. This is a panethnic condition.

D. Clinical manifestations

1. Hurler-Scheie syndrome is characterized by obstructive airway disease, valvular heart disease, corneal opacity, retinal degeneration, deafness, hepatomegaly, and neurologic deficits from spinal cord compression.

   2. Musculoskeletal manifestations are the progressive limitation in range of joint motion, short stature, dysostosis multiplex, and hip dysplasia.
E. Diagnostic investigations
   1. Laboratory tests. Diagnosis is confirmed by decreased α-L-iduronidase activity in peripheral blood leukocytes or cultures of skin fibroblasts. Urine analysis reveals excessive dermatan and heparin sulfate.
   2. Imaging studies
      a. Dysostosis multiplex is the term describing a constellation of radiographic findings. These bone abnormalities include a large skull with a thickened calvarium and J-shaped sella tursica, paddlelike ribs, anteroinferior beaking of the lower thoracic vertebrae, and upper lumbar vertebral bodies that are hypoplastic.
      b. Plain radiographs demonstrate constrictive iliac bodies, diaphyseal expansion of the long bones, central pointing of proximal metacarpals, and bulletlike proximal phalanges.
F. Treatment
   1. Treatment currently consists of enzyme therapy with the recombinant enzyme laronidase. Bone marrow transplant can lead to positive changes but does not impact on skeletal problems.
   2. Palliative and symptomatic treatments include surgery to relieve upper airway obstruction and splenectomy for severe anemia or bleeding complications. Surgical intervention includes orthopedic surgery for genu valgum, acetabular hip dysplasia, kyphoscoliosis, carpal tunnel syndrome, and trigger digits.
G. Prognosis
   1. The major cause of death is usually related to cardiac involvement and upper airway obstruction. Life expectancy varies from 5 years and into the fifth decade.
   2. The skeletal and joint complications are major sources of morbidity.
III. FABRY'S DISEASE
   A. Fabry's disease is a lysosomal lipid storage disease in which glycosphingolipids accumulate in nerve cells, organs, skin, and osteoarticular tissue. It is a sex-linked disease caused by deficiency of the enzyme α-galactosidase.
   B. Rheumatologic symptoms include painful crises of burning paresthesias of the extremities, and degenerative changes and flexion contractures of the distal interphalangeal (DIP) joints of the fingers.
   C. Systemic features include renal disease with progressive renal failure and cardiovascular, cerebrovascular, and ocular disease.

 SARCOIDOSIS

I. INTRODUCTION
   A. Sarcoidosis is a systemic disease of unknown etiology characterized by the presence of noncaseating granulomas in the involved tissue. The disease generally involves the lung, although any organ may be affected.
   B. The sarcoid granuloma may arise in the lung (86% of patients); lymph nodes (86%); liver (86%); spleen (63%); heart, kidney, or bone marrow (17% to 20%); or pancreas (6%).
II. Etiopathogenesis is unknown, but it appears that cellular immune mechanisms play a significant role.
III. PREVALENCE
   The disease is most common in African Americans (prevalence 40/100,000) and whites of northern European descent. The usual age of onset is from 20 to 40 years, occurring in women slightly more often than in men.
IV. CLINICAL MANIFESTATIONS
   A. The most frequent clinical manifestations are pulmonary symptoms, asymptomatic hilar adenopathy, constitutional symptoms, and extrathoracic manifestations that may include rheumatologic musculoskeletal disorders.
   B. Pulmonary symptoms include dry cough, dyspnea, and chest pain. Pleural effusions are rare.

C. **Early acute polyarthritis** is the most common, and is often the first manifestation, of the disease. **Erythema nodosum** is strikingly associated with early arthritis. Acute arthritis or periarthritis is usually symmetric and generally involves the larger joints, especially the ankles and knees, although fingers, hands, feet, shoulders, hips, wrist, and elbow can also be affected. Periarticular swelling is more common than joint effusions, and the inflammatory disease around the ankles is often confluent with that of erythema nodosum in the anterior calf.

D. **Löfgren's syndrome** is the constellation of acute arthritis, erythema nodosum, and bilateral hilar adenopathy in sarcoidosis.

E. **Arthritis occurring 6 months or later after onset of disease**
  1. The knee is the most frequently involved joint, followed by the ankles and PIP joints.
  2. Monarthritis may occur. This arthritis may be transient or chronic, and is not associated with erythema nodosum.
  3. The chronic form may manifest as dactylitis, characterized by the sausagelike swelling of the soft tissue over the affected digits, which is at times associated with redness, tenderness, pain, and stiffness.

F. **Myopathy is rare,** but the affected patients, mainly women, may have a chronic, progressive proximal muscle weakness.

G. **Parotid gland enlargement and keratoconjunctivitis** may be seen.

H. **Upper airway disease** may be seen in the form of sinusitis, laryngeal inflammation, or a saddle nose deformity.

I. **Eye involvement** is seen in approximately 22% of patients, with anterior uveitis being more common than posterior uveitis.

J. **Peripheral lymphadenopathy, renal, and central nervous system (CNS) involvement** are rare, but CNS involvement can be quite severe.

K. **Hepatic disease.** Most patients have hepatic granulomas, but only 20% have hepatomegaly or elevated liver enzymes.

L. **Constitutional symptoms** such as malaise, fever, and fatigue are often present.

M. **Dermatologic manifestations** may be erythema nodosum, papules, nodules, plaques, and lupus pernio.

V. **DIAGNOSTIC INVESTIGATIONS**
  A. **Laboratory tests**
    1. **Joint effusions,** when present, show noninflammatory synovial fluid.
    2. **Serum angiotensin-converting enzyme,** produced by the cells of the granuloma, is elevated in two-thirds of patients.
    3. **Synovial, muscle, skin, lymph node, bone marrow, and liver biopsies** may show the characteristic **noncaseating granulomas**. However, the histologic finding of noncaseating granulomas is quite nonspecific and can be found in patients with lymphomas or other malignancies, autoimmune disorders, infections, and allergic reactions. Therefore, the results of the biopsy must be placed in the context of the clinical presentation.
    4. **Bronchoalveolar lavage** specimens show an increased number of T lymphocytes during active disease.
  B. **Imaging studies**
    1. **There are four possible findings on chest x-ray:** type 0, no abnormalities; type 1, enlargement of the hilar and mediastinal lymph nodes; type 2, adenopathy and pulmonary infiltrates; type 3, fibrotic infiltrates without adenopathy.
    2. **Radiographic changes of the joints are uncommon, but cystic bone changes can occur** especially in the site of dactylitis.
    3. **Gallium citrate scan** may show increased uptake in the pulmonary parenchyma; this is not specific, but is helpful in following disease activity and course, as well as the effects of therapy.

VI. **DIFFERENTIAL DIAGNOSIS**
  A. **The joint disease** may mimic RA.
  B. **The disease overall may mimic** many infectious, allergic, autoimmune, and neoplastic diseases; hence tissue biopsy is very helpful to make the diagnosis.
  C. **The myopathy** may resemble polymyositis or muscular dystrophy.

D. The parotid gland involvement and **keratoconjunctivitis** may mimic Sjögren's syndrome.

E. The upper airway involvement may mimic Wegener's granulomatosis with sinusitis, inflammation of the larynx, and saddle nose deformity.

VII. TREATMENT

    A. Corticosteroids are the mainstay of treatment. Short courses of moderate dose steroids (20 to 40 mg prednisone daily) are used. Methotrexate and hydroxychloroquine can be used as corticosteroid-sparing agents in patients with chronic disease. Rarely, cyclophosphamide has been employed in refractory or severe cases.

    B. Anti-tumor necrosis factor-α (anti-TNF-α) agents have been effective in severe cases, with good results.

    C. NSAIDs may be used for acute episodes of arthritis.

VIII. PROGNOSIS

    A. The disease course is generally mild and treatment usually results in long-term remission.

    B. Chronic or aggressive disease develops in only a small number of patients and may demand equally aggressive immunosuppressive therapy.

 PIGMENTED VILLONODULAR SYNOVITIS

I. INTRODUCTION
PVNS is a rare disorder of unknown etiology characterized by a slowly progressive, yet potentially invasive, "benign" proliferation of the synovial tissue.

II. ETIOPATHOGENESIS

    A. Etiology is unknown. The histology demonstrates deposition of hemosiderin and the infiltration of histiocytes and giant cells in a fibrous stoma within the synovium of the tendon sheaths and large joints.

    B. Chronic inflammation, trauma, hemarthrosis, and chromosomal disorders may be the possible causes for PVNS.

III. PREVALENCE
The disease is more common in women than in men and typically presents during the third and fourth decade of life.

IV. CLINICAL MANIFESTATIONS

    A. Pigmented villonodular tenosynovitis (giant cell tumor of the tendon sheath), is the most common expression of PVNS. The lesion is isolated, discrete, and usually painless, but is slowly progressive and may cause erosion of the adjacent bone. The hand, especially the fingers, is the most common site of involvement.

    B. Diffuse intra-articular PVNS primarily affects young adults. It takes the form of a chronic monarticular arthropathy, with the knee being the most commonly involved joint (80%), followed by the hip (15%), and the ankle (5%). Less frequently, the hand, shoulder, wrist, or vertebrae may be affected.

    Progression is slow, with joint swelling and pain that is initially intermittent and later, persistent. A bloody joint effusion is usually present.

    C. Localized pedunculated villonodular synovitis is the least common presentation of PVNS. The knee is the most frequently involved joint and the lesion is localized to the medial or lateral compartment. The patient presents with mechanical symptoms of locking and clicking. Synovial effusions may be slightly bloody.

V. DIAGNOSTIC INVESTIGATIONS

    A. Laboratory tests
        1. There are no characteristic laboratory tests.
        2. Surgical biopsy confirms the diagnosis.

    B. Imaging studies
        1. MRI typically demonstrates nodular foci of decreased signal on both T_H1 and T_H2 weighted images due to deposition of hemosiderin. It may also show a diffuse synovial proliferation or localized mass.
        2. Radiographs may show soft-tissue swelling without calcifications.

VI. DIFFERENTIAL DIAGNOSIS

   A. Differential diagnosis consists of other nodular diseases of the synovium, including primary and secondary neoplasms.

   B. Diffuse intra-articular disease may mimic the chronic synovitis of RA.

VII. TREATMENT

   A. PVNS may be treated surgically, but recurrences are frequent. Radiotherapy alone or in association with synovectomy can reduce the risk of recurrence.

   B. Surgical excision is more successful in the localized form involving the knee. Open synovectomy or arthroscopic surgery may be used in both diffuse and localized disease.

   C. Total joint arthroplasty is required when extensive joint destruction is present.

VIII. PROGNOSIS

   A. The disease is limited locally, but may erode into adjacent bone causing damage.

   B. Localized disease has a good prognosis after surgical management, with very low recurrence.

   C. Diffuse disease of the knee can be refractory to treatment and also difficult to treat.

 REFLEX SYMPATHETIC DYSTROPHY

I. INTRODUCTION

   A. Reflex sympathetic dystrophy (RSD) (now more commonly called complex regional pain syndrome type 1) is a painful, disabling disorder often triggered by an inciting noxious event. The most common inciting event is injury to an extremity from trauma, surgery, or other events.

   B. RSD is defined by a constellation of signs and symptoms in a regional distribution. The symptoms are out of proportion to the apparent precipitating event.

II. ETIOPATHOGENESIS

   A. RSD results from conditions that cause regional tissue damage, pain and immobilization, and direct injury to the central nervous system. Local or central nervous system injury and immobilization lead to long-lasting changes.

   B. Trauma is the most common inciting event and it may be of a very minor nature. Fractures or their improper casting is a common cause. Many other minor injuries, procedures, metastatic cancer, pregnancy, and certain medications have also been implicated.

III. PREVALENCE

   RSD has been seen to affect all races in all geographic locations, although, due to variation in diagnostic criteria, its prevalence is difficult to assess.

IV. CLINICAL MANIFESTATIONS

   A. Pain is the predominant and disabling feature of RSD. The constellation of symptoms and signs for RSD are as follows:

   1. Pain may occur spontaneously, or as an exaggerated response to mild pain (hyperalgesia), or in response to ordinarily non-noxious stimulation (allodynia).

   2. Swelling (may be pitting, later brawny) and stiffness.

   3. Vasomotor and sudomotor changes causing alterations in skin temperature, alteration in skin color, hyperhidrosis, anhidrosis, and piloerection.

   4. Trophic skin changes with nails that may become brittle and ridged, have abnormal color, and show increased curvature. Skin may be thin and atrophied or hyperkeratotic.

   5. Functional disability initially resulting from pain, edema, and stiffness; but later from less reversible fibrotic changes.

   B. Hands and feet are typically affected. RSD is increasingly recognized in other areas, particularly the knee, and after arthroscopic surgery.

   C. There are localized variants ("segmental forms") limited to individual rays of the hand, foot, or parts of a joint.

   D. The manifestations of RSD may spread to affect contiguous and even contralateral areas. Movement disorders (resting tremor, postural tremor, action tremor, spasms, myoclonus, and apraxia) and psychiatric disturbances (affective disorders and behavioral disturbances) frequently develop.

E. Three stages have been defined (Steinbrocker classification), although all patients may not have evolved through the stages or proceed in a temporal fashion.

  1. **Stage 1 (acute).** Pain, tenderness, edema, and temperature changes predominate.
  2. **Stage 2 (dystrophic).** Pain extends beyond the area affected; loss of hair and dystrophic nails become apparent. Muscle wasting, osteoporosis, and decreased range of motion may occur.
  3. **Stage 3 (atrophic or chronic).** Atrophy, demineralization, functional impairment, and irreversible damage are present.

V. DIAGNOSTIC INVESTIGATIONS

  A. Laboratory tests. There are no diagnostic tests specific for RSD. Acute-phase reactants are abnormal only if they are secondary to an associated illness.

  B. Imaging studies

  1. **Plain radiographs** may show osteopenia, with a pattern that may be patchy or bandlike.
  2. **Technetium bone scan** may show increased uptake in periarticular tissues in the third phase (delayed images).

VI. DIFFERENTIAL DIAGNOSIS

Differential diagnosis includes conditions that themselves cause pain, immobility, and swelling with or without inflammation.

  A. Injuries like crush wounds, fractures, stress fractures, and osteonecrosis.

  B. Infections of both bone and soft tissue.

  C. Other conditions like thromboangiitis obliterans, Raynaud's syndrome, and inflammatory disorders such as RA.

  D. Thoracic outlet syndrome and cervical or thoracic spine disorders.

VII. TREATMENT

  A. General concepts of therapy. Early diagnosis and aggressive multimodal treatment, by a multidisciplinary treatment team (including anesthesiologist and physical therapist), are important for treatment.

  B. Treatment is focused on restoring function as rapidly as possible while avoiding an increase in pain. Pain and edema should be well controlled in order to pursue range of motion and strengthening.

  1. NSAIDs and analgesics are often insufficient for pain control (although the combination of ketorolac and amitriptyline may be efficacious). There has been an increase in the use of narcotics.
  2. Transcutaneous electronerve stimulator (TENS) may be helpful for pain control and vasomotor phenomena.
  3. Physical therapists should be utilized, especially ones that are experienced in this disorder. The following modalities are employed:
     a. Heat, cold, and contrast baths may all be utilized.
     b. Elevation, decongestive massage, and intermittent pneumatic compression are helpful in reducing edema.
     c. Range-of-motion exercises.
     d. Dynamic or static splinting may be helpful.
     e. Ultrasonography.
     f. Biofeedback.
  4. Ganglionic blocks with local anesthetics, epidural blocks, and regional intravenously catecholamine depletion (regional "chemical sympathectomy") can be helpful for assessment and treatment. Physical therapy should be instituted immediately after these blocks to improve the outcome.
  5. Surgical or chemical sympatholysis is controversial because of technical considerations, because the results are irreversible, and because pain may paradoxically recur or increase.
  6. Somatic blocks may be used if other blocks result in suboptimal pain relief. This may be used to facilitate physical therapy.
  7. Oral adrenergic receptor antagonists (prazosin, phentolamine, and others) have been reported as useful.

   8. Clonidine, through its agonist effect on inhibitory receptors, decreases the release of norepinephrine.
   9. Anticonvulsants such as carbamazepine (Tegretol), phenytoin, valproate, and gabapentin (Neurontin) have been used, as well as tricyclic antidepressants.
   10. Use of corticosteroids is controversial. One protocol consists of 4 days of treatment, but must be carefully considered in the light of the paucity of controlled trials regarding their benefit.
   11. Miscellaneous agents like calcium channel blockers, calcitonin, alendronate, pamidronate, and spinal cord stimulators have been reported as useful therapies.

 HEREDITARY PERIODIC FEVERS

Hereditary periodic fevers (or systemic autoinflammatory diseases) are a group of disorders characterized by unprovoked inflammatory episodes without high-titer autoantibodies. The majority of these exhibit mendelian patterns, some with specifically defined single gene defects, and present with recurrent attacks of fever, serosal inflammation, and muscular, articular, and cutaneous involvement. They are to be distinguished from autoimmune disorders such as RA and systemic lupus erythematosus (SLE) in that the autoinflammatory disorders are related to activation of the innate immune system while SLE and RA are caused by perturbations of the adaptive immune system.

Hereditary periodic fevers that will be discussed here include familial Mediterranean fever (FMF), hyperimmunoglobulin D syndrome (HIDS), and tumor necrosis factor receptor-associated periodic syndrome (TRAPS).

A periodic fever is a recurrent fever lasting from a few days to a few weeks, with symptomfree intervals. Periodic fevers lasting longer than 2 years, with a predictable course and family history, often suggests a noninfectious etiology.

I. FMF
   A. Introduction. FMF is a recessive autoinflammatory disease characterized by short attacks of serositis (peritonitis, pleuritis, or arthritis) and recurrent episodes of fever lasting 1 to 3 days.
   B. Etiopathogenesis
      1. The gene involved (*MEPV*, on the short arm of chromosome 16) encodes the protein pyrin, or marenostrin, whose precise function is still unknown.
      2. Affected patients lack a specific protease that is typically found in serosal fluids, which can inactivate both interleukin-8 and the chemotactic complement factor Va inhibitor.
      3. This is a disorder of the innate immune system as opposed to SLE and RA, which involve the adaptive immune system.
   C. Prevalence. More than 10,000 patients are affected worldwide. Patients are predominantly from the Mediterranean basin (Sephardic Jews, Arabs, Turks, and Armenians). It has also been described as affecting Greeks, Italians, Cubans, and Belgians. The frequency of the susceptibility gene varies widely among ethnic groups.
   D. Clinical manifestations
      1. Abdominal pain of 1 to 2 days' duration occurs in 95% of patients. Most patients present with an acute abdomen or peritonitis.
      2. The arthritis is typically acute monarticular or pauciarticular, occurring as the sole manifestation in 75% of patients. Chronic destructive arthritis and migratory arthritis are rare.
      3. Cutaneous manifestation is most commonly erysipeloid erythema, often on the shins or feet (7% to 40% of patients).
      4. Pleurisy is reported in 30% of patients; less than 1% has pericarditis. Male patients may present with acute scrotal swelling and tenderness.
      5. Characteristically, the symptoms are accompanied by **fever,** although patients may present with fever alone.
      6. Amyloid A amyloidosis is regarded as the main complication of the disease, with deposits in the kidneys, gastrointestinal tract, liver, spleen, heart, testes, and thyroid, most commonly occurring in Sephardic Jews.

E. Diagnostic investigations
   1. Laboratory tests
      a. There is no specific biological marker that is clinically available currently.
      b. During acute febrile attacks, the inflammatory mediators (amyloid A, fibrinogen, and C-reactive protein) are typically elevated.
      c. Proteinuria is highly suggestive of amyloidosis.
   2. Imaging studies. Radiologic studies are nonspecific, and even after many attacks radiographs may typically remain normal.
F. Differential diagnosis. Differential diagnosis includes other causes of periodic fever such as juvenile idiopathic arthritis, adult-onset Still's disease, Crohn's disease, and Behçet's syndrome.
G. Treatment
   1. The mainstay of treatment is daily colchicine prophylaxis to prevent acute attacks and also to prevent amyloidosis. Adult dose is 1.2 to 1.8 mg/day.
   2. There is some evidence that IL-1 is involved downstream in FMF. IL-1 or TNF-α inhibitors may be useful in the future for treatment of this disease.
H. Prognosis is linked to presence or absence of amyloid A amyloidosis.
   1. If amyloidosis is not present, life expectancy is normal.
   2. Treatment with colchicine arrests the amyloidosis and reverses proteinuria.

II. HYPERIMMUNOGLOBULIN D SYNDROME
A. Introduction. HIDS is a recessively inherited autoinflammatory disease primarily found in patients of northern European descent. It is characterized by onset in children younger than 1 year and accompanied by periodic fever and symptoms typically lasting 3 to 7 days.
B. Etiopathogenesis. The *MVK* gene on chromosome 12q24 encoding mevalonate kinase has been found to be the cause of the syndrome. The activity of mevalonate kinase is reduced to 5% to 15% of normal, with resultant increased serum cholesterol and increased urinary excretion of mevalonic acid.
C. Prevalence
   1. The median age of onset is 6 months. Most patients are white from western European countries, with 60% being Dutch or French.
   2. The HIDS registry in the Netherlands has data on 170 published and unpublished cases.
D. Clinical manifestations
   1. Clinical manifestations consist of an attack usually preceded by chills, with gradual defervescence. Cervical lymphadenopathy and abdominal pain with vomiting and/or diarrhea are very common. Peritonitis is rare.
   2. Other symptoms include hepatosplenomegaly, headache, arthralgias, erythematous, macules and papules, and urticaria.
   3. Arthritis is typically symmetric, polyarticular, and nondestructive.
   4. The attacks typically recur in a 4- to 6-week cycle, but vary widely for individual patients and from one patient to another.
E. Diagnostic investigations
   1. Laboratory tests
      a. Serum testing shows continuously high IgD values (more than 100 IU/mL); although in very young patients, the level may be normal. More than 80% of patients have high IgA levels as well.
      b. Acute-phase reactants (amyloid A, C-reactive protein, and white counts) are elevated during the attacks.
      c. Disease activity correlates with urinary excretion of neopterin, a marker of activated cellular immune response.
   2. Imaging studies. There are no specific imaging studies.
F. Differential diagnosis. Differential diagnosis includes other causes of periodic fever such as juvenile idiopathic arthritis, adult-onset Still's disease, Crohn's disease, and Behçet's syndrome.
G. Treatment. Currently, there is no uniform treatment of HIDS. Benefit has been reported from NSAIDs, corticosteroids, intravenous immunoglobulin (IVIG), colchicine,

and cyclosporine. TNF inhibitors and 3-hydroxy-3-methylglutaryl coenzyme A (HMG CoA) reductase inhibitors are under investigation.

H. Prognosis
1. The disease does not have any major effect on life span.
2. In some patients, the attacks due to the disease ameliorate in adulthood.
3. Amyloid has not been associated with HIDS.

III. TRAPS
A. Introduction. TRAPS is an autosomal dominant disorder, first described in 1982, with recurrent fever and symptoms typically lasting more than 1 week.
B. Etiopathogenesis. TRAPS is associated with mutations in the *TNFRSF1A* gene on the short arm of chromosome 12, which encodes a receptor for TNF. It has been suggested that structural changes in the TNF receptor may result in continuous TNF-α signaling through defects in receptor shedding, resulting in uncontrolled inflammation. Inconsistent with this theory is that two mutations are not associated with defects of shedding of the TNF receptor.
C. Prevalence. More than 20 families in Ireland, Australia, France, Puerto Rico, the United States, Finland, and the Netherlands have been affected.
D. Clinical manifestations
1. **Patients have recurrent fever with localized migratory myalgia (80% of patients) and painless erythema,** typically on the trunk.
2. **Abdominal pain** is common, often with associated diarrhea or constipation, nausea, and vomiting.
3. **Ocular manifestations** include painful conjunctivitis, periorbital edema, or both.
4. **Chest pain** may be due to sterile pleurisy or local myalgia.
E. Diagnostic investigations
1. **Laboratory tests**
   a. During attacks, patients have neutrophilia, increased C-reactive protein, and mild complement activation.
   b. Polyclonal Ig levels (especially IgA) may be elevated; IgD may also be elevated.
   c. Patients have low serum level of soluble type 1 TNF receptor.
2. **Imaging studies.** There are no characteristic imaging studies.
F. Differential diagnosis
1. TRAPS can be differentiated from the other periodic diseases by the length of time of the attacks, conjunctivitis, and localized myalgias.
2. Differential diagnosis includes other causes of periodic fever such as juvenile idiopathic arthritis, adult-onset Still's disease, Crohn's disease, and Behçet syndrome.
G. Treatment
1. Patients typically respond to high doses of oral steroids (>20 mg of prednisone). Increasing doses may be needed over time based on the disease activity for the same effect.
2. Small studies have been done with TNF-α inhibitors that are very promising.
3. A case report has been published with an IL-1 inhibitor as treatment that is promising.
H. Prognosis. TRAPS is also associated with amyloidosis, the most serious consequence of the disease, occurring in approximately 25% of affected families.

MULTICENTRIC RETICULOHISTIOCYTOSIS

I. INTRODUCTION
A. Multicentric reticulohistiocytosis (MR) is a systemic disorder of unknown etiology primarily affecting the skin (nodules), mucous membranes, and joints (destructive polyarthritis).
B. The disease usually begins during the fourth decade of life with polyarthritis, cutaneous lesions, or concurrent arthritis and skin manifestations. The onset is typically insidious, with articular involvement as the first symptom. Up to

25% of cases have been associated with malignancies, but the condition is not considered to be paraneoplastic. MR has been associated with other conditions such as hyperlipidemia, autoimmune diseases, and pregnancy as well.

II. **ETIOPATHOGENESIS.** Histologic analysis reveals multinucleated foreign body-type giant cells that stain positive for lipids and glycoproteins (periodic acid-Schiff's) and smaller histiocytes. The etiology of the disease is still unknown, although hidden malignancy and tuberculosis have been implicated.

III. **PREVALENCE. The disease is very rare.** The disease occurs in all parts of the world, and women are affected three times more often than are men.

IV. **CLINICAL MANIFESTATIONS**
   A. **The polyarthritis is symmetric, progressive, and destructive.** The small and large peripheral joints are involved. The joints most frequently affected are the interphalangeal (IP) joints of the hands including the DIP joints, shoulder, knee, wrist, hip, elbow, and spine.
   B. **Severely deforming arthritis mutilans** may develop in about half the patients.
   C. **The skin lesions** are usually asymptomatic, discrete, firm, pinkish brown or purple, hemispheric, nonpruritic papulonodules that occasionally coalesce.
      1. The nodules are most numerous over the dorsum of the hands, on the face, and behind the ears.
      2. Lesions occur on the buccal mucosa, nasal septum, or lips in about half the patients with skin nodules.
   D. **Bone, tendon sheath, muscle, liver, and lung** involvement have been reported, but are not common.

V. **DIAGNOSTIC INVESTIGATIONS**
   A. **Laboratory tests**
      1. Synovial fluid findings may be quite variable; most often, the effusions are inflammatory.
      2. The erythrocyte sedimentation rate is normal or slightly raised, and rheumatoid factor is absent.
      3. Nodule biopsy yields the diagnosis due to the finding of infiltration by histiocytes and large, multinucleated giant cells with a ground-glass appearance, which stain positively for lipids and glycoproteins (periodic acid-Schiff's).
   B. **Imaging studies.** Radiographs show extensive bone destruction rather than articular cartilage loss, and very mild osteopenia around the affected joints.

VI. **DIFFERENTIAL DIAGNOSIS**
   The disease may present very similar to RA. The skin lesions and DIP joint involvement help in this differential diagnosis.

VII. **TREATMENT**
   A. **Flares and spontaneous remissions** characterize this disease; therefore, the efficacy of different therapies is difficult to assess.
   B. **Immunosuppressive drugs** such as corticosteroids and cyclophosphamide have been effective. Low-dose methotrexate has also been shown to be useful as a maintenance therapy.
   C. **TNF antagonists.** Immunohistochemical analysis of skin nodules demonstrate TNF-α, supporting the use of anti-TNF-α therapy. Bisphosphonates have also been suggested as possible therapy.

VIII. **PROGNOSIS**
   The course of disease is not well-defined; it may be either mild and slow in progression or aggressive. Spontaneous remissions may be seen.

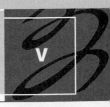

Orthopedic Surgery and Rehabilitation: Principles and Practice

V

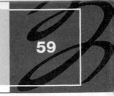

PROSTHETIC JOINT REPLACEMENT

Mark Figgie and Harry E. Figgie, III

59

INTRODUCTION

I. **Total joint arthroplasty** consists of resecting a damaged joint and replacing the articulating surfaces with prosthetic components. The convex side is usually a titanium alloy or a chrome–cobalt alloy that articulates with a concave surface made of high-density polyethylene. The polyethylene component is usually reinforced by a metal tray, which consists of titanium or chrome cobalt alloy. Traditionally, polymethylmethacrylate bone cement has been used as a grout between the implant and the bone. This material provides fixation by filling the irregular interstices of the bone and closely contacting the prosthetic surfaces. Recent prosthetic designs and technology have allowed the prosthesis to be attached to the bone without cement.

II. **Resection arthroplasty** consists of excision of the damaged joint for pain relief or control of infection. Stability and motion are achieved by the scar tissue that grows between the bone ends.

III. **Interposition arthroplasty** consists of excision of the damaged joint and interposition of a biologic or foreign nonarticular material between two bones. Commonly interposed materials include fascia, muscle, or silicone spacers. Relief of pain is the primary goal. Motion and stability are variable, depending on the joint involved and the material used.

VI. **Arthrodesis** or fusion is obtained by denuding the articular cartilage and shaping the subchondral bone to maximize bone-to-bone contact. The process of fusion is similar to the healing of a fracture. When solid bony fusion is achieved, no motion is possible.

RECONSTRUCTIVE ALTERNATIVES

The optimal artificial joint must allow for a stable, painfree, functional arc of motion. Additionally, its expected longevity should be adequate with regard to material properties and security of fixation. In general, the performance of the more common types of joint replacement is superior to that of resection arthroplasty, interposition arthroplasty, or arthrodesis.

443

I. **ARTHRODESIS.** In arthrodesis, the elimination of joint motion places abnormal stress on the joint above and below the fusion and on the contralateral extremity. In addition, arthrodesis may be difficult to achieve when metaphyseal bone loss is present. Fusion is used predominantly in the ankle, wrist, and hip and as salvage for a failed arthroplasty of the knee.

II. **Resection arthroplasty or interpositional arthroplasty** provides unpredictable pain relief, motion, and stability. It has been virtually abandoned in the knee and hip, except in salvage procedures, and is used most commonly in the wrist, carpometacarpal joint of the thumb, metacarpophalangeal joints of the hands, and metatarsophalangeal joints of the feet.

III. **Total joint replacement** usually provides a stable, painfree, functional arc of motion. Joint replacements of the hip and knee provide the most predictable results and have demonstrated adequate performance for more than 10 years. A small percentage of patients will require reoperation after 10 years, usually for loosening of prosthetic fixation.

INDICATIONS FOR TOTAL JOINT REPLACEMENT

Indications for total joint replacement are severe, unremitting pain with loss of joint function and radiographic evidence of articular damage. The degree of joint dysfunction is evaluated by using one of the several quantitative scoring systems with numeric grades for preoperative pain, motion, stability, and activity levels. Postoperatively, the same system can be used to evaluate the degree and the durability of improvement.

CONTRAINDICATIONS TO TOTAL JOINT REPLACEMENT

I. **ABSOLUTE CONTRAINDICATIONS.** Active local or remote sepsis.
II. **RELATIVE CONTRAINDICATIONS**
    A. Neurologic disorders, including hemiparesis, parkinsonism, and Charcot joint.
    B. Technical considerations.
        1. Severe loss of bone stock.
        2. Poor soft-tissue coverage.
        3. Multiple revision procedures.
    C. Systemic illness precluding elective surgery.
    D. Nutritional factors.

EXPECTED BENEFITS OF TOTAL JOINT REPLACEMENT

I. **PAIN RELIEF.** Replacement arthroplasty has given excellent pain relief, and hence, this becomes the primary choice for surgery in all joints.
II. **MOTION.** Range of motion following arthroplasty is closely related to the preoperative arc of motion.
III. **Stability** is related to the joint being replaced, type of prosthesis used, amount of bone resected, and the degree to which periarticular ligaments are preserved and balanced.

COMPLICATIONS OF TOTAL JOINT REPLACEMENT

Complications of total joint replacement are as follows (also see Chapter 60):
I. **Systemic complications** include the risks of general or regional anesthesia, myocardial infarction, pneumonia, and urinary tract infection.
II. **JOINT-SPECIFIC COMPLICATIONS**
    A. Deep venous thrombosis. All surgeries lead to a hypercoagulable state. The incidence of deep venous thrombosis may be as high as 60% in the setting of knee replacements and is approximately 10% to 15% in the case of hip replacements. Most of them are calf clots but the more dangerous proximal clots can exist as

well. Pulmonary embolism occurs in 1% to 4% of cases and is the leading cause of mortality following elective total joint arthroplasty. Some form of anticoagulation or mechanical prophylaxis is indicated for all patients undergoing total hip or total knee arthroplasty, but the type, duration, and time of initiation of the anticoagulation regimen is usually defined by the characteristics of the individual patient and the decisions of the orthopedist and internist.

B. Fat embolism. Bone marrow–derived fat is liberated in the process of all joint replacements but rarely leads to the fat embolism syndrome. This syndrome occurs mostly in bilateral joint replacements and varies from a mild elevation in the pulmonary artery pressure detected during monitoring for the procedure, to a life-threatening illness manifested by hypoxemia due to extensive pulmonary infiltrates, neurologic abnormalities, and disseminated intravascular coagulation. The care is supportive with appropriate respiratory care, often in an intensive care unit (ICU) setting, and at times requiring intubation and avoidance of large amounts of fluids that can shift into the lung because of a capillary leak syndrome.

C. Infection (see Chapter 46)

    1. Acute infection results from bacterial inoculation of the wound at the time of surgery. This is treated with open debridement, irrigation, most commonly, removal of the prosthesis, and closure over drains and is followed by approximately 6 weeks of antibiotic administration in preparation for reimplantation. Appropriate parenteral antibiotic therapy depends on obtaining accurate culture and sensitivity reports and adequate blood levels of the antibiotic selected.

    2. Late infection that occurs 6 to 12 months postoperatively arises, most likely, from the hematogenous spread of bacteria from a site of active infection to the prosthesis. The most common sources of such a bacteremia are the genitourinary tract, colorectum, teeth, and skin. Late infection usually results in prosthetic removal and in either immediate exchange with use of an antibiotic-impregnated cement or delayed exchange following 6 weeks of parenteral antibiotic therapy. In order to prevent such disastrous infections, antibiotic prophylaxis is mandatory for dental work, colonoscopy, cystoscopy, and other procedures in a manner similar to that needed for a prosthetic heart valve.

JOINT REPLACEMENT IN THE LOWER EXTREMITY

It is necessary to evaluate the status of all the joints of a lower extremity when replacement of one of them is planned. Correcting one problem may create another (e.g., correcting a valgus knee may accentuate a fixed varus ankle deformity).

I.   **Total hip replacement** is the procedure with the most predictable and reliable results. A metal femoral component is anchored into the femoral canal with acrylic cement, and a polyethylene acetabular component is similarly fixed into the acetabulum. Newer techniques utilizing an uncemented prosthesis rely on tissue ingrowth into irregularities in the prosthetic surfaces for fixation. The efficacy of tissue ingrowth in preventing late loosening, the most common problem encountered with cemented implants, is not yet known.

II.   **Total knee replacement** utilizes polyethylene tibial and patellar components and metal femoral components that are either cemented or uncemented. Recent reports of long-term follow-up of patients with cemented implants have shown knee replacement to be as predictable and reliable as total hip replacement, although technically more difficult. Close attention must be paid to the alignment and the ligamentous balancing during this procedure. Depending on the degree of deformity and ligamentous laxity or contracture, varying degrees of linkage between the tibial and femoral components may be selected in different prosthetic systems. In general, a completely constrained hinged implant will create high torsional stresses at the interface between prosthesis and bone and, therefore, will have unacceptably high rates of loosening or failure of prosthetic material. In most cases, less constrained systems are used that depend on either ligaments or augmented prosthetic surfaces for stability.

III. **Total ankle replacement** has a limited application. It is useful in a patient with se-vere arthritis of both the ankles and the subtalar joints, when an ankle fusion would be severely disabling. Ankle replacement usually provides an arc of motion at the ankle that allows a more physiologic gait cycle than would a fusion. Because of the high loads that cross the relatively thin components and cement, loosening may be a problem. Total ankle replacement, technically a difficult procedure, is reserved prima-rily for less active patients with polyarticular arthritis.

 JOINT REPLACEMENT IN THE UPPER EXTREMITY

Planning any joint replacement in an upper extremity must be directed at relieving pain and providing a functional hand. When several joints in the upper extremity are involved, the wrist and hand should receive primary attention, unless severe pain demands the replace-ment of a more proximal joint first.

I. **Total wrist replacement** usually provides a functional range of motion in addition to pain relief. It is therefore superior to arthrodesis from a functional standpoint, but its long-term efficacy has not been proved. The high loads that cross the small prosthesis are capable of causing loosening in the cemented replacements or excessive wear de-bris and secondary synovitis in silicone interposition arthroplasty. If a patient is active and expects to perform significant manual labor, an arthrodesis is the treatment of choice.

II. **FINGER IMPLANT ARTHROPLASTY.** Silicone interposition arthroplasty has been used successfully at the metacarpophalangeal joints in patients with arthritis. Pain re-lief, functional motion, and good stability may be obtained routinely, provided the preoperative deformity is not too great and that the functioning muscle–tendon units are still operative. Recent advances in cemented arthroplasty of small joints have made possible the replacement of proximal interphalangeal joints, but the surgical re-sults have not been evaluated during a long-enough period to demonstrate a clear and long-lasting advantage over arthrodesis.

III. **TOTAL ELBOW REPLACEMENT.** The elbow is an especially complex joint because of its crucial role in moving the hand in space throughout a wide range and the re-quirements for stability that are placed on it. Loads of up to six times one's body weight cross the elbow during the activities of daily living. An arthritic elbow can be severely painful and stiff and, in some cases, unstable. This presents significant disabil-ity to a patient with polyarticular rheumatoid arthritis who uses a cane or crutches. Re-placement of the elbow joint is a technically demanding procedure that may produce significant, long-lasting relief of pain in a relatively inactive patient. The linked pros-theses have built-in stability against varus–valgus stress and can be used in severe joint deformity. Minimally constrained surface replacements require the integrity of liga-mentous structures around the elbow for success.

VI. **TOTAL SHOULDER REPLACEMENT.** The replacement of the humeral head with a stemmed metallic prosthesis and the glenoid with a polyethylene component provides the patients with arthritis with relief from pain and, in many cases, restores a func-tional range of glenohumeral motion. Postoperative range of motion is largely deter-mined by the preoperative condition of the rotator cuff. Therefore, patients with rheumatism who have atrophic cuffs are less likely to gain significant motion than are patients with post-traumatic arthritis or avascular necrosis of the humeral head.

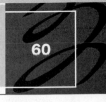

INTRODUCTION

Patients with rheumatic disease frequently require surgery for problems arising in the course of their chronic condition or in the acute setting of trauma or bone fracture. Therefore, rheumatologists, internists, and primary care physicians are often asked to evaluate patients in the perioperative setting. This chapter reviews the basic concepts that underlie perioperative medical care and management, emphasizing problems that are relatively specific to the patient with rheumatic disease.

The purpose of the preoperative medical and subsequent perioperative management are as follows:

- Identification of comorbid conditions that may affect perioperative clinical decision-making.
- Assessment of risk (both in magnitude and type).
- Anticipation of potential postoperative complications.

COMPONENTS OF A PREOPERATIVE MEDICAL EVALUATION

The preoperative evaluation should take place, whenever possible, in the office setting several weeks before surgery. Although not always possible (e.g., as in the setting of acute injury requiring immediate surgical intervention), such anticipatory evaluation allows for sufficient time for discourse with other physicians involved in the patient's care, for additional consultation and further investigation and, if necessary, for the institution of therapy directed at optimizing the patient's medical status prior to the contemplated surgery. The preoperative evaluation should serve as a focal point of an up-to-date medical assessment and communication among all members of the medical team who will be caring for the patient.

I. **MEDICAL EVALUATION.** No consensus exists regarding what constitutes the optimal preoperative medical evaluation. The nature and extent of the preoperative evaluation of the patient depends on such factors as age, functional capacity, existing comorbidity, the type of anesthesia, and the type of surgery to be performed. However, some general guidelines as given here can provide a useful framework for such evaluations.

A. **History and physical examination.** Except for young patients and those undergoing only minor surgical procedures, most other patients should undergo a complete medical history and physical examination immediately prior to the surgical procedure.

B. **Laboratory studies.** Although it has never been demonstrated that preoperative laboratory testing improves surgical outcome, a number of investigations may be considered appropriate and are commonly performed on patients prior to major surgical procedures. Depending on the nature of the problem and the magnitude of surgery required to correct it, as well as the nature and severity of coexisting diseases, such testing might include the following:

1. Complete blood count.
2. Urinalysis and culture (for those patients undergoing total joint arthroplasty).
3. Complete blood chemistries.
4. Prothrombin [international normalized ratio (INR)] and partial thromboplastin time (while these are not demonstrated to be of value as preoperative

447

investigations, they are of reasonable value in patients requiring anticoagulants after surgery, i.e., total joint arthroplasty).

5. A 12-lead electrocardiogram (ECG).

6. Chest radiograph (particularly in the elderly patients and those undergoing major joint or spine surgery).

II. **COORDINATION OF CARE.** At times, it is necessary to bring together the internist, orthopedist, and anesthesiologist preoperatively in a conference setting to address the conditions of very high-risk patients such as those undergoing bilateral joint procedures or extensive and prolonged spine surgery. This type of approach can often prevent significant cardiac, pulmonary, and neurologic problems, as well as problems with clotting postoperatively. This "ounce of prevention" usually pays off handsomely.

 ## ASSESSMENT OF SURGICAL RISK

A primary purpose of the preoperative medical evaluation is the identification of patients who are at higher risk for postoperative complications. Although the standard history and physical examination remain the principal screening method for the detection of conditions likely to affect the outcome of surgery, there are two rating systems that are useful in identifying patients who are most likely to develop postoperative complications.

I. The best known and most widely used is the **American Society of Anesthesiologists' (ASA) Physical Status Scale,** which has a high correlation with the patient's postoperative course. The ASA consists of five levels of risk, which are based on the presence of a systemic disturbance; absent (I), mild (II), moderate (III), severe (IV), and virtually certain to cause death (V); the subdesignation E denotes emergency surgery.

II. A second system, focused on the risk of cardiac complications after surgery, is the **Goldman Cardiac Risk Index** (or subsequent modifications of the index). This system is somewhat more complex, emphasizes recent myocardial infarction and decompensated congestive heart failure as risk factors, and is the foundation upon which much of the current perioperative cardiac risk assessment is based.

 ## ANESTHESIA IN PATIENTS WITH RHEUMATIC DISEASE

A variety of issues, which include airway considerations, the site and anticipated duration of surgery, existing comorbidity, and the patient's emotional state are important determinants for the type of anesthesia to be used, to decide whether invasive monitoring will be necessary, and to determine the length of time the patient will spend in the recovery room after surgery.

I. **TYPE OF ANESTHESIA.** Both general and regional anesthesia are commonly used in the surgical treatment of patients with rheumatic disease. General anesthesia with endotracheal intubation may present a particular danger in patients with rheumatoid arthritis or ankylosing spondylitis in which cervical spine and/or cricoarytenoid disease may be present. In patients with cervical spine instability or a rigid airway, fiberoptic intubation may be required. Regional anesthesia may take the form of limited local anesthesia for minor procedures, peripheral nerve block for surgery of the upper and lower extremity, and epidural/spinal anesthesia for arthroplasty in the lower extremity.

II. **MONITORING TECHNIQUES.** Patients undergoing major surgical procedures should have continuous electrocardiographic and pulse oximeter monitoring intraoperatively. At the discretion of the anesthesiologist, central venous pressure, arterial pressure, and Swan-Ganz catheter monitoring may be helpful in select patients. Such monitoring is often employed in patients undergoing bilateral joint replacement surgery and in those with a history of prior cardiac disease.

III. **POSTOPERATIVE ANALGESIA.** A number of options exist for the control of postoperative pain, including the traditional intravenous or intramuscular routes (systemic) versus the administration of epidural analgesia. Patient-controlled analgesia via an epidural route of administration is a very effective method of pain control postoperatively and often facilitates postoperative physical therapy, which is important in the restoration of range of motion in patients undergoing orthopedic surgery. This technique also reduces the systemic absorption of analgesics, thereby minimizing the problem of narcotic-induced respiratory depression, sedation, or cognitive problems in the elderly patients, or bowel problems such as ileus. Parenterally administered nonsteroidal anti-inflammatory drugs (NSAIDs), such as ketorolac (Toradol), are a useful alternative to traditional analgesia after surgery and can be used to reduce the requirement of narcotics after major surgery. These drugs should not be given to patients with the usual contraindications to NSAIDs such as peptic ulcer disease, renal disease, and the concomitant use of anticoagulants.

PERIOPERATIVE MANAGEMENT OF COMORBID MEDICAL CONDITIONS

The following discussion addresses the important comorbidities encountered in the perioperative setting. Table 60-1 summarizes medication concerns and reminders related to comorbid conditions.

I.   CARDIAC DISEASE AND HYPERTENSION

   A. Coronary artery disease

   1. **Introduction.** The presence and extent of cardiovascular disease in assessing the risk of noncardiac surgery cannot be overstated and is, fortunately, the most investigated and well-documented arena of perioperative medicine. A large subset of patients who undergo orthopedic procedures such as joint replacements and hip fracture repair are older individuals, or have a systemic joint disease such as rheumatoid arthritis. Both the older individuals and patients with rheumatoid arthritis have an increased incidence of coronary artery disease, the former because of age-related phenomena and the latter because of the inflammatory state itself.

   Practical guidelines for the physicians involved in the assessment and care of patients with cardiac disease are widely recognized. The predictive value of the routine clinical assessment, including medical history, physical examination, ECG, and chest x-ray is well established, at least with respect to the identification of the presence of pre-existing cardiac disease. However, it is also important to define disease severity and stability, as well as prior treatment received. The factors that work in concert with other clinical characteristics and ultimately define postoperative risk include the following:
      a. Age.
      b. Functional capacity (as determined by simple activity questionnaires).
      c. Comorbidity (particularly diabetes mellitus, peripheral vascular disease, and chronic pulmonary disease).
      d. Type of surgery to be performed (major orthopedic procedures tend to be of intermediate risk).
      e. A series of factors may predict postoperative myocardial infarction, congestive heart failure, and death after orthopedic surgery.

   2. **Major predictors** of increased perioperative cardiac risk are as follows:
      a. Recent myocardial infarction (<30 days).
      b. Unstable or severe angina.
      c. Poorly compensated congestive heart failure.
      d. Significant arrhythmias.
      e. Severe valvular disease.

   3. **Intermediate predictors** of increased perioperative cardiac risk are as follows:
      a. Mild angina.
      b. Prior myocardial infarction determined from history or by pathologic Q waves.
      c. Compensated or prior congestive heart failure.
      d. Diabetes.

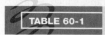

TABLE 60-1	Perioperative Evaluation and Care	
Category	**Medications**	**Reminders**
Cardiac	■ Continue medications through surgery ■ May have to change to transdermal, intravenous, or sublingual equivalents ■ Avoid abrupt withdrawal ■ Avoid rapid diuresis before surgery	■ Bacteremia during surgery may seed endocardium ■ Consider whether β-blockers should be used ■ Stop clopidogrel (Plavix) 10 d before surgery
Hypertension	■ Continue most medications through surgery, using nonoral forms if necessary ■ Change ganglionic blockers and MAOIs to other agents	■ Only severe (diastolic higher than 110) or malignant hypertension needs control preoperatively in most cases
Endocrine	**Diabetes:** ■ Stop oral hypoglycemics 1 d before surgery; discontinue chlorpropamide and glyburide 3 d before surgery ■ For insulin users, halve the usual insulin dose before surgery with dextrose and water and sliding scale insulin; for prolonged NPO or brittle diabetes, insulin drip **Thyroid disease:** ■ Continue thyroid supplements during surgery ■ Reduce L-thyroxine dose by 20% for long-term parenteral use **Corticosteroids:** ■ Stress doses if used regularly within a y of surgery, tapering over 3–4 d to maintenance after surgery	■ Even young patients with diabetes have autonomic insufficiency ■ Prolonged anesthetic effect after surgery may suggest hypothyroidism
Gastrointestinal and Hepatic	■ Cimetidine may precipitate confusion, delirium in the older individuals ■ Malabsorption, dysmotility of bowel, hepatic dysfunction may significantly alter pharmacodynamics of perioperative medications, including anesthetic	■ Nutritional assessment, vitamins ■ History of risk factors for hepatitis B or C ■ History of alcohol use ■ Watch for bleeding diathesis ■ Theophylline clearance may be decreased by cimetidine, erythromycin, ciprofloxacin
Renal	■ Caution with nephrotoxins, including acetaminophen	■ Don't feed too quickly for fear of ileus

(continued)

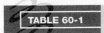

TABLE 60-1	Perioperative Evaluation and Care (*Continued*)	
Category	**Medications**	**Reminders**
Rheumatologic	■ NSAIDs: stop 5–7 d before surgery (reversible platelet function) ■ Hold anti-TNF biologics 1–2 wk preoperative and start again 1–2 wk postoperative when wound is clean and healing	■ Cervical spine disease may compromise safe intubation ■ RA patients with cervical spine disease should wear cervical collar to the OR ■ Treat asymptomatic bacteriuria in patients undergoing total joint arthroplasty ■ Patients with severe sicca syndrome require lubricant eye drops
Hematology	■ Hold cytotoxic or immunosuppressive drugs before surgery	■ Consider autologous blood transfusion requirements well in advance of surgery
Neurology	■ Continue anticonvulsant therapy	■ Phenothiazines may lower seizure threshold ■ Atropine may precipitate delirium in Parkinson's disease
Geriatrics	■ Polypharmacy common in the older individuals; continue medications only if indicated	■ Nutritional assessment ■ Delirium may be caused by sundowning, infection, ischemia, drug effect (sedatives especially), alcohol withdrawal, electrolyte imbalance, hypoxia ■ Discharge planning essential preoperatively ■ Advance directives should be discussed well before surgery
Miscellaneous	■ Ask about nonprescription drugs and supplements ■ Alcohol and illicit drug use should be considered possible	■ HIV risk factors ■ Patient may be unaware of pregnancy ■ Patient fears and expectations ■ Vaccination status

HIV, human immunodeficiency virus; MAOIs, monoamine oxidase inhibitors; NPO, nothing by mouth; NSAIDs, nonsteroidal anti-inflammatory drugs.
Adapted from MacKenzie CR, Sharrock NE. Perioperative medical considerations with rheumatoid arthritis. Perioperative medical considerations in patients with rheumatoid arthritis. *Rhem Dis Clin North Am.* 1998; 24(1):1–17, with permission.

   4. Minor predictors of increased perioperative risk are as follows:
   a. Advanced age.
   b. Abnormal ECG.
   c. Rhythm other than sinus rhythm.
   d. Low functional capacity.
   e. Prior stroke.

     f. Poorly controlled hypertension.

     g. Prior cardiac revascularization, currently asymptomatic.

5. Cardiac testing. The indications for preoperative exercise stress testing with or without nuclear scanning or ambulatory electrocardiography (Holter monitoring) are not clear. Ultimately, the decision will depend on the physician's estimates of the effectiveness, risk, and costs of such evaluations. Feasibility also may come into play in patients with chronic rheumatic diseases and orthopedic conditions, given the functional compromise that is attendant to such conditions. This is also an issue when there is the need to perform relatively urgent surgery, as in the case of fracture. Nonetheless, guidelines have emerged from a large body of clinical data.

     a. Patients who have had no clinical markers of risk, as well as those who have had coronary revascularization within the preceding five years and remain asymptomatic, are at such low risk for postoperative cardiac complications that further screening appears unjustified.

     b. In the remaining patients, mainly those with some risk factors for coronary artery disease, the issue of screening is particularly relevant. Exercise stress testing may be indicated and ultimately helpful in select patients. Such decisions can be reached in consultation with the cardiologist. The decision to further evaluate cardiac risk depends on the nature of surgery, but is seldom necessary before minor surgical procedures.

6. The use of β-blockers. The relevant therapeutic considerations mainly relate to medication management. Recognition of the protective role of β-blockade in the perioperative setting is perhaps the most significant advance in perioperative medical care. On the basis of several definitive studies and general consensus, β-blockade in patients undergoing major noncardiac surgery has been shown to reduce the risk for postoperative cardiac complications (myocardial ischemia and infarction) and mortality. Questions relevant to this issue are as follows:

     a. Which patients should receive β-blockers perioperatively?

     Criteria for deciding which patients should be treated with β-blockers are summarized in Table 60-2.

     b. Timing and choice of perioperative β-blockers

        i. The administration of these agents may be started a week or more prior to surgery, on the morning of surgery, in the holding area, or intraoperatively. If the patient has started receiving oral β-blockers prior to admission, they should take their oral dose on the morning of surgery. In patients receiving hypotensive epidural anesthesia, the anesthesiologist may prefer starting the β-blocker in the recovery room rather than in the operating room.

        ii. Atenolol (Tenormin) and metoprolol (Lopressor) are the recommended oral agents. In elderly patients, it is advisable to administer a lower dose (e.g., atenolol 12.5 to 25 mg/day, metoprolol 12.5 to 25 mg twice daily).

        iii. The optimal duration of β-blockade postoperatively has not been established in the literature. A minimum of 1 week is suggested, and most patients should be treated for 1 month or until follow-up by their internist or cardiologist. The dose of β-blocker should be appropriately tapered when discontinuing.

     c. Which β-blocking agent should be used?

     Studies demonstrating the benefits of β-blockade have used β_1-selective agents, and no advantage for any specific agent has been shown within this group of medications. Atenolol or metoprolol appear to be suitable and are considered equivalent choices.

     d. When should the use of β-blockers be started preoperatively?

     Physicians should attempt to begin therapy early enough in order to achieve a degree of β-blockade, which would generally require several days. Nonetheless, if it is not possible to initiate treatment in this time frame, the medication can be given intravenously by the anesthesiologist at

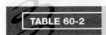

TABLE 60-2	Recommendations for the Use of Perioperative β-blockers

Perioperative β-blockers should be used in patients with *any* of these criteria:
- Ischemic heart disease, defined as:
  - History of myocardial infarction **or** Q waves on ECG
  - History of angina pectoris
  - Positive stress test
  - History of angioplasty or coronary artery bypass graft
- Cerebrovascular disease, defined as history of transient ischemic attack **or** cerebrovascular accident
- Diabetes mellitus requiring insulin therapy
- Chronic renal insufficiency, defined as baseline creatinine ≥2.0

Perioperative β-blockers should be used in patients meeting *any two* of the following criteria:
- Age 65 or older
- History of hypertension (treated or untreated)
- Current smoker
- History of hypercholesterolemia (treated or untreated)
- Diabetes mellitus not requiring insulin therapy

Possible contraindications for β-blockade (often such patients may still cautiously receive β-blockade on a case-by-case basis):
- Bradycardia, defined as a heart rate <60
- Congestive heart failure if uncontrolled
- Asthma/COPD history, especially if severe and/or uncontrolled
- History of intolerance of β-blockers

COPD, chronic obstructive pulmonary disease; ECG, electrocardiogram.
From Auerbach AD, Goldman L. Beta blockers and reduction of cardiac events in noncardiac surgery: scientific review. *JAMA.* 2002;287:1435–1444, with permission.

the time of initiation of anesthesia. Patients already taking β-blockers prior to surgery should be advised to continue the medication up to and including the morning of surgery.

e. **Other cardiac medications.** Other medications are also commonly employed in the treatment of chronic cardiac disease. Patients taking long-acting nitrates should be given the drug on the morning of surgery as well; cutaneous nitrates can be continued postoperatively until the patient resumes oral intake. Patients taking angiotensin-converting enzyme (ACE) inhibitors are at increased risk of circulatory instability, especially if the medication is taken immediately prior to surgery. Therefore, the administration of preoperative cardiac medication should be discussed and coordinated with the anesthesiologist prior to surgery.

f. **Postoperative monitoring for cardiac instability.** As with risk assessment, the optimal surveillance strategy for detecting postoperative myocardial infarction has not been well-studied. In patients with no preoperative evidence of coronary disease, detection strategies can be restricted only to those patients who develop signs or symptoms of cardiac dysfunction or ischemia. In those at greater risk for postoperative cardiac complications, surveillance for ischemic events should begin with an ECG immediately after surgery, with additional testing on each of the first two postoperative days. Although creatine phosphokinase (CPK) levels are usually elevated due to the muscle trauma associated with surgery, cardiac isoenzymes and, more recently, serial serum troponins are useful in the detection of myocardial infarction, particularly in those patients whose surveillance ECGs reveal changes suggestive of ischemia.

B. Hypertension. Blood pressure measurements should be taken in the lying and sitting position to determine the maximal orthostatic fall in blood pressure as well as the degree of blood pressure control. Patients are then classified as untreated, hypertensive controlled on medication, or hypertensive despite therapy. As the perioperative morbidity that is associated with chronic hypertension is largely a function of the presence of complications of the major end organs (cardiac, neurologic, and renal), the preoperative examination should focus on the assessment of these consequences of poorly controlled hypertension. Such determinations are relatively easily made from the common preoperative laboratory studies, chest radiograph, and ECG.

Controversy exists about whether mild to moderate hypertension (diastolic = 110 mm Hg) increases the risk of surgery. Patients whose blood pressure is higher than this are considered at greater risk and should be stabilized with antihypertensive therapy prior to surgery. Patients who are in satisfactory control of hypertension preoperatively should continue their medication, taking it on the morning of surgery and subsequently throughout the postoperative period, if their blood pressure allows. However, because of bed rest, fluid losses, and the hypotensive influences of various medications employed in the postoperative setting, some patients may temporarily require less (or no) antihypertensive medication. Because of their volume-depleting and potassium-depleting properties, it may be prudent to discontinue diuretics on the morning of surgery or potentially earlier.

C. Valvular heart disease. Surgical risks in patients with valvular heart disease depend on the valve affected as well as the nature and severity of the valvular lesion. The lesion conferring the highest perioperative risk is hemodynamically significant aortic stenosis. Mitral valve disease and aortic insufficiency, if not severe, are usually well tolerated, although any valvular disease associated with significant left ventricular dysfunction [New York Heart Association (NYHA) Class III or IV] increases the risk of surgery. Therefore, patients with a significant cardiac murmur, accompanied by signs or symptoms of left ventricular dysfunction, should undergo an echocardiographic assessment preoperatively, particularly if a major procedure is planned. Invasive hemodynamic monitoring perioperatively may be indicated in patients at higher risk.

D. Cardiomyopathies. The chronic cardiomyopathies, whether of the dilated or hypertrophic type, are associated with an increased incidence of postoperative congestive heart failure. Indeed, the hypertrophic cardiomyopathies generally are considered a relative contraindication to epidural or spinal anesthesia.

E. Arrhythmias and conduction abnormalities. Arrhythmias and conduction diseases may be markers for underlying cardiac or pulmonary disease, metabolic abnormalities, or drug toxicity. Therefore, the clinician should search for such conditions preoperatively and institute corrective action, if possible, before surgery.

A problem that arises with some frequency is the case of a patient with chronic atrial fibrillation who is given long-term anticoagulation. As the risk of embolic stroke in such patients who are not given anticoagulation is low, it is safe to temporarily discontinue warfarin (Coumadin) for a sufficient period of time preoperatively to allow for normalization of the prothrombin time and INR. Five days are generally sufficient.

II. PULMONARY DISEASE

Chronic obstructive pulmonary disease (COPD) (e.g., chronic bronchitis and emphysema) and asthma are the two most prevalent forms of chronic pulmonary disease and are the pulmonary problems seen most frequently in the preoperative setting. They are also demonstrated to be important predictors of postoperative complications, which may be pulmonary or nonpulmonary.

A. Minor pulmonary complications (atelectasis and bronchitis) are increased in patients who smoke, who have a chronic cough, or have abnormal spirometry. The risk of severe postoperative pulmonary complications (pneumonia and respiratory failure) is increased mainly in those patients with marked impairment in lung function [forced expiratory volume in one second (FEV$_1$) <1.5 L]. Among the nonpulmonary factors which contribute to the risk of postoperative complications are age, obesity, longer duration of anesthesia, oversedation, and poor patient effort.

B. **The risk of perioperative lung dysfunction depends, in large part, upon the type of surgery performed.** Patients with severe lung impairment can tolerate minor procedures, even under general anesthesia. The risk of pneumonia after major peripheral limb surgery (such as hip or knee surgery) is low, even in the patients with chronic lung disease. This is in marked contrast to intra-abdominal or intrathoracic surgery, which is associated with a high risk of atelectasis or pneumonia in patients, particularly in patients with severe COPD. Regional anesthesia for surgery on the extremities circumvents many of these problems. However, an interscalene block may transiently paralyze the ipsilateral diaphragm and reduce the forced vital capacity (FVC) by 30% to 40%. Therefore, patients with COPD undergoing shoulder surgery, in which interscalene block is frequently employed, should have pulmonary function studies performed preoperatively. In patients with severely impaired pulmonary function ($FEV_1 < 1$ L), interscalene block should be avoided altogether. Otherwise, patients with COPD fare well with this anesthesia, especially in the sitting position.

C. **Patients who have been using bronchodilators** on a chronic basis before surgery should be given their standard dose the night before surgery; bronchodilator therapy should be administered postoperatively either systemically or by nebulizer. Incentive spirometry equivalent to ten deep breaths/hour and early mobilization are helpful in the prevention of postoperative atelectasis.

D. **Patients with obstructive sleep apnea** pose significant challenges during the perioperative period. Most of these patients are obese and may remain undiagnosed preoperatively. They can be difficult to intubate and are particularly sensitive to the respiratory depressant effects of narcotics and benzodiazepines. There may be coexistent hypertension and ischemic heart disease, increasing the likelihood of postoperative respiratory arrest or sudden death. Use of epidural analgesia, regional blocks, and NSAIDs tend to preserve normal sleep patterns, improve analgesia, and reduce the risk of postoperative respiratory depression. Systemic narcotics should be used cautiously. If patients tolerate Continuous Positive Airway Pressure (CPAP), this should be used postoperatively at night. These patients should remain in a monitored unit for 12–24 hours following major surgery.

III. ENDOCRINE DISEASE

A. **Diabetes mellitus.** Diabetes is the most important endocrine disorder encountered in patients undergoing surgery. Patients with diabetes are at a slightly greater risk of postoperative death, a consequence of the greater prevalence of ischemic heart disease in them. Further, patients with diabetes and with autonomic insufficiency (manifested by postural hypotension, impotence, and nocturnal diarrhea) may be at risk for sudden cardiopulmonary arrest postoperatively.

The control of the serum glucose levels tends to be the focus of medical management postoperatively, and various effective approaches to diabetic therapy have been reported. A common approach for insulin users is the so-called "sliding scale" regimen; half to two-thirds the dose of the patient's usual morning long-acting insulin is given on the morning of surgery together with 5% dextrose. Supplemental short-acting insulin is then given as dictated by finger stick blood sugar values that are recorded four times a day. This regimen is continued until the patient resumes oral intake. A different regimen is indicated for patients taking oral hypoglycemic agents; these medications can be taken the day before surgery and resumed when the patient resumes eating. The only exception is chlorpropamide (Diabinese), which should be discontinued several days before surgery because of its long half-life.

B. **Chronic corticosteroid therapy**

1. **Since many patients with rheumatic disease take corticosteroids, prophylaxis against adrenal insufficiency and management of the patient's corticosteroid therapy in the perioperative setting are critically important.** Patients believed to be at increased risk for adrenal insufficiency include those currently taking more than 20 mg hydrocortisone or 5 mg prednisone/day, those who have taken such doses for more than 2 weeks in the preceding year, and those who are receiving replacement corticosteroid therapy for known adrenal insufficiency. When undergoing major surgical procedures, such patients have traditionally been given a so-called intravenous "stress-dose" therapy as follows:

    a. A dose of 100 mg of hydrocortisone prior to surgery.

    b. A second dose of 100 mg administered intraoperatively.

    c. A dose of 100 mg intravenously every 8 hours for the 24 hours after surgery.

    d. A dose of 50 mg intravenously every 8 hours the next postoperative day.

    e. A single intravenous dose of 100 mg on the third postoperative day.

    f. Revert to the patient's usual oral dose of corticosteroid on the fourth postoperative day if the patient is consuming food orally.

  2. This approach, however, has been called into question recently by a study done on patients undergoing orthopedic procedures. In this small, nonrandomized study, patients given only their baseline doses of glucocorticoid demonstrated no clinical or laboratory evidence of adrenocortical insufficiency postoperatively, suggesting that the commonly employed "stress doses" of corticosteroid may be unnecessary in patients undergoing orthopedic surgery as opposed to patients undergoing general surgery. In patients undergoing minor procedures (i.e., surgery on the distal extremities) or those requiring regional or local anesthesia, a single preoperative dose of 100 mg can be considered sufficient coverage, because the normal metabolic response (i.e., additional adrenocorticoid secretion) to minor surgery is minimal. Otherwise, we recommend giving 100 mg hydrocortisone every 8 hours followed by 50 to 75 mg every 8 hours, by which time the patients are usually able to take oral medications and can be reverted to their regular preoperative oral dose.

IV. GASTROINTESTINAL DISEASE

Gastrointestinal problems, both exacerbations of chronic conditions or problems arising *de novo*, may complicate the postoperative period and produce significant morbidity.

  A. Peptic ulcer disease, a reasonably common problem in the population with orthopedic/rheumatic disease conditions due to the high usage of NSAIDs, may become active after surgery; it is particularly problematic in patients who require anticoagulation prophylaxis, such as those who have undergone total joint arthroplasty. Therefore, patients with a history of peptic ulcer disease, gastrointestinal bleeding, or active dyspepsia should receive prophylactic histamine-2 blocker (H2-blocker) therapy or proton pump inhibitors throughout the postoperative period. In the presence of a strong clinical suspicion that an active peptic process is ongoing, the surgery should be canceled, a workup performed, and treatment instituted before proceeding with the surgery. In patients at risk for the development of gastrointestinal bleeding after surgery, serial stool guaiacs are a good surveillance approach.

  B. Ileus. Development of an abdominal ileus is a relatively common postoperative complication. Abdominal examination and questioning regarding the passing of gas and stool are mandatory for identifying early warning signs of problems. An important predisposing factor is the postoperative use of aggressive narcotic-based analgesics, coupled with an overzealous reintroduction of oral intake in the early postoperative period. Careful consideration should be given as to the optimal timing of the resumption of oral intake of both liquids and solids. Patients should be weaned off potent narcotic therapy as quickly as possible and appropriate stool softeners and cathartics given, particularly in patients with chronic gastrointestinal complaints and conditions.

V. GENITOURINARY CONDITIONS

  A. Catheter care. As a consequence of the need for bed rest, the use of narcotics and epidural anesthesia, and the presence of prostatic disease, urinary catheters are frequently placed in patients after major surgery. In general, such catheters should be removed as early as possible and a surveillance urine culture performed to rule out the development of a urinary tract infection. If urinary catheters are removed within 48 hours of surgery and urinary retention is avoided, the risk of urinary tract infection is small.

B. **Prostatic disease leading to urinary outflow obstruction is a common problem in men** after surgery. In patients with significant chronic symptomatology, urologic consultation should be obtained prior to surgery and therapy [including transurethral resection of the prostate (TURP) if deemed necessary] should be instituted. In patients with a propensity to urinary retention and those with enlarged prostate glands who report obstructive symptomatology, therapy with agents such as terazosin (Hytrin) and tamsulosin (Flomax) could be instituted before or at the time of surgery. In patients with a history of nephrolithiasis, dehydration should be rigorously avoided to help prevent the development of acute renal colic.

C. **Patients with chronic renal insufficiency are at increased risk of developing renal failure** postoperatively. This is usually due to periods of hypovolemia with reduced renal perfusion. These patients require careful attention in respect of fluid management. Patients on dialysis preoperatively should have their care coordinated with a nephrologist and dialysis unit.

VI. **INFECTIOUS COMPLICATIONS**

The risk of infection in a prosthetic joint is of great concern in patients undergoing total joint arthroplasty. Efforts to preoperatively prevent, detect, and treat any infectious process are of utmost importance. The skin, gums and teeth, and urinary tract are sites of specific concern, and infection can be ruled out by a careful physical examination and routine preoperative urine culture. In addition, formal dental consultation may be appropriate in patients with poor oral hygiene and dentition.

Prophylactic antibiotic therapy for patients undergoing total joint arthroplasty should begin less than 2 hours before surgery and continue for 24 hours. The recommended protocol at Hospital for Special Surgery involves cefazolin (Ancef) 1 g every 8 hours (total of three doses) or, in patients who are allergic to penicillin, vancomycin 1 g every 12 hours (total of two doses). Vancomycin should not be infused in less than 1 hour to avoid the "red man" syndrome.

VII. **NEUROLOGIC PROBLEMS**

A. **Confusional states.** Elderly patients are at significant risk for the development of confusional states after surgery due to a confluence of factors arising in the perioperative setting. These risk factors include the use of sedatives, analgesics, anesthesia, fever, metabolic derangements, sleep deprivation, hypoxemia, and the disorienting effects of an unfamiliar environment. For example, in patients undergoing emergent surgical repair of a fractured hip, 30% to 50% have been reported to develop significant changes in cognitive functioning. Although such changes are usually a transient phenomenon, clinicians should focus on the detection and treatment of correctable causes that may present in this unusual fashion, particularly in the geriatric patient population. Such causes include metabolic disturbances (hyponatremia and hypoxemia); offending medications (which might well be discontinued); infection; and acute conditions (respiratory failure, myocardial infarction, cardiac arrhythmias, congestive heart failure, pulmonary embolism syndrome, fat embolism syndrome, and so on). Likewise, elderly patients and patients with underlying neurologic dysfunction (e.g., alcoholism, dementia, and parkinsonism) are at increased risk for postoperative delirium. Formal neurologic consultation and workup is occasionally necessary although generally unrevealing.

B. **Neuropraxias.** Neuropraxias arise more often after upper and lower extremity surgery, as they are generally a compression or stretch phenomenon resulting from prolonged positioning of the extremity during surgery, casting, or regional anesthesia. Early detection and intervention is critical to the ultimate outcome in these circumstances. Patients with antecedent neurologic disease are at increased risk of neuropraxia.

C. **Emotional/psychiatric problems.** Patients who live with the consequences of chronic rheumatic diseases or disabling orthopedic conditions may have emotional difficulties due to chronic pain, disability, and limitations in career opportunities, social interactions, and personal relationships. Because surgery is a significant life stress, such individuals may require additional emotional support perioperatively. Further, some patients may be taking or may require antidepressant or antianxiolytic medication. In the patient who is being treated with monoamine oxidase inhibitors (MAOIs), which is now rare, it is recommended that the medication be discontinued 10 to 14 days before surgery and the anesthesiologist alerted to the situation. Patients who are given these agents are at risk of marked circulatory instability when given general anesthesia and certain narcotics, especially meperidine. If there is a significant psychological or substance abuse problem, the patient should be seen or spoken to by a psychiatrist who can follow up on the patient through the surgery. Specific treatments may be started before surgery and added postoperatively, depending on the course of the disease in the patient.

VIII. COAGULATION DISTURBANCES

Patients with disturbances of coagulation should be carefully assessed preoperatively. Those with a genetic disease, for example, hemophilia or von Willebrand's disease, should have coagulation factors administered preoperatively, preferably guided by formal consultation with a hematologist. Acquired coagulation disturbances due to warfarin, clopidogrel (Plavix), or the various heparin preparations require the cessation of these medications preoperatively. In general, it is safe to perform anesthesia and surgery with an INR of ≤1.5. With clopidogrel and heparin, there are no reliable tests to guide therapy. For this reason, it is often considered prudent to discontinue clopidogrel 10 days and heparin 24 to 36 hours before surgery or before the administration of regional anesthesia.

MANAGEMENT OF SPECIFIC CLINICAL PROBLEMS

Specific clinical problems that may be encountered and which may benefit by perioperative management are discussed here roughly in order of how often they are encountered.

I. VENOUS THROMBOEMBOLISM

A. Prevention. Prevention of venous thromboembolic phenomenon after orthopedic surgery is the most thoroughly studied of potential postoperative complications. Pulmonary embolism, perhaps the most dreaded complication of orthopedic surgery, remains an important cause of postoperative mortality. Numerous protocols have documented efficiency in minimizing this risk.

All surgery is associated with a hypercoagulable state. Thus, prevention begins at the time of the procedure. Expeditious surgery reduces the risk of deep venous thrombosis (DVT) after operations such as total hip replacement. The type of anesthesia employed is also important; epidural anesthesia reduces the risk of proximal DVT after total hip replacement by twofold to threefold and also reduces the overall risk of DVT by at least 30% to 40%; epidural anesthesia also reduces the risk of DVT after total knee replacement, but to a lesser extent. Other intraoperative interventions, such as hypotensive anesthesia and intraoperative heparin administration, further reduce thrombogenesis.

B. Mechanical methods of reducing risk of thromboembolism also have proven to have efficacy and include pneumatic compression boots, foot pumps, compression stockings, foot flexion/extension exercises, and early ambulation. These maneuvers are safe, effective, and do not increase the risk of bleeding.

C. Anticoagulation. Because all types of surgery, large or small, cause a hypercoagulable state, the mainstay of treatment is anticoagulation, although its cost–benefit profile continues to be controversial. Prophylactic anticoagulation is begun immediately following surgery. Regimens include warfarin (Coumadin) with a target INR in 2 to 2.5 range, formerly subcutaneous heparin 5,000 units twice a day or three times a day, and more recently low-molecular-weight heparin (LMWH). A new selective inhibitor of factor Xa, fondaparinux (Arixtra/Xantidar), has been reported to be even more effective in the prevention of venous thrombosis than enoxaparin (Lovenox) in patients undergoing total joint arthroplasty and after hip fracture repair. Aspirin is also effective when combined with other modalities and continues to have its proponents.

A multimodal approach, relying on a combination of intraoperative modalities, postoperative mechanical devices, early ambulation, and low-intensity postoperative anticoagulation, is preferred for most patients by most experts and clinicians. See the HSS thromboembolic prophylaxis guidelines at www.hss.edu.

II. FAT EMBOLISM SYNDROME

Fat embolism syndrome is not uncommon after total joint arthroplasty, particularly in patients undergoing bilateral joint replacement procedures. Time of onset is variable; hemodynamic instability may develop almost immediately (presaged by a rise in pulmonary artery pressure when the prosthesis is cemented) or more insidiously over the first 2 to 3 postoperative days. In the latter group, it is often very unclear what is happening early on, because patients gradually become moderately to severely hypoxemic after surgery, may be hypotensive and, in the case of the elderly patients, often become confused. Hematologic abnormalities such as transient thrombocytopenia are commonly seen. Frank adult respiratory distress syndrome may develop and may become life-threatening, requiring aggressive supportive measures (i.e., intubation).

Treatment is supportive and includes the administration of increased concentrations of inspired oxygen (possibly via ventilator); the prevention of pulmonary hypertension by fluid restriction, the use of diuretics, and venodilators; and the prevention of pain. Corticosteroid and heparin therapy have not been demonstrated to be of benefit and are not recommended.

Pulmonary artery catheterization may be helpful to guide therapy; if the pulmonary artery diastolic pressure is maintained at less than 20 mm Hg, respiratory insufficiency is usually prevented. In severe cases, systemic manifestations of fat embolization may occur and become associated with myocardial infarction or severe brain injury. Whether this represents transpulmonary transfer or passage of fat through a patent foreman ovale is unknown.

III. ANTIPHOSPHOLIPID SYNDROME (APS) AND SYSTEMIC LUPUS ERYTHEMATOSUS (SLE)

A. APS is a condition consisting of vascular thrombosis and/or pregnancy-related morbidity arising as a consequence of the presence of antiphospholipid antibodies (aPL), most often the lupus anticoagulant or anticardiolipin antibodies. This syndrome may exist in a primary form, unassociated with an underlying connective tissue disease, or is considered secondary when it arises in the setting of such conditions as SLE. As a consequence of their general hypercoagulability, patients with APS are at increased risk of postoperative thrombosis. Their need for long-term anticoagulation results in challenges in perioperative management, specifically managing the often delicate balance between the patient's propensity to thrombosis against the risk of postoperative bleeding due to the need for anticoagulation.

Although fraught with potential risk, surgery may be necessary in patients with APS and recommendations have been published to guide medical management. First, the important, adjunctive role of physical methods in the prevention of venous thrombosis should not be forgotten. Therefore, such methods as intermittent venous compression should be aggressively employed preoperatively and postoperatively. Second, the perioperative period without anticoagulation should be kept to a minimum. Therefore, for patients on chronic warfarin therapy, the medication should be stopped 3 to 4 days before surgery to allow for normalization of the INR, and concomitant therapy with LMWH instituted at therapeutic dosages (1 mg/kg, every 12 hours) and continued until the night before surgery when it should be stopped. For many surgical procedures, particularly orthopedic surgery, warfarin can be restarted the night of the surgical procedure. If there is no contraindication, LMWH in prophylactic dosages (30 mg, every 12 hours) can be restarted simultaneously with warfarin and maintained until a therapeutic INR has been achieved. It should be remembered that conventional dosages of these agents may result in "undercoagulation" in patients with APS, and larger dosages, if feasible, may be considered necessary postoperatively, irrespective of the risk of bleeding that such therapy confers.

Given the frequent use of epidural and spinal anesthesia in patients undergoing orthopedic surgery, the risk of epidural and spinal hematoma as a complication of such anesthesia should be noted. The avoidance of this serious complication is, in part, the rationale for omitting the heparin dose on the night before surgery. In addition, at our institution, heparin is not restarted until at least 4 hours after the removal of the epidural/spinal needle. There are important and recent guidelines regarding anticoagulation in the setting of epidural catheters, wherein Plavix has to be stopped 10 days before surgery, and so on.

B. SLE. The patient with SLE has specific perioperative medical issues that are outside of the APS noted in the preceding text. These include the following:

1. The potential for surgery-related disease flares.
2. Increased risk for infection due to treatment with long-term immunosuppressant medications.
3. Raynaud's-related finger spasms and possible visceral vasospasm due to cold intravenous fluids; thus, fluids should be warmed prior to infusion.
4. Premature coronary artery disease is present in over 40% of patients with SLE.
5. Diabetes due to steroid treatment can be exacerbated by surgery.
6. Hypertension either due to steroids or renal disease.
7. Presence of renal disease with a need to avoid nephrotoxins and severe blood pressure shifts.

IV. HIP FRACTURE

Hundreds of thousands of patients are admitted to hospitals in the United States annually for treatment of a fractured hip, resulting in major costs to society, to patients, and to their families. Within the first year of fracture, 20% of elderly patients with hip fracture die, compared to 9% of age-matched subjects without a fracture. Further, one-sixth of patients who survive one year after fracture are confined to long-term care facilities, while another one-third continue to require assistive devices or the help of others to manage their daily activities. Therefore, after a fracture of the hip, most patients experience permanent impairment in functional capacity and the rates of permanent institutionalization are high. Risk factors thought to increase the need for admission to a nursing home include living alone prior to the fracture, having no children, and being of the female gender.

Most hip fractures occur in frail, elderly women with osteoporosis, who have sustained a fall. Indeed, falls are the most common antecedent event in these circumstances, and fractures are the most common serious fall-related injury. Risk factors for hip fracture include increasing age, poor general health, maternal history of hip fracture, a history of hyperthyroidism, poor depth perception, use of psychoactive medication, sedentary lifestyle, low bone mineral density and, of course, osteoporosis. Actually, the predisposition to hip fracture is thought to represent the integral part of the patient's overall disease-related or age-related medical problems.

Hip fractures can be divided into two major categories—intracapsular fractures of the femoral head and extracapsular fractures (intertrochanteric or subtrochanteric). The current approach to treatment is surgical, utilizing either internal fixation (pinning) or prosthetic joint replacement. Although a matter of ongoing debate, more severe (i.e., displaced) intracapsular fractures of the femoral head are often treated with joint replacement because they may result in a serious compromise to the blood supply of the femoral head leading to osteonecrosis, collapse of the femoral head, and secondary osteoarthritis. Internal fixation is the usual surgical approach to displaced femoral neck fractures. However, in the frail, elderly patient with lower anticipated functional requirements and life expectancy, such fractures may be treated with total joint arthroplasty as well.

Specific issues that must be addressed preoperatively and postoperatively include: approaches to anticoagulation, anticipation of the prevalent cognitive problems that arise in elderly patients after surgery, as well as the range of potential cardiac, pulmonary, genitourinary, and neurologic problems that are frequently encountered. The medication-related side effects that reflect the changes in the functions of their organ systems due to senescence are also important considerations.

V. THE DIFFICULT NECK

Some patients with rheumatoid arthritis, generally those with advanced and aggressive disease, may manifest significant cervical spine involvement with instability arising from atlantoaxial or subaxial subluxation. This complication presents both important risks to the patient undergoing surgery and significant challenges for the anesthesiologist, particularly if endotracheal intubation is required. These patients have an increased risk for cord compression during intubation or from uncontrolled neck movement during positioning for surgery.

Cervical spine instability should be ruled out prior to surgery with flexion/extension radiographs in those patients with neck pain or crepitus on range-of-motion testing, radicular symptoms, or arm and/or leg weakness. Affected patients should wear a soft cervical collar to the operating room, both for neck immobilization and as a warning to all involved not to overmanipulate the neck. When possible, epidural or spinal anesthesia should be employed.

Additional problems arising from the rheumatoid disease process include involvement of the temporomandibular joint, which may limit jaw opening, and arthritis of the cricoarytenoid joints. Because these problems also may influence the choice of airway management, the anesthesiologist as well should be informed preoperatively about these manifestations of the disease process.

The converse situation arises in the patients with ankylosing spondylitis, where the patient's rigid cervical spine may also present technical challenges for the anesthesiologist during intubation. In such a setting, a fiberoptic method is often employed in this clinical context.

VI. IMMUNOSUPPRESSIVE/ANTI-INFLAMMATORY THERAPY

In patients with rheumatic disease, the question often arises as to what, if anything, should be done about their regimens of methotrexate, tumor necrosis factor inhibitors, and other immunosuppressive agents. Few data exist to guide recommendations for immunosuppressive therapy in the perioperative setting. Whether or not such agents increase the potential for infection or delay wound healing is uncertain, but it has become common practice and seems prudent to discontinue such therapy 1 to 2 weeks prior to surgery and restart them approximately 1 to 2 weeks postoperatively, or when the surgeon feels the wound is clean and healing optimally. Acute disease flares resulting from the abrupt discontinuation of immunosuppressive therapy for such brief periods are unusual and can usually be managed with corticosteroids.

Anti-inflammatory therapy, particularly aspirin, should be discontinued at least 5 days before the surgical procedure because their antiplatelet effects may increase the risk of bleeding. This does not appear to be necessary with the cyclooxygenase-2 inhibitors. The latter agents, in high doses, may be associated with an increased risk of myocardial infarction and stroke and this needs to be taken into consideration in patients who are already at high risk for coronary artery disease.

VII. THE INTEGUMENT

As a result of chronic therapy (i.e., corticosteroids and immunosuppressive agents) or as a manifestation of the debilitating consequences of underlying rheumatic disease (i.e., decubitus ulceration) or orthopedic condition, skin integrity may be compromised before and after the surgical procedures in patients undergoing orthopedic surgery. In addition, delayed wound healing and a propensity to infection may result from these influences. The early institution of preventive measures to combat the development of decubitus ulcers (particularly of the heels and buttock region) is vital to an uncomplicated postoperative course.

VIII. THE EYE

Patients taking long-term optic medication should have their eye drops instilled prior to surgery, especially if a prolonged procedure is anticipated. The one exception to this recommendation involves the use of phosphodiesterase inhibitors in the treatment of glaucoma. These agents may prolong the action of the neuromuscular blocker, succinylcholine. This is particularly pertinent in patients with Sjögren's syndrome who require artificial tears to prevent perioperative conjunctival injury.

Patients in the prone position are at risk for ocular injury secondary to external pressure. Patients with underlying vasculitis of the optic vessels are at particular risk of ischemic injury to the eye. Therefore, the anesthesiologist must take particular care to position the patient carefully, avoiding excessive pressure on the eye, and keep appropriate eye protection.

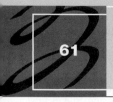

61 PHYSICAL THERAPY
Sandy B. Ganz and Louis L. Harris

 INTRODUCTION

Management of the physical therapy for patients with musculoskeletal and rheumatic diseases is a challenging task, even for the most astute clinician.

I. **The goals of physical therapy** in the treatment of patients with rheumatic diseases are fourfold:
    A. Preventing disability.
    B. Restoring function.
    C. Relieving pain.
    D. Educating the patient.

II. **EVALUATION.** Before these goals can be achieved, a thorough evaluation of the patient for physical therapy is performed, which includes the following:
    A. **Functional assessment**
        1. **Bed mobility.** Observe the patient performing functional movements.
            a. Turning over from a supine position to the side and then to a prone position.
            b. Moving up and down in bed.
            c. Moving from a supine to a sitting position.
        2. **Transfer status.** Observe the patient transfer to and from various surfaces (i.e., bed, chair, and toilet).
        3. **Gait analysis**
            a. **Observational.** Watch the patient ambulate with or without assistive devices on level surfaces and stairs.
            b. **Instrumented** gait analysis with a foot switch stride analyzer or computerized video analysis.
    B. **Range of motion (ROM) assessment of all joints**
    C. **Strength assessment**
        1. Manual muscle test of trunk, neck, and proximal and distal muscles to determine weak musculature.
        2. Instrumental biomechanical muscle test.
        3. Isometric/isokinetic objective strength measurement, recorded of select muscle groups, performed with an isokinetic dynamometer (i.e., Cybex[1], Lido[2]).
    D. **Posture assessment.** Observe the patient in both standing and ambulating postures during functional activities.
    E. **Respiratory status.** Chest evaluation consists of the following:
        1. Auscultation.
        2. Chest expansion.
        3. Description of cough.
        4. Inspirometry.

III. **COMPONENTS OF TREATMENT.** After the physical therapy evaluation has been performed, the clinician has baseline data for future comparison and a basis for determining treatment goals. These specific goals are achieved through therapeutic exercise, other modalities, functional activities, and perhaps the most important aspect of treatment, patient education (Table 61-1).

---

[1]Cybex, Ronkonkoma, NY
[2]Loredon, Davis, CA

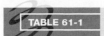 TABLE 61-1	Components of Treatment in Musculoskeletal and Rheumatic Disorders

Therapeutic exercise	Modalities
Range of motion	Heat
Strengthening	Cold
Endurance	Relaxation
Breathing	Electrotherapy
Massage and mobilization	Hydrotherapy, traction
Functional activities	Patient education
Gait training	Joint protection
Transfer and bed mobility	Home program
Activities of daily living	Body mechanics

IV. THERAPEUTIC EXERCISE

A. Goals of exercise
1. Maintain or improve ROM.
2. Strengthen weak muscles.
3. Increase endurance.
4. Enhance respiratory efficiency through breathing exercises.
5. Improve balance and coordination.
6. Enable joints to function better biomechanically (Table 61-2).

B. Therapeutic exercises used in the treatment of musculoskeletal and arthritic conditions are as follows:
1. **ROM.** Excursion of a joint through its available range.
2. **Passive range of motion (PROM).** Without active muscle contraction around the joint, the joint is moved through available ROM by another individual, object, or by the use of the other extremity.
3. **Active assisted range of motion (AAROM).** The patient performs ROM exercises with the assistance of another individual, object, or the use of another extremity.
4. **Active range of motion (AROM).** The patient performs ROM exercises without assistance.
5. **Active resisted range of motion (ARROM).** The patient performs ROM exercises with some form of resistance (manual or mechanical resistance, elastic bands, or weights).

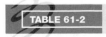 TABLE 61-2	Treatment Goals

Stages of disease	Treatment goals	Exercise
Acute	Control inflammation	Passive range of motion
	Maintain ROM	AAROM
	Minimize loss of function	
Subacute	Increase ROM	AROM
	Maintain strength	Isometric
Chronic	Increase ROM	AROM
	Increase strength	AAROM
	Increase endurance	Isokinetic
		Aerobic

AAROM, active assisted range of motion; AROM, active range of motion; ROM, range of motion

6. Strengthening exercises
  a. Static. Isometric exercises in which the patient contracts or tightens the muscle around the joint without producing any joint motion.
  b. Dynamic. Some form of resistance is used for the patient to work against, either manually or with an externally applied load (i.e., weight).
      i. Isotonic. Concentric or eccentric contractions of variable speed with use of a set weight or resistance throughout the full ROM.
      ii. Isokinetic. A concentric or eccentric contraction at a set speed with use of a set weight or resistance throughout the full ROM.
C. General instructions to patients
  1. Use pain as your guide. Pain or discomfort should not last longer than one hour after exercise.
  2. Make the exercise a part of your daily routine.
  3. Try to do a complete set of exercises at least twice a day at a time convenient to you.
  4. Prescribed medication and heat or cold applications may precede exercise to enhance relaxation and decrease pain.
  5. Perform only those exercises prescribed for you by your physician or therapist.
  6. Perform exercises on a firm surface.
  7. Exercise slowly with a smooth motion. Do not rush.
  8. Avoid holding your breath while exercising.
  9. Modify the exercise regimen during an acute attack of the disease, and contact your physician or physical therapist if you have any complaints or problems with the exercises.

V. PHYSICAL AGENTS (MODALITIES). Various modalities/treatments are employed by the physical therapist, including the application of heat, cold, electrical stimulation, mechanical traction, and mobilization/massage. These are generally provided as an adjunct to a total rehabilitative program.
A. Superficial heating
  1. Hot packs contain a silica gel that absorbs water. These packs are kept in thermostatically controlled water at 175°F (79.4°C). The literature demonstrates that hot-pack effectiveness reached at a depth of 1 cm increases skin temperature by 10°C.
    a. Indications. Relief of pain, muscle spasm, and decreased ROM.
    b. Contraindications. Sensory involvement, open lesions, and malignancy.
  2. Paraffin bath. Paraffin wax is mixed with mineral oil and maintained at 118°F (48°C) to 126°F (52°C). It is most useful in the treatment of hands. The wax mold conforms to the hand and provides heat to all joint surfaces. The heating benefits are similar to those obtained with hot packs.
    a. Indications. Relief of pain, muscle spasm, and decreased ROM.
    b. Contraindications. Sensory involvement and open lesions.
  3. Hydrotherapy (whirlpool, therapeutic pool). Water is maintained at 94°F (34°C) to 96°F (36°C). Coupled with its ability to partially eliminate the effect of gravity (buoyancy), heated water can provide excellent moist heat and exercise, simultaneously. Whirlpools are also beneficial to promote wound cleaning and healing. Hydrotherapy is a related form of heat treatment.
    a. Indications
      i. Muscle spasms, relief of pain, and decreased ROM.
      ii. Whirlpool. Open lesions.
    b. Contraindications
      i. Patients with decreased heat tolerance.
      ii. Therapeutic pool. Open lesions, urinary tract infection, diarrhea; extreme care should be taken in patients with cardiopulmonary involvement.
  4. Fluidotherapy is a dry application of heat. A bed of finely ground solids (e.g., glass beads with an average diameter of 0.0165 in.) are blown with thermostatically controlled warm air. This creates a warm, semifluid mixture

for treatment of the hand or foot. The temperatures are within the same ranges as the paraffin wax.

   a. Indications. Relief of pain, muscle spasm, and decreased ROM.

   b. Contraindications. Sensory involvement and open lesions.

B. Deep-heating ultrasound. The application of high-frequency sound waves to the musculoskeletal system causes a deep-heating response. This response is deeper than that induced by other physical agents, and it has been demonstrated that the intra-articular temperature of the hip joint rises by 1.43°C after a properly applied therapeutic dose. Typical patient exposure is 1 to 2 W/cm² for 5 to 10 minutes. Ultrasound can also be combined with electrical stimulation.

   1. Indications. Pain relief, muscle spasm, and decreased ROM.

   2. Contraindications. Local malignancy, unstable vertebrae (after laminectomy), pregnancy, and spinal cord disease; ultrasound should not be applied directly over the eyes, brain, or spinal cord.

C. Cold. Cryotherapy is very effective in promoting vasoconstriction, thereby decreasing restricted joint ROM resulting from an inflammatory process and aiding pain relief. Cold modalities include ice packs, frozen gel packs (cold packs), and ice massage.

   1. Indications. Swelling and inflammatory reactions, spasms, contusions, and traumatic arthritis.

   2. Contraindications. Decreased sensation, sensitivity to cold, and Raynaud's phenomenon.

D. Mobilization generally means moving the joints, including spinal joints, through an ROM designed to stretch the joint capsule and, in some instances, to move the joint beyond the norm of its associated muscles. The technique is primarily used in patients with musculoskeletal pain.

   1. Indications. Joint hypomobility, decreased proprioception, restriction of accessory joint motion, ligamentous tightness, adhesions, and joint dysfunction.

   2. Contraindications. Ligamentous laxity and unstable joints.

E. Massage is a widely practiced modality. It is intended to relieve pain, soft-tissue tightness, and muscle spasm. It is often used in conjunction with heat or cold applications. Other forms of massage include acupressure, connective tissue massage, postural integration (rolling), and deep friction massage.

   1. Indications. Muscle spasm and decreased extensibility of soft tissues.

   2. Contraindications. Cellulitis, malignancy, and phlebitis.

F. Electrical stimulation is one of the oldest and most effective physical agents. Its purpose is to contract or re-educate muscle, relax muscle spasms, stimulate nerves to promote motion and pain relief, and generally improve circulation. A wide range of gadgets using different current types (AC and DC) and a wide variety of electrical generators [low-volt, high-volt, biofeedback, transcutaneous electrical nerve stimulation (TENS)] are available. No individual system or model is ideal for all clinical situations, and the therapist's choice depends on the desired therapeutic response.

   1. Indications. Muscle re-education, denervated muscles, pain relief, decreased general circulation, decreased muscle strength during immobilization, and decreased ROM.

   2. Contraindications. Phlebitis, demand pacemakers, hemorrhage, and recent fractures.

G. Mechanical traction. Intermittent traction is utilized for spinal disorders, generally in conjunction with other modalities. The amount of traction prescribed depends on the area being treated and on the patient's tolerance. Its effectiveness in promoting relaxation through muscle stretching, relieving nerve compression, and relieving pain has been demonstrated. Patients receive intermittent traction two to three times/week on average for 20 minutes.

   1. Indications. Muscle spasm, mild nerve compression, and vertebral osteoarthritis.

   2. Contraindications. Unstable vertebrae, local malignancy, spinal cord disease, osteoporosis, osteomyelitis, and pregnancy.

GENERAL GUIDELINES FOR REHABILITATION OF SPECIFIC RHEUMATOLOGIC DISORDERS AND AREAS OF THE BODY

I. **Systemic rheumatic diseases** including rheumatoid arthritis, juvenile idiopathic arthritis, progressive systemic sclerosis, and systemic lupus erythematosus are characterized by multisystem involvement. All are chronic, remitting, and relapsing with variable clinical courses that result in myriad clinical manifestations. Comprehensive rehabilitative management is necessary in the treatment of such systemic inflammatory diseases. Rest is essential in the management of active inflammatory joint or soft-tissue disease, and the amount of rest versus activity is the subject of extensive debate. Peripheral joint involvement in psoriatic arthritis, reactive arthritis, and colitic arthropathies should be treated in a similar manner to that in rheumatoid arthritis and juvenile idiopathic arthritis, as noted in the subsequent text. The proper balance between rest and exercise is the key to successful treatment.

   A. **Aims of treatment**
      1. Preserve or increase functional level.
      2. Decrease pain.
      3. Improve joint mechanics.
      4. Decrease joint inflammation.
      5. Improve ROM, strength, and endurance.

   B. **Therapy**
      1. **Active inflammatory disease**
         a. Rest
            i. Systemic (body) rest.
            ii. Articular (joint) rest.
            iii. Emotional rest.
         b. Joint protection
            i. Splinting.
            ii. Assistive devices.
            iii. Ambulatory aids.
         c. Techniques for relaxation and stress reduction.
         d. Education of the patient.
      2. **Pain**
         a. Superficial heat.
         b. Cryotherapy.
         c. TENS.
      3. **Decreased ROM**
         a. PROM.
         b. AAROM.
         c. Stretching.
      4. **Weakness.** Muscle strengthening with the following:
         a. Isometric.
         b. Isotonic.
         c. Isokinetic.
      5. **Ambulation**
         a. Ambulatory aid.
         b. Orthotic.
      6. **Decreased endurance techniques**
         a. Energy conservation.
         b. Aerobic exercise program.
      7. **Difficulty with activities of daily living (ADL)**
         a. Adaptive equipment.
         b. Assistive devices.

II. **SPONDYLOARTHROPATHIES (SPINAL AND SACROILIAC DISEASE)**
   A. Maintenance of an erect posture is critical for all ADL, including sitting, standing, walking, and sleeping. Patients should sleep in a prone or supine position on a firm

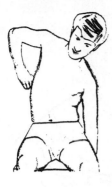

Figure 61-1. Chest mobilization (inspiration). Bend away from right side during inspiration.

mattress with one small pillow or no pillow. (Pillows under the knees should be avoided at all times to prevent flexion deformities.) Breathing and chest expansion exercises are extremely important. In addition, stretching exercises that facilitate extension of the neck, spine, and peripheral joints should be taught and diligently followed.

B. Aims of treatment
   1. Facilitate skeletal mobility.
   2. Prevent contractures.
C. Exercises. Figures 61-1–61-7 are examples of appropriate exercises used in the treatment of patients with back involvement in ankylosing spondylitis and other spondyloarthropathies.

III. OSTEOPOROSIS
   A. Weight-bearing activities such as brisk walking, biking, jogging, and working with a select group of exercise machines can be an effective way to maintain and strengthen muscles while stimulating bone formation. These types of exercises and activities are referred to as impact-loading or weight-bearing exercises. An exercise program should consist of postural retraining, education in proper body mechanics, deep breathing, stretching, strengthening, and impact-loading activities. Extreme caution should be taken during forward flexion exercises of the spine because of the longer lever arm produced with increased flexion. An osteoporotic vertebral body may not be able to tolerate this load, and compression fracture with wedging may occur.

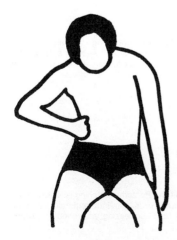

Figure 61-2. Chest mobilization (expiration). Bend toward right side during expiration. Push fisted hand into the lateral aspect of chest as you bend toward the right side.

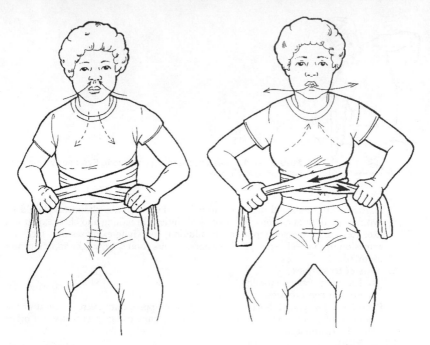

Figure 61-3. Belt exercises for lateral costal expansion. Reinforce lateral costal expansion during inspiration. Assist with pressure along the rib cage during expiration. (Reprinted from the Saunders Group, Inc. © 1996.)

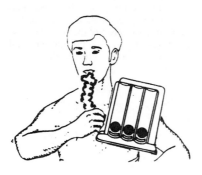

Figure 61-4. Deep breathing with an incentive inspirometer. For inspiration, use right side up and breathe in. For expiration, use upside down and breathe out.

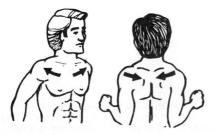

Figure 61-5. Pectoral stretching (shoulder blade pinch). Stand or sit straight and tall. Pull your shoulders back, squeezing your shoulder blades together.

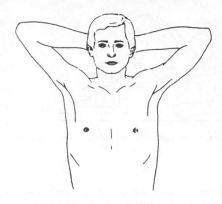

Figure 61-6. Pectoral stretching (hands behind head). Stand or sit. Place your hands behind your head with elbows in front. Move your elbows back as far as possible.

B. Aims of treatment
   1. Strengthen abdominal muscles and extensor musculature of the spine.
   2. Pectoral stretching.
   3. Increase weight-bearing activities of lower extremities.
C. Exercises. See Figures 61-8–61-10 for appropriate exercises used in the treatment of patients with osteoporosis.
IV. **POLYMYOSITIS AND DERMATOMYOSITIS**
   A. The degree of muscle weakness can be quite variable because muscle destruction during the acute inflammatory phase is variable, as is muscle regeneration during

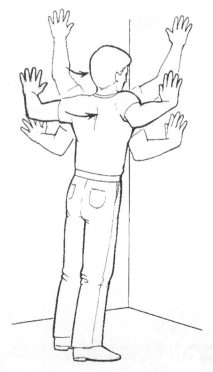

Figure 61-7. Pectoral stretching (standing). Stand facing a corner. Put the palms of your hands on the wall. Slowly lean your chest into the corner. (Reprinted from the Saunders Group, Inc. © 1996.)

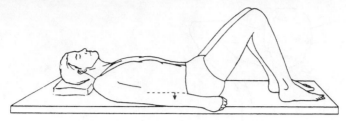

Figure 61-8. Lying on your back with knees bent, press the small of your back into the bed. Tighten your abdominal and buttock muscles.

the recovery phase. Patients exhibit difficulty climbing stairs, rising from low surfaces, and performing various aspects of ADL. The emphasis of rehabilitation is on progressive proximal muscle-strengthening exercises. Vigorous exercise of any type that is injudicious may be associated with a rise in serum enzyme levels, increased fatigue, and a decrease in function and strength. Therefore, a balance between rest and exercise must be achieved. Overall, disease assessment involves a myositis functional assessment (Appendix D), a biomechanical muscle test with isokinetics (Cybex or Lido), and monitoring of creatinine kinase. Physical therapy management and type of exercise are determined from the results of the above tests. It remains controversial whether exercise should be avoided during an increase in creatine kinase levels or an increase in overall disease activity.

B. Aims of treatment
    1. Increase proximal muscle strength.
    2. Improve function.
    3. Decrease pain.
C. Exercises. See Figures 61-11–61-28 for appropriate exercises used in the treatment of patients with polymyositis and dermatomyositis.

V. SCLERODERMA (SYSTEMIC SCLEROSIS)
    A. Prevention of joint contractures is the primary goal in the physical therapy management of patients with progressive systemic sclerosis. A ROM program designed to stretch soft-tissue contractures should be instituted immediately. Passive stretching of all joints, soft-tissue mobilization, and massage are highly recommended. In addition, paraffin is used on the hands in an effort to decrease pain and increase finger ROM. Skin tightness around the jaw is extremely common. A series of temporomandibular joint exercises are routinely performed to increase jaw excursion. Deep breathing, use of incentive inspirometer, and mobilization of the chest wall to increase chest expansion should be incorporated into the physical therapy program. To assist with feeding and chewing activities, speech therapy is often instituted.
    B. Aims of treatment
        1. Increase ROM.
        2. Prevent contractures.
        3. Improve chest expansion.

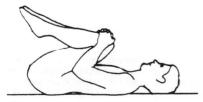

Figure 61-9. Knees to chest. Lying on your back, slowly bring both knees up to your chest.

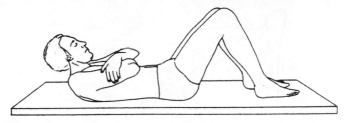

Figure 61-10. Partial sit-ups. Lie on your back with knees bent and arms crossed. With chin tucked, slowly lift your head and shoulders toward your knees.

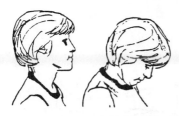

Figure 61-11. Neck flexion. Sitting or standing with your back straight, bend your head forward and tuck your chin in toward your chest.

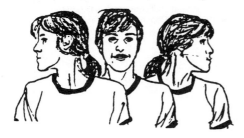

Figure 61-12. Neck rotation. Sitting or standing with your back straight, tuck your chin in toward your chest. Look over your right shoulder, then over your left shoulder.

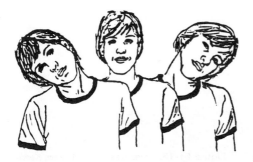

Figure 61-13. Neck lateral flexion. Sitting or standing with your back straight, tuck your chin in. Bend your head toward your shoulder.

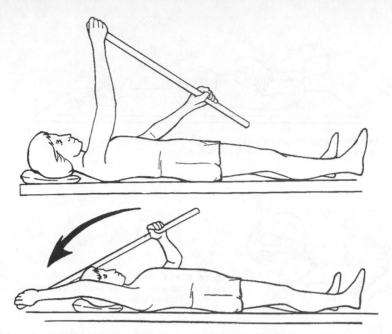

Figure 61-14. Shoulder flexion. Lie on your back while holding a rod, with one hand at the top and the other near the bottom. Pull the rod back toward your head until your arm holding onto the top is straight. Return to starting position. Switch hands and repeat. (Reprinted from the Saunders Group, Inc. © 1996.)

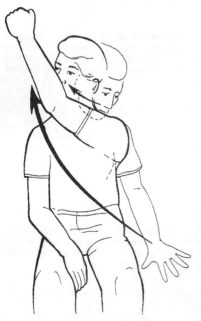

Figure 61-15. Diagonal shoulder flexion. Keeping your elbow straight, bring your left arm down across your body with your thumb pointing toward your right hip. (Reprinted from the Saunders Group, Inc. © 1996.)

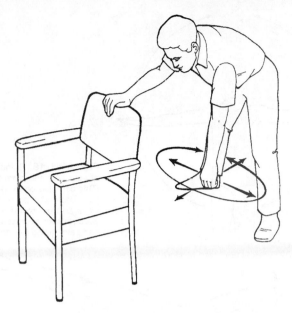

Figure 61-16. Pendulum exercises. Stand holding on to a sturdy chair with your uninvolved arm. Bend forward at the waist and bend your knees to help protect your back. Let your involved arm hang limp. Keep your shoulder relaxed, and use your body motion to swing your arm in a circle. (Reprinted from the Saunders Group, Inc. © 1996.)

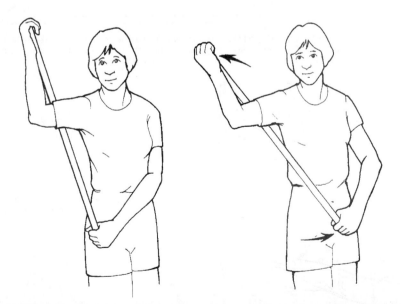

Figure 61-17. Shoulder rotation exercise. While standing, hold a stick or towel as illustrated, with the uninvolved arm over your shoulder and holding the top and the involved arm holding the bottom. Slowly pull the top of the stick or towel with your uninvolved arm as shown. (Reprinted from the Saunders Group, Inc. © 1996.)

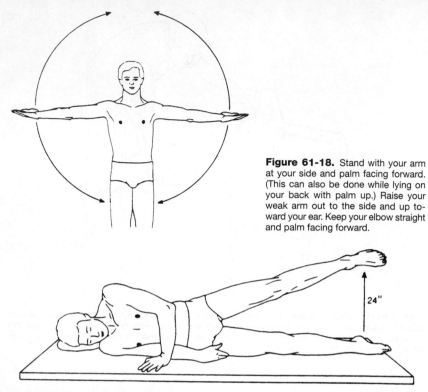

Figure 61-18. Stand with your arm at your side and palm facing forward. (This can also be done while lying on your back with palm up.) Raise your weak arm out to the side and up toward your ear. Keep your elbow straight and palm facing forward.

24"

Figure 61-19. Leg lifts while lying on side. Lie on your side, weak leg on top. The lower leg should be bent to help balance. Keep the top leg straight and in line with your body. Stay on your side and lift your leg up toward the ceiling. Do not bring your leg forward. Slowly lower it.

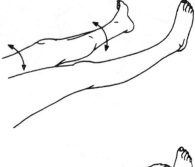

Figure 61-20. Hip external rotation. Lying on your back with your leg straight, roll entire leg outward.

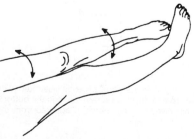

Figure 61-21. Hip internal rotation. Lying on your back with your leg straight, roll entire leg inward.

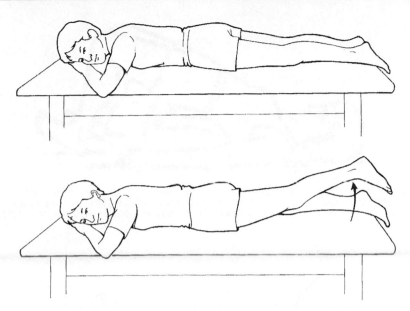

Figure 61-22. Prone hip extension. Lie on your stomach with both legs straight. Lift one leg up toward the ceiling, keeping your knee straight. Slowly lower it. (Reprinted from the Saunders Group, Inc. © 1996.)

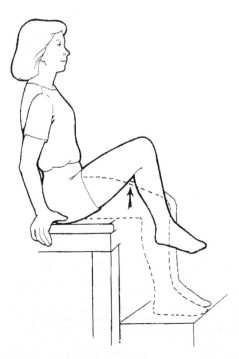

Figure 61-23. Hip flexion. Sitting on stairs or a chair with both feet flat on the floor, raise one knee up toward your chest as high as possible. Slowly lower it. (Reprinted from the Saunders Group, Inc. © 1996.)

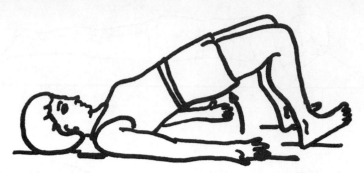

Figure 61-24. Bridging exercise. Lie on your back with knees bent and arms straight. Pull toes up toward the ceiling and push heels into the floor. Tighten buttocks and slowly lift up until hips are fully extended. Return to the starting position and repeat. (Reprinted from the Saunders Group, Inc. © 1996.)

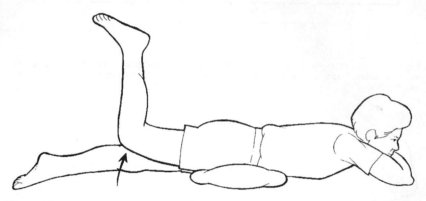

Figure 61-25. Gluteal contraction. Lying prone, with pillow under abdomen, bend one knee and lift toward ceiling. Slowly lower to starting position and repeat. (Reprinted from the Saunders Group, Inc. © 1996.)

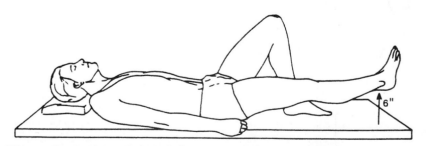

Figure 61-26. Lie on your back with your weak leg as straight as possible. Bend the other leg as illustrated to protect your back. Tighten your thigh muscle. Raise your leg while keeping it straight. Keep your thigh muscles tight and leg straight as you slowly lower it.

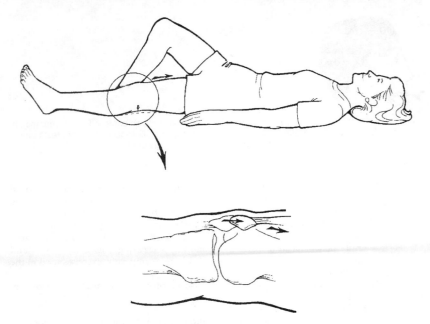

Figure 61-27. Quad set. Half sitting with your involved leg straight, bend your other leg as illustrated. Tighten the muscles on the top of your thigh. This will make your kneecap move toward your hip. (Reprinted from the Saunders Group, Inc. © 1996.)

   C. Exercises. Figures 61-1–61-4, 61-29, and 61-30 are appropriate exercises used in the treatment of systemic sclerosis, in addition to PROM for all joints.
VI. NECK PAIN
   A. Aims of treatment
      1. Decrease pain.
      2. Increase muscle relaxation.
      3. Improve head and neck posture.
   B. Therapy
      1. The **modalities** available to the physical therapist include heat and electrical stimulation.

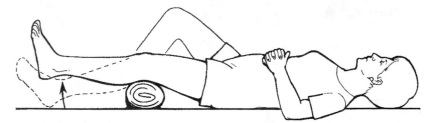

Figure 61-28. Terminal knee extension. Lying on your back with a firm pillow under your involved knee, slowly lift your foot up. Your knee should remain on the pillow. Try to keep your leg as straight as possible. (Reprinted from the Saunders Group, Inc. © 1996.)

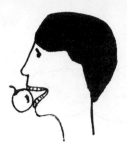

Figure 61-29. Jaw excursion. Hold an apple in front of your mouth. Gradually open your mouth, sliding your top and bottom teeth on the apple and increasing the jaw's range of motion.

2. **Specific manual mobilization techniques** include manual and motorized intermittent cervical traction, which provide muscle and soft-tissue stretching to promote relaxation of the neck and upper back, and pain relief.
3. An **exercise program** consisting of gentle active exercises progressing to isometric exercises in the supine position, or with the head supported, are generally beneficial in increasing circulation, decreasing muscular tension, and improving posture. Figures 61-11–61-13 are examples of exercises used in the treatment of neck pain.
4. An educational component should also be provided to ensure the following:
   a. Proper postural awareness.
   b. Body mechanics.
   c. Preventive measures, which include an explanation of home or work activities to be avoided because they may contribute to the patient's complaints (e.g., driving, computer terminal/typewriter operation, sleeping postures).

VII. SHOULDER
   A. Aims of treatment
      1. Improve joint ROM.
      2. Increase muscle strength.
      3. Decrease pain.
   B. Therapy
      1. **Exercise program.** An ROM program initially consisting of manual joint mobilization and passive ROM should be instituted. As ROM increases, the patient is instructed in active exercise, progressing to a strengthening program as tolerated. As the patient progresses, an individualized program can be planned, guided by the needs of the patient. Figures 61-14–61-18 are examples of exercises used in the treatment of shoulder pain.

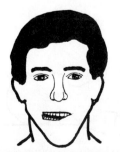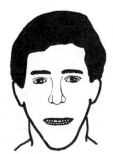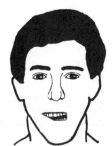

Figure 61-30. Lateral jaw excursion. Smile so that your top and bottom teeth are touching. Move your mouth from right to left.

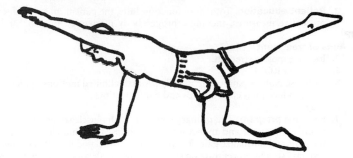

Figure 61-31. Bobath exercise. Assume position as illustrated. While keeping your back level, raise one arm and opposite leg as shown. Repeat with opposite arm and leg. (Reprinted from the Saunders Group, Inc. © 1996.)

2. **Physical agents** that can be an adjunct to the exercise program are various heat modalities and electrical stimulation to decrease pain. Cryotherapy may also be utilized following an exercise session to decrease any physiologic response to treatment.

3. **Patient education.** It is essential that the patient be educated regarding the goals of physical therapy and be given a daily home exercise program. A pulley system is an excellent device to include in this exercise program.

VIII. **LOW-BACK PAIN**

   A. **Aims of treatment**

   1. Decrease pain.
   2. Increase muscle relaxation.
   3. Strengthen abdominal muscles.
   4. Normalize low-back joint motion and posture.

   B. **Therapy**

   1. **Physical agents** (modalities) are available that can be incorporated to decrease pain. These include hot packs, ultrasound, and electrical stimulation. When indicated, passive joint and soft-tissue mobilization are also effective manual techniques to further decrease pain, increase circulation, and aid in restoring normal joint motion.

   2. An **exercise program** consists of exercises designed to stretch the pelvis, low back, and hamstrings and to strengthen the abdominal muscles. As the patient progresses, an individualized program can be guided by the patient's tolerance and need. Figures 61-8–61-10, 61-19–61-24, 61-31, and 61-32 are examples of exercises used in the treatment of low-back pain.

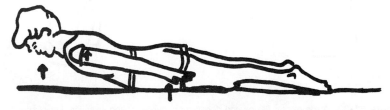

Figure 61-32. Lower back strengthening. Lie on belly with forehead resting on floor or small towel roll. Raise head, shoulders, chest, belly, and hands off floor as shown. Return to starting position and repeat. (Reprinted from the Saunders Group, Inc. © 1996.)

        3. Patient education. To restore function fully, the patient must be educated in preventive measures, including proper body mechanics, posture, and ADL.

IX. HIP

A. Aims of treatment
1. Increase muscle strength.
2. Maintain ROM.
3. Decrease pain. A painful hip usually results in limited motions, which can further produce joint contractures and gait deviations.

B. Therapy
1. **Exercise program.** The primary emphasis with muscle strengthening is to optimize the extensor and abductor muscle groups. These muscles help to stabilize the joint and normalize gait. ROM activities associated with this strengthening program should concentrate on stretching the hip flexors and adductors and ensuring functional rotational ROM. See Figures 61-19–61-24 for examples of exercises used in the treatment of hip pain.
2. **Heat modalities** such as hot packs and ultrasound can be employed to complement the exercise program and promote pain relief.

X. KNEE

A. Aims of treatment
1. Increase ROM.
2. Improve muscle strength of the quadriceps and hamstrings.
3. Normalize ambulation and function.
4. Decrease pain.

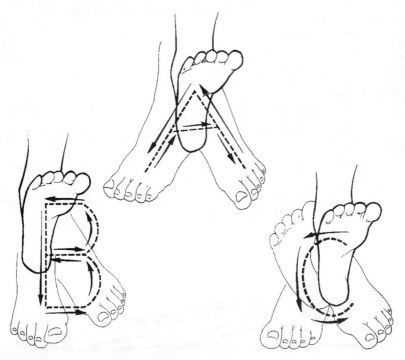

Figure 61-33. Ankle plantar flexion and dorsiflexion, eversion, and inversion. For plantar flexion and dorsiflexion, bring your toes down and then up toward your head. Also, try drawing an imaginary A. For eversion and inversion, push sole inward and then outward. Now, try drawing an imaginary B and C. (Reprinted from the Saunders Group, Inc. © 1996.)

B. Therapy

1. A **therapeutic exercise program** should be established that concentrates on AROM and AAROM and progresses to muscle strengthening as tolerated. Many resistive exercise programs are available that utilize free weights and various types of exercise equipment. Isometric quadriceps sets and straight leg raising are excellent exercises to initiate quadriceps control, followed by an individualized program to meet the patient's specific needs. Figures 61-25–61-28 are examples of exercises used in the treatment of knee pain.

2. **Physical agents.** Various heat modalities and forms of electrical stimulation can be employed to complement the exercise program by decreasing pain before an exercise session. Cryotherapy can also be an essential part of the total program, depending on the patient's needs and response to treatment.

XI. ANKLE. Treatment of the ankle during the acute stage focuses on the initial control of swelling. This is accomplished with rest, ice, compression, and elevation (RICE). If no severe instability is present, the patient may be referred for physical therapy.

A. Aims of treatment

1. Increase muscle strength and function.
2. Increase and maintain ROM.
3. Decrease pain.
4. Normalize gait.

B. Therapy. An isometric program that progresses to active resistive exercises, encompassing functional and weight-bearing activities, is important. These help to improve balance and coordination, and aid in preparing the patient for gait training and normalizing the ankle motion during ambulation. Figures 61-33–61-35 are examples of exercises used in the treatment of ankle pain.

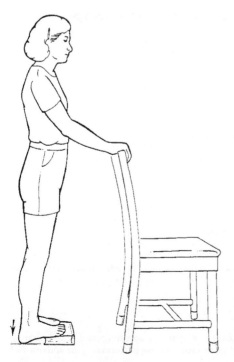

Figure 61-34. Heel cord stretching. Stand with the ball of your foot on a book. Hold on to a firm chair or surface. Try to place your heel on the floor. Gently lean forward, keeping your knee straight. Hold, then stand on your toes, and return to starting position. (Reprinted from the Saunders Group, Inc. © 1996.)

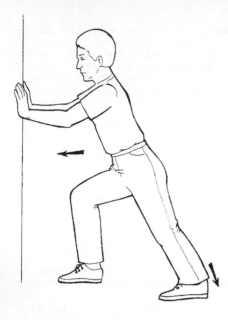

Figure 61-35. Gastrocnemius (calf) stretch. Stand in front of a wall and bend one leg while keeping the other leg back. Lean forward and push against the wall and you will feel the stretch in your calf muscle, or gastrocnemius. (Reprinted from the Saunders Group, Inc. © 1996.)

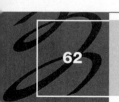

62 OCCUPATIONAL THERAPY: THERAPIST'S MANAGEMENT OF RHEUMATOLOGIC DISORDERS OF THE HAND
Aviva Wolff

$\mathcal{R}$heumatic diseases such as rheumatoid arthritis, osteoarthritis, and post-traumatic arthritis commonly affect the small joints of the hand, wrist, elbow, and shoulder. With these pathologies, the intricate biomechanics of the hand is altered, and hand function is affected. Therefore, the prevention of hand deformities, and the preservation or restoration of hand function are fundamental components of the treatment process. The form of therapeutic intervention that is crafted depends on the specific pathology, the deformity with which each patient presents, and one's goals and functional needs. Hand therapy intervention in rheumatic disease falls into one of two categories, conservative treatment and postoperative management. Surgical intervention to correct hand deformities is performed to relieve pain, correct deformity, and improve function. Postoperative management of common hand surgeries is specific to the operative procedure performed and is beyond the scope of this manual. Common upper extremity surgeries performed for rheumatic disease include arthroplasties, fusions, synovectomies, and correction of deformities. This chapter will focus on the conservative management of rheumatic conditions of the hand.

 GOALS

Hand therapy intervention has evolved over the years to accommodate new research, ideas, and information. The primary goal is to facilitate the performance of activities of daily living (ADL) by overcoming barriers. This is accomplished by maintaining or improving abilities and compensating for decreased ability. Therefore, the goals of conservative management are as follows:

- Increase functional abilities.
- Correct and maintain joint alignment to reduce progression of deformity.
- Reduce joint stress.
- Reduce stiffness, pain, and inflammation.
- Increase joint range of motion.

 ## ASSESSMENT

Hand assessment includes physical examination, evaluation of symptoms, and the assessment of function. The International Classification of Functioning, Disability and Health (ICF) defines function as the ability to perform tasks by participating in activities within the environment. In recent years, health care providers have placed a strong emphasis on a person's ability to function within his or her environment. Hand therapists have always focused on ability to function within the environment, and the hand assessment reflects this emphasis.

I. **Physical examination** involves a detailed assessment of the nature of the anatomical abnormality, such as swan neck deformity or ulnar drift. Photographs and video imaging provide visual representation of the structural changes in the hand. Although the assessment of the anatomical position is important, the evaluation of function is critical. Often, what appears as severe deformity is not accompanied by great loss of function.

II. **EVALUATION OF SYMPTOMS.** Physical impairment measures of grip and pinch strength, range of motion (goniometric measurements), edema (circumferential and volumetric), and pain (visual analog scale) are used to quantify symptoms of weakness, stiffness, swelling, and pain. Administration of measures follows the guidelines described in the American Society for Hand Therapist's (ASHT's) Clinical Assessment Recommendations manual. Specific attention is given to the following aspects when measuring range of motion in the joints of the hand: degree of hyperextension; degree of ulnar drift; composite joint motion; whether the neutral or anatomic position of the joint can be obtained; and, if it cannot be obtained, the number of degrees by which it cannot. Although these measurements provide some useful information in assessing physical changes in the hand, they do not accurately assess functional ability or quality of life. Clinical studies have proven that decreased function is associated more with pain and discomfort than with stiffness and decreased motion.

III. **FUNCTIONAL ASSESSMENT.** Standardized outcome measures have been developed for arthritic conditions to assess the combined measurements of range of motion, strength, and functional tasks. These are useful tools of assessment for hand-related function in ADL in patients with rheumatic disease. In recent years, several additional tests have been developed, which are self-administered and allow the patients to report on their level of function. These instruments are standardized, well validated, and provide quantitative information. Following is a brief description of performance-based measures that are available for the assessment of hand impairment in rheumatic conditions. These instruments are particularly valuable in establishing a baseline and documenting change. Selection of the appropriate instrument is based on the relevant clinical characteristics of the patient.

   A. **Selected objective tests for the assessment of hand function**
      1. **Hand functional index (HFI).** The HFI assesses the movement and malpositioning of the thumb, fingers, and wrist by movement tasks. Each hand is assessed separately. Nine different movement tasks are included. This test can be administered in less than 1 minute.
      2. **Arthritis hand function test (AHFT).** The AHFT assesses hand strength and dexterity by measurements of strength and functional tasks. Both hands are assessed together. Components of the test include five bilateral dexterity tasks, two bilateral strength tasks, three measurements of strength (grip,

two point pinch, and three point pinch), and one measurement of dexterity (nine hole peg test).

3. **Sequential occupational dexterity assessment (SODA).** The SODA is a dexterity test that was designed specifically for patients with rheumatoid arthritis to measure bimanual hand dexterity. The SODA combines objective assessment with a self-report component. Four unilateral and eight bilateral ADL tasks assess dexterity. Patients rate their perception of difficulty and pain with each task. Estimated time of completion is 20 minutes. A short version of six items is also available.

B. **Self-reported performance-based measures**

1. **Australian/Canadian (AUSCAN) Osteoarthritis Hand Index.** The AUS-CAN Osteoarthritis Hand Index is a three-dimensional self-administered questionnaire for patients with osteoarthritis of the hand. A total of 15 items are grouped into three categories; pain, stiffness, and physical disabilities. A five point Likert-scale is used to record responses. Psychometric properties have been well established. The index is available in English, French, and Spanish.

2. **Arthritis Impact Measurement Scales 2-Short Form (AIMS2-SF).** The AIMS2-SF is a multidimensional self-administered questionnaire that is widely used for patients with arthritis, and has been translated into many languages. The original index, the **Arthritis Impact Measurement Scales** (AIMS), used 45 items that span nine domains including mobility, physical activity, dexterity, ADL, social role, social activity, depression, and anxiety. Responses are recorded using a five-point Likert scale. It has since undergone several revisions and reductions resulting in the most recent short form, developed in 1997. The shorter version contains 26 items that focus on physical activity and function, and has psychometric properties similar to those of the AIMS and the AIMS2.

3. **Western Ontario Osteoarthritis of the Shoulder (WOOS) Index.** The WOOS is an instrument developed specifically for osteoarthritis of the shoulder. It is a self-administered questionnaire containing 19 items in four domains (pain, physical symptoms, lifestyle function, and sport/recreation/leisure). The patient's response to each item is noted on a 100-mm visual analog scale. Psychometric properties are well documented.

4. **Cochin Rheumatoid Hand Disability Scale.** The Cochin scale is a self-report questionnaire that assesses hand function in ADL. It is a hand-specific instrument that was designed for the hand affected with rheumatic arthritis. Eighteen items are assigned to five categories: kitchen, dressing, hygiene, office, and others. The right and left hand are assessed separately.

5. **Other self-report instruments** that assess hand function and have been validated in patients with arthritis, although not designed specifically for arthritic conditions, include the disabilities of the arm, shoulder, and hand (DASH) index, the Michigan hand outcomes questionnaire (MHQ), and the patient-rated wrist/hand evaluation (PRWHE).

 TREATMENT

The overall goal of therapeutic intervention is to improve functional ability. This is accomplished by a variety of methods that include provision/fabrication of splints, education on joint protection principles, provision of assistive devices, use of modalities, and instruction on exercises. Armed with the baseline data collected during the evaluation process, the therapist establishes a treatment plan.

I. **SPLINTING.** The purpose of splinting arthritic joints is to reduce pain and inflammation, to reduce progression of deformity, to improve function by increasing support and stability, and to prevent repetitive stress on the joint during activity. Common problems that require splinting are discussed in the subsequent text.

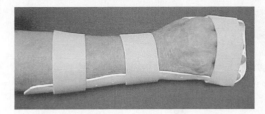

Figure 62-1. Resting hand splint.

A. **Wrist and hand synovitis.** Nighttime resting hand splints are beneficial to increase comfort (Fig. 62-1). The splints are designed to decrease inflammation and pain by providing support to the wrist, metacarpophalangeal (MP), and interphalangeal (IP) joints. The joints are supported in a position opposite to the direction of potential deformity. Arthritis pain has been found to decrease with night splinting. This is particularly helpful in inflammatory joint disorders such as rheumatoid arthritis.
B. **Wrist synovitis.** A volar-based wrist immobilization splint that provides support to the wrist and allows motion of the digits is provided for wear during acute inflammatory episodes and for the treatment of carpal tunnel syndrome (Fig. 62-2).
C. **MP ulnar deviation and palmar subluxation.** MP ulnar deviation deformities are splinted at night to position the MP joints in radial alignment. When fabricating the splint the wrist radial deformity is addressed along with the MP ulnar deformity. The splint must provide proper wrist ulnar alignment and supportive strapping (Fig. 62-3). Hand-based functional splints that support the digits in radial alignment are provided for use during functional activities. These are made of soft and light material and/or are hinged at the MP joints to allow function (Fig. 62-4). Soft material is chosen to increase comfort and tolerance.
D. **Swan neck deformity.** Swan neck deformities are splinted with lightweight finger splints that prevent proximal interphalangeal (PIP) joint hyperextension and allow PIP flexion. Custom thermoplastic splints in a figure-of-eight design may be fabricated. However, because these splints are needed for a long term, a high temperature thermoplastic option, the Oval 8 splint, is a good alternative. It is available from 3-Point Products, Inc. (Annapolis, Maryland) (Fig. 62-5). A silver ring splint that is custom fitted, the SIRIS splint (Silver Ring Splint Company, Charlottesville, Virginia), is also available, and preferred for its esthetic appeal. A recent study reported increased dexterity in 17 patients with swan neck deformities following the use of silver ring splint.
E. **Boutonniere deformity.** The PIP joint is splinted in extension at night (Fig. 62-6) to prevent progression of the deformity. This position is often not well tolerated during the day, because PIP flexion is blocked and function is limited.
F. **Carpometacarpal (CMC) joint synovitis.** A forearm-based thumb immobilization splint that immobilizes the CMC and MP joints in functional opposition is

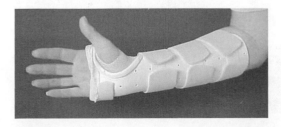

Figure 62-2. Volar-based wrist immobilization splint.

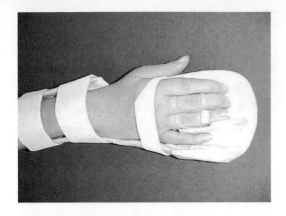

Figure 62-3. Resting hand splint (with wrist ulnar alignment and supportive strapping).

fabricated to reduce the stress on the joint during activities (Fig. 62-7). The IP joint of the thumb is free to allow functional use. There is supporting evidence for use of either hand-based or forearm-based splints in the treatment of pain due to osteoarthritis of the first CMC joint. It has been our experience that the forearm-based splint provides increased comfort and pain relief in relation to the hand-based version.

II. **PATIENT EDUCATION.** Education of the patient is a critical component of intervention in patients with rheumatoid arthritis. Patients are instructed on basic principles of joint protection, energy conservation, and activity modification. Joint protection principles were first described by Cordery in 1965 to decrease stress on joints with rheumatoid arthritis, and have since been modified for osteoarthritic joints as well. The general principles of joint protection are listed in the subsequent text. Comprehensive resources and instruction booklets are available from national arthritis organizations. Contact information is provided at the end of this chapter.

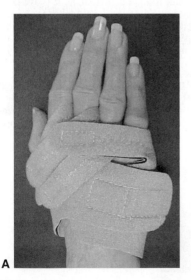

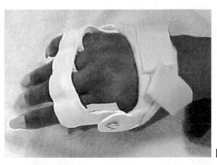

Figure 62-4. A: Hand-based antiulnar deviation splint. **B:** Hinged antiulnar deviation splint.

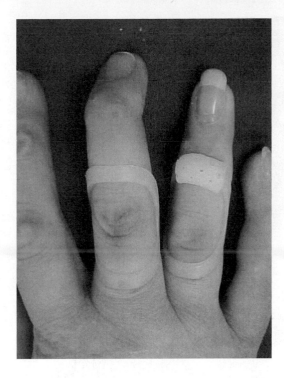

Figure 62-5. Oval 8 Splint—PIP joint extension block splint. (Photo courtesy of A. Griffith.)

A. Joint protection principles

1. Distribution of pressure over large surface areas is encouraged. Examples for this include: using both hands when possible; using large joints instead of smaller joints; sliding objects instead of lifting; and using the palms, in place of fingers, to lift and to push.

2. Maintaining one stationary position for long periods of time is discouraged.

3. Positions that promote deformity are avoided, such as bending the elbows.

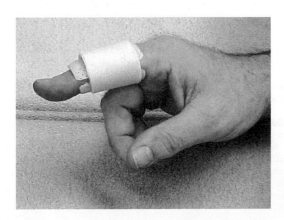

Figure 62-6. PIP joint extension splint. (Photo courtesy of A. Barenholtz.)

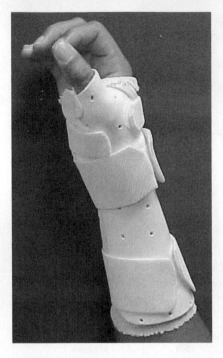

Figure 62-7. Forearm-based thumb CMC joint immobilization splint.

   4. Excessive load on the joints can be avoided by using raised handles, nonslip surfaces, and by resorting to techniques that assist the affected patient (such as using a toothpaste pump as opposed to a squeeze tube).
B. Energy conservation principles
   1. Balancing of rest along with activity is encouraged. Frequent, short breaks are recommended. Light activities should be alternated with heavier activities. Patients are taught to recognize early signs of fatigue so that they can rest before reaching the point of exhaustion. Extra time should be allowed for completion of tasks.
   2. Painful activities are avoided. Patients are instructed to end an activity prior to the onset of pain. Ability for early recognition of the signs of discomfort is reinforced to avoid straining the joints. Activities are adapted to eliminate pain.
   3. Techniques to minimize the amount of energy expenditure are encouraged, such as using disposable dishes, buying prepared food, and conveniently storing frequently used utensils to minimize effort to gain access to them.
   4. General muscle strengthening/conditioning and physical fitness is promoted. Aerobic exercise has been found to be an effective method for the reduction of pain, and yoga programs are beneficial in reducing stiffness and joint pain in the hands.
III.   TREATMENT OF STIFFNESS AND LOSS OF MOTION. General range of motion exercises are performed for the wrists, hands, and digits within a pain-free range. Exercise will help maintain the range of motion, but usually does not improve motion that is already limited. Strengthening programs should be used with extreme caution to avoid worsening the deformities and aggravating the condition of painful joints. Strengthening exercises that are deemed appropriate are performed in a pain-free range. Isometric exercises may be appropriate to strengthen the thenar muscles and the rotator cuff.

SUMMARY

Treatment of the patient with arthritis requires a thorough knowledge of the disease process, the potential deformities, and the specific needs of the individual. A comprehensive evaluation is performed to develop an appropriate treatment plan based on the principles described.

Patient and Organization Resources:

Arthritis Foundation
1330 W Peachtree Street
Atlanta, Georgia 30309
Phone: 404-872-7100; toll-free 800-283-7800
Website: www.arthritis.org

The Arthritis Society, National Office
250 Bloor Street East, Suite 901
Toronto, Ontario M4W 3P2 Canada
Phone: 416-967-1414; fax 416-967-7171
Website: www.arthritis.ca

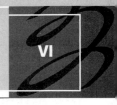

Complementary and Alternative Medicine

VI

Gina Kearney and C. Ronald MacKenzie

 INTRODUCTION

Complementary and alternative medicine (CAM) refers to a diverse group of medical and health care systems, practices, and products, which are not currently considered to be a part of conventional medicine, or medicine as practiced by physicians (MD or DO) and other traditionally trained allied health professionals. Therefore, until recently, CAM therapies and holistic philosophy in general were practiced outside the domain of traditional medicine. They were not part of US medical school curricula and were even less prominent in U.S. hospitals. These divisions, however, are gradually disappearing as the prevalence and use of CAM has risen steadily over the last decade. Use of at least one of the 16 alternative therapies by the general public increased from 33.8% in 1990 to 42.1% in 1997. During the same 7-year period, CAM expenditures increased 45.2% and have been estimated at $27 billion.

It is clear that the upward trend in the use of CAM is continuing, spurred on mainly by the use of CAM therapy initiated by the patient. Results from the National Health Interview Survey (NHIS) in 2000 revealed that 62% of those surveyed used some form of CAM therapy during the 12 months preceding the survey, generally for conditions such as back pain, head/chest colds, neck pain, joint pain or stiffness, and anxiety or depression. The primary reason for the use of CAM is its "perceived efficacy," with 55% of those surveyed in the NHIS reporting they believed that CAM would improve health when used in combination with conventional medical treatments.

 TERMINOLOGY

When describing various modalities, **complementary therapies** generally refer to those therapies that are **used with** conventional medicine, and **alternative** medicine/therapies are those that are **used in place of** conventional medicine. The term **integrative** is being used more often to better illustrate the "complementary" nature of care; however, most people are more familiar with CAM. Although some scientific evidence exists regarding some select modalities of CAM, for most modalities there are questions that are yet to be answered through well-designed scientific studies. Safety and efficacy are at the core of most debates because these issues will shape the future of CAM research.

COMPLEMENTARY AND ALTERNATIVE MEDICINE AND RHEUMATIC DISEASE

Conventional medicine usually offers symptomatic relief for patients with rheumatic disease, but for a significant number of those affected, cure is not a reasonable goal that can be hoped for or an expected clinical outcome. Because of this constrained expectation, it is not surprising that many individuals with rheumatic disease have incorporated CAM into their health care regimen. Estimates of CAM use among this population are generally higher than among patients with other conditions. Studies have reported the use of CAM by patients with rheumatic disease to be ranging from 63% to as much as 94% among those surveyed. Severe pain, arthritis (both rheumatoid arthritis and osteoarthritis), and fibromyalgia are among the rheumatologic conditions particularly amenable to CAM intervention, with exercise, over-the-counter products (topical remedies), spiritual aids (prayer, meditation, and relaxation), and dietary recommendations (vitamins, herbs, and supplements) being the most commonly selected CAM modalities.

Although most conventional practitioners are not adequately trained to provide CAM therapies for their patients directly, there exists a responsibility, at a minimum, to be prepared to discuss and guide patients to appropriate resources and/or to refer them to qualified CAM practitioners. Of the numerous CAM therapies, the following represents an overview of select CAM modalities that may be of interest (and potential benefit) for the patient with rheumatism.

ALTERNATIVE MEDICAL SYSTEMS

Alternative medical systems are built upon complete systems of theory and practice. As stated by the National Center for Complementary and Alternative Medicine (NCCAM) of the National Institutes of Health (NIH), alternative medical systems may be unfamiliar to many; however, many of these systems have evolved separately from and earlier than the large number of conventional approaches commonly utilized. Listed in the subsequent text are some examples.

I.   **AYURVEDA.** Ayurveda is Sanskrit for **the science of life** and is a form of medicine that has been practiced in India for thousands of years. Ayurvedic medicine places equal emphasis on the body, mind, and spirit and uses herbs, yoga, diet, meditation, massage, exposure to the sun, and breathing exercises to restore natural harmony and balance to the body. An ayurvedic doctor identifies an individual's "constitution" or overall health profile by determining his or her metabolic body type (Vata, Pitta, or Kapha) through an assessment of personal history. The individual's "constitution" then becomes the foundation for a specific plan of treatment designed to guide the individual back into balance with the environment.

II.   **TRADITIONAL CHINESE MEDICINE.** The roots of Chinese medicine, on which acupuncture, massage, and herbal therapy are based, date back as far as to the Shang dynasty (1000 B.C.). One of the major underpinnings of traditional Chinese medicine (TCM) is the belief that there are patterns of energy flow (Qi or chi) present in all living things, which are essential for health and well-being. When these patterns of energy flow become disrupted or blocked, illness and/or disease results. Within the system of energy pathways, or meridians, there are over 1,000 acupoints that can be stimulated through the insertion of needles. Hence, the practice of **acupuncture** is believed to help correct and rebalance the flow of energy and restore health. Acupuncture is frequently used to treat both acute conditions and chronic pain, and has shown promise in treating arthritis, fibromyalgia, lupus, chronic fatigue syndrome, and low-back pain.

III. **HOMEOPATHY.** This system of medical practice is based on the **Law of Similars,** or the theory that any substance that can produce symptoms of disease or illness in a healthy individual can cure those symptoms in a sick individual. Administered in diluted form, homeopathic remedies are derived from plant, animal, and mineral sources. Numbering in the thousands, these over-the-counter natural remedies have been used to treat a variety of ailments including allergies, asthma, influenza, headaches, and indigestion. Homeopathy offers a low-risk, affordable approach to many acute and chronic conditions. Although individuals have used homeopathy for self-care/healing for many years, the optimal effect is realized only when the "proper" remedy is selected. Homeopathic remedies are now widely available in drug stores and health food stores, but are often marketed as standard drugs, meaning, a specific remedy or combination of remedies is indicated for each condition. However, the classic prescribing of homeopathic remedies is based on the personal characteristics and symptoms of the particular individual rather than the specific condition, which is extremely important in treating serious health conditions. Although not harmful, selection of an incorrect remedy will simply have no effect, often resulting in the dismissal of this treatment approach prematurely. For this reason, it is best to consult a well-trained and experienced homeopath for the best results. Keeping this in mind, a listing of some of the homeopathic remedies commonly recommended for specific rheumatic conditions are given here (dosages are indicated by letters and numbers, such as "12 C").

    A. **Ankylosing spondylitis.** *Tuberculinum* nosode, 12 C (only in the early stages of the disease).

    B. **Fibromyalgia.** *Cimicifuga racemosa*, 9 C.

    C. **Rheumatoid arthritis (RA).** *Streptococcin* nosode, 12 C (only in the early stages of the disease).

    D. **Rheumatic joints.** *Apis mellifica*, 9 C (for painless swelling) and *Bryonia alba*, 9 C (for painful swelling).

IV. **NATUROPATHY.** This broad system of medicine is based on the theory that the body is a self-regulating mechanism with the natural ability to maintain a state of health and wellness. Emphasis is placed on employing healthy practices (prevention) and self-healing. Practitioners of naturopathy generally elect to avoid invasive procedures and the use of synthetic drugs, and try to cure illness and disease by harnessing the body's natural healing powers. This is accomplished by the use of a combination of modalities from practices such as herbal medicine, homeopathic treatment, massage, dietary supplements, and other physical therapies. Causes of the illness, or root causes as they are sometimes referred to, are identified and treated using a holistic approach. The doctor assumes the role of an educator and a motivator to enable individuals to take responsibility for their own health. The relationship between the physician and patient, in essence, becomes part of the therapy.

MANIPULATIVE AND BODY-BASED THERAPIES

I. **CHIROPRACTIC.** The third largest independent health profession in the United States, this treatment modality involves adjustment of the spine and joints to influence the body's nervous system and natural defense mechanisms to alleviate pain and improve general health. Chiropractors make their diagnosis based on physical examination, history, palpation of the spine, and often x-rays. An assumption of chiropractic is that health is a state of balance, particularly of the nervous and musculoskeletal systems. When the spine is fully aligned, nerve energy flows freely to every cell and organ in the body. This free flow of energy nurtures the innate ability of the body to work optimally and coordinate normal body functions. There are three primary treatment goals: (a) to reduce or eliminate pain; (b) to correct the subluxation (or misalignment) of the spine; and (c) to offer preventive maintenance so that the problem does not recur. For the patient with rheumatism, chiropractic can be an effective adjunctive therapy for the back, neck, and shoulder syndromes, sciatica, muscle spasms, headaches, and arthritic conditions.

II.   MASSAGE AND BODYWORK. Therapeutic massage is a means of manipulating muscles and other soft tissues by rubbing, kneading, rolling, pressing, and tapping movements, causing them to relax and lengthen, thereby allowing for pain-relieving oxygen and blood to flow to the affected area(s). Benefits of massage can be experienced on physical, mental, and emotional levels. Massage relieves muscle tension and stiffness, reduces muscle spasm, speeds recovery from exertion, improves joint flexibility and motion, increases ease and efficiency of movement, improves posture, improves local circulation, induces a relaxed state of alertness, reduces anxiety, increases the feeling of well-being, and raises awareness of the mind–body connection. There are four major categories of massage and bodywork (with over 75 different methods).

A.   European. Uses long strokes, kneading, and friction (Swedish massage).

B.   Deep tissue. Deep manipulation of the fascia (Rolfing/structural integration, myofascial release, trigger point massage).

C.   Pressure point. Application of pressure to unblock meridians (Shiatsu, Amma, acupressure, Jin Shin Do, reflexology).

D.   Movement integration. Consists of bodywork (not necessarily massage) that teaches methods for rebalancing and new/better ways to move (Feldenkrais, Alexander technique, and Trager).

Care should be taken to seek out a licensed professional wherever possible, and it should be noted that for some situations [phlebitis/thrombosis, severe varicose veins, acute inflammation of the skin, soft tissue, or joints (including acute RA), and some types of cancer] massage may be contraindicated.

BIOLOGICALLY BASED THERAPIES

I.   DIET-BASED INTERVENTIONS. There are no specific diets for patients with arthritis, primarily because of the fact that there are so many types of arthritis and related conditions. A well-balanced diet consisting of whole foods is the best recommendation for the general population as well as those with rheumatic conditions. Listed here are some guidelines that will often make significant improvements in the control of symptoms; however, it should be understood that these guidelines cannot be substituted for the expertise of a registered dietitian or nutritionist.

A.   Eat lots (and a variety) of fruits and vegetables—at least five servings per day. Whole foods are best and have the highest concentration of phytochemicals, which have antioxidant, anti-inflammatory, antiallergic, and antiviral properties. Fruit juices should be avoided due to the high content of sugar and number of calories. For example, it would be a better choice to eat an apple rather than drink a glass of apple juice.

B.   Eat fish three to five times per week. Fish oils have shown a great deal of promise in combating the inflammation associated with many conditions, particularly RA, and represent the fastest growing category of supplements. The omega-3 fatty acids make up the anti-inflammatory fats whereas the omega-6 fatty acids comprise the proinflammatory fats. The goal is to have an intake of both in a balanced ratio of 1:1. Fish oils can be added to the diet by consuming fish or taking supplements. A recent study has reported that fish oil supplements were generally safer than fish because of the potential for the presence of mercury and polychlorinated biphenyls (PCBs) in whole fish. Although supplements may be considered safer, one must take care to purchase them from a reputable supplier to ensure that they contain what has been claimed and that they are fresh (fish oils can become rancid). When consuming fish, it should be noted that omega-3 fatty acids are mostly found in mackerel, salmon, tuna, bluefish, sturgeon, anchovy, trout, sardines, herring, and mullet.

C.   Include olive oil in the diet. Olive oil contains phytochemicals and also has antioxidant properties. There is some speculation that it may also influence inflammation.

D.   Reduce the consumption of animal proteins/fats. Animal proteins and fats are contained in meat, poultry, cheese, butter, and other animal products. Reduction in their consumption will aid in balancing fats and cholesterol. Evidence has shown that the vegetarian diet can significantly improve arthritic/inflammatory symptoms as it reduces the intake of the proinflammatory fatty acids.

E. Eat less. One should reduce the intake of sugary foods and avoid fried foods. Calories should be reduced or maintained at a lower level in order to control body weight. This is particularly important for patients with osteoarthritis (OA) of the knees, and for all those wishing to prevent other health problems associated with excess weight/obesity. This is consistent with the current concept of the pathogenesis of OA of the knee, one that includes joint trauma and mechanical imbalance as triggers for enzymatic breakdown of cartilage.

F. Identify and avoid foods that are problematic. Some food items clearly act as triggers of inflammation for some individuals. Testing for skin allergy, fasting, trying out diets by eliminating food items that are suspect, or simply keeping a food diary/journal are useful measures to identify problematic foods.

II. VITAMINS, OTHER SUPPLEMENTS, AND HERBS. The recommended daily allowances (RDAs) of the most important vitamins (B, C, D, and E) are found in a good multivitamin tablet. Reading the label will reveal the ingredients and amounts contained. In addition to taking a multivitamin, there are some additional supplements that may warrant consideration.

A. Selenium. This essential trace mineral is needed to make the antioxidant glutathione peroxidase, which seems to be present in lower levels in patients with OA. Some studies have suggested that selenium has both anti-inflammatory and analgesic benefits in patients with arthritis. The US RDA for adults is 70 μg, but intake of up to 200 μg is considered safe. As with all supplements, one should buy organic items wherever possible.

B. Zinc. The diet of a patient with arthritis is often deficient in zinc. Zinc is important because it may be helpful in inhibiting the release of the inflammatory mediator histamine from immune cells. One clinical study indicated that zinc decreased inflammation and stiffness in patients with RA who failed to benefit from nonsteroidal anti-inflammatory drugs (NSAIDs) as well as other anti-inflammatory drugs. The RDA of zinc for adults in the United States is 12 to 15 mg, with a safe upper threshold of 30 mg.

C. Boswellia serrata. This ancient herb, often used in Ayurveda, is a very safe botanical extract and is both cartilage protective and anti-inflammatory. A safe dosage of this herb consists of 600 mg/day (in three divided doses), and is based on products that contain approximately 65% boswellic acids.

D. Ginger. Inexpensive and widely available, ginger has been shown to be an effective reliever of inflammation-induced pain and also has other health benefits with no side effects. Ginger inhibits the 5-lipoxygenase enzyme and its inflammatory cascade reaction. It also partially blocks the cyclooxygenase (COX) enzymes, but unlike synthetic NSAIDs, does not fully block COX-1 and does not create gastric bleeding, stomach upset, or any other untoward effects. Fresh ginger is best, and consumption of three to 50 g will have beneficial effects without any side effect.

 MIND–BODY THERAPIES

The "mind–body connection" is well documented, and teaches that we are not without any control over our body's functioning. There are a number of relatively simple, yet powerful modalities that can be utilized to foster self-care and self-healing in patients with rheumatism.

I. MEDITATION. Meditation is a process of suspending the stream of thoughts by focusing on the present and thereby calming the mind. Deep breathing is often a means to relax and allow the individual to silence inner chatter. Generally performed once or twice daily for 20 to 30 minutes, meditation is used to reduce stress, alter hormone levels, and elevate one's mood. Meditation has been shown to lower blood pressure, adrenaline levels, heart rate, and skin temperature. Meditation has been identified as an effective means for reducing the intensity of pain and improving adaptive functioning. There are several approaches to the practice of meditation.

    A. Concentrative meditation. Attention is focused on breathing, an image, or a sound (such as a mantra or chant).

    B. Mindfulness meditation. Attention is given to the sensations, sounds, smells, thoughts, and feelings that are being experienced without becoming involved in those experiences and letting thoughts flow; they are simply "seen" and acknowledged, much like a passing parade.

    C. Transcendental meditation. Introduced by Maharishi Mahesh Yogi, this form of meditation involves the body reaching a level of profound relaxation while the mind achieves a more alert state.

While meditation in any of its many forms can be a wonderful means for relaxation and stress management, it takes practice and consistency to avail of its greatest benefit. Many commercial recordings on tape are available to guide in the practice of meditation and can be helpful for those who are initially learning to meditate.

II.   **BIOFEEDBACK.** This technique teaches individuals to learn how to consciously regulate normally unconscious body functions such as breathing, heart rate, and blood pressure. Biofeedback training used with simple electronic monitoring devices enables individuals to identify changes associated with targeted symptoms and to develop measures to alter those changes. Biofeedback has been used to reduce stress, eliminate headaches, recondition injured muscles, control asthma attacks, and relieve pain. Additionally, research has shown biofeedback to have improved the symptoms associated with Raynaud's phenomenon, lupus, and scleroderma.

III.   **EXERCISE AND MOVEMENT.** Maintaining mobility is a major goal for individuals with arthritis and many other rheumatic conditions. It is natural that individuals experiencing pain in a joint want to avoid using it. When a joint is not used, muscles and connective tissues weaken and contract. The result is an increased loss of mobility and function, and subsequently, increased pain. The goals of exercise are threefold, and are to (a) maintain flexibility, stability, and strength of the joint and its supportive structures; (b) promote overall health and well-being; and (c) prevent obesity. Exercise is one of the most effective complementary strategies for rehabilitation as it up-regulates anti-inflammatory, health promoting processes in nearly all body tissues. It can also help maintain joint range of motion and enhance overall strength and endurance. Yoga and Tai Chi are both gentle forms of exercise that are particularly helpful for patients with arthritis. Check with local chapters of the Arthritis Foundation for a class called PACE (People with Arthritis Can Exercise), which they developed and have found to be beneficial for individuals with all forms of arthritis. Dance therapy has been shown to help increase range of motion and decrease symptoms of RA as well as other associated symptoms of depression, anxiety, fatigue, and tension.

IV.   **GUIDED IMAGERY/VISUALIZATION.** This method involves a series of relaxation techniques followed by the visualization of detailed images that are calming and peaceful. It is on the basis of the principle that images in the mind can create specific responses in the body. When fully relaxed, the patient develops an image that depicts the desired state of healing and/or recovery.

    A. To achieve relaxation, patients may imagine being in a peaceful, beautiful, safe place (either an actual scene that has been experienced or one that is created in the mind).

    B. To facilitate the healing of broken bones, patients may imagine bridges being built across bones to connect and strengthen them.

    C. To reduce painful inflammation, one might visualize the affected area being bathed in healing, cool, blue water.

Books and tapes are readily available to assist (or guide) imagery practice. The number of training/certification programs for health care professionals has grown significantly in recent years and, because of this, many practitioners now use some form of imagery work with their patients.

V.   **RELAXATION/STRESS MANAGEMENT.** Although the cause of arthritis is not known, in some forms of the condition it is believed to be a disturbance of the immune system. The effects of stress on the immune system are well documented, so it is possible that by reducing one's stress, arthritic symptoms would also be diminished. The same holds true for inflammation, which is also aggravated by stress. Direct anatomical connections have been demonstrated to exist between dendritic cells in the skin and nerves, supporting the mind–body hypothesis of disease. When confronted by stressors, the body responds by defensively preparing for "fight or flight." This is an important and necessary response in acute situations, but when the stress response continues over a long period (as in chronic illness), the body ultimately becomes fatigued, less resilient, and may encounter additional problems such as gastrointestinal disturbances, increased susceptibility to infections, and even some forms of mental illness. Effective stress management and relaxation may: (a) strengthen the immune system that helps the body resist factors that can cause complications; (b) aid in decreasing pain intensity; (c) decrease muscle tension; (d) decrease anxiety and depression; (e) enhance an individual's ability to maintain control of chronic disease and cope with it; (f) promote a sense of well-being; and (g) facilitate healing.

VI. **PRAYER.** Most individuals believe in the healing power of prayer. As mentioned earlier, the NHIS reported that 62% of those surveyed used CAM during the 12 months preceding the survey, **when prayer made specifically for health reasons was included in the definition of CAM.** Without the inclusion of prayer as a component of CAM, this figure dropped to 36%. Whether it is prayer for someone else's health or for one's own health, prayer has the ability to create a sense of strength, purpose, hope, and ability to manage and cope with life's challenges. The sense of a connection to God or simply a "higher power" differentiates spirituality from religion, although for some, there may be no distinction.

VII. **MISCELLANEOUS THERAPIES/FOLK REMEDIES**

   A. **Copper bracelets.** Copper bracelets, worn on the wrist, are one of the most well known and widely used folk remedies for inflammatory types of arthritis. There is no scientific evidence that they work, but hundreds of anecdotal reports hail their efficacy. Given their low cost and the absence of risk, they may be worth trying.

   B. **Magnet therapy.** Most magnets marketed to consumers for health purposes are of a type called static (or permanent) magnets, meaning they have magnetic fields that do not change. Products that are used in magnet therapy and which may contain static magnets include shoe insoles, heel inserts, mattress pads, bandages, belts, pillows and cushions, and bracelets (and other jewelry). Scientific research does not yet firmly support a conclusion that magnets of any type can relieve pain, although many individuals do experience and report relief. Various theories have been proposed as to why this may happen, but clinical trials have produced conflicting results. The U.S. Food and Drug Administration (FDA) has not approved the marketing of products for magnet therapy with claims of benefits to health (such as "relieves arthritis pain").

   C. **Bee venom.** Use of bee venom, or "apitherapy," for arthritis dates back by many centuries. When used, indications for treatment include inflammatory autoimmune disorders. Although there is some positive (anecdotal) evidence, much more research will need to be done to draw any firm conclusion. One must also be aware that some individuals (approximately one in 50) are highly allergic to bee venom. For this reason, one should be tested in a doctor's office for allergic reactions, where an antidote is available, prior to trying this therapy.

   While there is much research that needs to be done to ensure efficacy of many CAM modalities, many show promise in their application and assistance in caring for patients with rheumatism. The following comprises a list of resources for a more detailed look at the various systems and therapies discussed.

 RESOURCES

Complementary/Alternative Medicine

- Altmednet.com: www.altmendnet.com (many CAM links)
- Arthritis Foundation: www.arthritis.org
- Cochrane Collaboration: www.cochrane.org (evidence-based research/systematic reviews)

- Integrative Medicine/Care: www.forhealers.com (information network and professional resources including research)
- National Center for Complementary and Alternative Medicine: www.nccam.nih.gov (affiliated with NIH, conducts and supports research and provides clearinghouse for CAM information)

Healing Systems

- Ayurvedic Institute: www.ayurveda.com
- Traditional Chinese Medicine: www.acupuncture.com
- American Academy of Medical Acupuncture: www.medicalacupuncture.org
- American Association of Oriental Medicine: www.aaom.org
- Naturopathic Medicine/American Association of Naturopathic Physicians: www.naturopathic.org
- Homeopathic Medicine/National Center for Homeopathy: www.homeopathic.org or www.healthy.net/nch
- Chiropractic Medicine/American Chiropractic Association: www.amerchiro.org
- Association for Integrative Medicine: www.integrativemedicine.org

Meditation, Biofeedback, Imagery, Stress Reduction

- The Mind–Body Medical Institute: www.mindbody.harvard.edu (information and referrals)
- Association for Applied Psychophysiology and Biofeedback: www.aapb.org
- Insight Meditation Society: www.dharma.org (information and links)

Prayer and Spirituality

- International Center for the Integration of Health Spirituality: www.nihr.org

Exercise and Movement

- Tai Chi: www.taichichih.org
- Yoga/American Yoga Association: www.americanyogaassociation.com
- Yoga Research Center: www.yrec.org

Massage and Bodywork

- Alexander Technique: www.alexandertechnique.com
- Feldenkrais Educational Foundation of North America (FEFNA): www.feldenkrais.com
- Feldenkrais Resources: www.feldenkrais-resources.com
- National Certification Board for Therapeutic Massage and Bodywork: www.ncbtmb.com (referral list)
- American Massage Therapy Association: www.amtamassage.org (information about massage and locator service for referrals)
- American Reflexology Certification Board: www.arcb.net (information and referral list)

Vitamins, Supplements, and Herbs

- U.S. Food and Drug Administration: www.fda.gov (access to MEDWATCH as well as warnings on herbal products)
- American Botanical Council: www.herbalgram.org (information about herbs)
- ConsumerLab.com: www.consumerlab.com (consumer information and independent evaluations/reviews of products that affect health and nutrition)
- Herb Research Foundation: www.herbs.org
- HerbMed: www.amfoundation.org (Alternative Medicine Foundation Herbal Database)
- NIH Office of Dietary Supplements: http://dietary-supplements.info.nih.gov
- American Dietetic Association: www.eatright.org (referrals to registered dietitians)
- American Herbalists Guild: www.americanherbalistsguild.com (referrals to herbal practitioners)

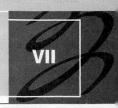

Formulary

VII

Arthur M. F. Yee and Jane E. Salmon

Recent progress in the understanding of the pathophysiology of rheumatic diseases and in the development of new therapeutic approaches has greatly expanded the pharmacologic armamentarium with which to treat these illnesses. Moreover, the spectrum of conditions which falls under the realm of rheumatology increasingly overlaps with that of other medical specialties, so previously known medicines have frequently found new applications. Thorough appreciation of the indications, contraindications, goals of therapy, and potential adverse effects of any medicine is essential for its appropriate administration. Nonetheless, while the need for a given therapeutic category may be defined by the clinical situation, the use of a specific agent is often determined by an empiric trial that considers patient response, tolerance, and compliance, as well as by drug expense. As with all medications, recognition of contraindications and careful monitoring of potentially adverse effects is of paramount importance, especially in children, older individuals, and women who are contemplating conception, are pregnant, or are breast-feeding.

 PREGNANCY AND MEDICATIONS

Many rheumatic diseases affect women of childbearing age, and hence, the clinician should be keenly aware of the many possible complications of medications and their effects on fertility, fetal development, and breast-feeding. A frank and thorough discussion with the patient is paramount **even before** pregnancy is attempted.

Although it is impossible to create absolute rules about the management of medications, the overriding principle will always be to weigh the potential benefits of any drug against its potential risks, which is to be considered on an individual case basis. Although minimizing drug intervention during pregnancy is always desired, there is very strong evidence for discontinuing the use of some drugs such as cyclophosphamide, methotrexate, or leflunomide, both before and during gestation, and effective contraceptive techniques must be implemented when prescribing such drugs to women of childbearing age. For other medications such as azathioprine (AZA) or hydroxychloroquine, the evidence is not as clear, although they are probably relatively safe. Warfarin should be discontinued because of its known teratogenic effects and should be substituted with heparin. Aspirin and nonsteroidal anti-inflammatory drugs (NSAIDs) should be discontinued in the latter part of pregnancy because of the potential premature closure of the ductus arteriosus, and yet, in the antiphospholipid syndrome, low-dose aspirin is an important treatment option in ensuring a successful pregnancy. Prednisone and methylprednisolone at low to moderate doses will not cross the placenta and are considered to be safe for fetal development. In contrast, the fluorinated corticosteroids (e.g., dexamethasone and betamethasone) will cross the placenta. (See Chapter 38 for further information on this topic.)

NONSTEROIDAL ANTI-INFLAMMATORY DRUGS

NSAIDs exhibit antipyretic, anti-inflammatory, and analgesic properties through their ability to inhibit the production of proinflammatory prostaglandins by the enzyme cyclooxygenase-2 (COX-2). They are used for degenerative musculoskeletal problems, systemic inflammatory illnesses, crystalline diseases, soft-tissue injuries, and certain hypercoagulable states, between other conditions. NSAIDs are essentially equipotent, although responses and tolerances may vary between individual patients. If an inadequate therapeutic response or intolerance occurs, a trial of an alternative agent, especially from a different chemical class, is often worthwhile. Compliance may be related to schedule of administration (Table 1). Concurrent use of multiple NSAIDs does not enhance efficacy and increases toxicities and is not generally recommended. In all patients being treated with NSAIDs for a long term, particularly the older individuals and those with impaired liver or kidney function, regular monitoring of hepatic and renal function is essential.

Traditional NSAIDs, such as ibuprofen and naproxen, also inhibit COX-1, the function of which includes constitutive "housekeeping" functions such as the production of gastroprotective prostaglandins. Accordingly, gastrointestinal toxicities (e.g., bleeding, ulcerations, and perforations) are a major morbidity associated with their use. If NSAIDs are indicated in individuals at a high risk of gastrointestinal complications, gastroprotective agents such as misoprostol or proton pump inhibitors should be concurrently used.

Aspirin and the traditional NSAIDs inhibit platelet function and, in general, should be discontinued before major elective procedures. Because aspirin irreversibly inhibits platelet function, it must be withdrawn for at least 7 to 10 days (the lifespan of a circulating platelet) before such procedures. NSAIDs reversibly inhibit platelets and should be stopped four to five half-lives before surgeries if necessary (approximately 3 to 5 days for medicines that are administered three or more times daily or 5 to 7 days for medicines that are administered

---

| TABLE 1 | Nonsteroidal Anti-inflammatory Drugs |

Drug, available dosages (mg)	Frequency	Maximum daily dosage (mg)
Aspirin, 81, 325, 500, 650	q.i.d.	6,000
Celecoxib, 100, 200, 400	q.d.–b.i.d.	400
Diclofenac,[a] 25, 50, 75	b.i.d.–q.i.d.	200
Etodolac, 200, 300, 400, 500	b.i.d.–t.i.d.	1,200
Fenoprofen, 300, 600	t.i.d.–q.i.d.	3,200
Flurbiprofen, 50, 100	t.i.d.–q.i.d.	300
Ibuprofen, 200, 300, 400, 600, 800	t.i.d.–q.i.d.	2,400
Indomethacin,[a] 25, 50	t.i.d.	150
Ketoprofen,[a] 25, 50, 75	t.i.d.–q.i.d.	300
Ketorolac, 10	t.i.d.–q.i.d.	40
Meclofenamate, 50, 100	t.i.d.–q.i.d.	400
Mefenamic acid, 250	q.i.d.	1,000
Meloxicam, 7.5, 15	q.d.	15
Nabumetone, 500, 750	q.d.–b.i.d.	2,000
Naproxen,[a] 250, 375, 500	b.i.d.–t.i.d.	1,500
Oxaprozin, 600	q.d.	1,800
Piroxicam, 10, 20	q.d.	20
Salsalate, 500, 750	b.i.d.–t.i.d.	4,000
Sulindac, 150, 200	b.i.d.	400
Tolmetin, 200, 400	t.i.d.	1,800

[a]Sustained-release formulations are available.
b.i.d., twice daily; q.d., every day; q.i.d., four times daily; t.i.d., three times daily.

once or twice daily). Intriguingly, ibuprofen, and probably other NSAIDs as well, mitigate the cardioprotective effects of aspirin. If concomitant NSAID and aspirin therapy is desired, it is recommended that the aspirin be administered at least 2 hours before the NSAID is ingested.

Major recent scientific advances have led to the development of a new generation of NSAIDs (known as coxibs) that preferentially inhibit the activity of COX-2. Because of their relative sparing of constitutive COX-1 activity, coxibs have been shown to have fewer adverse gastrointestinal effects than traditional NSAIDs. Clinically, however, this benefit has not been as great as initially hoped for. Moreover, serious concerns have been recently raised over the cardiovascular safety of coxibs. Coxibs appear to actually promote thromboembolic vascular disease (e.g., myocardial infarctions, cerebrovascular accidents) in a dose-dependent manner, probably owing to the unopposed production of thromboxane, which is procoagulant. High and especially supratherapeutic doses of rofecoxib have been associated with an increased risk of myocardial infarctions. The cardiovascular risks are likely enhanced further by aggravated hypertension and fluid retention common to all classes of NSAIDs. Rofecoxib and Valdecoxib have been withdrawn from the market because of these concerns, and there are data that suggest that celecoxib and all NSAIDs may also present considerable dangers in certain high-risk patient populations and should be avoided in patients with significant cardiovascular risk factors (e.g., known coronary artery disease, diabetes, and dyslipidemias). NSAIDs differ in their selectivity for COX-1 and COX-2, and it is possible that adverse effects seen clinically may, in fact, reflect their relative degrees of selectivity (Table 2).

Aspirin, traditional NSAIDs, and coxibs have potential nephrotoxicities. COX-2–mediated prostaglandins have vasodilatory effects on the afferent arterioles in the kidneys and are necessary to maintain renal perfusion, particularly in low flow states, so NSAIDs are relatively contraindicated in patients with any degree of renal insufficiency. Hypertension and fluid retention are relatively common problems, but frank deterioration of renal function is not rare.

Asthmatic attacks, urticaria, and angioedema may be related to enzymatic inhibition of prostaglandin synthesis in susceptible individuals or to immunoglobulin E (IgE)-mediated reactions. Patients who have these reactions to aspirin or other NSAIDs may be sensitive to all NSAIDs, although some studies indicate that coxibs can be safe in this regard. Rashes are not uncommon, but recent postmarketing surveillance has identified rare, severe, cutaneous reactions to valdecoxib including exfoliative dermatitis, Stevens-Johnson syndrome, and toxic epidermal necrolysis, possibly related to sulfonamide reactivity.

Pregnancy is another relative contraindication to the use of NSAIDs because NSAIDs may cause hemorrhagic complications or premature closure of the ductus arteriosus in the third trimester. The benefit of NSAIDs in pregnant women must be weighed very carefully against these risks.

TABLE 2	Relative Cyclooxygenase-2 (COX-2) Selectivity of Selected Agents

Drug	IC_{50} COX-1/COX-2 ratio[a]
Rofecoxib[b]	35
Valdecoxib[b]	30
Celecoxib	7.6
Diclofenac	3
Etodolac	2.4
Meloxicam	2
Indomethacin	0.4
Ibuprofen	0.2
Piroxicam	<0.1

[a]Defined as the ratio of the concentration of drug needed to provide 50% inhibition of COX-1 to the concentration of drug needed to provide inhibition of COX-2. Higher ratios reflect greater COX-2 selectivity.
[b]Rofecoxib and valdecoxib are no longer commercially available.

Aspirin

Action
Inhibits prostaglandin synthesis.

Metabolism
Aspirin (acetylsalicylic acid) is metabolized in the liver and excreted by the kidney. Its half-life increases with increasing dose. It is highly bound to albumin in plasma and widely distributed to all tissues, including synovium.

Adverse Reactions
Gastrointestinal discomfort with nausea and dyspepsia is common, especially in the older individuals. Gastrointestinal blood loss may occur. Tinnitus, decreased hearing acuity, or both are related to mild toxicity and are reversible with a decrease in dosage but may be easily missed in the older individuals with baseline presbycusis. Central nervous system symptoms such as headache, vertigo, and irritability can occur in the older individuals. Aspirin may induce mild, reversible hepatocellular injury in patients being treated for acute rheumatic fever, juvenile idiopathic arthritis, and active systemic lupus erythematosus (SLE) and can be associated with Reye's syndrome. Platelet adhesiveness, aggregation, and adenosine diphosphate release are irreversibly inhibited.

Caution
Idiosyncratic reactions such as asthma occur in 0.02% of individuals. Patients with asthma and nasal polyps are at a higher risk for this reaction. Cross-reactivity exists with other NSAIDs but has not been reported with sodium or magnesium salicylates. Aspirin is uricosuric at high dosages (>4 to 5 g/day), but low dosages (<2 g/day) may lead to urate retention. Aspirin may displace other drugs bound to albumin, thereby potentiating the effects of oral hypoglycemics, warfarin, and other medications. Because aspirin inhibits platelet aggregation and prolongs bleeding time, it should be avoided or used with great caution in patients receiving heparin or warfarin anticoagulants. Some patients may be resistant to aspirin but the clinical significance of laboratory aspirin resistance requires further research.

Supply
Available as tablets, 325, 500, and 650 mg. Buffered tablets, formulated with either absorbable (bicarbonate) or nonabsorbable antacids, are not associated with reduced gastrointestinal bleeding. Enteric-coated tablets are often better tolerated, with less dyspepsia and occult gastrointestinal blood loss, but also have more variable absorption rates than either buffered or nonbuffered tablets. Rectal suppositories are incompletely absorbed. Time-released tablets have delayed absorption with possibly more sustained plasma levels. The physician should be aware of the fact that many over-the-counter drug combinations containing aspirin are widely available.

Dosage
A dosage of 600 to 1,200 mg every 4 to 6 hours, preferably with meals. For optimal anti-inflammatory effects, blood levels between 20 and 30 mg/dL and a total daily dosage of 3 to 6 g are usually required. Dosages necessary to achieve adequate therapeutic concentrations vary with the individual patient. Maximum tolerated dose may be reached slowly; therefore, waiting for 1 week between dosage changes is appropriate. Salicylate levels are routinely available and may be useful to determine adequacy of dosage, patient compliance, and toxicity.

Celecoxib (Celebrex)

Action
Inhibits prostaglandin synthesis via preferential inhibition of COX-2.

Metabolism
Celecoxib is a diaryl-substituted pyrazole. Celecoxib may be generally administered without considering the timing of meals and will achieve peak plasma levels within 3 hours, although high-fat meals may delay peak plasma levels. Approximately 97% of the drug is protein bound, primarily to albumin. Metabolism is largely mediated via cytochrome P-450 2C9,

and excretion is through both the feces and urine. The effective half-life is approximately 11 hours. Celecoxib has cross-reactivity with sulfonamide medications.

Adverse Reactions
Dyspepsia and gastrointestinal intolerance are common, and vigilance for gastrointestinal hemorrhage is necessary. The renal effects are similar to other NSAIDs. Higher dosages may be associated with an increased risk for thrombotic vascular disease. Other intolerances include hypertension, edema, and dermatologic reactions.

Caution
Lower initial doses are recommended in the geriatric population and in the setting of hepatic insufficiency. Potential drug interactions have been identified with lithium and fluconazole. Celecoxib may be taken with low-dose aspirin and warfarin and appears to have no effect on platelet function at therapeutic levels. The drug is contraindicated in patients with known allergies to other NSAIDs or to sulfonamides and should also be avoided during pregnancy.

High-dose celecoxib (800 mg/day) has been associated with an increased risk of myocardial infarction in a population of patients using it to prevent colon polyps. All NSAIDs and celecoxib may have increased cardiovascular toxicity in high-risk patients. Careful risk-benefit decisions must be made in all patients.

Supply
Capsules, 100, 200, and 400 mg.

Dosage
A dosage of 200 to 400 mg in single or divided doses daily. Maximum daily dosage is 400 mg.

Diclofenac (Cataflam, Voltaren, Arthrotec)

Action
Inhibits prostaglandin synthesis.

Metabolism
Diclofenac is a phenylacetic acid derivative. Absorption is delayed by food. Peak plasma level after administration occurs in 2 to 3 hours. Ninety-nine percent is reversibly bound to plasma albumin. The half-life is approximately 2 hours. It is metabolized and excreted through urine (65%) and bile (35%).

Adverse Reactions
Gastrointestinal ulceration, bleeding, and perforation occur in 1% of patients. Headaches and dizziness are common. Elevation in levels of transaminases is present in 2% of patients and is generally reversible, although severe hepatotoxicity has been reported. Cross-reactivity occurs in patients with aspirin sensitivity.

Caution
Owing to potential hepatotoxicity, liver function test results should be followed up closely. Signs and symptoms of gastrointestinal bleeding and renal dysfunction should also be monitored. Diclofenac displaces albumin-bound drugs, which may lead to interaction with other drugs. Renal prostaglandin effects may increase toxicity of methotrexate, digoxin, and cyclosporine. Extreme caution should be exercised or this drug should be avoided in patients taking anticoagulants.

Supply
Tablets, 25, 50, and 75 mg. The 50- and 75-mg preparations are also available in combination with misoprostol (200 µg).

Dosage
A dosage of 50 to 75 mg twice daily, which may be increased to a maximum of 200 mg/day.

Diflunisal (Dolobid)

Action
Inhibits prostaglandin synthesis.

Metabolism
Diflunisal is a difluorophenyl derivative of salicylic acid that is not metabolized to salicylic acid. Peak plasma level occurs 2 to 3 hours after ingestion. Ninety percent is excreted through the urine as glucuronides. The plasma half-life is 8 to 12 hours.

Adverse Reactions
See section Aspirin. Diflunisal may cause less gastrointestinal irritation than aspirin. The dose-related effect on platelet function is reversible.

Caution
See section Aspirin. More than 99% of diflunisal is protein bound and may displace other protein-bound drugs, with resultant drug interactions. Serious interaction with indomethacin has been reported.

Supply
Tablets, 250 and 500 mg.

Dosage
A dosage of 250 to 500 mg twice daily An initial loading dose of 1,000 mg may accelerate attainment of steady state serum levels. Maximum dose is 1,500 mg.

Etodolac (Lodine)

Action
Inhibits prostaglandin synthesis.

Metabolism
Etodolac is an indole acetic acid derivative. Food or antacids do not appear to compromise gastrointestinal absorption, although peak serum concentrations and time to attain peak concentrations may be affected.

Adverse Reactions
Dyspepsia and gastrointestinal intolerance are common. Hepatic and renal toxicities are of concern. Other intolerances include hypertension, edema, malaise, depression, and dermatologic reactions.

Caution
Hepatic and renal function should be monitored closely with long-term use.

Supply
Capsules, 200 and 300 mg; tablets, 400 mg and 500 mg.

Dosage
A dosage of 200 to 300 mg twice daily or three times daily Maximum daily dosage is 1,200 mg.

Fenoprofen Calcium (Nalfon)

Action
Inhibits prostaglandin synthesis.

Metabolism
Fenoprofen is a propionic acid derivative. It is rapidly absorbed, with peak plasma levels in 90 minutes and a half-life of 160 minutes; concomitant food ingestion decreases rate and extent of absorption. The drug undergoes enterohepatic circulation. Ninety percent is excreted through the urine as glucuronides. Aspirin decreases the peak blood levels.

Adverse Reactions
Dyspepsia and gastrointestinal bleeding occur less commonly than with aspirin. Rash, headache, sodium retention, and, rarely, interstitial nephritis and nephrotic syndrome may occur.

Caution
Fenoprofen is 90% protein bound and may displace other protein-bound drugs with resultant drug interactions. Cross-reactivity occurs in patients with aspirin sensitivity.

Supply
Tablets, 600 mg; capsules, 200 and 300 mg.

Dosage
A dosage of 300 to 600 mg four times daily. Maximum daily dosage is 3.2 g.

Flurbiprofen (Ansaid)

Action
Inhibits prostaglandin synthesis.

Metabolism
Flurbiprofen is a phenylalkanoic acid derivative. It is well absorbed, with peak levels in 1.5 hours, and has an elimination half-life of 5.7 hours. It is extensively metabolized and excreted primarily through the urine. It is 99% protein bound.

Adverse Reactions
Dyspepsia, nausea, diarrhea, and abdominal pain are common. Gastrointestinal ulceration and bleeding may occur. Headaches and fluid retention are also common. Renal and hepatic dysfunction may occur but usually are reversible upon discontinuation of the drug.

Caution
Flurbiprofen is protein bound, it may modify levels of other protein-bound drugs. It may affect bleeding parameters and should be used with caution in patients receiving anticoagulants.

Supply
Tablets, 50 and 100 mg.

Dosage
A dosage of 200 to 300 mg/day administered in three to four divided doses.

Ibuprofen (Advil, Motrin, Nuprin, Vicoprofen)

Action
Inhibits prostaglandin synthesis.

Metabolism
Ibuprofen is a propionic acid derivative. It is 38% protein bound, and the half-life is 2 hours. It is primarily metabolized by the liver. Approximately equivalent amounts of the metabolized drug are excreted through urine and feces.

Adverse Reactions
Dyspepsia is common. Occult gastrointestinal bleeding may be less common than with aspirin. Occasionally, headaches, rashes, and salt retention occur. Aseptic meningitis and hypersensitivity reactions, notably in patients with SLE, have been reported.

Caution
Ibuprofen decreases platelet aggregation and prolongs bleeding time. Caution must be exercised in patients taking anticoagulants. Concomitant use with aspirin may decrease the effect of the aspirin. Cross-reactivity occurs in patients with aspirin sensitivity. It is not recommended during pregnancy. There is no clear evidence of effectiveness when the daily dosage is increased to 2,400 mg.

Supply
Tablets, 300, 400, 600, and 800 mg (200 mg available over-the-counter). Also available in combination with hydrocodone bitartrate (7.5 mg).

Dosage
A dosage of 1,200 to 2,400 mg in three to four divided doses.

Indomethacin (Indocin)

Action
Inhibits prostaglandin synthesis.

Metabolism
Indomethacin is an indoleacetic acid and is 90% bound to albumin. The kidneys excrete 65% of the metabolized drug. Probenecid may increase plasma levels of indomethacin by interfering with its excretion.

Adverse Reactions
Gastrointestinal side effects (dyspepsia, bleeding, nausea, and vomiting) occur in 10% to 40% of patients on prolonged use. Central nervous system side effects, occurring in 10% to 25% of patients, include headaches, vertigo, dizziness, blurred vision, and psychiatric disturbances. Less common problems include sodium retention, exacerbation of hypertension, hepatitis, and bone marrow suppression.

Caution
Indomethacin is not recommended for pregnant women or breast-feeding mothers. It antagonizes the natriuretic and antihypertensive effects of furosemide. Indomethacin should be used cautiously in patients with coagulation defects or in patients receiving anticoagulants because it does inhibit platelet aggregation. Cross-reactivity occurs in patients with aspirin sensitivity.

Supply
Capsules, 25 and 50 mg; sustained-release, 75 mg; oral suspension, 25 mg/mL; and rectal suppositories, 50 mg.

Dosage
A dosage of 25 mg three times daily or four times daily, taken with meals. Dosage can be gradually increased by 25-mg increments to 150 to 200 mg/day. The sustained-release preparation may be taken once or twice daily to a maximum of 150 mg/day.

Ketoprofen (Orudis, Oruvail, Actron)

Action
Inhibits prostaglandin synthesis.

Metabolism
Ketoprofen is a propionic acid derivative that is well absorbed after oral administration, but delayed and reduced peak concentrations occur when administered with food. Peak plasma levels are reached at 0.5 to 2 hours with a half-life of 2 to 4 hours. The drug is 99% bound to protein. Kidneys excrete 60% of drug as glucuronide, and enterohepatic recirculation accounts for the other 40%.

Adverse Reactions
Dyspepsia, gastrointestinal ulceration, bleeding, and perforation may occur in up to 1% to 2% of patients with long-term use. Central nervous system side effects such as headache, dizziness, and drowsiness are the second most common adverse reactions. Impaired renal function [edema, increased blood urea nitrogen (BUN)] and interstitial nephritis may occur. Reversible mild elevation of transaminase levels may be seen in up to 15% of patients, but marked elevations are seen in less than 1%. Cross-reactivity occurs in patients with aspirin sensitivity.

Caution

Ketoprofen displaces albumin-bound drugs, which may lead to interactions with methotrexate and other protein-bound drugs. It decreases platelet adhesion and aggregation and should be used with caution in patients on anticoagulation.

Supply

Capsules, 25, 50, and 75 mg; sustained-release capsules, 100, 150, 200 mg (12.5 mg tablets are available over-the-counter).

Dosage

Starting dosage of 75 mg three times daily or 50 mg four times daily. Daily dose is 150 to 300 mg in three or four divided doses.

Ketorolac (Toradol)

Action

Inhibits prostaglandin synthesis.

Metabolism

Ketorolac, a pyrrolizine carboxylic acid derivative, is available as a trimethamine salt. It is the only NSAID available in the United States that can be administered orally or parenterally (intramuscular or intravenous). The bioavailability of the drug is very high regardless of the route of administration, although the rate of absorption is slowest following intramuscular injection. When administered orally, the rate of absorption, but not the extent of absorption, may be diminished with food. The rate of absorption is also reduced in the geriatric patient or in the setting of hepatic or renal impairment. Peak plasma concentrations may be achieved within 3 minutes after intravenous administration. The drug is hydroxylated in the liver and mainly excreted through urine.

Adverse Reactions

Adverse nervous system reactions including headache, somnolence, and dizziness have been reported in up to 23% of patients. Gastrointestinal intolerance is reported in 13% of patients, regardless of the route of administration, but is probably even more common in elderly patients in whom the drug is commonly prescribed to avoid the use of narcotics. Borderline elevations of serum liver enzymes may be detected in up to 15% of patients, although less than 1% have elevations more than three times of normal limits. Anaphylactoid reactions have been rarely reported.

Caution

Ketorolac is bound tightly to serum proteins. However, it does not displace digoxin and only slightly displaces warfarin. Gastrointestinal hemorrhage is a significant concern, and it is recommended that the use of ketorolac be limited to acute and severe pain and to not exceed 5 consecutive days. Dosage adjustment is necessary with renal or hepatic impairment.

Supply

Tablets, 10 mg; injectable 15 and 30 mg/mL.

Dosage

Oral dosage is 10 mg up to four times daily. The initial intravenous and intramuscular doses are 15 to 30 mg and 30 to 60 mg, respectively. Up to 30 mg can then be used for maintenance of parenteral administration every 6 hours.

Meclofenamate Sodium (Meclomen)

Action

Inhibits prostaglandin synthesis.

Metabolism

Meclofenamate sodium is an anthranilic acid derivative. Peak plasma levels occur in 30 to 60 minutes with a half-life of approximately 3 hours; concomitant antacid administration does not interfere with absorption. Approximately two-thirds is excreted through the urine, mostly as the glucuronide conjugate, while approximately one-third appears in the feces.

Adverse Reactions
Gastrointestinal reactions occur more frequently than with aspirin. Diarrhea may occur in up to one-third of patients; nausea in approximately 10% of patients. Headache, dizziness, rash, and other reactions associated with NSAIDs may also occur.

Caution
Meclofenamate sodium enhances the effect of warfarin but has a smaller effect than aspirin on platelet aggregation. The drug is not recommended for use during pregnancy. Cross-reactivity occurs in patients with aspirin sensitivity.

Supply
Capsules, 50 and 100 mg.

Dosage
A dosage of 50 to 100 mg four times daily.

Mefenamic Acid (Ponstel)

Action
Inhibits prostaglandin synthesis.

Metabolism
Mefenamic acid is an anthranilic acid derivative, which is rapidly absorbed after oral administration. After metabolism in the liver, approximately two-thirds of the drug is excreted through urine, while the remaining one-third is eliminated through the feces.

Adverse Reactions
Gastrointestinal adverse reactions are the most common and include diarrhea, nausea, dyspepsia, and peptic ulcer disease. Mild reversible liver enzyme abnormalities are frequent (up to 15%).

Caution
Mefenamic acid is highly protein bound. It enhances the effects of warfarin and can elevate serum lithium concentrations.

Supply
Capsules, 250 mg.

Dosage
A dose of 500 mg loading dose followed by 250 mg every 6 hours.

Meloxicam (Mobic)

Action
Meloxicam is a derivative of oxicam and inhibits prostaglandin synthesis.

Metabolism
The absorption of meloxicam appears to be insignificantly affected by coadministration with food. Peak blood levels occur at approximately 5 hours. The mean half-life is between 15 and 20 hours. The drug is primarily metabolized by the cytochrome P-450 system (2C9 and 3A4), and the metabolites are excreted fecally and renally.

Adverse Reactions
Gastrointestinal bleeding, peptic ulceration, dyspepsia, tinnitus, dizziness, headache, edema, and other reactions generally associated with NSAIDs may occur.

Caution
Meloxicam can inhibit platelet aggregation; therefore, although not shown to greatly affect the effects of warfarin, concomitant use is discouraged. The drug is not recommended for use during pregnancy. Cross-reactivity may occur in aspirin-sensitive patients. Like for other drugs with long half-lives, special care should be provided for the older individuals.

Supply
Tablets, 7.5 and 15 mg.

Dosage
A dosage of 7.5 to 15 mg/day.

Naproxen (Naprosyn, Naprelan, Aleve)

Action
An arylalkanoic derivative that inhibits prostaglandin synthesis.

Metabolism
Absorption is not significantly delayed by food. Ninety-eight percent is protein bound. The half-life is 12 to 15 hours. Kidneys excrete 80% to 90% in conjugated form. Aspirin decreases peak plasma levels.

Adverse Reactions
Gastrointestinal bleeding, dyspepsia, headache, dizziness, and sodium retention occur less frequently than with aspirin. Interstitial nephritis rarely occurs.

Caution
Naproxen displaces albumin-bound drugs, which may lead to drug interactions. It inhibits platelet aggregation and should be used with caution in patients taking anticoagulants. Cross-reactivity occurs in patients with aspirin sensitivity.

Supply
Tablets, 250, 375, and 500 mg. Single daily dosage, sustained-release formulations are available. Nonprescription strength tablets are also available.

Dosage
A dosage of 250 mg twice daily, which may be increased to 500 mg twice daily. Up to 1,000 mg of the sustained-release formulation may be taken once a day.

Oxaprozin (Daypro)

Action
Inhibits prostaglandin synthesis.

Metabolism
Oxaprozin is a propionic acid derivative. The rate but not the extent of gastrointestinal absorption is reduced by food, and not by antacids.

Adverse Reactions
Gastrointestinal precautions should be observed as with other NSAIDs.

Caution
Geriatric patients may tolerate the drug less well because of the long half-life of the drug. Modification of the dosage is necessary in the setting of renal impairment and significant liver disease.

Supply
Tablets, 600 mg.

Dosage
A dosage of 600 to 1,800 mg/day in single doses.

Piroxicam (Feldene)

Action
Inhibits prostaglandin synthesis.

Metabolism
Piroxicam is an oxicam derivative that is well absorbed after oral administration with no effect of antacids on plasma levels. Peak levels are achieved 3 to 5 hours after administration with a long but variable half-life (range 30 to 86 hours). The drug is excreted through urine and feces (approximately 2:1), with less than 5% of it being unchanged by biotransformation. Piroxicam is highly protein bound.

Adverse Reactions
Gastrointestinal bleeding, peptic ulceration, dyspepsia, tinnitus, dizziness, headache, edema, and other reactions generally associated with NSAIDs may occur.

Caution
Piroxicam can displace other protein-bound drugs, such as warfarin. Platelet aggregation may be affected. The drug is not recommended for use during pregnancy. Cross-reactivity occurs in aspirin-sensitive patients. Like for other drugs with long half-lives, special care should be provided for the older individuals.

Supply
Capsules, 10 and 20 mg.

Dosage
A dosage of 20 mg/day. Higher doses are not recommended and may be associated with increased gastrointestinal side effects.

Salicylate Salts (Trilisate)

Action
Inhibit prostaglandin synthesis.

Metabolism
See section Aspirin.

Adverse Reactions
Salicylates other than aspirin may cause less gastrointestinal disturbance and less gastrointestinal bleeding than aspirin. They have fewer inhibitory effects on platelet function.

Caution
Sodium salicylate may constitute a substantial sodium load for patients with heart failure or hypertension. Hypermagnesemic toxicity may develop with magnesium salicylate in patients with renal insufficiency.

Supply
Sodium salicylate tablets 325 and 650 mg; choline salicylate liquid, 870 mg/5 mL; magnesium salicylate tablets, 325, 500, 545, 600 mg; choline magnesium trisalicylate tablets, 293 mg/363 mg, 440 mg/544 mg, 587 mg/725 mg; choline magnesium trisalicylate liquid, 293 mg/5 mL choline salicylate and 362 mg/5 mL magnesium salicylate; trolamine salicylate 10% cream or lotion.

Dosage
Sodium salicylate 325 to 650 mg every 4 hours, maximum of 5,400 mg/day.
Choline salicylate 435 to 870 mg every 4 hours, maximum of 7,200 mg/day.
Magnesium salicylate 300 to 600 mg every 4 hours, maximum of 3,500 mg/day.

Choline magnesium trisalicylate, maximum 4,500 mg total salicylate, daily in divided doses. Trolamine salicylate 10% cream or lotion, two to four times daily for topical use.

Salsalate (Disalcid, Argesic, Salflex, Salsitab)

Action
Inhibits prostaglandin synthesis.

Metabolism
Salsalate is the salicylate ester of salicylic acid and is activated after hydrolysis to salicylate. It is completely absorbed by the gastrointestinal tract, mostly in the small intestine. However, because up to 13% of the drug is conjugated with glucuronic acid in the liver and not hydrolyzed to active metabolites, the bioavailability of salsalate is less than that of a theoretically equivalent intake of salicylate. The drug is almost exclusively excreted through urine.

Adverse Reactions
See section Salicylate Salts.

Caution
See section Salicylate Salts.

Supply
Capsules, 500 mg; tablets, 500 and 750 mg.

Dosage
A dosage of 500 to 750 mg twice daily; maximum daily dosage 4,000 mg.

Sulindac (Clinoril)

Action
Inhibits prostaglandin synthesis.

Metabolism
An indene acetic derivative of indomethacin, sulindac requires hepatic activation to the active sulfide metabolite. The half-life of sulindac is approximately 8 hours, whereas the half-life of the active sulfide metabolite is 16 to 18 hours. It is tightly protein bound. Metabolites are excreted largely in the kidney, with 25% to 30% being found in feces.

Adverse Reactions
Dyspepsia, nausea, gastrointestinal bleeding, tinnitus, headaches, dizziness, hepatitis, rash, and edema may occur. There are reports of relative sparing of renal function when compared to other NSAIDs, but these remain subject to debate and do not justify unmonitored use in patients at risk for renal impairment.

Caution
Sulindac may potentiate oral hypoglycemic agents, anticoagulants, and other protein-bound drugs. It prolongs bleeding time and should be used with caution in patients receiving anticoagulants. Cross-reactivity may occur in patients with aspirin sensitivity.

Supply
Tablets, 150 and 200 mg.

Dosage
A dosage of 150 mg twice daily. The dosage may be increased to 200 mg twice daily.

Tolmetin Sodium (Tolectin)

Action
Inhibits prostaglandin synthesis.

Metabolism

The half-life of this pyrrole acetic acid derivative is 60 minutes. Ninety-nine percent of the drug is excreted through urine and 99% is protein bound.

Adverse Reactions

Peptic ulcers occur in 2% to 3% of patients. Gastrointestinal bleeding occurs in another 1%. Other reactions include diarrhea, abdominal pain, nausea, dyspepsia, rash, sodium retention, light-headedness, headache, and dizziness.

Caution

False-positive tests for urinary protein are noted when sulfosalicylic acid, but not tetrabromophenol-blue (Albustix), is used. It may decrease platelet adhesiveness and prolong bleeding time. Cross-reactivity occurs in patients with aspirin sensitivity.

Supply

Tablets, 200 and 600 mg; capsules, 400 mg.

Dosage

A dosage of 400 mg three times daily, preferably including doses on waking up and at bedtime. Dosages higher than 1,800 mg/day are not recommended. Tolmetin is approved for use in children.

CORTICOSTEROIDS AND CORTICOTROPIN

Corticosteroids are potent anti-inflammatory agents capable of quickly suppressing many disease manifestations of systemic, autoimmune, and inflammatory disorders, and are available in forms suitable for topical, locally injectable, and systemic use. Corticotropin or adrenocorticotropic hormone (ACTH) has been used for the treatment of acute crystalline arthritides. Although their ability to modify the ultimate course of disease varies from disease to disease, their side effects with prolonged use are incontrovertible. Among the plethora of adverse effects associated with corticosteroid use, hypertension, weight gain, Cushing's syndrome, glucose intolerance, osteoporosis, osteonecrosis, emotional lability, premature atherosclerosis, immunosuppression, and others are included. Strong efforts should be made to employ disease-modifying agents to ensure that corticosteroids play as minimal a role as possible in the management of inflammatory arthritis. Similarly, long-term use of agents with long half-lives (e.g., dexamethasone) is generally not favored by rheumatologists because of their increased propensity to cause these adverse effects.

Corticosteroids differ in relative anti-inflammatory (glucocorticoid) potency and relative mineralocorticoid potency. A comparison of the properties of different selected corticosteroids is given in Table 3.

Corticosteroids

Action

Corticosteroid agents suppress inflammation, as well as humoral and cell-mediated immune responses.

Metabolism

Corticosteroids are well absorbed from the gastrointestinal tract. Prednisone is a prodrug, which is hepatically metabolized to prednisolone, the active compound. Further hepatic metabolism results in the inactivation of corticosteroids. Corticosteroids are 90% protein bound.

Adverse Reactions

Systemic corticosteroid therapy is associated with numerous potential adverse effects that are more likely to occur with prolonged or high-dose use. Cutaneous side effects include acne, hirsutism, striae, purpura, thinning of the skin, and impaired wound healing. Osteoporosis, myopathy, and aseptic necrosis of bone may occur. Gastrointestinal side effects

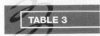

TABLE 3	Comparison of Selected Corticosteroids		
Drug	Equivalent dose[a]	Relative anti-inflammatory potency	Relative mineralocorticoid potency
Cortisone	25	0.8	2
Hydrocortisone	20	1	2
Prednisone	5	4	1
Prednisolone	5	4	1
Methylprednisolone	4	5	0.5
Triamcinolone	4	5	0
Paramethasone	2	10	0
Dexamethasone	0.75	25	0
Betamethasone	0.6	30	0

[a] Based on anti-inflammatory effects.

include peptic ulceration with bleeding or perforation, especially when administered with NSAIDs. Hypertension and edema, secondary to fluid retention occur commonly. Steroid psychosis and benign intracranial hypertension are the central nervous system adverse reactions. Ocular effects include cataracts and glaucoma. Patients may experience growth arrest, secondary amenorrhea, impotence, and suppression of the hypothalamic–pituitary–adrenal axis. Glucose intolerance, hyperosmolar nonketotic coma, and centripetal obesity occur. There is increased susceptibility to bacterial, fungal, mycobacterial, and viral infections.

Intra-articular corticosteroids may cause a crystal-induced transient synovitis. NSAIDs, rest, and cold compresses will facilitate resolution of condition; persistence of the synovitis beyond 24 hours raises the possibility of an arthrocentesis-introduced infectious arthritis. Topical corticosteroids, especially the more potent fluorinated compounds, may cause cutaneous telangiectasia, striae, epidermal and dermal atrophy, rosacealike facial eruptions, and senile-type purpura. When used with occlusive dressings, infection, folliculitis, and decreased heat exchange may occur.

Caution
Blood sugar levels, complete blood counts, stool guaiacs, and blood pressure should be periodically determined. Diabetes mellitus, hypertension, pregnancy, and psychosis are relative contraindications. Patients receiving steroids for a long term have a suppressed hypothalamic–pituitary–adrenal axis and require glucocorticoid supplementation during surgical procedures or other physiologic stress. Repeated administration of intra-articular and periarticular injections of corticosteroids may lead to disruption of cartilage and supporting soft-tissue structures. Long-term steroid usage demands appropriate immunizations and measures to ensure protection against osteoporosis.

Systemic absorption of topical steroid preparations may occur. Prolonged use, especially of the more potent compounds, can lead to suppression of the hypothalamic–pituitary–adrenal axis.

Dosage
The safest steroid regimen is characterized by the lowest, effective dosage for the shortest period. Numerous schedules for administering corticosteroids have been developed to limit side effects and maximize therapeutic response. Prednisone and methylprednisolone are the most widely used preparations for systemic use and are typically administered once to four times daily. Alternate-day regimens may possibly decrease the incidence of side effects but often are insufficient to suppress disease activity adequately.

Intra-articular corticosteroids are useful in patients with only one or a few symptomatic joints. Dosages vary from 5 mg of methylprednisolone for small joints of the hand to up to 80 mg for large joints such as the knee.

The efficacy of topical steroids is related to both potency and percutaneous penetration. Adequate hydration of the skin, inflammation, and occlusion with plastic wraps enhance penetration. Better biologic activity is often obtained with ointment rather than cream or lotion preparations. As a general principle, therapy is started with stronger preparations and later switched over to less-potent strengths once control of skin manifestations is achieved.

Supply

I. **SELECTED ORAL PREPARATIONS.** Prednisone tablets, 1, 2.5, 5, 10, 20, and 50 mg. Prednisolone tablets, 1, 2.5, and 5 mg. Methylprednisolone tablets, 2, 4, 8, 16, 24, and 32 mg. Dexamethasone tablets, 0.25, 0.5, 0.75, 1.5, and 4 mg.

II. **SELECTED PARENTERAL PREPARATIONS.** Hydrocortisone vial, 100, 250, 500, and 1,000 mg. Methylprednisolone vial, 40, 125, 500, and 1,000 mg.

III. **SELECTED INTRA-ARTICULAR PREPARATIONS.** Methylprednisolone acetate, 20 and 40 mg/mL suspension in 1-, 5-, and 10-mL containers. Triamcinolone acetonide, 40 mg/mL suspension in 1-, 5-, and 10-mL vials; 10 mg/mL suspension in 5-mL vials. Triamcinolone hexacetonide, 20 mg/mL suspension in 1- and 5-mL vials. Prednisolone tertiary butylacetate, 20 mg/mL suspension in 1-, 5-, and 10-mL vials.

IV. **SELECTED TOPICAL PREPARATIONS**

    A. Very high strength. Betamethasone dipropionate 0.05% (Alphatrex, Diprolene, Maxivate, Psorion), clobetasol propionate 0.05% (Temovate), diflorasone diacetate 0.05% (Psorcon), halobetasol propionate 0.05% (Ultravate).

    B. High strength. Desoximetasone 0.25% (Topicort), fluocinolone acetonide 0.2% (Synalar-HP), fluocinonide 0.05% (Lidex), halcinonide 0.1% (Halog), triamcinolone acetonide 0.1% (Aristocort A).

    C. Moderate strength. Betamethasone valerate 0.1% (Valisone), fluocinolone acetonide 0.025% (Synalar), flurandrenolide 0.05% (Cordran), hydrocortisone valerate 0.2% (Westcort), triamcinolone acetonide 0.025% (Kenalog, Aristocort).

    D. Low strength. Hydrocortisone 0.25%, 0.5%, and 1.0%. Other preparations with cortisone, prednisolone, methylprednisolone acetate.

Corticotropin

Action

Corticotropin stimulates secretion of cortisol by the adrenal glands. However, because corticotropin is beneficial even in patients with adrenal suppression being treated for crystal-induced arthritis, other mechanisms of action are also postulated.

Selected Indications

Acute crystal-induced arthritides.

Metabolism

Corticotropin is a polypeptide usually extracted from the porcine pituitary gland and is administered either intramuscularly or intravenously. Peak plasma cortisol levels are achieved usually within 1 hour of injection. The metabolism of corticotropin is not fully known, but it is rapidly removed from plasma by many tissues.

Adverse Reactions

Corticotropin may cause immediate hypersensitivity reactions even without previous exposure, which may range from minor skin reactions to anaphylaxis. With prolonged use, typical toxicities associated with corticosteroid use may occur. Moreover, suppression of endogenous corticotropin release by the pituitary may result in hypothalamic-pituitary insufficiency.

Caution

Corticotropin is contraindicated in patients with known previous hypersensitivity reactions to the medication or to porcine proteins.

Supply
A dose of 25 or 40 units for intramuscular, intravenous, or subcutaneous injection.

Dosage
A dosage of 25 to 40 units every 8 hours for up to 2 days.

DISEASE-MODIFYING ANTIRHEUMATIC DRUGS

Disease-modifying antirheumatic drugs (DMARDs) are much more readily and promptly utilized for the treatment of systemic rheumatic illnesses than before. Also called slowly acting antirheumatic drugs (SAARDs) or remittive agents in the medical literature, these drugs certainly are slowly acting but probably do not induce indefinite remissions in most cases. In rheumatoid arthritis, for example, the capacity of these agents to modify disease varies greatly from drug to drug and from patient to patient. As a group, their modes of action are quite varied but often poorly understood. Some are clearly immunosuppressive or cytotoxic, whereas others may act on reducing systemic inflammation. Their potential for and spectrum of adverse effects are diverse, so careful monitoring for toxicities is crucial. Although their clinical effect generally becomes apparent only after several weeks to months, they appear capable of ameliorating the course of disease in a significant percentage of patients and reducing cumulative corticosteroid use. Accordingly, DMARDs are also commonly used and known as steroid-sparing agents. Moreover, there appears to be advantages in using combinations of DMARDs to maximize benefit without the development of increasing toxicities.

Azathioprine (AZA) (Imuran) and 6-mercaptopurine (Purinethol)

Action
Inhibition of purine synthesis.

Selected Indications
Rheumatoid arthritis, SLE, vasculitis.

Metabolism
AZA is a prodrug, which is converted to the active compound 6-mercaptopurine. However, because of better gastrointestinal absorption, AZA is more widely used. Urinary excretion, partial hepatic metabolism, and tissue uptake account for its clearance from the blood.

Adverse Reactions
Hematologic toxicity is usually mild leukopenia and thrombocytopenia; aplastic anemia is rare. Drug fever and a severe systemic allergiclike reaction may occur. Hepatitis and pancreatitis may also occur. Nausea, especially during initiation of therapy, is common. Stomatitis may be seen. An increased incidence of late lymphoreticular and hematopoietic malignancy is possible. The immunosuppressive effects of these drugs increase susceptibility to infections.

Caution
Complete blood counts and platelet counts should be obtained on a weekly basis at the outset of therapy and then on a monthly basis when a stable dosage is determined. A rapid fall in leukocyte count requires a decrease in dosage or discontinuation of the drug. Liver function tests should be obtained periodically. Allopurinol inhibits the metabolism of both AZA and 6-mercaptopurine, causing high levels to accumulate; therefore, concomitant use of allopurinol should either be avoided or a significant reduction in the dosage of AZA dose by 75% is appropriate. AZA has been used safely during pregnancy, but as with any medication, discontinuation of the drug, if possible, is preferable. Dosages must be adjusted in patients with hepatic or renal impairment.

Supply
AZA tablets, 50 mg. 6-mercaptopurine tablets, 50 mg.

Dosage
AZA, 2 to 3 mg/kg/day. 6-mercaptopurine, 1 to 2 mg/kg/day.

Chlorambucil (Leukeran)

Action
Alkylating agent that interferes with cell function and mitotic activity by inhibition of intracellular macromolecules.

Selected Indications
Severe rheumatoid arthritis, SLE, vasculitis.

Metabolism
Oral absorption is generally reliable. There is incomplete information about metabolism and excretion.

Adverse Reactions
Myelosuppression is usually moderate, gradual, and rapidly reversible. Gastrointestinal discomfort, dermatitis, and hepatotoxicity occasionally occur.

Caution
Complete blood counts should be frequently obtained. Delayed occurrence of acute leukemia is reported. Infertility may occur in both sexes.

Supply
Tablets, 2 mg.

Dosage
A dosage of 0.05 to 0.2 mg/kg/day. Total daily dosage (usually 4 to 10 mg) is administered as a single dose.

Chloroquine (Aralen)

Action
The mode of action of chloroquine is unknown. Potential actions include binding nucleic acids, stabilization of lysosomal membranes, and trapping of free radicals.

Selected Indications
Rheumatoid arthritis, SLE, cutaneous lupus erythematosus.

Metabolism
Chloroquine is well absorbed from the gastrointestinal tract. The drug is concentrated and retained in body tissues. Peak plasma concentrations are attained within 2 hours, which may be facilitated by coadministration with food. Chloroquine and its metabolites are slowly excreted by the kidneys. Unabsorbed drug is eliminated through the feces.

Adverse Reactions
Most common side effects are allergic eruptions and gastrointestinal disturbances (e.g., anorexia, nausea, cramps, diarrhea). The most serious, potential complication is ocular toxicity that appears to be dose-dependent but more common than with hydroxychloroquine. Reversible corneal deposits of the drug are detectable by slit-lamp examination, but retinopathy affecting macular pigmentation may be irreversible. Less common side effects include hyperpigmented rash, hypopigmentation of hair, neuropathy, ototoxicity, and cardiomyopathy. Hematologic toxicity is rare.

Caution

Ophthalmologic examination (color testing, visual fields, funduscopy, slit-lamp examination) should be performed every 4 to 6 months. Complete blood count should be performed periodically. At the first sign of visual disturbance, the drug should be discontinued. Chloroquine may cause hemolytic anemia in patients with glucose-6-phosphate dehydrogenase (G-6-PD) deficiency. The drug is contraindicated in patients with significant visual, hepatic or renal impairment, porphyria, and in patients who are pregnant.

Supply

Tablets, 250 and 500 mg.

Dosage

A dosage of 250 mg/day.

Cotrimoxazole (Bactrim, Septra)

Action

Cotrimoxazole is a fixed combination of sulfamethoxazole (SMX) and trimethoprim (TMP), both of which are synthetic folate antagonists. Although most widely used as an anti-infective, it has found use in some cases of limited Wegener's granulomatosis,

Selected Indications

Mild Wegener's granulomatosis, prophylaxis against *Pneumocystis carinii* infections.

Metabolism

Cotrimoxazole is rapidly absorbed after oral administration, and peak plasma levels of both components are reached within 4 hours. The liver converts TMP to oxide and hydroxylated metabolites, and acetylates and conjugates SMX to its metabolites. Almost all of these metabolites are excreted through the urine. Elimination of cotrimoxazole is highly dependent on the renal function.

Adverse Reactions

Gastrointestinal intolerances and hypersensitivity skin reactions of all degrees account for most adverse effects. Hypersensitive reactions may occur more commonly in patients with SLE. Cytopenias may occur, especially in individuals with underlying hematologic abnormalities. Patients with renal impairment may develop potentially life-threatening electrolyte abnormalities, particularly hyperkalemia.

Caution

Cotrimoxazole should be used with caution in the setting of liver or kidney impairment, underlying hematologic problems, and possibly folate or G-6-PD deficiency. Patients with sulfa allergies should not receive cotrimoxazole.

Supply

Tablets, TMP 80 mg/SMX 400 mg and TMP 160 mg/SMX 800 mg.

Dosage

For limited Wegener's granulomatosis, TMP 160 mg/SMX 800 mg twice daily. For prophylaxis against *P. carinii*, TMP 160 mg/SMX 800 three times a week.

Cyclophosphamide (Cytoxan)

Action

Cyclophosphamide is an alkylating agent that structurally damages nucleic acids and proteins, resulting in immunosuppressive effects.

Selected Indications

Severe rheumatoid arthritis, SLE, systemic vasculitis, systemic sclerosis, and interstitial lung disease.

Metabolism

The drug is well absorbed from the gastrointestinal tract. It requires activation by the liver to produce active metabolites. Genitourinary exposure to unchanged drug and metabolites excreted through the urine results in significant toxicities.

Adverse Reactions

Anorexia, nausea, and vomiting are common complaints but can be treated with antiemetic agents. More seriously, bone marrow depression and predisposition to infection can be life-threatening but are generally reversible with discontinuation of the drug. Alopecia, infertility in both sexes (amenorrhea or defective spermatogenesis), hemorrhagic cystitis (in up to 25% of patients), fibrosing cystitis, carcinoma of the bladder, hematopoietic malignancies, and pulmonary fibrosis can occur. Antidiuretic hormonelike activity may occur with large doses and result in clinically significant hyponatremia.

Caution

Cyclophosphamide is relatively contraindicated in pregnant women and in patients with hepatic impairment. Dosage requires adjustment in the setting of renal insufficiency. Complete blood counts, platelet counts, and urine analysis must be frequently obtained. Maintenance of high urine output and the use of 2-mercaptoethane sulfonate (MESNA) may reduce bladder complications. Hormonal therapy or cryopreservation of sperm, fertilized or unfertilized ova, or ovarian tissue may be considered to address issues of cyclophosphamide-induced infertility.

Supply

Tablets, 25 and 50 mg; vials, 100, 200, and 500 mg for intravenous injection.

Dosage

Oral route: 0.5 to 3.5 mg/kg/day administered as single morning dosage. Intravenous route: For treatment of diffuse proliferative glomerulonephritis in SLE or systemic vasculitides, begin with monthly intravenous treatments at an initial dose of 0.5 g/m^2; subsequent dosages can be increased by 25% if the 7- to 10-day postinfusion leukocyte count is greater than 5,000/mL or decreased by 25% if the 7- to 10-day postinfusion leukocyte count is less than 3,000/mL. After 6-monthly treatments, the treatment interval is reduced to every 2 to 3 months for the second 6 months. Further treatments are defined by the clinical course. Adequate hydration and pretreatment with MESNA reduces the risks of bladder toxicities associated with intravenous use.

Cyclosporine A (Sandimmune, Neoral)

Action

Cyclosporine A is a nonpolar, cyclic oligopeptide. It is a potent inhibitor of early steps in T-cell activation via suppression of early gene transcription.

Selected Indications

Rheumatoid arthritis, psoriatic arthritis, other autoimmune diseases.

Metabolism

The unmetabolized drug is active. Absorption of cyclosporine A is variable after oral administration, averaging approximately 30% of the ingested dose but varying from 2% to 89%, and is reduced by coadministration of food. Serum levels may be followed up if desired. Cyclosporine A is available in two oral formulations, which differ in bioavailability and, therefore, do not exhibit equivalent dosing. The nonaqueous liquid formulation (Neoral) immediately forms an emulsion in aqueous fluids and has a bioavailability of 1.2 to 1.5 times that of the conventional liquid preparation (Sandimmune). Peak levels appear between 3 and 4 hours, and the drug is metabolized on first-pass through the liver. More than 90% of cyclosporine A is protein bound and bound mostly to lipoproteins. It crosses the placenta and into the breast milk. Approximately 95% is eliminated via feces.

Adverse Reactions

Nephrotoxicity is the most frequent and clinically significant adverse effect. In clinical trials, more than half of patients with rheumatoid arthritis treated with cyclosporine experienced significant elevation in serum creatinine levels, although less than 10% required discontinuation of the drug. New or exacerbation of pre-existing hypertension is also frequently observed. Other common side effects include gastrointestinal intolerance, infections, gout, hypertrichosis, hyperesthesias, paresthesias, gingival hyperplasia, abnormal results of liver function tests, and potential oncogenicity.

Caution

Daily dosage should not exceed 5 mg/kg body weight; the usual starting dose in rheumatoid arthritis is usually 2.5 mg/kg body weight daily. Careful monitoring of renal function and arterial blood pressure tests should be performed. The serum creatinine levels should not be allowed to increase to more than 50% of baseline. Hypertension may be controlled with nifedipine or isradipine, but not with verapamil or diltiazem, both of which interfere with the hepatic metabolism of cyclosporine A. Special caution should be exercised with concomitant use of methotrexate which can decrease the elimination of cyclosporine A. Other medications to be avoided because of drug interactions include antifungal azole derivatives (ketoconazole, fluconazole, itraconazole), macrolide antibiotics (erythromycin, clarithromycin), and allopurinol, among many others. Grapefruit juice increases the bioavailability of the drug. Cyclosporine A is contraindicated in premenopausal women who do not practice effective contraception, in pregnant women, and in breast-feeding mothers.

Supply

Capsules (Sandimmune), liquid filled, 25, 50, 100 mg; Capsules (Neoral), liquid filled, for emulsion, 25, 100 mg; Solution (Sandimmune), 100 mg/mL; Solution (Neoral), for emulsion, 20 mg.

Dosage

A dosage of 2 to 5 mg/kg body weight daily in twice a day dosing.

Dapsone

Action

Possible anti-inflammatory effects due to inhibition of prostaglandin synthesis, complement activation, and myeloperoxidase-mediated pathways.

Selected Indications

Cutaneous lupus erythematosus, SLE.

Metabolism

Dapsone is easily absorbed within the gastrointestinal tract. Peak levels are attained within 2 to 8 hours. The half-life of the drug is approximately 1 day. Dapsone is partially acetylated by the liver. The drug with its metabolites are mostly excreted through urine, approximately 20% of which is unchanged drug.

Adverse Reactions

Dose-dependent hemolytic anemia and methemoglobinemia are the most frequent serious adverse effects. Hemolysis may occur in patients with or without G-6-PD deficiency but is more severe in patients with G-6-PD deficiency. Supplementation with ascorbic acid, folic acid, and iron may prevent some of the hematologic effects. Cutaneous hypersensitivity and gastrointestinal intolerances may occur. Elevated results of liver function tests are common, but toxic hepatitis and cholestatic jaundice have been only rarely reported.

Caution

Patients with significant anemia should not receive dapsone, and G-6-PD screening may be indicated in individuals with a suspected high risk for hemolysis (e.g., concurrent medications with adverse hematologic effects) or myelosuppression. Complete blood counts and liver function tests should be followed weekly for the first month and then regularly thereafter with long-term administration.

Supply

Tablets, 25 and 100 mg.

Dosage

Initial dosage 50 mg/day; increases titrated to response to a maximum of 400 mg/day.

Intravenous Gammaglobulin

Action

Intravenous preparations of gammaglobulin contain modified polyvalent antibodies with intact opsonic activity, but with few or no aggregates. Action in thrombocytopenia may involve blockade of macrophage Fc receptors. Other proposed mechanisms of action include the activity of anti-idiotypic antibodies, effects on cytokine production and on cytokine receptors, and induction of increased catabolism of pathogenic immunoglobulin.

Selected Indications

Inflammatory myositis, immune thrombocytopenia purpura, SLE, Kawasaki's disease, and vasculitis.

Metabolism

It is evenly distributed in the intravascular and extravascular spaces after 6 days. The half-life is 3 weeks. Disaccharides used for stabilization are excreted through the urine.

Adverse Reactions

Less than 1% of patients develop reactions, including flushing, fever, dizziness, nausea, and hypotension, 30 to 60 minutes after infusions are begun. All patients should be observed carefully and vital signs monitored during infusions, but because of the high fluid load, particular caution should be taken in patients with congestive heart failure.

Caution

Patients with selective IgA deficiency may possess antibodies to IgA and should not receive intravenous gammaglobulin that has not been depleted of IgA molecules.

Supply

A dose of 1-, 3-, and 6-g vials with sodium chloride for reconstitution. IgA-depleted preparations are available.

Dosage

For treatment of inflammatory myositis or idiopathic thrombocytopenic purpura, 2 g/kg body weight (cumulative) in divided doses over 3 to 5 days.

Gold Compounds (Ridaura, Aurolate, Myochrysine)

Action

Mode of action of gold compounds in rheumatoid arthritis is unknown. Alters macrophage and complement functions.

Selected Indications

Rheumatoid arthritis, psoriatic arthritis.

Metabolism

Approximately half of the administered intramuscular dose is excreted within 1 week, 30% through the urine and the remainder through the stool. Gold in the circulation rapidly equilibrates with synovial fluid. It is stored by the reticuloendothelial system. It is 90% protein bound.

Approximately 25% of oral gold (auranofin) is absorbed and metabolized, with 15% being excreted through urine and the remainder through feces. In blood, it is 60% protein bound and 40% associated with red blood cells.

Adverse Reactions

Forty percent of patients experience some toxicity. Eosinophilia, although common, does not necessarily predict toxicity. The most common reaction is dermatitis, which may be heralded by pruritus or eosinophilia, or both. Both dermatitis and stomatitis are reversible with discontinuation of the drug or reduction of dosage, and except for the rare instances of exfoliative dermatitis, lower dosages are tolerated. Hematologic abnormalities occur in 1% to 2% of patients. Thrombocytopenia is most common, followed by leukopenia, agranulocytosis, and pancytopenia. Gold should not be restarted in patients with hematologic complications. Proteinuria may be seen in 4% of patients, but nephrotic syndrome with membranous glomerulonephritis is much less common. Proteinuria of greater than 0.5 g/day requires cessation of therapy. Proteinuria, hematuria, or leukocyturia is a signal to interrupt therapy until urinalysis gives normal results. Nitritoid reactions characterized by self-limited episodes of sweating, flushing, dizziness, nausea, and shortness of breath after administration of gold may occur with the thiomalate preparation. Unusual problems include enterocolitis, intrahepatic cholestasis, skin hyperpigmentation, peripheral neuropathy, pulmonary infiltrates, and deposits of gold in the cornea.

Adverse reactions to oral gold (auranofin) are similar to but are generally less frequent than that with intramuscular gold. The only exceptions are that abdominal discomfort and diarrhea are more common for oral gold.

Caution

Gold is contraindicated in patients with previous gold allergy and in patients with previous severe dermatologic, renal, or hematologic complications caused by gold. Relative contraindications include functional impairment of the kidneys or the liver. Agents with a potential to suppress the bone marrow should not be administered along with gold. Regular monitoring of complete blood counts and urine analysis, especially during the onset of therapy and at times of dose escalation, is required.

Dosage

An initial intramuscular 10-mg dose of gold should be administered to assess idiosyncratic reactions, followed by a 25-mg dose the second week, and 50-mg weekly doses thereafter. If clinical improvement is achieved, the dosing interval can be increased gradually. Long-term therapy can typically be maintained at 50 mg every 4 to 6 weeks. Clinical response is gradual and usually occurs when the cumulative dose is 300 to 700 mg. Dosage for children and adolescents is 1 mg/kg up to 25 mg/injection. Auranofin is initially administered at 3 mg/day and increased to a maximum of 9 mg/day for maintenance therapy.

Supply

Gold sodium thiomalate (Aurolate, Myochrysine), 10, 25, 50, 100 mg/mL in 1-mL ampules; 50 mg/mL in 10-mL ampules. Auranofin (Ridaura), tablets, 3 mg.

Hydroxychloroquine (Plaquenil)

Action

Mode of action is unknown. Potential actions include binding nucleic acids, stabilization of lysosomal membranes, and trapping of free radicals.

Selected Indications

Rheumatoid arthritis, SLE, sarcoidosis, dermatomyositis, and cutaneous lupus erythematosus.

Metabolism

Hydroxychloroquine is well absorbed from the gastrointestinal tract. The drug is concentrated and retained in body tissues. Detectable amounts of the drug are excreted by the kidney months after the therapy is discontinued.

Adverse Reactions

Most common side effects are allergic eruptions and gastrointestinal disturbances (e.g., anorexia, nausea, cramps, diarrhea). The most serious complication is ocular toxicity. Reversible corneal deposits of the drug are detectable by slit-lamp examination. Although retinopathy affecting macular pigmentation may be irreversible, it is extremely rare in patients with normal renal function receiving no more than the recommended dosages. Less common side effects include hyperpigmented rash, hypopigmentation of hair, neuropathy, ototoxicity, and cardiomyopathy. Hematologic toxicity is rare.

Caution

When administered in daily dosages of less than 6.5 mg/kg body weight in patients with normal renal function, serious adverse effects are uncommon. Ophthalmologic examination (e.g., color testing, visual fields, funduscopy, slit-lamp examination) should be performed every 6 to 12 months. Complete blood count should also be performed periodically. At the first sign of visual disturbance, the drug should be discontinued, and a formal ophthalmologic examination obtained. Hydroxychloroquine may cause hemolytic anemia in patients with G-6-PD deficiency. The drug is contraindicated in patients with significant visual, hepatic, or renal impairment, and porphyria. Hydroxychloroquine during pregnancy is regarded by many rheumatologists as generally safe. There are anecdotal reports of exacerbations of psoriasis with hydroxychloroquine.

Supply

Tablets, 200 mg.

Dosage

Initially 400 mg in single or divided doses; after good response (4 to 12 weeks), maintain at 200 mg/day.

Leflunomide (Arava)

Action

Inhibition of pyrimidine synthesis.

Selected Indications

Rheumatoid arthritis.

Metabolism

Following oral administration, leflunomide is converted into its active metabolite M1, which reaches peak levels after 8 to 12 hours. Administration of cholestyramine or charcoal reduces plasma titers of M1. The metabolite is extensively bound to albumin, and its half-life is approximately 2 weeks. M1 is excreted through both feces and urine.

Adverse Reactions

Gastrointestinal effects including diarrhea occurred in more than one-fourth of patients, and elevated results of liver function studies were conduced in 10% of the patients. The effects on the liver may be compounded by concurrent use of other hepatotoxic agents such as methotrexate. Postmarketing surveillance reports have identified several fatalities owing to liver failure, notably in patients receiving concomitant methotrexate. Rash and alopecia are not uncommon.

Caution

Leflunomide can cause fetal harm and is contraindicated during pregnancy and in breast-feeding mothers. Women of childbearing potential should use reliable modes of contraception. Significant hepatic insufficiency is also a relative contraindication, and liver function tests should be followed up regularly, especially during the initial part of therapy. Although coadministration with methotrexate does not demonstrate pharmacokinetic interactions, there may be additive hepatotoxic effects. In patients with renal insufficiency, the levels of M1 may be doubled. Cholestyramine or activated charcoal may be administered to accelerate the elimination of M1.

Supply
Tablets, 10, 20, 100 mg.

Dosage
Loading dose of 100 mg/day for 3 days, followed by 10 to 20 mg/day maintenance dose. Many rheumatologists forego the loading dose because of patient intolerance.

Methotrexate (Rheumatrex, Trexall)

Action
Methotrexate is a folate antagonist that inhibits dihydrofolate reductase, resulting in pleiotropic effects including immunosuppressive and anti-inflammatory properties.

Selected Indications
Rheumatoid arthritis, psoriatic arthritis, vasculitis, inflammatory myositis, uveitis, sarcoidosis.

Metabolism
Methotrexate is readily absorbed from the gastrointestinal tract in dosages of less than 0.1 mg/kg body weight. Approximately 50% is protein bound and is susceptible to displacement by sulfonamides, salicylates, NSAIDs, and other drugs. Fifty percent to 80% is rapidly excreted renally, which is enhanced by urine alkalinization. Impaired renal function considerably affects elimination of methotrexate.

Adverse Reactions
Patients should be observed for marrow suppression (leukopenia, thrombocytopenia, or complete aplasia) and gastrointestinal injury (ulcerative stomatitis, diarrhea, hemorrhagic enteritis, hepatic dysfunction including cirrhosis). Pulmonary infiltrates and eosinophilic pneumonitis, osteoporosis, rashes, and alopecia may occur. Many of the mucocutaneous toxicities may be prevented by a daily intake of 1 mg folic acid.

Caution
Methotrexate is an abortifacient and a teratogen and is absolutely contraindicated during pregnancy. Women of childbearing age considering its use must practice effective birth-control techniques. Use in nonmalignant disease requires emphasis on long-term side effects. The risk of hepatic cirrhosis supports weekly administration of the drug and careful monitoring of hepatic function, which may include liver biopsy. Renal function, pulmonary function, and complete blood count should also be monitored. Every six weeks, CBC, differential, platelet counts, AST, ALT, and albuminare are recommended. Although pretreatment and serial liver biopsies are no longer universally recommended in patients with rheumatoid arthritis, their utility remains a subject of debate in other diseases such as psoriatic arthritis. A baseline chest x-ray is suggested, along with hepatitis A, B, and C screening.

Supply
Tablets, 2.5, 5, 7.5, 10, 15 mg; vials, 5 and 50 mg for parenteral use.

Dosage
For rheumatoid arthritis and for psoriatic arthritis, 7.5 to 10 mg may be used on a weekly basis initially, administered orally or parenterally, and dosage increased as clinically indicated typically by 2.5 mg increments. The optimal dose for rheumatoid arthritis falls in the range of 15 to 25 mg weekly. For inflammatory polymyositis and vasculitides, initial therapy with 10 to 15 mg orally or parenterally weekly is recommended, with gradual increases in 5-mg increments to 30 to 50 mg weekly.

Minocycline (Dynacin, Minocin)

Action
Semisynthetic tetracycline derivative that probably inhibits proteolytic enzyme activity in rheumatoid arthritis.

Selected Indications
Rheumatoid arthritis.

Metabolism
Gastrointestinal absorption is excellent in the fasting state but is reduced with intake of food and antacids. Peak serum levels are reached within 4 hours. The serum half-life is 11 to 26 hours and does not appear to be affected by mild hepatic or renal dysfunction, although dose adjustment may be necessary in severe renal impairment. Elimination is through both urinary and fecal excretion.

Adverse Reactions
Like other tetracyclines, a photosensitive skin rash may occur. Long-term use may result in hyperpigmentation of the skin. Lightheadedness and dizziness may occur especially early on in therapy. Gastrointestinal intolerances are very common. Because minocycline is also an antibiotic, long-term use may result in overgrowth of nonsusceptible organisms such as fungus or *Clostridium difficile*. A lupuslike syndrome with arthralgias and myalgias has been reported in association with long-term minocycline use.

Caution
Minocycline causes discoloration of dentin and should be avoided in children, pregnant women, and lactating mothers.

Supply
Tablets and capsules, 50 and 100 mg. Suspension, 50 mg/5 mL.

Dosage
A dosage of 100 mg twice daily.

Mycophenolate Mofetil (CellCept)

Action
Immunosuppression via inhibition of guanosine synthesis.

Selected Indications
SLE, vasculitis, other autoimmune disorders.

Metabolism
Mycophenolate mofetil is rapidly absorbed and then hydrolyzed to its active metabolite mycophenolic acid (MPA). Food does not affect absorption. MPA is later inactivated by hepatic glucuronidation. The inactive metabolites are mostly excreted through urine (93%), with the remaining excreted through feces.

Adverse Reactions
Gastrointestinal effects including nausea, diarrhea, mucosal hemorrhage, and ulceration can occur. Leukopenia and infections, especially by opportunistic organisms, are also potential problems. In the population undergoing renal transplantation, there may be an increased risk of lymphoproliferative and nonmelanoma skin carcinomas.

Caution
Complete blood counts should be obtained initially on a weekly basis and then on a monthly basis. A rapid fall in leukocyte count requires a decrease in dosage or discontinuation of the drug. Liver function tests should be performed periodically. Vigilance for infection and malignancy should be maintained. Mycophenolate should be avoided in pregnant and breast-feeding women. Dose adjustment is necessary in patients with severe renal insufficiency.

Supply
Tablets, 250 and 500 mg.

Dosage
Initially 500 mg twice daily; can increase as indicated to 1,500 mg twice daily.

D-Penicillamine (Cuprimine, Depen)

Action
Mode of action in rheumatoid arthritis is largely unknown. D-Penicillamine decreases circulating immune complexes and rheumatoid factor titer and inhibits lymphocyte responsiveness to mitogens. In systemic sclerosis, inhibition of collagen cross-linking has been hypothesized as the mechanism of action.

Selected Indications
Rheumatoid arthritis, systemic sclerosis, Wilson's disease.

Metabolism
The drug is well absorbed from the gastrointestinal tract and rapidly excreted through urine. It should be administered on an empty stomach (1 to 2 hours before a meal) to avoid interference of absorption by dietary metals.

Adverse Reactions
Pruritus and skin rash represent the most common side effects and can occur at any time. They can be treated either by lowering the dosage of penicillamine or by administering antihistamines. Stomatitis also occurs. Alteration of taste is frequent, independent of dosage, and self-limited, with resolution in 2 to 3 months despite continued drug administration. Bone marrow depression may occur precipitously at any time. If the platelet count falls below $75,000/\mu L$, therapy must be discontinued. The most common late toxic effect is immune complex nephropathy. Proteinuria may be seen in 20% of patients. If proteinuria exceeds 1 g/day, the dosage should be reduced. Nephrotic syndrome, hypoalbuminemia, or hematuria requires discontinuation of the drug. Less common side effects include autoimmune syndromes (e.g., drug-induced lupus, Goodpasture's syndrome, myasthenia gravis, pemphigus, stenosing alveolitis, polymyositis), which necessitate prompt discontinuation of the drug.

Caution
D-Penicillamine administration is relatively contraindicated in patients who are receiving other myelosuppressive agents such as gold compounds or immunosuppressants. Renal insufficiency and pregnancy are other contraindications. A history of penicillin allergy does not preclude use of penicillamine. All patients should have complete blood counts with platelets and urinalysis at 2-week intervals for the first 6 months of therapy and monthly thereafter.

Supply
Capsules, 125 and 250 mg.

Dosage
Initially, a single daily dose of 250 mg, which can be increased in 2 to 3 months to 375 or 500 mg/day if clinical response is insufficient. Further increases to a maximum dose of 750 mg/day may be made after an additional 2 to 3 months.

Protein A Immunoadsorption Column (Prosorba)

Action
Protein A immunoadsorption column consists of protein A from *Staphylococcus* bound to a silica matrix. Employing apheresis technology, potentially pathogenic IgG and IgG-containing immune complexes are removed.

Selected Indications
Refractory rheumatoid arthritis, immune thrombocytopenia purpura.

Metabolism
Extracorporeal passage of plasma through the immunoadsorption column is performed using an apheresis machine. The treated plasma is then transferred back to the patient.

Adverse Reactions
The most common adverse effects are joint pains and swelling, fatigue paresthesias, headache, hypotension, anemia, nausea, sore throat, edema, abdominal pain, hypertension, rash, dizziness, diarrhea, hematoma, flushing, chills, dyspnea, chest pain, and fever. Other complications associated with any procedure involving apheresis may occur, including blood loss, damage to blood cells, and problems arising from fluid balance mismanagement (e.g., hypertension, hypotension, arrhythmias). In patients with rheumatoid arthritis, there is an incidence of infection and/or local thrombosis at the site of central venous catheters.

Caution
A full discussion with the patient covering reasonable expectations and potential adverse effects of treatment is mandatory before initiating therapy. This device should only be used at facilities with extensive experience in apheresis. Strict sterile technique is essential, and careful monitoring of vital signs and fluid status is crucial. Concurrent use of angiotensin-converting enzyme (ACE) inhibitors is contraindicated, and withdrawal of the drug at least 3 days before the procedure is recommended by the manufacturer. Patients with previous intolerance to apheresis procedures, hypercoagulable states, or conditions that may become exacerbated by apheresis should not undergo treatment. Treatment may not be advisable in individuals with poor peripheral access, impaired renal function, relative hypotension, significant vascular disease, intracranial disease, severe anemia, systemic infections, or significant risk for congestive heart failure and fluid overload. Patients with rheumatoid arthritis may be at a particular risk for developing severe anemia.

Supply
Prepackaged sterile polycarbonate columns containing 200 mg of protein A covalently bound to 300 mL of silica matrix.

Dosage
Individualized according to patient status. In general, weekly apheresis may be performed.

Quinacrine Hydrochloride (Atabrine)

Action
Mode of action is unknown. Potential actions include binding nucleic acids, stabilization of lysosomal membranes, and trapping of free radicals.

Selected Indications
Rheumatoid arthritis, SLE, cutaneous lupus erythematosus.

Metabolism
Quinacrine is well absorbed from the gastrointestinal tract and widely distributed into body tissues where it is concentrated and retained. Detectable amounts of the drug are excreted by the kidney months after the therapy is discontinued.

Adverse Reactions
Common side effects include nausea, vomiting, anorexia, abdominal cramps, rash, and a reversible yellow discoloration of skin. Less common reactions include central nervous system stimulation, emotional changes, altered pigmentation of skin and nails (black and blue), and cardiomyopathy. Reversible corneal edema and deposits have been reported, but retinopathy is rare. Rare toxicity includes psychosis and aplastic anemia.

Caution
Ophthalmologic examination should be performed every 6 months during long-term therapy. At any sign of visual disturbance, the drug should be discontinued. Quinacrine may cause hemolytic anemia in patients with G-6-PD deficiency. It is contraindicated during pregnancy.

Supply
Tablets, 100 mg.

Dosage
A dose of 100 mg/day.

Sulfasalazine (Azulfidine)

Action
Exact mechanism is unknown, but there is evidence for anti-inflammatory, immunomodulatory, antibacterial, and antifolate effects.

Selected Indications
Rheumatoid arthritis, spondyloarthropathies, inflammatory bowel diseases.

Metabolism
Sulfasalazine is partially absorbed (one-third) from the small intestines and extensively metabolized. It is split into 5-amino salicylic acid and sulfapyridine; the latter is metabolized in the liver. The metabolic products are excreted through the urine.

Adverse Reactions
The most common side effects occurring in up to one-third of patients include anorexia, headache, nausea, vomiting, gastric distress, and reversible oligospermia. Rash, oral ulcers, pruritus, urticaria, fever, and hemolytic anemia are less frequent. Blood dyscrasias (especially leukopenia) can occur at any time, but especially at the initiation of the therapy and during dose escalation. Hypersensitivity reactions and central nervous system effects have been reported rarely.

Caution
Azulfidine is contraindicated in patients with porphyria and should be administered with caution in patients with hepatic or renal disease, blood dyscrasias, or allergies. Complete blood counts and liver function tests should be done frequently. Urine analysis should also be followed up. Adequate fluid intake must be maintained to prevent crystalluria and renal stones. Patients with G-6-PD deficiency should be followed up closely for signs of hemolysis. Azulfidine should be avoided in patients with sulfa allergies and should not be given simultaneously with sulfa drugs.

Supply
Tablets, 500 mg.

Dosage
A dosage of 1 to 1.5 g twice daily with meals is gradually attained by 500 mg increments on a weekly basis.

Thalidomide (Thalomid)

Action
Thalidomide is an immunomodulatory agent with anti-inflammatory and antiangiogenic properties. Its effect is partly, but not exclusively, due to modulation of tumor necrosis factor-α (TNF-α) expression.

Selected Indications
Cutaneous manifestations of SLE, sarcoidosis, juvenile idiopathic arthritis, Behçet's disease.

Metabolism
Thalidomide is slowly absorbed in the gastrointestinal tract, reaching peak plasma levels 2.5 to 6 hours after ingestion. Fat intake delays absorption. The elimination half-life is 3 to 7 hours. Metabolism of the drug is primarily via spontaneous nonenzymatic hydrolysis, and the excretion of metabolites in humans is not known.

Adverse Reactions

Teratogenicity is the most important adverse effect of thalidomide. Central nervous system effects include sedation and the lowering of seizure thresholds; concomitant use of other central nervous system depressants should be avoided. A dose-dependent peripheral neuropathy, sometimes painful, is relatively common and often irreversible. Discontinuation of the medication should be considered at the earliest symptom or sign of peripheral neuropathy. Neutropenia can occur at any time during treatment, and complete blood counts need to be monitored every 4 to 6 weeks.

Caution

Because of extreme teratogenicity, thalidomide is absolutely contraindicated during pregnancy. Pretreatment counseling is mandatory for patients of both genders. Women of childbearing potential should use two forms of contraception for 4 weeks before initiating thalidomide, while using thalidomide, and for 4 weeks after stopping thalidomide. A baseline blood pregnancy test is required before the initiation of therapy and periodically during therapy in these patients. Thalidomide is also contraindicated during breast-feeding. Because thalidomide can be found in the semen, a man having sexual intercourse with a woman of childbearing potential should use a latex condom. Men wishing to conceive a child should stop thalidomide therapy at least 4 weeks before trying to conceive. A special registration process is required in order for physicians to prescribe this medication and for patients to receive it (www.cellgene.com).

Supply

Capsules, 50, 100, 200 mg.

Dosage

Initially 50 mg/day. If indicated and tolerated, can increase to 200 mg/day.

 ## BIOLOGIC AGENTS

Although biologic agents may be broadly defined and will certainly be subject to redefinition as their use evolves, they generally describe specific antibodies or recombinant forms of natural inhibitors against modulatory molecules of immunity or inflammation. These agents have been most widely studied in the setting of rheumatoid arthritis, but represent a new approach to the treatment of all systemic inflammatory rheumatic diseases.

Adalimumab (Humira)

Action

Inhibition of TNF-α.

Selected Indications

Rheumatoid arthritis, psoriatic arthritis, psoriasis ankylosing spondylitis.

Metabolism

Adalimumab is a recombinant human IgG1 monoclonal antibody specific for human TNF-α that inhibits TNF binding to cell surface receptors. After subcutaneous injection, peak serum levels are reached after 131 hours, and the mean half-life is approximately 2 weeks. No pharmacokinetic data in the setting of renal or hepatic impairment is available.

Adverse Reactions

Local injection site reactions occur in more than one-third of patients but generally do not result in discontinuation. As with other immunomodulatory agents, vigilance for both common and atypical (e.g., mycobacteria, fungi) infections should be maintained, and discontinuation of the drug is recommended when severe infections are identified. The effects of adalimumab in patients with history of malignancies or on the risk of new malignancies are not clear, but the development of lymphomas has been reported in association with its use, thought to be related to RA itself. Rare autoimmune phenomena have been associated with the use of adalimumab, including a lupuslike syndrome and demyelinating disorders. Some data suggest an association with congestive heart failure.

Caution

Serious infections and sepsis, with rare fatalities, have been reported as adverse reactions of adalimumab therapy. Cases of tuberculosis, including disseminated disease, have also been seen, and pretreatment screening with intradermal tuberculin testing and chest radiography is recommended. Latent tuberculosis should be treated before considering adalimumab therapy. Concurrent live vaccinations should not be given. Concomitant use of other immunosuppressants likely increases the risks of infection. Multiple TNF inhibitors should not be administered simultaneously, and concurrent use of anakinra is not recommended. Adalimumab should be used with caution in patients with cardiomyopathies.

Supply

A dose of 40 mg in prefilled syringes.

Dosage

A dosage of 40 mg subcutaneously, once every 1 or 2 weeks.

Anakinra (Kineret)

Action

Competitive inhibition of interleukin-1 (IL-1).

Selected Indications

Rheumatoid arthritis, autoinflammatory disorders.

Metabolism

Anakinra is a recombinant structural analog of IL-1 receptor antagonist that competes with IL-1 by binding to the IL-1 receptor on cell surfaces. After subcutaneous injection, peak serum levels are reached between 3 and 7 hours. The terminal half-life is approximately 5 hours. Dose adjustments are recommended in the setting of severe renal insufficiency (creatinine clearance <30 mL/minute) and end-stage renal disease. No data on the effects of hepatic impairment are available.

Adverse Reaction

Local injection site–reactions are very common and often result in the discontinuation of the therapy. The most serious adverse effects are leukopenia with neutropenia and increased propensity for infections. As with other immunomodulatory agents, vigilance for both common and atypical (e.g., mycobacteria, fungi) infections should be maintained, and discontinuation of the drug is recommended when severe infections are identified. The effects of anakinra in patients with history of malignancies or on the risk of new malignancies are not clear, but the development of lymphomas has been reported in association with its use.

Caution

Serious infections and sepsis, with rare fatalities, have been reported with anakinra therapy. Patients with asthma may be at particular risk. Concurrent live vaccinations should not be given. Concomitant use of other immunosuppressants likely increases the risks of infection. In particular, the combination of anti-TNF medications and anakinra increases the risk of neutropenia and infection and is not recommended.

Supply

A dose of 100 mg in prefilled syringes.

Dosage

A dosage of 100 mg subcutaneously, once a day.

Etanercept (Enbrel)

Action
Inhibition of TNF-α.

Selected Indications
Rheumatoid arthritis, psoriatic arthritis, psoriasis, juvenile idiopathic arthritis, ankylosing spondylitis.

Metabolism
Etanercept is a dimeric recombinant protein consisting of two ligand-binding domains of the human 75-kDa (p75) TNF-α receptor fused to the Fc domain of human IgG1. After subcutaneous injection in patients with rheumatoid arthritis, the median half-life is approximately 102 hours. Maximum serum concentration is reached in 69 hours. Pharmacokinetic differences have not been noted between male and female patients, or between adult and pediatric patients. The effects of hepatic and renal impairment are not known.

Adverse Reactions
Local injection site–reactions occur in more than one-third of patients but may respond to topical corticosteroids and generally do not result in discontinuation. As with other immunomodulatory agents, vigilance for both common and atypical (e.g., mycobacteria, fungi) infections should be maintained, and discontinuation of the drug is recommended when severe infections are identified. The effects of etanercept in patients with history of malignancies or on the risk of new malignancies are not clear, but the development of lymphomas has been reported in association with its use, thought to be related to RA itself. Rare autoimmune phenomena have been associated with the use of etanercept, including a lupuslike syndrome and demyelinating disorders. Some data suggest an association with congestive heart failure.

Caution
Serious infections and sepsis, with rare fatalities, have been reported with etanercept therapy. Cases of tuberculosis, including disseminated disease, have also been seen, and pretreatment screening with intradermal tuberculin testing and chest radiography is recommended. Latent tuberculosis should be treated before considering etanercept therapy. Concurrent live vaccinations should not be given. Concomitant use of other immunosuppressants likely increases the risks of infection. In particular, concurrent use of anakinra has not been shown to increase therapeutic efficacy and is associated with greater propensity to infection. Multiple TNF inhibitors should not be administered simultaneously, and concurrent use of anakinra is not recommended. Etanercept should be used with caution in patients with cardiomyopathies.

Supply
Sterile lyophilized powder, 25 mg for reconstitution with 1.0 mL sterile water; 50 mg in prefilled syringes.

Dosage
A dosage of 25 mg subcutaneously, twice weekly; or 50 mg subcutaneously, once weekly.

Infliximab (Remicade)

Action
Inhibition of TNF-α.

Selected Indications
Rheumatoid arthritis, Crohn's disease, psoriatic arthritis, psoriasis, ankylosing spondylitis.

Metabolism
Infliximab is a chimeric monoclonal antibody comprising antigen-binding sequences of murine origin specific for human TNF-α and constant regions of human IgG1κ. After

intravenous infusion, the mean half-life is approximately 8 to $9\frac{1}{2}$ days. No pharmacokinetic data in the setting of renal or hepatic impairment is known.

Adverse Reactions

Minor infusion reactions occur within 1 to 2 hours in 20% of patients. Serious reactions, including anaphylaxis and hypotension, occur in less than 1%. As with other immunomodulatory agents, vigilance for both common and atypical (e.g., mycobacteria, fungi) infections should be maintained, and discontinuation of the drug is recommended when severe infections are identified. The effects of infliximab on patients with history of malignancies or on the risk of new malignancies are not clear, but the development of lymphomas has been reported in association with its use, thought to be related to RA itself. Rare autoimmune phenomena have been associated with the use of etanercept, including a lupuslike syndrome and demyelinating disorders. Some data suggest an association with congestive heart failure.

Caution

Serious infections and sepsis, with rare fatalities, have been reported with infliximab therapy. Cases of tuberculosis, including disseminated disease, have also been seen, and pretreatment screening with intradermal tuberculin testing and chest radiography is recommended. Latent tuberculosis should be treated before considering infliximab therapy. Concurrent live vaccinations should not be given. Concomitant use of other immunosuppressants likely increases the risks of infection. Multiple TNF inhibitors should not be administered simultaneously, and concurrent use of anakinra is not recommended. Infliximab should be used with caution in patients with cardiomyopathies.

Supply

A dose of 100 mg, lyophilized concentrates for reconstitution just before infusion.

Dosage

For rheumatoid arthritis, the dosage is 3 mg/kg by intravenous infusions at weeks 0, 2, and 6 and then every 8 weeks thereafter. Concomitant methotrexate therapy is formally recommended. The dosage can be increased to 10 mg/kg or the interval reduced to every 4 weeks, as clinically indicated. In the setting of congestive heart failure, the maximum dosage is 5 mg/kg.

For Crohn's disease, the dosage is 5 mg/kg by intravenous infusions at weeks 0, 2, and 6 and then every 8 weeks thereafter. The dosage can be increased to up to 10 mg/kg, as clinically indicated. In the setting of congestive heart failure, the maximum dosage is 5 mg/kg.

For ankylosing spondylitis, the dosage is 5 mg/kg by intravenous infusions at weeks 0, 2, and 6 and then every 6 weeks thereafter.

MEDICATIONS FOR CRYSTALLINE ARTHRITIDES

NSAIDs and corticosteroids are the mainstays in the treatment of acute gout and crystalline arthritides. Although colchicine may also be used in the acute setting, it is more widely used for prophylaxis. Hypouricemic agents reduce serum uric acid levels by either inhibiting production or increasing excretion of uric acid and are used primarily in patients with chronic, recurrent gouty arthritis, tophaceous gout, nephrolithiasis, and urate nephropathy.

Allopurinol (Zyloprim, Lopurin)

Action

Allopurinol, an analog of the purine hypoxanthine, inhibits the enzyme xanthine oxidase, which converts hypoxanthine to xanthine, and xanthine to uric acid. Plasma and urine concentrations of uric acid are lowered. Allopurinol also acts by a feedback mechanism to inhibit *de novo* purine synthesis.

Selected Indications

Refractory/recurrent gouty arthritis, tophaceous gout, nephrolithiasis, urate nephropathy, prevention of tumor lysis syndrome.

Metabolism
Twenty percent is excreted through the urine unchanged, with the remainder excreted through the urine as alloxanthine. The half-life of the major metabolite oxypurinol, which also inhibits xanthine oxidase, is 30 hours. The efficacy of allopurinol decreases when the creatinine clearance falls below 20 mL/minute.

Adverse Reactions
A maculopapular rash is the most common side effect and occurs in 3% of patients. For minor allergic reactions, desensitization protocols are available. Allopurinol can paradoxically trigger gouty attacks, especially during the initiation of therapy or during dose adjustments. Allopurinol therapy should not be given for several weeks, until an acute flare of gout has resolved for several weeks. Immune complex dermatitis and hepatitis, occasionally with vasculitis and nephritis, can occur; pruritus is an important warning symptom. Side effects from allopurinol are increased in the presence of marked renal failure (creatinine clearance <20 mL/minute).

Caution
Allopurinol inhibits the oxidation of 6-mercaptopurine. Because 6-mercaptopurine is the active metabolite of AZA, concomitant use of either AZA or 6-mercaptopurine should be avoided with allopurinol. Alternatively, 75% dosage reductions should be made. Allopurinol inhibits hepatic microsomal enzymes for drug metabolism; warfarin derivatives and other drugs metabolized by these enzymes should be administered in lower dosages. Concurrent administration of ampicillin and allopurinol leads to a threefold higher incidence of drug rash. The toxicity of cytotoxic agents, such as cyclophosphamide, appears to be enhanced by concomitant administration of allopurinol. The dosage of allopurinol should be reduced in patients with renal insufficiency and failure.

Supply
Tablets, 100 and 300 mg.

Dosage
For mild disease, 200 to 300 mg/day is usually adequate, but the dosage should be individualized to achieve the desired serum urate level of less than 6 mg/dL. It is advisable to start with 100 mg/day and gradually build toward full dosage to lessen the probability of acute gout attacks that may be precipitated by the sudden lowering of the serum uric acid levels. Allopurinol is counterproductive and is to be avoided in acute attacks of gout. For severe tophaceous gout, 400 to 600 mg/day in divided doses can be used. The maximum single dose should be 300 mg. Total daily doses in excess of 600 mg are associated with increased toxicity. It is advisable to prescribe colchicine (0.6 mg/day or twice daily) as prophylaxis against acute gout during the first 6 months of therapy.

To prevent uric acid nephropathy when treating neoplastic disease, a daily dosage of 600 to 800 mg (in divided doses) may be required, with the maintenance of large volumes of alkalinized urine.

Colchicine (ColBenemid, Proben-C, Col-Probenecid)

Action
Colchicine inhibits microtubule assembly, which interferes with granulocyte mobility and the inflammatory response to precipitated crystals.

Selected Indications
Acute crystal-induced arthritis, prophylaxis for crystal-induced arthritis, autoinflammatory disorders.

Metabolism
Although complete metabolism is unknown, colchicine is deacetylated in the liver to inactive metabolites; 10% is excreted unchanged by the kidney. The drug half-life is 90 minutes and is prolonged in patients with renal insufficiency.

Adverse Reactions

Gastrointestinal irritation producing nausea, vomiting, and abdominal pain occurs in up to 80% of patients receiving oral colchicine for acute gout. Bone marrow depression, renal dysfunction, and hemorrhagic colitis may occur, especially with overdose or in the setting of liver or renal disease.

Caution

Intravenous colchicine should be diluted in normal saline (10 to 15 mL) and administered slowly over 5 minutes through a free-flowing intravenous route to decrease the chance of infiltration and soft-tissue necrosis. Fatalities have been reported with intravenous administration. Reduction in dosage is necessary in patients with liver or renal impairment.

Supply

Tablets, 0.6 mg. Intravenous ampules, 2 mL containing 1 mg of colchicine. Also available in combination with probenecid (ColBenemid), tablets, colchicine 0.5 mg/probenecid 500 mg.

Dosage

For maintenance prophylaxis, 0.6 mg/day or twice daily. For acute attacks, oral colchicine, 0.6 to 1.2 mg initially, followed by 0.6 mg hourly until symptoms abate or toxicity occurs. In patients with normal renal function, the total cumulative dose should not exceed 8 mg. Intravenous colchicine, 1 to 2 mg initially, followed by 0.5 mg every 6 to 8 hours up to a total of 4 mg. Dosage should be reduced significantly or this drug avoided in the presence of renal or hepatic disease.

Probenecid (Benemid, ColBenemid, Proben-C, Col-Probenecid)

Action

Probenecid is a uricosuric agent that inhibits renal tubular resorption of organic acids, including uric acid. It is not effective with creatinine clearances less than 40 mL/minute.

Selected Indications

Hyperuricemia associated with refractory/recurrent gouty arthritis.

Metabolism

Probenecid is excreted through urine in the glucuronide form and as oxidized metabolites. The half-life is dose-dependent and ranges from 6 to 12 hours.

Adverse Reactions

Gastrointestinal irritation occurs in 10% of patients, whereas systemic hypersensitivity characterized by fever and rash is seen in approximately 3%.

Caution

Large alkaline urine output should be maintained, especially during the first week of therapy, to prevent the formation of urate renal stones. A history of renal calculi is a relative contraindication. Probenecid may alter the metabolism of other drugs by decreasing their excretion (indomethacin, ampicillin), reducing their volume of distribution (ampicillin), or delaying metabolism (heparin). Probenecid is antagonized by low-dose salicylates (<3 g/day).

Supply

Tablets, 500 mg. Also available in combination with colchicine (ColBenemid, Proben-C, Col-Probenecid), tablets, colchicine 0.5 mg/probenecid 500 mg.

Dosage

A dosage of 250 mg twice daily for 1 week, then 500 mg twice daily. Maintenance colchicine should be given during the first 3 months of probenecid therapy and then can be stopped if the patient is asymptomatic. Probenecid is not useful in acute attacks of gout.

Sulfinpyrazone (Anturane)

Action
A uricosuric that inhibits renal tubular reabsorption of organic acids.

Selected Indications
Hyperuricemia associated with refractory/recurrent gouty arthritis.

Metabolism
The drug is rapidly and completely absorbed with peak plasma levels in approximately 1 hour. Sulfinpyrazone is 98% protein bound. The kidney excretes approximately 40% unchanged.

Adverse Reactions
Gastrointestinal irritation is common. Because sulfinpyrazone has structural similarities to phenylbutazone, it should be avoided in patients with known sensitivity to phenylbutazone.

Caution
Large alkaline urine output should be maintained, especially during the first week of therapy, to decrease risk of urate calculi formation. Sulfinpyrazone inhibits platelet aggregation and potentiates the action of protein-bound drugs such as oral hypoglycemics and oral anticoagulants. The action of sulfinpyrazone is antagonized by low-dose salicylates and is ineffective in the presence of renal failure.

Supply
Tablets, 100 mg; Capsules, 200 mg.

Dosage
Start with 50 to 100 mg twice daily with meals and increase gradually over several weeks to a maintenance dosage usually of 300 to 400 mg/day in 3 to 4 divided doses. The maximum recommended daily dosage is 800 mg. Maintenance colchicine should be given for the first 3 months of therapy to prevent precipitation of an acute attack of gouty arthritis.

 ANALGESICS

Acetaminophen

Action
Centrally acting analgesia.

Metabolism
Acetaminophen is rapidly absorbed in the gastrointestinal tract and reaches peak levels within 1 hour. The drug is metabolized by the liver largely to the glucuronide conjugate and then excreted through urine.

Adverse Reactions
Although rare, hepatic toxicity including hepatic failure is the most dangerous potential adverse effect.

Caution
Alcohol use or abuse, fasting, concurrent use of medications that induce cytochrome P-450 activity, and pre-existing liver disease increase risk of liver toxicity. Reduced doses are necessary in children.

Supply
Tablets, caplets, gelcaps, 160, 325, 500 mg; Liquid, 500 mg/15 mL; Multiple combinations with other medications are available.

Dosage
A dosage of 325 to 1,000 mg every 6 hours as necessary. Maximum adult daily dosage is 4 g.

Amitriptyline (Elavil)

Action
Amitriptyline is a tricyclic antidepressant (TCA), which is thought to block reuptake of a variety of neurotransmitters. This and other TCAs have been used for the adjuvant treatment of neuropathic pain and in patients with fibromyalgia.

Metabolism
Amitriptyline is rapidly absorbed by the gastrointestinal tract. The plasma half-life can range from 10 to 50 hours. Amitriptyline and its metabolites are primarily excreted through urine.

Adverse Reactions
The most common adverse effects are related to anticholinergic activity such as xerostomia, mydriasis, constipation, and urinary retention, especially in geriatric patients. Central nervous system and neuromuscular symptoms are also common, including cognitive changes, somnolence, and exacerbations of underlying psychiatric disorders. Extrapyramidal symptoms ranging from minor involuntary movements and tardive dyskinesia to parkinsonianism may occur. Cardiovascular effects include conduction disturbances and arrhythmias and postural hypotension.

Caution
Acute toxicities relate to extensions of adverse reactions. An acute withdrawal syndrome may result after the sudden discontinuation of longstanding therapy. A baseline electrocardiogram is generally recommended. This drug should be used with extreme caution in the geriatric population. Concomitant use of monoamine oxidase inhibitors (MAOIs), hypotensive agents, central nervous system depressants, sympathomimetics, and anticholinergic medications should be avoided.

Supply
Tablets, 10, 25, 50, 75, 100, 150 mg.

Dosage
For neuropathic pain and fibromyalgia, initially 10 mg at bedtime, with escalating doses to a maximum of 300 mg/day.

Capsaicin (Zostrix, Dolorac)

Action
Inhibition of substance P.

Metabolism
No information is available.

Adverse Reactions
Capsaicin may cause local skin irritation, burning, and erythema.

Caution
Capsaicin is meant for external use only and should not be used on open wounds. Contact with eyes should be avoided, and hands should be washed immediately after application. Dried material may cause irritation to nasal and respiratory mucosa and should not be inhaled.

Supply
Cream, 0.025%, 0.075%, and 0.25%.

Dosage
At lower doses, apply topically on skin, up to four times daily; 0.25%, apply topically to skin up to twice daily.

Gabapentin (Neurontin)

Action
Gabapentin is a structural analog of γ-aminobutyric acid (GABA), which has been used to treat neuropathic pain syndromes. Although designed to mimic GABA activity at inhibitory neuronal synapses, gabapentin does not bind to GABA receptors, and its precise mechanism of action is not known.

Metabolism
At therapeutic doses, the bioavailability of gabapentin is approximately 60%. It is not significantly metabolized in humans and is excreted almost exclusively by the kidneys.

Adverse Reactions
Gabapentin is well tolerated. Nervous system effects are the most common intolerances and include somnolence, dizziness, ataxia, and fatigue.

Caution
Concurrent use with other central nervous system depressants should be avoided. Dose adjustment is necessary in the setting of severe renal insufficiency.

Supply
Capsules, 100, 300, and 400 mg; Tablets, 600 and 800 mg scored; Solution, 250 mg/5 mL.

Dosage
Initially, 300 mg/day in divided doses to be titrated up to 2,400 mg/day in divided doses.

Tramadol Hydrochloride (Ultram, Ultracet)

Action
Tramadol is a synthetic, centrally acting analgesic. Although it is not an opiate derivative, it is a selective opiate μ-receptor agonist. It may also have additional analgesic properties through inhibition of synaptic monoamine reuptake.

Metabolism
Drug absorption is good and is not affected by food. Tramadol is partially metabolized by the liver. Approximately 90% of the drug and its metabolites are excreted through the urine.

Adverse Reactions
Tramadol shares similar adverse reactions with true opiates, including central nervous system effects (e.g., lightheadedness, somnolence), nausea, constipation, xerostomia, and pruritus. It may also potentially cause respiratory depression when administered at high doses and may lower seizure threshold. Tolerance, addiction, and manifestations of withdrawal may also occur, but risks are thought to be relatively small when compared to other opiate agonists.

Caution
Tramadol should be used with extreme caution in conjunction with other medications that may depress the central nervous system, such as other opiates, alcohol, sedatives, and hypnotics, or with those that may reduce seizure threshold such as MAOIs and antipsychotic agents. Patients receiving MAOIs should not receive tramadol also because of the drug's inhibitory effects on monoamine reuptake. Less frequent dosing should be considered in patients with renal or hepatic impairment.

Supply
Tablets, 50 mg. Also available as 37.5 mg in combination with acetaminophen 325 mg (Ultracet).

Dosage
A dosage of 50 to 100 mg every 4 to 6 hours as needed.

DRUGS FOR OSTEOPOROSIS AND METABOLIC BONE DISEASES

Alendronate (Fosamax)

Action
Alendronate is a bisphosphonate, which inhibits osteoclast activity and bone resorption but does not interfere significantly with bone mineralization.

Selected Indications
Osteoporosis prevention and treatment, Paget's disease of the bone.

Metabolism
Alendronate is poorly absorbed by the gastrointestinal tract, especially when taken with food. Calcium-, aluminum-, and magnesium-containing supplements and antacids interfere with absorption. Absorbed drug is tropic for bone and will persist within the bony skeleton for years. The terminal half-life is approximately 11 years. Excretion is through the urine.

Adverse Reactions
Gastrointestinal intolerances are the most common adverse effects and include diarrhea, nausea, abdominal pain, and, most importantly, esophagitis and esophageal ulcerations. Adequate calcium repletion before the initiation of therapy may reduce the risk of arthralgias and other musculoskeletal complaints.

Caution
Alendronate must be taken on an empty stomach, after which the patient should not eat or lie down for at least half an hour. Patients with pre-existing esophageal reflux or inflammation may not be good candidates for alendronate therapy. It is contraindicated in women of childbearing potential.

Supply
Tablets, 5, 10, 35, 40, 70 mg.

Dosage
For osteoporosis prevention or osteopenia, 5 mg/day or 35 mg weekly. For osteoporosis treatment, 10 mg/day or 70 mg weekly. For Paget's disease, 40 mg/day with reassessment after 6 months.

Calcitonin (Calcimar, Miacalcin)

Action
Inhibits osteoclast activity and bone resorption.

Selected Indications
Osteoporosis prevention and treatment, Paget's disease of the bone, analgesia for acute vertebral fractures, hypercalcemia.

Metabolism
Calcitonin is a protein, which is rapidly metabolized to smaller, inactive fragments in the kidneys.

Adverse Reactions

Nausea and vomiting occurs in 10% of patients with either intranasal or subcutaneous route. Flushing of face and hands, peripheral paresthesias, urticaria, altered taste, and local skin reactions may be more common with subcutaneous calcitonin. Low-dose skin testing is recommended by some before full-dose subcutaneous treatment. Irritation of the nasal mucosa, epistaxis, and perforation can be seen rarely with the nasal inhaler, so periodic nasal examinations are indicated.

Caution

Neutralizing antibodies may develop with partial loss of effectiveness.

Supply

Nasal spray, 200 units/spray (14 dose canisters). Sterile injectable solution, 1 mL vials.

Dosage

For postmenopausal osteoporosis, 100 units/day by subcutaneous or intramuscular injection or 200 units/day intranasally alternating nostrils with each dose. For Paget's disease, 100 units daily by subcutaneous or intramuscular injection.

Calcium Preparations

Action

Increased calcium pool available for gastrointestinal absorption.

Selected Indications

Osteoporosis prevention and treatment.

Metabolism

Renal excretion of absorbed fraction.

Adverse Reactions

Nausea, constipation, and gastrointestinal irritation may occur.

Caution

Hypercalcemia may occur, especially in patients receiving concomitant vitamin D. Calcium carbonate is ineffective in patients with achlorhydria.

Supply

Many different preparations and dosages of calcium carbonate, calcium citrate, calcium gluconate, and calcium lactate are available, frequently in combination with vitamin D.

Dosage

Supplement dietary calcium intake to achieve total elemental calcium: 1,000 mg/day in divided doses for men and premenopausal women; 1,500 mg/day in divided doses for postmenopausal women.

Estrogens

Action

Estrogens are bound by nuclear receptors in various tissues and ultimately affect the transcription of genes, which bear the estrogen response element. In bone, inhibition of osteoclast activity is the eventual effect resulting in reduced bone resorption.

Selected Indications

Prevention and treatment of postmenopausal osteoporosis.

Metabolism

Unconjugated estrogens are rapidly inactivated by the liver after oral administration and so are usually given parenterally. By contrast, conjugated estrogens may be administered orally. Estrogens accumulate in body fat and so may be cleared more slowly in obese patients. Steroidal estrogens are metabolized primarily by the liver via conjugation and then excreted through the urine. A substantial amount is recirculated through the liver from bile for further metabolism.

Adverse Reactions

Malignancies are the most feared potential complication of estrogen therapy (see section Caution). It is clear that unopposed prolonged estrogen use increases the risk of endometrial carcinoma in postmenopausal women, and recent data also strongly support a link with the development of breast cancers. Although estrogens often improve the condition in hypercholesterolemia, evidence suggests that the risk of coronary and cerebrovascular disease is increased with their use. Other potential adverse effects are manifold and include hypertension, hypercoagulability and thromboembolic disorders, fluid retention, nausea, vomiting, pancreatitis, skin rashes, glucose intolerance, hypercalcemia, hypertriglyceridemia, abnormal results of liver function tests, cholestasis, gall bladder disease, breakthrough vaginal bleeding, menstruallike cramping, fibroid enlargement, changes in affect, migraine headaches, mastodynia, and breast secretions.

Caution

Estrogens increase the risk of breast cancers. Most physicians consider a past or current history of breast cancer as a contraindication for estrogen therapy. Use in women without a personal history but with a close family history of breast cancer requires careful discussion of risks and benefits of initiating or withholding therapy. Estrogens also increase the risk of endometrial carcinoma in postmenopausal women; coadministration of progestin in women with intact uteri is recommended to reduce this risk. Estrogens are associated with developmental defects in fetal reproductive organs and are contraindicated in pregnancy. Other contraindications to estrogen therapy include undiagnosed abnormal vaginal bleeding, active or past thrombophlebitis, and severe liver disease. Caution should also be taken in individuals with pre-existing uncontrolled hypertension, cardiovascular disease, asthma, migraine headaches, seizure disorders, renal dysfunction, depression, gall bladder disease, hypercoagulable states, and fibroids.

Supply

Estradiol:
- Tablets, 0.5, 1, 2 mg.
- Transdermal patch, 0.025, 0.05, 0.075, 0.1 mg/24 hour.

Estradiol/norethindrone acetate combinations:
- Transdermal patch, estradiol 0.05 mg and norethindrone acetate 0.14 mg or 0.25 mg/24 hour.

Conjugated estrogens:
- Tablets, 0.3, 0.625, 0.9, 0.125 mg.

Conjugated estrogens/medroxyprogesterone combinations:
- Monophasic regimen, conjugated estrogens 0.625 mg and medroxyprogesterone 2.5 mg.
- Monophasic regimen, conjugated estrogens 0.625 mg and medroxyprogesterone 5 mg.
- Biphasic regimen, conjugated estrogens 0.625 mg in 28 tablets with medroxyprogesterone 5 mg in 14 tablets.

Estropipate:
- Tablets, 0.75, 1.5, 3.0 mg.

Esterified estrogens:
- Tablets, 0.3, 0.625, 1.25, 2.5 mg.

Dosage

Recommended initial dosages for prevention and treatment of postmenopausal osteoporosis are administered. Women with intact uteri should receive concomitant cyclical or continuous progestin therapy; for example, oral medroxyprogesterone may be administered either in a cyclic manner (5 mg/day during the last 2 weeks of a 4-week cycle) or continuously (2.5 mg/day). Women who have undergone hysterectomies may be given estrogen therapy without progestin.

Estradiol:
- Oral regimen: 0.5 mg/day.
- Transdermal regimen: 0.05 mg/24-hour patch applied twice weekly. (Note: Combination patches containing norethindrone acetate 0.14 mg or 0.25 mg/24 hour are available.)

Conjugated estrogens:
- A dosage of 0.625 mg orally each day. (Note: Combination regimens for concomitant continuous or cyclical medroxyprogesterone are available.)

Estropipate:
- A dosage of 0.75 mg orally each day.

Esterified estrogens:
- A dosage of 0.3 mg/day orally each day.

Etidronate Disodium (Didronel)

Action
Etidronate disodium is a bisphosphonate compound, which may inhibit osteoclast and osteoblast activity and diminish bone resorption and new bone formation.

Selected Indications
Osteoporosis prevention and treatment, Paget's disease of the bone.

Metabolism
Etidronate must be taken 2 hours before eating to ensure adequate absorption. It is adsorbed to developing apatite crystals during bone formation. It is excreted unchanged by the kidneys.

Adverse Reactions
Defective mineralization of bone, with accumulation of unmineralized osteoid, and possible onset of new bone pain and pathologic fractures can occur. Mild abdominal cramps, nausea, and diarrhea are common.

Caution
Patients with renal insufficiency should be treated cautiously. Like other bisphosphonates, etidronate is contraindicated in women of childbearing potential.

Supply
Tablets, 200, 400 mg.

Dosage
For Paget's disease, 400 mg/day given as a single dosage 2 hours before meals. Reassessment is indicated after 6 months of therapy. Dosages above 10 mg/kg/day should be used cautiously and reserved for suppression of rapid bone turnover or for prompt reduction in elevated cardiac output. For treatment of postmenopausal osteoporosis, the dosage is etidronate, 400 mg/day (2 hours before or after a meal) for 14 days every 3 months.

Fluoride, Sodium

Action
Fluoride incorporates into the bone, rendering it less soluble; stimulates new bone formation.

Selected Indications
Osteoporosis prevention and treatment.

Metabolism
Absorbed from gastrointestinal tract and incorporated into bone.

Adverse Reactions

Occasional gastrointestinal upset. Excessive doses can cause mottling of teeth and formation of thickened bones of poor quality (osteomalacia and osteosclerosis). Therefore, despite apparent improvement in bone density, the risk of fractures may increase.

Caution

To prevent precipitation of calcium fluoride, calcium supplements and sodium fluoride are given at separate times of the day. Fluoride supplements should not be given to patients with renal insufficiency.

Supply

Tablets, 1 mg. Larger capsules and oral solution are also available in some pharmacies.

Dosage

A dosage of 10 mg elemental fluoride, twice daily.

Pamidronate (Aredia)

Action

Pamidronate is a bisphosphonate, which inhibits osteoclast activity.

Selected Indications

Paget's disease of the bone, osteoporosis.

Metabolism

After intravenous administration, pamidronate is immediately retained in bone, preferentially in areas of high turnover. The drug is then slowly cleared by the kidney, with a terminal half-life of approximately 300 days.

Adverse Reactions

Most adverse effects appear to be dose-related. These include fatigue, somnolence, infusion site reactions, anorexia, nausea, gastrointestinal hemorrhage, and electrolyte abnormalities (e.g., hypocalcemia, hypokalemia, hypomagnesemia, hypophosphatemia). Cardiopulmonary effects such as hypertension, atrial fibrillation, tachycardia, syncope, and rales may occur with the highest doses. Fever occurs in approximately one-fifth of patients. Cytopenias may occur rarely.

Caution

Serum electrolytes should be followed up closely. In patients with pre-existing hematologic conditions, complete blood counts should also be followed up. Pamidronate should not be given to women of childbearing potential.

Supply

Vials of lyophilized powder, 30 mg, 60 mg, and 90 mg, for reconstitution with sterile water.

Dosage

For Paget's disease, 30 mg/day intravenously given over 4 hours for 3 days. Higher doses are recommended for hypercalcemia associated with malignancies. For osteoporosis treatment and prevention, 30 mg intravenous.

Raloxifene (Evista)

Action

Raloxifene is a benzothiophene compound and is a selective estrogen receptor modulator. It has estrogen agonist activity on bone and antagonist activity on breast and uterine tissue. Its antiosteoporotic effects are probably due to inhibition of osteoclast activity.

Metabolism

Sixty percent of ingested drug is absorbed. It is glucoronidated on first pass in the liver and excreted almost entirely through the feces. Its half-life is approximately 27 hours.

Adverse Reactions
Hot flashes and leg cramps occur. Like other estrogens, there is an increased risk of venous thromboembolism.

Caution
Men and premenopausal women are not good candidates for raloxifene therapy. Raloxifene is absolutely contraindicated in pregnant women. The drug is contraindicated in patients with histories of thromboembolic disease and in patients with known hypersensitivity to the drug or components of the tablets. Cholestyramine causes a 60% reduction in absorption and should not be coadministered with raloxifene. Risks of breast and gynecologic malignancies have not been adequately studied.

Supply
Tablets, 60 mg.

Dosage
A dosage of 60 mg/day.

Risedronate (Actonel)

Action
Risedronate is a bisphosphonate, which inhibits osteoclast activity and bone resorption but does not interfere with bone mineralization.

Selected Indications
Osteoporosis treatment and prevention, Paget's disease of the bone.

Metabolism
Risedronate is poorly absorbed by the gastrointestinal tract especially when taken with food; fasting absorption is less than 1%. Calcium-, aluminum-, and magnesium-containing supplements and antacids interfere with absorption. Absorbed drug is tropic for bone. The terminal half-life is 480 hours. Excretion is through the urine.

Adverse Reactions
Gastrointestinal intolerances are the most common adverse effects and include diarrhea, nausea, abdominal pain, and esophagitis. Approximately one-third of patients may experience arthralgias, but adequate calcium repletion before the initiation of therapy may reduce the risk of musculoskeletal discomfort.

Caution
Risedronate must be taken on an empty stomach, after which patients should not eat at least for 30 minutes or lie down. Risedronate is contraindicated in women of childbearing potential.

Supply
Tablets, 5, 30, 35 mg.

Dosage
For osteoporosis prevention or treatment, 5 mg/day or 35 mg weekly. For Paget's disease, 30 mg/day, with reassessment after 2 months of therapy.

Teriparatide (Forteo)

Action
Teriparatide is a recombinant N-terminus fragment of human parathyroid hormone, which stimulates new bone formation.

Selected Indications
Osteoporosis treatment.

Metabolism

After subcutaneous injection, maximum plasma concentrations are reached within 30 minutes, and the drug becomes undetectable within 4 hours. Elimination is thought to be by nonspecific enzymatic metabolism by the liver and excretion in the kidneys, but the effects of hepatic and renal insufficiency are not clear.

Adverse Reactions

The most common side effects are nausea, dizziness, leg cramps, and headaches. Injection site reactions are rare. Hypercalcemia and hypercalciuria can occur.

Caution

Teriparatide should not be prescribed to patients at increased risk for osteosarcoma, including patients with unexplained elevations in bone alkaline phosphatase concentration, Paget's disease, prior skeletal irradiation, or open epiphyses (i.e., children, adolescents, and young adults). Serum calcium level should be monitored periodically. Bisphosphonates may interfere with the action of teriparatide, and concurrent use is not recommended.

Supply

A dose of 750 μg in a reusable 3 mL-pen injector.

Dosage

A dosage of 20 μg subcutaneously, once a day; a full treatment course is typically no more than 2 years.

Vitamin D

Action

Vitamin D belongs to the family of sterol derivatives, which increases intestinal absorption of calcium and may increase mobilization of mineral from bone.

Selected Indications

Prevention and treatment of postmenopausal osteoporosis, prevention of drug-induced osteoporosis, osteomalacia, rickets, hypoparathyroidism, hypocalcemia, renal osteodystrophy.

Metabolism

The activation of vitamin D is effected via sequential hepatic and renal hydroxylation. The metabolites of vitamin D are mostly excreted in bile.

Adverse Reactions

Vitamin D toxicity may produce hypercalcemia and hyperphosphatemia, causing renal failure, hypertension, drowsiness, abdominal discomfort, and metastatic calcifications.

Caution

Calcium supplementation may be necessary to optimize vitamin D therapy. Monitoring of serum and urinary calcium to assess for vitamin D toxicity on a monthly basis is recommended. If urinary calcium levels rise above 120 mg/day, the dosage of vitamin D should be reduced.

Supply

Many options are available including the following:
- Vitamin D_3, 200 to 400 IU (contained in many multivitamin preparations).
- Ergocalciferol (vitamin D_2), 25,000 and 50,000 IU.
- Calcitriol capsules, 0.25 and 0.5 μg.
- Calcifediol capsules, 20 and 50 μg.
- Dihydrotachysterol tablets, 0.125, 0.2, and 0.4 μg.

Dosage

Postmenopausal osteoporosis: at least 400 IU of vitamin D_3 daily. Prevention of drug-induced osteoporosis: vitamin D_3 400 IU twice daily. Appropriate agent and dosing for other conditions should be adjusted on a clinical basis.

ANTICOAGULANTS

Indications for the use of anticoagulation have grown. In rheumatology, specifically, some situations in which anticoagulants are widely utilized include primary treatment in the antiphospholipid syndrome and other hypercoagulable states, adjuvant therapy in Raynaud's phenomenon and other low-flow states, and in prophylaxis against deep venous thrombosis (DVT). Warfarin and heparins remain the primary agents that are currently available.

Major recent advances have been in the development and use of low-molecular-weight heparin (LMWH) preparations, which appear to be equally effective as, safer, and more easy to use than traditional unfractionated heparin. All heparins act by enhancing the activity of antithrombin III, which neutralizes thrombin and factor Xa. Several preparations of LMWH (e.g., dalteparin, enoxaparin, tinzaparin) are currently available in the United States. They are all depolymerized heparins, but they differ in the degradation process by which they are obtained. One major difficulty in the current use of these preparations is the lack of standardization of activity. The drugs are not interchangeable on a milligram-for-milligram basis, and even attempts to standardize according to biochemical activity (e.g., antifactor Xa activity) have been unsatisfactory.

Although these LMWHs are effective via the subcutaneous route and do not require monitoring of prothrombin time (PT) nor partial thromboplastin time (PTT), physicians must appreciate that when used at therapeutic doses, they do induce full anticoagulation. Therefore, as with intravenous heparin, significant risks of hemorrhage do exist. Moreover, although thrombocytopenia is less frequent, it can still occur.

Dalteparin (Fragmin)

Action

Dalteparin is a depolymerized heparin prepared by nitrous acid degradation of porcine intestinal heparin. It potentiates antithrombin III activity.

Selected Indications

Prophylaxis of DVT, hypercoagulable states.

Metabolism

The metabolic fate of dalteparin is not fully known. Most of it is probably removed by the reticuloendothelial system and by vascular endothelium. Some of the drug may be excreted through urine.

Adverse Reactions

Hematoma at injection sites is the most common adverse effect. Hemorrhage, although much less frequent than with unfractionated heparin, is still a concern. Hematomas at the site of epidural or spinal anesthesias may result in potentially devastating neurologic compromise including permanent paralysis. Allergic reactions and skin necrosis are rare. Thrombocytopenia is much less common than with unfractionated heparin.

Caution

Monitoring of PT or PTT is not necessary. Use in patients with underlying thrombocytopenia or other potential bleeding diathesis should be monitored closely. Regular monitoring of hemoglobin and platelet counts is required. Careful consideration of use in the setting of epidural or spinal anesthesia must be taken. Dalteparin is contraindicated in patients with active hemorrhaging or in those with allergies to porcine products. It should not be administered intramuscularly. This drug should be used cautiously in the setting of renal insufficiency.

Supply

Disposable prefilled syringes, 2,500, 5,000, 7,500, and 10,000 anti-factor Xa units. Multidose vials, 10,000 and 25,000 anti-factor Xa units/mL.

Dosage
For DVT prophylaxis, 5,000 antifactor Xa units injected subcutaneously, once daily.

Enoxaparin (Lovenox)

Action
Enoxaparin is a depolymerized heparin prepared by the alkaline degradation of porcine intestinal heparin. It potentiates antithrombin III activity.

Selected Indications
Prevention or treatment of DVT and pulmonary embolism, hypercoagulable states.

Metabolism
The metabolic fate of enoxaparin is not fully known. Most of it is probably removed by the reticuloendothelial system and by vascular endothelium, but there is some clinically significant clearance through the kidneys, so dose adjustment in the setting of renal insufficiency is necessary.

Adverse Reactions
Hematoma at injection sites is the most common adverse effect. Hemorrhage, although much less frequent than with unfractionated heparin, is still a concern. Hematomas at the site of epidural or spinal anesthesias may result in potentially devastating neurologic compromise including permanent paralysis. Allergic reactions and skin necrosis are rare. Thrombocytopenia is much less common than with unfractionated heparin.

Caution
Monitoring of PT or PTT is not necessary. Use in patients with underlying thrombocytopenia or other potential bleeding diathesis should be monitored closely. Regular monitoring of hemoglobin and platelet counts is required. Careful consideration of use in the setting of epidural or spinal anesthesia must be taken. Enoxaparin is contraindicated in patients with active hemorrhaging or in those with allergies to porcine products. It should not be administered intramuscularly. Dose adjustment in the setting of renal dysfunction is necessary.

Supply
Disposable prefilled syringes, 30, 40, 60, 80, 100, 120, 150 mg. Multidose vial, 300 mg/3 mL.

Dosage
For DVT prophylaxis, 0.5 mg/kg injected subcutaneously, twice daily. For treatment of DVT or pulmonary embolism, 1 mg/kg injected subcutaneously, twice daily.

Fondaparinux (Arixtra)

Action
Fondaparinux is a synthetic inhibitor of factor Xa.

Selected Indications
Prevention of DVT and pulmonary embolism.

Metabolism
Fondaparinux is excreted primarily through the urine and is contraindicated in patients with creatinine clearances less than 30 mL/minute.

Adverse Reactions
Hematoma at injection sites is the most common adverse effect. Hemorrhage, although much less frequent than with unfractionated heparin, is still a concern. Hematomas at the

site of epidural or spinal anesthesias may result in potentially devastating neurologic compromise including permanent paralysis. Allergic reactions and skin necrosis are rare. Thrombocytopenia is much less common than with unfractionated heparin.

Caution
Monitoring of PT or PTT is not necessary. Use in patients with underlying thrombocytopenia or other potential bleeding diathesis should be monitored closely. Careful consideration of use in the setting of epidural or spinal anesthesia must be taken. Fondaparinux is contraindicated in patients with active hemorrhage. It should not be administered intramuscularly. Alternative agents or dose adjustment in the setting of renal dysfunction is recommended.

Supply
Prefilled syringes, 2.5 mg.

Dosage
For DVT prophylaxis, 2.5 mg subcutaneously, once a day.

Heparin, Unfractionated

Action
Heparin is a heterogeneous mixture of anionic sulfated glycosaminoglycans, usually extracted from porcine intestinal mucosa or bovine lung. It potentiates antithrombin III activity.

Selected Indications
Prevention and treatment of DVT and pulmonary embolism, hypercoagulable states.

Metabolism
The metabolic fate of heparin is not fully known. Most of it is probably removed by the reticuloendothelial system and by the vascular endothelium. A small amount may be excreted through urine.

Adverse Reactions
Hemorrhage and hematomas are the most common adverse effects. Hematomas at the site of epidural or spinal anesthesias may result in potentially devastating neurologic compromise including permanent paralysis. Thrombocytopenia may occur in 15% of patients treated with bovine heparin and in 5% of patients treated with porcine heparin. Two reversible mechanisms of thrombocytopenia are identified, both of which are idiosyncratic and not dose-dependent: (i) a direct nonimmunologic effect and (ii) a heparin-dependent IgG platelet-aggregating phenomenon. Rarely, a paradoxical thrombogenic "white clot" syndrome may occur with local or systemic manifestations. Prolonged heparin use may cause osteoporosis.

Caution
Although the PTT is most sensitive to heparin and is used for dose adjustment, the prothrombin time (PT)/international normalized ratio (INR) may also be affected, especially at high dosages. Baseline PTT and PT/INR should be obtained before continuous intravenous therapy. Use in patients with underlying thrombocytopenia or other potential bleeding diathesis should be monitored closely. Regular monitoring of hemoglobin and platelet counts is required. The use of this drug in the setting of epidural or spinal anesthesia must be considered carefully. Heparin is contraindicated in patients with active hemorrhaging or in those with allergies to porcine or bovine products. It should not be administered intramuscularly. Reversal of hemorrhagic complications may require protamine sulfate.

Supply
Bovine lung: Vials, 1,000, 5,000, 10,000 units/mL for subcutaneous injection.
Porcine intestine: Vials, 10, 20, 25, 30, 50, 100, 300, 1,000, 2,500, 5,000, 7,500, 10,000, 20,000 units/mL for subcutaneous injection.

In 5% dextrose, 40, 50, 100 units/mL for intravenous administration.
In normal saline, 2, 50, 100 units/mL for intravenous administration.

Dosage
General guidelines for DVT prophylaxis: 5,000 to 7,500 units injected subcutaneously, twice daily. Adjustments may be necessary as clinically indicated. General guidelines for full-dose continuous intravenous use: 50 to 100 units/kg body weight-loading dose followed by 10 to 15 units/kg body weight/hour continuous infusion. Rebolus and/or readjust infusion rate to desired PTT initially every 6 hours and then daily after a stable dose is achieved. Adjustments may be necessary as clinically indicated.

Tinzaparin (Innohep)

Action
Tinzaparin is a LMWH prepared by enzymatic digestion of porcine intestinal heparin. It potentiates antithrombin III activity.

Selected Indications
Prevention and treatment of DVT and pulmonary embolism, hypercoagulable states.

Metabolism
The metabolic fate of tinzaparin is not fully known. Most of it is probably removed by the reticuloendothelial system and by the vascular endothelium. Some may be excreted through urine.

Adverse Reactions
Hematoma at injection sites is the most common adverse effect. Hemorrhage, although much less frequent than with unfractionated heparin, is still a concern. Hematomas at the site of epidural or spinal anesthesias may result in potentially devastating neurologic compromise including permanent paralysis. Allergic reactions and skin necrosis are rare. Thrombocytopenia is much less common than with unfractionated heparin.

Caution
Monitoring of PT or PTT is not necessary. Use in patients with underlying thrombocytopenia or other potential bleeding diathesis should be monitored closely. Regular monitoring of hemoglobin and platelet counts is required. The use of this drug in the setting of epidural or spinal anesthesia must be carefully considered. Tinzaparin is contraindicated in patients with active hemorrhage or in those with allergies to porcine products. It should not be administered intramuscularly.

Supply
Multiuse vials, 20,000 antifactor Xa units/mL.

Dosage
For DVT prophylaxis, 50 units/kg subcutaneously, once a day. For DVT and pulmonary embolism treatment, 175 units/kg, subcutaneously, once a day.

Warfarin Sodium (Coumadin)

Action
Warfarin indirectly alters the synthesis of functional coagulation factors by interfering with vitamin K activity, which is required for γ-carboxylation of factors II, VII, IX, and X.

Selected Indications
Prophylaxis and treatment of DVT, hypercoagulable states, antiphospholipid syndrome, postcerebrovascular accident care.

Metabolism
Warfarin is generally well absorbed by the gastrointestinal tract, but the rate of absorption can be highly dependent on individual variability and the commercial source of the drug.

Although peak levels of warfarin occur within hours after ingestion, its antithrombogenic effects are not dependent on the plasma levels but rather on the levels of the vitamin K–dependent factors, which may not occur until at least 2 days after administration. Intravenous administration of warfarin does not hasten the onset of activity. The effects of warfarin may be potentiated or diminished by innumerable foods and medications, all of which should be taken into careful consideration during treatment. Warfarin is hepatically inactivated, and the metabolites are excreted through urine.

Adverse Reactions
Hemorrhage is the most common adverse effect of warfarin. Potentially fatal necrosis of the skin or other tissue is a rare complication, most commonly seen in individuals with defects or deficiencies in the antithrombotic factors protein C or protein S. This is seen usually early after initiation of therapy and is thought to be caused by the rapid depletion of the vitamin K–dependent protein C, resulting in a transient prothrombotic state. Another rare complication is cholesterol microembolization syndrome, which can result in systemic microvascular ischemia. Although the PT/INR is most sensitive to warfarin, the PTT can also be elevated at high doses.

Caution
Close monitoring of the PT/INR is required for appropriate dosing of warfarin, especially at the start of the therapy or when changes in concurrent medications are made. Familiarity with drugs, which may enhance or reduce the anticoagulant effects of warfarin, is advised. Warfarin is contraindicated during pregnancy and in breast-feeding women. Intramuscular injections should not be given to anticoagulated individuals.

Supply
Tablets, 1, 2, 2.5, 4, 5, 7.5, 10 mg. Injectable solution, 5 mg.

Dosage
Dosed daily as dictated by desired INR. For most indications (e.g., treatment of DVT, atrial fibrillation), an INR of 2.0 to 3.0 is generally recommended. For patients with mechanical heart valves, an INR of 2.5 to 3.5 should be maintained.

 VASOACTIVE AGENTS

Vasoactive agents are useful in the management of systemic and pulmonary hypertension, Raynaud's phenomenon, and congestive heart failure. Vascular tone may be relaxed by (i) inhibition of sympathetic function (e.g., prazosin), (ii) direct relaxation of smooth muscle (e.g., hydralazine), (iii) calcium channel blockade (e.g., amlodipine, diltiazem, nifedipine, verapamil), and (iv) inhibition of ACE (e.g., captopril, enalapril). The use of ACE inhibitors, in particular, has a drastically changed outcome in diffuse systemic sclerosis. Included in the subsequent text is a small sampling of available agents.

Amlodipine (Norvasc)

Action
Amlodipine is a calcium channel blocker that dilates the coronary and peripheral arteries and the arterioles.

Selected Indications
Hypertension, Raynaud's phenomenon.

Metabolism
Dose adjustment is not generally necessary in the setting of renal insufficiency. However, elimination can be reduced in the setting of hepatic impairment and in geriatric patients.

Adverse Reactions

Hypotension, bradycardia, dizziness, headache, congestive heart failure, pedal edema, nausea, and rash may occur. In Raynaud's phenomenon, all vasodilators may precipitate a vascular steal syndrome.

Caution

Amlodipine should be avoided in patients with sick sinus syndrome, atrioventricular conduction disturbances, severe congestive heart failure, or hypotension (systolic blood pressure <90 mm Hg).

Supply

Tablets, 2.5, 5, 10 mg.

Dosage

Initially 2.5 mg/day.

Bosentan (Tracleer)

Action

Bosentan is a specific and competitive antagonist of endothelin-1 (ET-1) at the site of ET receptors.

Selected Indications

Primary or secondary pulmonary hypertension.

Metabolism

In healthy individuals, peak plasma concentrations after oral administration are achieved within 3 to 5 hours, and the terminal half-life is approximately 5 hours. However, exposure in patients with pulmonary hypertension is probably increased. Bosentan induces cytochrome P-450 enzymes (CYP2C9, CYP3A4, and CYP2C19), and excretion of metabolites is primarily through the biliary system. No dose adjustment is generally necessary in the setting of renal dysfunction.

Adverse Reactions

Liver toxicity is the most clinically significant potential adverse effect and can occur at any point during therapy. Dose-related decreases in hemoglobin warrant regular monitoring of the complete blood count. Flushing, edema, hypotension, palpitations, dyspepsia, fatigue, and pruritus are common but are mild side effects.

Caution

Bosentan is a likely teratogen and is absolutely contraindicated during pregnancy. Women of childbearing age who are considering the use of this drug must be counseled on the effective means of contraception, and a negative pregnancy test should be confirmed before use. Cyclosporine A increases levels of bosentan, and concurrent use of these two medications is contraindicated. Liver function should be assessed before the therapy and closely thereafter. Bosentan should not be prescribed if baseline aminotransferases are greater than three times the upper limit of normal range. The drug should be discontinued if symptomatic hepatic impairment occurs, or if the serum bilirubin exceeds twice that of the upper limit of normal range. Concomitant use of glyburide increases the risk of liver enzyme abnormalities and is also contraindicated. In addition to liver function testing, complete blood counts should also be monitored closely to assess anemia.

Supply

Tablets, 62.5, 125 mg.

Dosage

A dosage of 62.5 mg twice daily for 4 weeks, and if indicated and tolerated, increased to 125 mg twice daily for maintenance.

Captopril (Capoten)

Action
ACE inhibitor that reduces peripheral vascular resistance and venous tone.

Selected Indications
Hypertension, treatment of scleroderma renal crisis, proteinuria.

Metabolism
Rapid oral absorption with peak blood levels at 1 hour. The drug should be taken 1 hour before meals, because food reduces absorption. Twenty-five percent to 30% of the drug is protein bound. Excretion is through urine.

Adverse Reactions
Rash occurs in 10%, dysgeusia in 7%, proteinuria in 2%, orthostatic hypotension in 2%, proteinuria in 1% to 2%, angioedema in 1%, cough in 0.5% to 2%, neutropenia in 0.3%, and renal failure in 0.1%. Gastric irritation and fever have been reported.

Caution
Severe hypotension may be seen in salt- or volume-depleted patients, such as those on diuretics. Patients with congestive heart failure may have elevations in BUN and serum creatinine levels. Neutropenia with myeloid hypoplasia occurred mainly in patients with SLE or other autoimmune diseases. Complete blood count, urinalysis, and renal (especially serum potassium and creatinine) parameters should be checked frequently. Renal function and electrolyte abnormalities in patients with SLE, in particular, should be watched closely. Dosage should be decreased in patients with renal dysfunction.

Supply
Tablets, 12.5, 25, 50, and 100 mg.

Dosage
Initial dosage is 12.5 mg three times daily, then 25 mg three times daily. After 1 to 2 weeks, dosage may increase to 50 mg three times daily, and then increase at 1- to 2-week intervals to a maximum of 150 mg three times daily.

Diltiazem (Cardizem)

Action
Calcium channel blocker that dilates the coronary and peripheral arteries and the arterioles.

Selected Indications
Hypertension, Raynaud's phenomenon.

Metabolism
Diltiazem is absorbed with peak level in 3 hours and has a half-life of 4 hours. It is 80% protein bound. There is extensive hepatic metabolism.

Adverse Reactions
Hypotension, bradycardia, dizziness, headache, congestive heart failure, pedal edema, nausea, and rash may occur. In Raynaud's phenomenon, all vasodilators may precipitate a vascular steal syndrome.

Caution
Diltiazem must be avoided in patients with sick sinus syndrome, atrioventricular conduction disturbances, severe congestive heart failure, or hypotension (systolic blood pressure <90 mm Hg). It should not be used with cyclosporine A. There are data that suggest that extended-release forms may be safer than rapid-release preparations.

Supply
Tablets, 30, 60, 90, 120 mg. Extended-release capsules, 120 mg, 180 mg, 240 mg, 300 mg.

Dosage
Initially 120 mg/day in single or divided doses. Can increase as tolerated to 480 mg/day in single or divided doses.

Enalapril/Enalaprilat (Vasotec)

Action
ACE inhibitors that reduce peripheral vascular resistance and venous tone.

Selected Indications
Hypertension, treatment of scleroderma renal crisis, proteinuria.

Metabolism
Enalapril is the ethylester of enalaprilat. Gastrointestinal absorption of enalapril is appreciable (approximately 55% to 75%) and does not appear to be affected by foods, in contrast to enalaprilat, which is poorly absorbed and is administered intravenously. Enalapril is a prodrug, which is activated by hepatic hydrolysis. Two-thirds of the drug and its metabolites are excreted through urine, while the remaining is eliminated through feces.

Adverse Reactions
Less than 5% of patients will discontinue enalapril for adverse effects. These may include neurologic complaints (dizziness, vertigo), postural hypotension, deterioration of renal function, hypersensitivity reactions, leukopenia, dysgeusia, hyperkalemia, and chronic cough.

Caution
Severe hypotension may be seen in salt- or volume-depleted patients, such as those on diuretics. Patients with congestive heart failure may have elevations in BUN and serum creatinine levels. Complete blood count, urinalysis, and renal (especially serum potassium and creatinine) parameters should be checked frequently. Renal function and electrolyte abnormalities in patients with SLE, in particular, should be watched closely. Conversion between intravenous and oral dosing requires careful attention.

Supply
Enalapril tablets, 2.5, 5, 10, 20 mg. Enalaprilat injectable solution for intravenous use, 1.25 mg/mL.

Dosage
The initial dosage of enalapril is 2.5 daily; maximum dosage is generally 40 mg/day in once or twice daily dosing. The initial dosage of enalaprilat is 1.25 mg every 6 hours, which can be raised to 5 mg every 6 hours, as indicated.

Nifedipine (Procardia, Adalat)

Action
Calcium channel blocker that causes coronary and peripheral arterial vasodilation.

Selected Indications
Hypertension, Raynaud's phenomenon.

Metabolism
Nifedipine is well absorbed, with peak levels attained within 2 hours. The drug is highly protein bound. It is completely metabolized in the liver before being excreted through urine.

Adverse Reactions

Hypotension, dizziness, headache, tachycardia, fatigue, edema, flushing, nausea, nasal congestion, and leg cramps have been noted. In Raynaud's phenomenon, all vasodilators may precipitate a vascular steal syndrome.

Caution

Close monitoring of blood pressure is recommended. There are data suggesting that extended-release forms of calcium channel blockers may be safer than rapid-release preparations.

Supply

Capsules, 10, 20 mg. Extended-release tablets, 30, 60, 90 mg.

Dosage

Initially, 30 mg/day in single or divided doses, which can be raised to 90 mg/day.

Prazosin (Minipress)

Action

Arterial and venous dilator, which may act via α-adrenergic receptor blockade.

Selected Indications

Hypertension, Raynaud's phenomenon.

Metabolism

Peak plasma levels are attained within 3 hours of ingestion, and the half-life is 2 to 3 hours. It is highly protein bound and extensively metabolized in the liver.

Adverse Reactions

Orthostatic hypotension, syncope, peripheral edema, fatigue, headache, dizziness, and nausea may occur. Rarely, urinary frequency, impotence, rash, and nasal congestion have been noted.

Caution

Symptomatic orthostatic hypotension with syncope may occur after the first dose. Therefore, the first dose should not exceed 1 mg and should be given at bedtime, with instructions to the patient to remain in bed at least 3 hours after the drug is administered. Dosage may be increased to 1 mg twice daily, then three times daily, with further gradual increments. Tolerance to hemodynamic effects may develop during long-term treatment.

Supply

Capsules, 1, 2, and 5 mg.

Dosage

A dosage of 1 mg three times daily, gradually increased to 20 mg/day in divided doses if necessary and if tolerated.

Verapamil (Calan, Covera, Isoptin, Verelan)

Action

Calcium channel blocker that reduces coronary and peripheral vascular resistance.

Selected Indications

Hypertension, Raynaud's phenomenon.

Metabolism

Gastrointestinal absorption is excellent, with peak serum levels occurring in 1 to 2 hours. Ninety percent of the drug is protein bound. The half-life is 3 to 6 hours, with marked prolongation in patients with hepatic dysfunction. There is extensive metabolism in the liver, and excretion of active metabolites is through urine.

Adverse Reactions
Hypotension, peripheral edema, bradycardia, heart block, congestive heart failure, headaches, dizziness, constipation, and abnormal results of liver function tests may occur. In Raynaud's phenomenon, all vasodilators may precipitate a vascular steal syndrome.

Caution
Verapamil increases digoxin levels by 50% to 70%. It should be avoided in patients with sick sinus syndrome, severe congestive heart failure, or hepatic or renal impairment. There are data suggesting that extended-release forms of calcium channel blockers may be safer than rapid-release preparations.

Supply
Tablets, 40, 80 and 120 mg. Extended-release tablets, 120, 180, and 240 mg.

Dosage
Initially, 120 mg/day in single or divided dose; can increase to up to 480 mg/day.

 ## MISCELLANEOUS
Cevimeline (Evoxac)

Action
Cevimeline is a cholinergic agonist that binds to muscarinic receptors on exocrine glandular cells, thereby stimulating glandular secretions.

Selected Indications
Xerostomia in primary and secondary Sjögren's syndrome.

Metabolism
Peak plasma levels can be reached within 2 hours, although concomitant food causes a slight delay in reaching peak concentrations. The mean half-life is approximately 5 hours. Hepatic mechanisms (CYP2D6 and CYP3A3/4) are primarily responsible for metabolism, and excretion is mostly through the kidneys. However, the effects of renal and hepatic impairment have not been fully evaluated.

Adverse Reactions
Cholinergic effects are responsible for many of the adverse reactions of cevimeline, such as sweatiness, visual disturbance, rhinitis, bronchial constriction, nausea, gastrointestinal discomfort, diarrhea, and blood pressure lability. Cardiac conduction disturbances and asthma exacerbations are of particular concern.

Caution
Patients with uncontrolled asthma or in whom miosis is undesired (e.g., iritis or closed-angle glaucoma) are not good candidates for cevimeline. β-adrenergic antagonists should be cautiously given concurrently for fear of cardiac dysrhythmias.

Supply
Capsules, 30 mg.

Dosage
A dosage of 30 mg three times daily, usually before meals.

Chondroitin Sulfate/Glucosamine Sulfate

In the United States, chondroitin sulfate and glucosamine sulfate are considered as nutritional supplements and not as medicines and so have not been rigorously studied for metabolism, efficacy, and toxicity.

Selected Indications
Osteoarthritis.

Action
Usually taken together, these agents are thought to possibly maintain synovial joint integrity by optimizing synthesis of collagen and glycosaminoglycans, stimulation of hyaluronic acid secretion by chondrocytes, and inhibition of degradative enzymes.

Metabolism
Both agents are absorbed in the gastrointestinal tract. At least some of the compounds can then be traced to synovial joints.

Adverse Reactions
Mild gastrointestinal intolerances such as bloatedness and flatus are common but generally do not result in discontinuation. Concern that glucosamine elevates blood glucose levels has not borne out in well-controlled clinical trials.

Caution
No data are available on effects on fertility, pregnancy, or lactation.

Supply
Glucosamine sulfate, capsules and tablets, 500 mg. Chondroitin sulfate, capsules and tablets, 400 mg. Also available in combined forms.

Dosage
Glucosamine sulfate, 1,500 to 2,000 mg/day in divided doses. Chondroitin sulfate, 1,200 to 1,600 mg/day in divided doses.

Cyclosporine Ophthalmologic Emulsion (Restasis)

Action
Cyclosporine is a potent inhibitor of early steps in T-cell activation via suppression of early gene transcription. When used topically in the eye, it is thought to suppress inflammation of the lacrimal glands.

Selected Indications
Keratoconjunctivitis sicca in primary and secondary Sjögren's syndrome.

Metabolism
No systemic absorption of cyclosporine is detectable after ophthalmologic topical application.

Adverse Reactions
The most common adverse event is ocular burning occurring in 17% of patients. Other local effects include conjunctival hyperemia, edema, discharge, epiphora, pain, itching, and foreign body sensation.

Caution
After application of the cyclosporine emulsion, patients should wait for at least 15 minutes before inserting contact lenses. The safety of use in patients with a history of herpetic keratitis has not been assessed.

Supply
A 0.05% emulsion in single-use vials, supplied as 32 vials/tray.

Dosage
After gentle agitation of the vial, one drop to each eye every 12 hours.

Hyaluronans (Hyalgan, Orthovisc, Supartz, Synvisc)

Action
Increases viscoelasticity of synovial fluid and possibly reduces chondrodegradation.

Selected Indications
Osteoarthritis.

Metabolism
High-molecular-weight fractions of sodium hyaluronate for sterile intra-articular injection are derived from chicken combs and are available in a buffered physiologic sodium chloride solution. The intra-articular half-life of sodium hyaluronate is less than 24 hours. Hyaluronans are degraded by intra-articular enzymes, free radicals, and sheer forces. The degradation products are removed through lymphatics and undergo hepatic catabolism.

Adverse Reactions
Most adverse effects are related to symptoms associated with the site of injection including pain, swelling, effusion, warmth, and redness. Some of these cases are exacerbations of gout or pseudogout and rarely introduced infections. Self-limited allergic reactions have been reported.

Caution
At present, hyaluronans are approved only for osteoarthritis of the knee. Increases in knee inflammation after administration in the setting of inflammatory arthritides (e.g., rheumatoid arthritis and gout) have been noted. Because the source of the agent is rooster combs, precaution should be taken in patients with allergies to avian proteins, feathers, and egg products. Strict sterile technique is to be observed, and no injection should be attempted through skin which appears infected. Disinfectants containing quaternary ammonium salts should not be used for skin preparation.

Supply
A dose of 2 mL prefilled syringes and vials.

Dosage
Removal of any knee effusion is recommended before administration of hyaluronans. A dosage of 2 mL administered weekly for 3 to 5 weeks, depending on specific preparation recommendations.

Lansoprazole (Prevacid)

Action
Lansoprazole is a substituted benzimidazole, which specifically inhibits the proton pump system on the secretory surface of the gastric parietal cell.

Selected Indications
Gastroesophageal reflux, gastroprotection against NSAIDs, systemic sclerosis.

Metabolism
Absorption of lansoprazole occurs after the drug leaves the stomach and is diminished when the drug is taken after intake of food. Lansoprazole is transformed into two active metabolites, which act locally at the parietal cell, so plasma levels do not reflect activity at the gastric mucosa. The drug is extensively metabolized by the liver, and its metabolites are excreted through both feces (67%) and urine (33%). Dose adjustment should be considered in patients with hepatic impairment.

Adverse Reactions
Lansoprazole is generally well tolerated. Minor adverse effects reported include gastrointestinal intolerance, diarrhea, nausea, vomiting, headache, dizziness, and rashes.

Caution
Lansoprazole may increase clearance of theophylline. It may also interfere with absorption of drugs (such as ketoconazole, ampicillin esters, and digoxin) in which gastric pH is an important determinant of bioavailability.

Supply
Delayed-release capsules, 15 and 30 mg.

Dosage
A dosage of 15 to 30 mg/day.

Metoclopramide (Reglan)

Action
Metoclopramide stimulates upper gastrointestinal peristalsis without stimulating gastric, biliary, or pancreatic secretions, possibly by sensitizing tissue to the effects of acetylcholine.

Selected Indications
Gastrointestinal dysmotility, systemic sclerosis.

Metabolism
Metoclopramide is rapidly absorbed via the gastrointestinal tract, and peak plasma levels are reached within 2 hours. The mean half-life is approximately 6 hours. It is partially metabolized by hepatic conjugation and is excreted primarily through urine. Patients with renal impairment may require dose adjustment.

Adverse Reactions
Central nervous system effects including sedation, headache, restlessness, cognitive, or affective changes may occur in more than 10% of patients. Extrapyramidal reactions including acute dystonic reactions, akathisia, parkinsonian symptoms, and tardive dyskinesia may occur.

Caution
Metoclopramide should not be used in patients with poorly controlled hypertension or in patients with pheochromocytoma. It is also contraindicated in patients where acceleration of gastrointestinal motility is undesired, such as acute hemorrhages. Patients at risk for extrapyramidal symptoms should not receive metoclopramide.

Supply
Tablets, 5 and 10 mg. Syrup, 1 mg/mL. Injectable, 5 mg/mL; 2-, 10-, and 30-mL vials.

Dosage
A dosage of 10 to 20 mg up to four times daily, taken orally 15 to 30 minutes before meals. Parenteral administration of 10 mg may be given intramuscularly, or intravenously over 1 to 2 minutes.

Misoprostol (Cytotec)

Action
Misoprostol is a synthetic analog of prostaglandin E_1, which has protective properties against gastric inflammation and ulceration induced by NSAIDs.

Selected Indications
Gastroprotection against NSAIDs.

Metabolism
Absorption of misoprostol is rapid but is diminished by food or antacids. It is converted into its active form via de-esterification. Most of the drug is excreted through urine, but dose adjustment is generally not necessary in the setting of renal impairment.

Adverse Reactions
Abdominal discomfort, flatulence, and diarrhea are commonly reported. Gynecologic symptoms including spotting, cramps, hypermenorrhea, and dysmenorrhea may also occur. Postmenopausal vaginal bleeding requires thorough evaluation.

Caution
Misoprostol has abortifacient properties and is contraindicated in pregnant women. Women of childbearing age must be warned of these properties and must comply with effective contraceptive methods before being prescribed misoprostol.

Supply
Tablets, 100 and 200 μg. Misoprostol 200 μg is also available in combination with diclofenac 50 and 75 mg.

Dosage
A dosage of 200 μg four times daily. May be reduced to 100 μg four times daily if the higher dose is not tolerated.

Omeprazole (Prilosec)

Action
Omeprazole is a substituted benzimidazole, which specifically inhibits the proton pump system on the secretory surface of the gastric parietal cell.

Selected Indications
Gastroesophageal reflux, gastroprotection against NSAIDs, systemic sclerosis.

Metabolism
Absorption of omeprazole occurs after the drug leaves the stomach. Although the drug is easily absorbed after oral administration, there is extensive first-pass hepatic metabolism, resulting in an absolute bioavailability of approximately 30% to 40% of an equivalent intravenous dose. Accordingly, bioavailability increases in individuals with chronic liver disease. Approximately three-fourths of the administered drug is excreted through urine, whereas the remainder is excreted through feces.

Adverse Reactions
Omeprazole is generally well tolerated. Minor reported adverse effects include gastrointestinal intolerance, diarrhea, nausea, vomiting, headache, dizziness, and rashes.

Caution
Omeprazole may interfere with the metabolism and increase plasma levels of warfarin, phenytoin, and diazepam. It may also interfere with absorption of drugs (such as ketoconazole, ampicillin esters, and digoxin) in which gastric pH is an important determinant of bioavailability.

Supply
Delayed-release capsules, 20 and 40 mg.

Dosage
A dosage of 20 to 40 mg/day.

Pilocarpine Hydrochloride (Salagen)

Action
Pilocarpine is a cholinergic parasympathomimetic, which increases salivary gland secretions in Sjögren's syndrome.

Selected Indications
Xerostomia in primary and secondary Sjögren's syndrome.

Metabolism
Peak levels are achieved within 1 hour after oral administration but are delayed with high-fat meals. Pilocarpine does not bind to serum proteins. It is thought to be inactivated at neuronal synapses and in plasma. Pilocarpine and its metabolites are excreted through urine.

Adverse Reactions

At dosages recommended for xerostomia, excessive sweating is the most commonly reported adverse effect, occurring in 40% of patients. Urinary frequency, flushing, and chills can also occur.

Caution

Pilocarpine is contraindicated and should be avoided in patients with underlying cardiovascular disease in which transient hemodynamic changes may not be tolerated and in patients with uncontrolled asthma or chronic obstructive pulmonary disease. It should also not be used when miosis is undesirable. Concomitant use of β-adrenergic antagonists may result in conduction disturbances. Toxicity is caused by exaggeration of parasympathetic and cholinergic effects and may require treatment with atropine and hemodynamic support. Pregnant and breast-feeding women should not be given pilocarpine. Pilocarpine should be avoided in patients with narrow-angle glaucoma.

Supply

Tablets, 5, 7.5 mg.

Dosage

A dosage of 5 to 7.5 mg four times daily, typically before meals.

Sunscreens

Action

Absorption of ultraviolet (UV) light. Medium-wave (UVB: 280 to 320 nm) light is the major cause of sunburn and, probably, lupus-related skin reactions. Long-wave light (UVA: 320 to 400 nm) is the major cause of photosensitivity reactions.

Selected Indications

SLE, cutaneous lupus erythematosus, prevention of sun exposure while on photoreactive medications.

Metabolism

Topical use only.

Adverse Reactions

Local hypersensitivity reactions to active compounds or vehicle, contact dermatitis, and photocontact dermatitis can occur. Sunscreens may prevent cutaneous synthesis of vitamin D, especially in the older individuals.

Caution

Patients allergic to thiazides, sulfa drugs, benzocaine, procaine, aniline dyes, and paraphenylene diamine may have allergic reactions to p-aminobenzoic acid (PABA), a common active ingredient. PABA-free preparations are available.

Dosage

Sunscreens are rated by sun protection factor (SPF). Higher values reflect greater degrees of protection. Preparations of at least SPF 30 are recommended. Sunscreen should be applied 1 to 2 hours before sun exposure and several times during exposure, especially after sweating or swimming. Reapplication does not extend the period of protection.

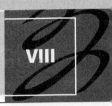

Appendices VIII

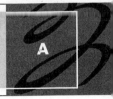

AMERICAN COLLEGE OF RHEUMATOLOGY CRITERIA FOR DIAGNOSIS AND CLASSIFICATION OF RHEUMATIC DISEASES
Allan Gibofsky

A

CRITERIA FOR THE CLASSIFICATION OF RHEUMATOID ARTHRITIS

For classification purposes, a patient is said to have rheumatoid arthritis if he/she has satisfied at least four of the following seven criteria. Criteria I through IV must have been present for at least 6 weeks. Patients with two clinical diagnoses are not excluded. Designation as classic, definite, or probable rheumatoid arthritis is not to be made.[1]

I.   **MORNING STIFFNESS.** Morning stiffness in and around the joints, lasting at least 1 hour before maximal improvement.

II. **ARTHRITIS OF THREE OR MORE JOINT AREAS.** At least three joint areas simultaneously have had soft-tissue swelling or fluid (not bony overgrowth alone) when observed by a physician. The 14 possible areas are right or left proximal interphalangeal (PIP), metacarpophalangeal (MCP), wrist, elbow, knee, ankle, and metatarsophalangeal (MTP) joints.

III. **ARTHRITIS OF HAND JOINTS.** At least one area is swollen (as defined in the preceding text) in a wrist, MCP, or PIP joint.

IV. **SYMMETRIC ARTHRITIS.** There is simultaneous involvement of the same joint areas (as defined in II) on both sides of the body (bilateral involvement of PIPs, MCPs, or MTPs is acceptable without absolute symmetry).

V.   **RHEUMATOID NODULES.** Subcutaneous nodules over bony prominences or extensor surfaces or in juxta-articular regions, observed by a physician.

VI. **SERUM RHEUMATOID FACTOR.** Demonstration of abnormal amounts of serum rheumatoid factor by any method for which the result has been positive in less than 5% of healthy control subjects.

VII. **RADIOGRAPHIC CHANGES.** Changes typical of rheumatoid arthritis on posteroanterior hand and wrist radiographs, which must include erosions or unequivocal bony

---

[1]Arnett FC, Edworthy SM, Bloch DA, et al. The American Rheumatism Association 1987 revised criteria for the classification of rheumatoid arthritis. *Arthritis Rheum* 1988;31:315–324.

decalcification localized in or most marked adjacent to the involved joints (osteoarthritis changes alone do not qualify).

CLASSIFICATION OF GLOBAL FUNCTIONAL STATUS IN RHEUMATOID ARTHRITIS

Usual self-care activities include dressing, feeding, bathing, grooming, and toileting. Avocational (recreational and/or leisure) and vocational (work, school, homemaking) activities are patient-desired and age- and sex-specific.

I.   **CLASS I.** Completely able to perform usual activities of daily living (self-care, vocational, and avocational).
II. **CLASS II.** Able to perform usual self-care and vocational activities, but limited in avocational activities.
III. **CLASS III.** Able to perform usual self-care activities, but limited in vocational and avocational activities.
VI. **CLASS IV.** Limited in ability to perform usual self-care, vocational, and avocational activities.

CRITERIA FOR THE CLASSIFICATION OF SYSTEMIC LUPUS ERYTHEMATOSUS

The proposed classification is based on 11 criteria. For the purpose of identifying patients in clinical studies, a person shall be said to have systemic lupus erythematosus (SLE) if any four or more of the 11 criteria are present, serially or simultaneously, during any interval of observation.[2]

I.   **MALAR RASH.** Fixed erythema, flat or raised, over the malar eminences, with a tendency to spare the nasolabial folds.
II. **DISCOID RASH.** Erythematous raised patches with adherent keratotic scaling and follicular plugging; atrophic scarring may occur in older lesions.
III. **PHOTOSENSITIVITY.** Skin rash as a result of unusual reaction to sunlight, determined by patient history or physician observation.
IV. **ORAL ULCERS.** Oral or nasopharyngeal ulceration, usually painless, observed by a physician.
V.   **ARTHRITIS.** Nonerosive arthritis involving two or more peripheral joints, characterized by tenderness, swelling, or effusion.
VI. **SEROSITIS**
     A. Pleuritis. Convincing history of pleuritic pain or rubbing, recorded by a physician, or evidence of pleural effusion **or**
     B. Pericarditis. Documented by electrocardiogram (ECG), rubbing, or evidence of pericardial effusion.
VII. **RENAL DISORDER**
     A. Persistent proteinuria greater than 0.5 g/day or greater than 3+ if quantitation not performed **or**
     B. Cellular casts. May be red cell, hemoglobin, granular, tubular, or mixed.
VIII. **NEUROLOGIC DISORDER**
     A. Seizures. In the absence of offending drugs or known metabolic derangements, such as uremia, ketoacidosis, or electrolyte imbalance **or**
     B. Psychosis. In the absence of offending drugs or known metabolic derangements, such as uremia, ketoacidosis, or electrolyte imbalance.
IX. **HEMATOLOGIC DISORDER**
     A. Hemolytic anemia. With reticulocytosis **or**
     B. Leukopenia. Leukocytes less than $4,000/\text{mm}^3$ total on two or more occasions **or**
     C. Lymphopenia. Lymphocytes less than $1,500/\text{mm}^3$ on two or more occasions **or**

[2]Tan EM, Cohen AS, Fries JF, et al. The 1982 revised criteria for the classification of systemic lupus erythematosus. *Arthritis Rheum* 1982;25:1271–1277.

D. Thrombocytopenia. Thrombocytes less than $100,000/mm^3$ in the absence of offending drugs.

X. IMMUNOLOGIC DISORDER

A. Positive lupus erythematosus (LE) cell preparation **or**

B. Antideoxyribonucleic acid (DNA). Antibody to native DNA in abnormal titer **or**

C. Anti-Sm. Presence of antibody to Smith nuclear antigen **or**

D. False-positive serologic test for syphilis known to be positive for at least 6 months and confirmed by *Treponema pallidum* immobilization or fluorescent treponemal antibody absorption test.

XI. ANTINUCLEAR ANTIBODY. An abnormal titer of antinuclear antibody by immunofluorescence or an equivalent assay at any point of time and in the absence of drugs known to be associated with "drug-induced lupus" syndrome.

CRITERIA FOR THE CLASSIFICATION OF CHURG-STRAUSS SYNDROME (TRADITIONAL FORMAT), THEIR SENSITIVITY AND SPECIFICITY VERSUS OTHER DEFINED VASCULITIS SYNDROMES

For classification purposes, a patient is said to have Churg-Strauss syndrome (CSS) if at least four of these six criteria are positive. The presence of any four or more of the six criteria yields a sensitivity of 85% and a specificity of 99.7%.[3]

I. ASTHMA.

II. EOSINOPHILIA GREATER THAN 10%.

III. NEUROPATHY, MONO OR POLY.

IV. PULMONARY INFILTRATES, NONFIXED.

V. PARANASAL SINUS ABNORMALITY.

VI. EXTRAVASCULAR EOSINOPHILS.

CRITERIA FOR THE CLASSIFICATION OF FIBROMYALGIA

For classification purposes, patients are said to have fibromyalgia if both criteria are satisfied. Widespread pain must have been present for at least 3 months. The presence of a second clinical disorder does not exclude the diagnosis of fibromyalgia.[4]

I. HISTORY OF WIDESPREAD PAIN. Pain is considered widespread when all of the following are present: pain in the left side of the body, pain in the right side of the body, pain above the waist, and pain below the waist. In addition, axial skeletal pain (cervical spine or anterior chest or thoracic spine or low back) must be present. In this definition, shoulder and buttock pain is considered as pain in each involved side. "Low-back" pain is considered lower segment pain.

II. PAIN IN 11 OF 18 TENDER POINT SITES ON DIGITAL PALPATION. Pain, on digital palpation, must be present in at least 11 of the following 18 sites. Digital palpation should be performed with an approximate force of 4 kg. For a tender point to be considered "positive," the subject must state that the palpation was painful. Tender is not to be considered "painful."

A. Occiput. Bilateral, at the suboccipital muscle insertions.

B. Low cervical. Bilateral, at the anterior aspects of the intertransverse spaces at C5-7.

C. Trapezius. Bilateral, at the midpoint of the upper border.

D. Supraspinatus. Bilateral, at origins, above the scapula spine near the medial border.

E. Second rib. Bilateral, at the second costochondral junction, just lateral to the junctions on upper surfaces.

---

[3]Masi AT, Hunder GG, Lie JT, et al. The American College of Rheumatology 1990 criteria for the classification of Churg-Strauss syndrome (allergic granulomatosis and angiitis). *Arthritis Rheum* 1990;33: 1094–1100.

[4]Wolfe F, Smythe HA, Yunus MB, et al. The American College of Rheumatology 1990 criteria for the classification of fibromyalgia: report of the multicenter criteria committee. *Arthritis Rheum* 1990;33:160–172.

F. Lateral epicondyle. Bilateral, 2 cm distal to the epicondyles.

G. Gluteal. Bilateral, in upper outer quadrants of buttocks in the anterior fold of muscle.

H. Greater trochanter. Bilateral, posterior to the trochanteric prominence.

I. Knee. Bilateral, at the medial fat pad proximal to the joint line.

CRITERIA FOR THE CLASSIFICATION OF WEGENER'S GRANULOMATOSIS

For purposes of classification, a patient is said to have Wegener's granulomatosis if at least two of these four criteria are present. The presence of any two or more criteria yields a sensitivity of 88.2% and a specificity of 92.0%.[5]

I.   NASAL OR ORAL INFLAMMATION. Development of painful or painless oral ulcers or purulent or bloody nasal discharge.

II. ABNORMAL CHEST RADIOGRAPH. Chest radiograph showing the presence of nodules, fixed infiltrates, or cavities.

III. URINARY SEDIMENT. Microhematuria (>5 red blood cells per hpf) or red cell casts in urine sediment.

VI. GRANULOMATOUS INFLAMMATION FOUND ON BIOPSY. Histologic changes showing granulomatous inflammation within the wall of an artery or in the perivascular or extravascular area (artery or arteriole).

CRITERIA FOR THE CLASSIFICATION OF GIANT CELL (TEMPORAL) ARTERITIS

For purposes of classification, a patient is said to have giant cell (temporal) arteritis if at least three of these five criteria are present. The presence of any three or more criteria yields a sensitivity of 93.5% and a specificity of 91.2%.[6]

I.   AGE AT DISEASE ONSET ≥50 YEARS. Development of symptoms or findings beginning at 50 years or older.

II. NEW HEADACHE. New onset of or new type of localized pain in the head.

III. TEMPORAL ARTERY ABNORMALITY. Temporal artery tenderness to palpation or decreased pulsation, unrelated to arteriosclerosis of cervical arteries.

IV. ELEVATED ERYTHROCYTE SEDIMENTATION RATE. Erythrocyte sedimentation rate greater than or equal to 50 mm/hour in the Westergren's method.

V.   ABNORMAL ARTERY BIOPSY. Biopsy specimen with artery showing vasculitis characterized by a predominance of mononuclear cell infiltration or granulomatous inflammation, usually with multinucleated giant cells.

CRITERIA FOR THE CLASSIFICATION OF ACUTE ARTHRITIS OF PRIMARY GOUT[7]

I.   MONOSODIUM URATE MONOHYDRATE MICROCRYSTALS IN JOINT FLUID DURING ATTACK.

II. TOPHUS CONTAINING URATE CRYSTALS OR

III. THE PRESENCE OF SIX OF THE FOLLOWING:

   A. MORE THAN ONE ATTACK OF ACUTE ARTHRITIS.

   B. MAXIMUM INFLAMMATION DEVELOPED WITHIN 1 DAY.

[5]Leavitt RY, Fauci AS, Bloch DA, et al. The American College of Rheumatology 1990 criteria for the classification of Wegener's granulomatosis. *Arthritis Rheum* 1990;33:1101–1107.

[6]Hunder GG, Bloch DA, Michel BA, et al. The American College of Rheumatology 1990 criteria for the classification of giant cell arteritis. *Arthritis Rheum* 1990;33:1122–1128.

[7]Wallace SL, Robinson H, Masi AT, et al. Preliminary criteria for the classification of the acute arthritis of primary gout. *Arthritis Rheum* 1977;20:895–900.

C. **MONOARTHRITIS ATTACK.**
D. **REDNESS OBSERVED OVER JOINTS.**
E. **FIRST MTP JOINT PAINFUL OR SWOLLEN.**
F. **UNILATERAL FIRST MTP JOINT ATTACK.**
G. **UNILATERAL TARSAL JOINT ATTACK.**
H. **TOPHUS (PROVEN OR SUSPECTED).**
 I. **HYPERURICEMIA.**
 J. **ASYMMETRIC SWELLING WITHIN A JOINT FOUND ON X-RAY.** This criterion could logically be found on examination as well as on x-ray. However, the protocol did not request this information in regard to examination.
K. **SUBCORTICAL CYSTS WITHOUT EROSIONS FOUND ON X-RAY.**
L. **NEGATIVE CULTURE OF JOINT FLUID FOR MICROORGANISMS DURING ACUTE ATTACK.**

 ## CRITERIA FOR THE CLASSIFICATION OF HENOCH-SCHÖNLEIN PURPURA

For purposes of classification, a patient is said to have Henoch-Schönlein purpura if at least two of these four criteria are present. The presence of any two or more criteria yields a sensitivity of 87.1% and a specificity of 87.7%.[8]

 I. **PALPABLE PURPURA.** Slightly raised "palpable" hemorrhagic skin lesions, not related to thrombocytopenia.
 II. **AGE LESS THAN OR EQUAL TO 20 YEARS AT DISEASE ONSET.** Patient 20 years or younger at onset of first symptoms.
 III. **BOWEL ANGINA.** Diffuse abdominal pain, worse after meals, or the diagnosis of bowel ischemia, usually including bloody diarrhea.
 IV. **WALL GRANULOCYTES FOUND ON BIOPSY.** Histologic changes showing granulocytes in the walls of arterioles or venules.

---

[8]Mills JA, Michel BA, Bloch DA, et al. The American College of Rheumatology 1990 criteria for the classification of Henoch-Schönlein purpura. *Arthritis Rheum* 1990;33:1114–1121.

NEUROLOGIC DERMATOMES
Allan Gibofsky

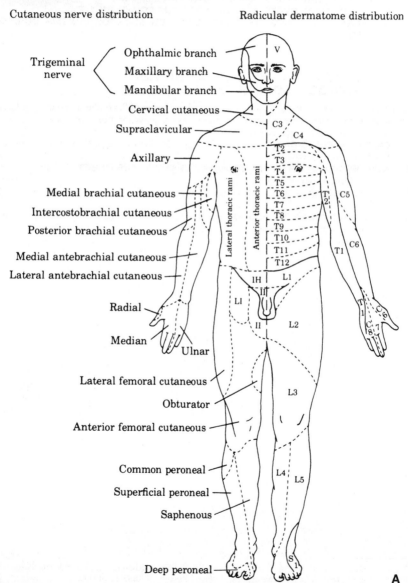

Cutaneous nerve distribution

Radicular dermatome distribution

Trigeminal nerve
- Ophthalmic branch
- Maxillary branch
- Mandibular branch

Cervical cutaneous

Supraclavicular

Axillary

Medial brachial cutaneous

Intercostobrachial cutaneous

Posterior brachial cutaneous

Medial antebrachial cutaneous

Lateral antebrachial cutaneous

Radial

Median

Ulnar

Lateral femoral cutaneous

Obturator

Anterior femoral cutaneous

Common peroneal

Superficial peroneal

Saphenous

Deep peroneal

Lateral thoracic rami

Anterior thoracic rami

V
C3
C4
T2
T3
T4
T5
T6
T7
T8
T9
T10
T11
T12
IH
IL
II
L1
L2
L3
L4 L5
T2
C5
C6
T1
C7
C6
C8
S1

A

Radicular dermatome distribution   Cutaneous nerve distribution

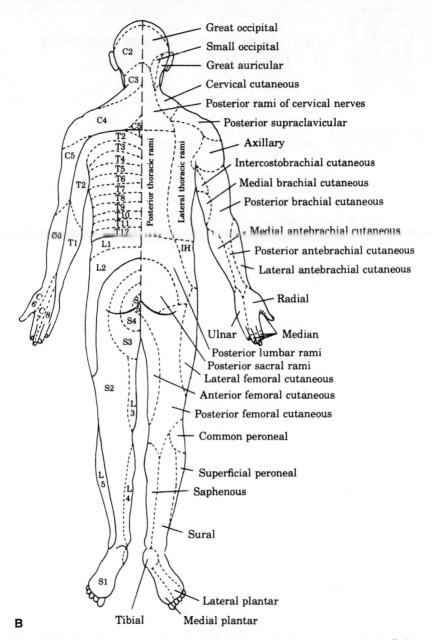

B

Figure B-1. A: Radicular dermatomes and cutaneous nerve distribution, anterior view. **B:** Radicular dermatomes and cutaneous nerve distribution, posterior view.
IH, iliohypogastric; II, ilioinguinal; LI, lumboinguinal.

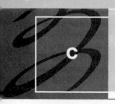

FUNCTIONAL OUTCOME INSTRUMENTS

Lisa A. Mandl and Melanie J. Harrison

TABLE C-1	Health Assessment Questionnaire (HAQ)

This questionnaire includes information from you to provide a record of your health status today. Please try to answer each question, even if you do not think it is related to your situation. There are no right or wrong answers. Please answer exactly as you think or feel. Thank you.

Please CIRCLE the ONE best answer for your abilities at this time for the following questions:

Answer choices:

1) Without ANY difficulty.
2) With SOME difficulty.
3) With MUCH difficulty.
4) UNABLE to do.
5) Not applicable.

AT THIS MOMENT, are you able to:

a) Dress yourself, including tying shoelaces and doing buttons?
b) Get in and out of bed?
c) Lift a full cup or glass to your mouth?
d) Walk outdoors on flat ground?
e) Wash and dry your entire body?
f) Bend down to pick up clothing from the floor?
g) Turn regular faucets on and off?
h) Get in and out of a car, bus, train, or airplane?
i) Run errands and shop?
j) Climb up a flight of stairs?
k) Walk 2 miles?
l) Run or jog 2 miles?
m) Drive a car 5 miles from your home?
n) Participate in sports and games as you would like?
o) Get a good night's sleep?
p) Deal with the usual stresses of daily life?
q) Deal with feelings of anxiety or being nervous?
r) Deal with feelings of depression or feeling blue?

TABLE C-2	**Western Ontario McMaster Universities (WOMAC) Osteoarthritis Index Version VA3.1**

Patients are instructed to answer as per the condition of the study joint in the last 48 hours.

SECTION A—PAIN

How much pain have you had...
a) when walking on a flat surface?
b) when going up or down stairs?
c) at night while in bed?
d) while sitting or lying down?
e) while standing?

SECTION B—STIFFNESS

How severe has your stiffness been...
a) after you first woke up in the morning?
b) after sitting or lying down or while resting later in the day?

SECTION C—DIFFICULTY PERFORMING DAILY ACTIVITIES

How much difficulty have you had...
a) when going down the stairs?
b) when going up the stairs?
c) when getting up from a sitting position?
d) while standing?
e) when bending to the floor?
f) when walking on a flat surface?
g) getting in or out of a car, or getting on or off a bus?
h) while going shopping?
i) when putting on your socks or panty hose or stockings?
j) when getting out of bed?
k) when taking off your socks or panty hose or stockings?
l) while lying in bed?
m) when getting in or out of the bathtub?
n) while sitting?
o) when getting on or off the toilet?
p) while doing heavy household chores?
q) while doing light household chores?

ANSWERS ARE GIVEN USING ONE OF THE FOLLOWING SCALES:

Visual analog scale: Patients are asked to mark their answers by putting an "X" through a horizontal line.
Example:

No |————————————————————————| Extreme
Pain   Pain

Likert Scale: Patients are asked to choose one of the following answers:
1) None
2) Slight
3) Moderate
4) Very
5) Extreme

TABLE C-3	Systemic Lupus Erythematosus Disease Activity Index (SLEDAI)

Trained assessor (e.g., physician) enters weight in score column if descriptor is present currently or in the preceding 10 days.

Weight	Score	Descriptor	Definition
8	____	Seizure	Recent onset. Exclude metabolic, infectious, or drug causes.
8	____	Psychosis	Altered ability to function in normal activity due to severe disturbance in the perception of reality. Include hallucinations; incoherence; marked loose associations; impoverished thought content; marked illogical thinking; bizarre, disorganized, or catatonic behavior. Exclude uremia and drug causes.
8	____	Organic brain syndrome	Altered mental function with impaired orientation, memory, or other Intellectual function, with rapid onset and fluctuating clinical features. Include clouding of consciousness with reduced capacity to focus, and inability to sustain attention to environment, plus at least two of the following; perceptual disturbance, incoherent speech, insomnia or daytime drowsiness, or increased or decreased psychomotor activity. Exclude metabolic, infectious, or drug causes.
8	____	Visual disturbance	Retinal changes of SLE. Include cytoid bodies, retinal hemorrhages, serous exudate or hemorrhages in the choroid, or optic neuritis. Exclude hypertensive, infectious, or drug causes.
8	____	Cranial nerve disorder	New onset of sensory or motor neuropathy involving cranial nerves.
8	____	Lupus headache	Severe, persistent headache; may be migrainous, but must be nonresponsive to narcotic analgesia.
8	____	CVA	New onset of cerebrovascular accident(s). Exclude arteriosclerosis.
8	____	Vasculitis	Ulceration, gangrene, tender finger nodules, periungual infarction, splinter hemorrhages, or biopsy or angiogram proof of vasculitis.
4	____	Arthritis	More than two joints with pain and signs of inflammation (e.g., tenderness, swelling, or effusion).
4	____	Myositis	Proximal muscle aching/weakness, associated with elevated creatine phosphokinase/aldolase or electromyogram changes or a biopsy showing myositis.
4	____	Urinary casts	Heme-granular or red blood cell casts.
4	____	Hematuria	>5 red blood cells/hpf. Exclude stone, infection, or other causes.
4	____	Proteinuria	>0.5 g/24 h. New onset or recent increases of more than 0.5 g/24 h.
4	____	Pyuria	>5 white blood cells/hpf. Exclude infection.
2	____	New rash	New onset or recurrence of inflammatory type rash.
2	____	Alopecia	New onset or recurrence of abnormal, patchy, or diffuse loss of hair.

(continued)

TABLE C-3		Systemic Lupus Erythematosus Disease Activity Index (SLEDAI) (*Continued*)	

Weight	Score	Descriptor	Definition
2	____	Mucosal ulcers	New onset or recurrence of oral or nasal ulcerations.
2	____	Pleurisy	Pleuritic chest pain with pleural rub or effusion, or pleural thickening.
2	____	Pericarditis	Pericardial pain with at least one of the following: rub, effusion, or electrocardiogram or echocardiogram confirmation.
2	____	Low complement	Decrease in CH50, C3, or C4 below the lower limit of normal for testing laboratory.
2	____	Increased DNA binding	>25% binding by Farr assay or above normal range for testing laboratory.
1	____	Fever	>38°C. Exclude infectious cause.
1	____	Thrombocytopenia	<100,000 platelets/mm^3, exclude drug causes.
1	____	Leukopenia	<3,000 white blood cells/mm^3, exclude drug causes.

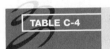

TABLE C-4	System Lupus International Collaborating Clinics/American College of Rheumatology Damage Index for Systemic Lupus Erythematosus

Directions:	Damage (nonreversible change, not related to active inflammation) occurring since onset of lupus, ascertained by clinical assessment and present for at least 6 mo unless otherwise stated. Repeat episodes must occur 6 mo apart to score 2. The same lesion cannot be scored twice.

Item	Score
Ocular (either eye, by clinical assessment)	
Any cataract ever	1
Retinal change or optic atrophy	1
Neuropsychiatric	
Cognitive impairment (e.g., memory deficit, difficulty with calculation, poor concentration, difficulty in spoken or written language, impaired performance levels) or major psychosis	1
Seizures requiring therapy for 6 mo	1
Cerebrovascular accident ever (score 2 >1)	1 (2)
Cranial or peripheral neuropathy (excluding optic)	1
Transverse myelitis	1
Renal	
Estimated or measured glomerular filtration rate <50%	1
Proteinuria >3.5 g/24 hours	1
or	
End-stage renal disease (regardless of dialysis or transplantation)	3

(continued)

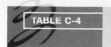

| TABLE C-4 | System Lupus International Collaborating Clinics/American College of Rheumatology Damage Index for Systemic Lupus Erythematosus (*Continued*) |

Item	Score
Pulmonary	
Pulmonary hypertension (right ventricular prominence, or loud P2)	1
Pulmonary fibrosis (physical and radiograph)	1
Shrinking lung (radiograph)	1
Pleural fibrosis (radiograph)	1
Pulmonary infarction (radiograph)	1
Cardiovascular	
Angina or coronary artery bypass	1
Myocardial infarction ever (score 2 if >1)	1(2)
Cardiomyopathy (ventricular dysfunction)	1
Valvular disease (diastolic murmur, or systolic murmur >3/6)	1
Pericarditis for 6 mo, or pericardiectomy	1
Peripheral vascular	
Claudication for 6 mo	1
Minor tissue loss (pulp space)	1
Significant tissue loss ever (e.g., loss of digit or limb) (score 2 if >1 site)	1 (2)
Venous thrombosis with swelling, ulceration, or venous stasis	1
Gastrointestinal	
Infarction or resection of bowel below duodenum spleen, liver, or gall bladder ever, for cause any (score 2 if >1 site)	1 (2)
Mesenteric insufficiency	1
Chronic peritonitis	1
Stricture or upper gastrointestinal tract surgery ever	1
Musculoskeletal	
Muscle atrophy or weakness	1
Deforming or erosive arthritis (including reducible deformities, excluding avascular necrosis)	1
Osteoporosis with fracture or vertebral collapse (excluding avascular necrosis)	1
Avascular necrosis (score 2 if >1)	1 (2)
Osteomyelitis	1
Skin	
Scarring chronic alopecia	1
Extensive scarring or panniculum other than scalp and pulp space	1
Skin ulceration (excluding thrombosis) for >6 mo	1
Premature gonadal failure	1
Diabetes (regardless of treatment)	1
Malignancy (exclude dysplasia) (score 2 if >1 site)	1 (2)

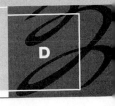

MYOSITIS FUNCTIONAL ASSESSMENT
Sandy B. Ganz and Louis L. Harris

D

NAME _____ DATE _____

THIS FORM IS DESIGNED TO EVALUATE LOWER EXTREMITY FUNCTION IN
PATIENTS WITH MYOSITIS. ALL ACTIVITIES SHOULD BE RATED ON THE
PATIENT'S ABILITY TO PERFORM A GIVEN TASK WITHOUT THE ASSISTANCE
OF THE EXAMINER.

TRANSFER FROM SUPINE TO SITTING (5)

A. (5) Spontaneously, normal; on request, use of upper extremity is not required.
B. (4) Spontaneously; but use of upper extremity is required.
C. (3) Tentatively; use of upper extremity is required.
D. (2) Laboriously; props up on both elbows.
E. (1) Laboriously; rolls to side while lying and pushes to sitting with arms.
F. (0) Unable to assume sitting position.

TRANSFER FROM SITTING TO STANDING (4)

A. (4) Rises from low chair (knees 2 in. higher than hips) without use of arms or compensatory movements.
B. (3) Rises from standard chair (knees at level with hips) spontaneously without use of arms or compensatory movements.
C. (2) Rises from standard chair tentatively; must use arms.
D. (1) Rises from standard chair laboriously; use of upper extremity, compensatory movements, or both are required for transfers.
E. (0) Unable to assume standing posture from a standard chair.

RISING FROM A LOW BENCH (9 IN.); TO BE EVALUATED ONLY IF SCORED A OR B ON TRANSFERS FROM SITTING TO STANDING (2)

A. (2) Able to sit and rise without difficulty; normal.
B. (1) Able to sit and rise, but with effort or difficulty.
C. (0) Unable to rise from a low bench.

STAIR CLIMBING—FOUR 6-IN. STEPS (14) UP/DOWN

A. (7) (7) Reciprocal (step over step), normal; on request, no use of arms.
B. (6) (6) Reciprocal; on request, no use of arms, but deviations present.
C. (5) (5) Nonreciprocal; on request, no use of arms.
D. (4) (4) Reciprocal; use of one arm is required.
E. (3) (3) Reciprocal; use of two arms is required.
F. (2) (2) Nonreciprocal; use of one arm is required.
G. (1) (1) Nonreciprocal; use of two arms is required.
H. (0) (0) Unable to negotiate stairs.

COMMENTS

_____

_____

_____

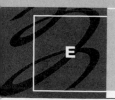

NORMAL LABORATORY VALUES

Allan Gibofsky and Stephen A. Paget

TABLE E-1	Normal Laboratory Values

Tests	Normal values	
Immunologic		
Rheumatoid factor		
Latex fixation	<1:160 titer	
Rate nephelometric	<30 IU/mL	
Anticyclic citrullinated peptide antibody	<20 U	
Serum complement		
Total hemolytic complement (CH_{50})	150–250 U/mL	
Complement components (immunoassays)		
C1q	11–22 mg/dL	
C2	1.6–3.6 mg/dL	
C3	64–210 mg/dL	
C4	11.5–50.0 mg/dL	
C5	7.1–20.4 mg/dL	
C1 esterase inhibitor	14–30 mg/dL	
Factor B	14.8–31.0 mg/dL	
Antinuclear antibody	Negative	
Anti-DNA antibody (*Crithidia* immunofluorescence)	Negative	
Anti-Ro antibody	Negative	
Anti-La antibody	Negative	
Anti-RNP antibody	Negative	
Anti-Sm antibody	Negative	
Antistreptolysin O	0–125 Todd units	
Serum immunoglobulins (immunoassay)		
IgG	723–1,685 mg/dL	
IgA	69–382 mg/dL	
IgM	63–277 mg/dL	
Hematologic		
Blood counts	**Male**	**Female**
WBC (includes five-part differential)	3.5–10.7	3.5–10.7
RBC $\times 10^{12}$/L	4.2–5.6	4.0–5.2
Hb (g/dL)	13–17	11.5–16.0
HcT (%)	38–52	34–46
MCV (fL)	82–98	82–98
PLT $\times 10^{9}$/L	160–400	
Differential	**%**	**Absolute**
Neutrophils	40.0–74.0	1.90–8.00
Lymphocytes	19.0–48.0	0.90–5.20
Monocytes	3.4–9.0	0.16–1.00

(continued)

TABLE E-1	Normal Laboratory Values *(Continued)*

Tests		Normal values
Eosinophils	0.0–7.0	0.00–0.80
Basophils	0.0–1.5	0.00–0.20
Larger unstained cells	0.0–4.0	—
Stained smears—bands	<10	
Sedimentation rate (Westergren's)		0–27 mm/h (female)
		0–12 mm/h (male)
C-reactive protein		0–1 mg/dL
Activated partial thromboplastin time		Upper limit 38.0 s
Prothrombin time (dependent on reagent lot no.)		Upper limit 13.0 s
Fibrinogen		200–400 mg/dL
Biochemistry		
Acid phosphatase		0–5.5 μ/L
Albumin		3.5–5.0 g/dL
Aldolase		0–7.4 μ/L
Alkaline phosphatase		30–110 μ/L
Amylase		25–125 μ/L
Bicarbonate		23–35 mEq/L
Bilirubin, total		0–1.0 mg/dL
Calcium		8.5–10.5 mg/dL
Chloride		97–107 mEq/L
Cholesterol		150–240 mg/dL
Creatine kinase		40–175 μ/L (female)
		40–225 μ/L (male)
Creatinine		0.4–1.2 mg/dL
GGTP		0–70 μ/L
Glucose		70–105 mg/dL
Iron		20–170 μg/dL (female)
		20–200 μg/dL (male)
Iron-binding capacity		250–450 μg/dL
LDH		80–200 μ/L
5'-NT		4–11.5 μ/L
Phosphorus, inorganic		2.5–5.0 mg/dL
Potassium		3.5–5.0 mEq/L
Protein, total		6.0–8.0 g/dL
Salicylate therapeutic level		6–20 mg/dL
SGOT (AST)		10–45 μ/L
SGPT (ALT)		0–40 μ/L
Sodium		135–145 mEq/L
Triglyceride		72–174 mg/dL
Urea nitrogen		5–25 mg/dL
Uric acid		2.0–9.0 mg/dL
Endocrine		
TSH		0.49–4.60 μIU/mL
T_4 (immunoassay)		4.9–10.7 μg/dL
T_3 uptake (immunoassay)		28%–36%
T_3 RIA (immunoassay)		
0–14 y		125–250 ng/dL
14–23 y		100–220 ng/dL
>24 y		80–180 ng/dL
Intact PTH (immunochemiluminescent assay)		1.0–5.0 pmol/L
N-terminal PTH (immunochemiluminescent assay)		0–6.1 pmol/L
C-terminal PTH (RIA)		0–50 mEq/mL

(continued)

Tests	Normal values
Quantitative urinary excretion	
Calcium	50–400 mg/24 h
Hydroxyproline, total	15–45 mg/24 h
Magnesium	75–150 mg/24 h
Sodium	43–217 mEq/24 h
Potassium	26–123 mEq/24 h
Phosphorus (inorganic)	340–1,100 mg/24 h
Amylase (enzymatic/kinetic)	1–17 U/h
Protein	10–100 mg/24 h
Creatinine	800–1,900 mg/24 h
Creatinine clearance	70–180 mL/min
Uric acid (diet-dependent)	250–750 mg/24 h

ALT, alanine aminotransferase; AST, aspartate aminotransferase; GGTP, γ-glutamyltranspeptidase; Hb, hemoglobin; HCT, hematocrit; Ig, immunoglobulin; LDH, lactate dehydrogenase; MCV, mean corpuscular volume; NT, nucleotidase; PLT, platelet; PTH, parathyroid hormone; RBC, red blood cells; RIA, radioimmunoassay; RNP, ribonucleoprotein; SGOT, serum glutamic-oxaloacetic transaminase; SGPT, serum glutamic-pyruvic transaminase; TSH, thyroid-stimulating hormone; WBC, white blood cells.

BASIC RHEUMATOLOGY LIBRARY AND INFORMATION WEB SITES
Theodore R. Fields

Textbooks
- Canale ST. *Campbell's Operative Orthopedics*, 10th ed. St. Louis, Mo: Mosby, 2003.
- Kelley WN, et al. *Textbook of Rheumatology*, 7th ed. Philadelphia, Pa: WB Saunders, 2004.
- Hochberg M. *Rheumatology*, 3rd ed. London: Mosby, 2003.
- Koopman WJ. *Arthritis and Allied Conditions*, 15th ed. Philadelphia, Pa: Lippincott Williams & Wilkins, 2004.
- Lahita RG. *Systemic Lupus Erythematosus*, 4th ed. San Diego, Calif: Academic Press, 2004.
- Isenberg DA, et al. *Oxford textbook of Rheumatology*. 3rd ed. Oxford, 2004.
- Wallace DJ, Hahn BH. *Dubois' Lupus Erythematosus*. 6th ed. Philadelphia, Pa: Lippincott Williams & Wilkins, 2002.
- Weisman MH, et al. *Treatment of Rheumatic Diseases: Companion to Kelley's Textbook of Rheumatology*. Philadelphia, Pa: WB Saunders, 2001.

References
- *AHFS Drug Information 2004*. Bethesda, Md: American Society of Health-System Pharmacists, 2004.
- Montvale NJ. *Physicians' Desk Reference*. 59th ed. Medical Economics Company, 2005.

Journals
- *Annals of the Rheumatic Diseases*. London: British Medical Association.
- *Arthritis and Rheumatism*. Atlanta: American College of Rheumatology.
- *Bulletin on the Rheumatic Diseases*. Atlanta: Arthritis Foundation.

- *Clinical and Experimental Rheumatology.* Pisa, Italy.
- *Current Opinion in Rheumatology.* Philadelphia: Lippincott Williams & Wilkins.
- *Journal of Rheumatology.* Toronto: Journal of Rheumatology.
- *Lupus.* London: Macmillan.
- *Rheumatic Disease Clinics of North America.* Philadelphia: WB Saunders.
- *Rheumatology International.* Heidelberg, Germany: Springer-Verlag.
- *Scandinavian Journal of Rheumatology* and supplements. Oslo: Scandinavian University Press.
- *Seminars in Arthritis and Rheumatism.* Philadelphia: WB Saunders.

Websites

- American College of Rheumatology. Site for rheumatology professional organization, with guidelines, position statements, links to Arthritis & Rheumatism Journal, etc. www.rheumatology.org
- Arthritis Foundation. www.arthritis.org
- Hospital for Special Surgery, Musculoskeletal Educational Site (Illustrated monographs on all aspects of musculoskeletal diagnosis and treatment, etc.). www.hss.edu
- Johns Hopkins Rheumatology Division Educational Site (Case studies, meeting summaries, special reports, information for physicians and patients, etc.). www.hopkins-arthritis.com
- NIH Information for Patients (NIH-selected material to educate your patients)–MedLine Plus. www.medlineplus.org
- PIER (Physician's Information and Education Resource—for members of the American College of Physicians) includes data on multiple rheumatic diseases. http://pier.acponline.org
- Scleroderma Foundation—information for patients and physicians. www.scleroderma.org
- Information for patients on lupus and latest research findings: Lupus Foundation: www.lupus.org; Alliance for Lupus Research: www.lupusresearch.org; Lupus Research Institute: www.lupusresearchinstitute.org
- Information for patients—Wegener's Granulomatosis Association. www.wgassociation.org

Page numbers followed by *f* indicate figures; numbers followed by *t* indicate tables.